HEALTH
THIRD EDITION

Benjamin A. Kogan, M.D., Dr. P.H.

HEALTH
THIRD EDITION

HARCOURT BRACE JOVANOVICH, INC.

New York San Diego Chicago San Francisco Atlanta
London Sydney Toronto

**What is best in this book is dedicated
to the memory of my parents.**

Cover: "Prehistorie," by Max Papart. Courtesy of the Nathan Galleries. Acknowledgments and copyrights for illustrations continue at the back of the book on page 503.

Printed in the United States of America

Library of Congress Catalog Card Number: 79-92816

ISBN: 0-15-535588-0

Preface

A decade has passed since the publication of the first edition of this book. To bring the massive amount of new material about health science within a limited number of pages required much selection, revision, and rewriting. The theme of the book, however, remains unchanged. The preface of the first edition pointed out that people were trapped in the web of their own technological triumphs. Never before had they known so much about their inner mechanisms and outer world. Yet never before had they been so threatened by the imbalances between them. "Since ecological balance is essential to human health," it was stated in 1970, "people need to know what is causing ecological imbalance. They must seek and find ways of achieving harmony between their slowly changing inner environment and their rapidly changing outer environment. This is the central and recurring theme of this book." As yet, it cannot be otherwise. The threat to our internal environment by our external environment remains perhaps the most persistent problem of our time. And, for this reason, the study of human inner and outer ecosystems continues to be the guiding principle in the structure of this book.

The first chapter explores the meanings of health for the individual within a community and relates those meanings to ecology and its numerous ecosystems. But human ecology includes more than interrelationships with other living communities, whether plant or other animal life. Human ecology also encompasses the varied facets of human culture. The next chapter describes some of the imbalances between people and their environment. The accumulating pollutions of this plundered planet are presented to the student as urgent business with which everyone must be involved. Continuing the ecological concept, the third chapter treats communicable disease as an invasion of our environment by agents of the outer environment—self versus nonself. This chapter includes the most recent information about sexually transmitted diseases; nonspecific urethritis and genital herpes receive the renewed emphasis they merit today; and current topics such as Legionnaires' disease, the newly discovered non-A, non-B hepatitis virus, and the swine influenza episode are discussed.

Chapter Four presents recent material concerning the causes of atherosclerosis, the nation's greatest killer. Happily, the U.S. death rates from heart disease and stroke are both declining, and health workers must be given due credit for this. Unfortunately, our experience with cancer, also covered in Chapter Four, is not so successful. A special insertion titled "Disease and Destiny" has been included as a way for the reader to trace the historical course of a disease (particularly plague) and the impact of individual illness (particularly Napoleon's) on human destiny. Disease has often twisted history, and the past provides lessons for the future. The fifth and sixth chapters are concerned with emotional life. New to this edition are the concepts of Maslow (now added to those of Erikson); recent research on the possibilities that some elements of personality problems are chemically related; and, for the first time, a discussion of aging and death as normal processes of life. Chapter Six on stress, anxiety, and depression gives strong attention to suicide and offers practical pointers to prevent it. The subject of Chapter Seven is drugs and their abuse. Alcoholism was not a major problem among teen-agers ten years ago, but today it is, and suggested here are several ways of dealing with it. Newer drugs of abuse—Dalmane, Valium, PCP, and Darvon—are introduced in this edition, as are current examinations of the older major drug problems.

Chapter Eight deals with general body health. Although it emphasizes physical fitness, it is extended to include fitness of special body structures—the eyes, ears, and teeth. The ninth chapter, about nourishment, has been brought up to date. Chapter Ten—on love and marriage—recognizes that courtship has changed dramatically in the past years and that marriage and divorce rates are increasing. This book takes a positive approach to marriage and gives some important practical factors to consider in choosing a partner. But there is a thorough discussion of ways to cope with divorce and, more importantly, ways to help children cope with it. Chapter Eleven realistically considers sexuality as an important part of the personality. The discussion explores sexual inadequacies, misconceptions about sexuality, recent findings on homosexuality, and the changing roles of women. All the material in Chapter Twelve—on reproduction, overreproduction, and birth control—has been brought up to date and a section on abortion has been added. Chapters Thirteen and Fourteen—on human beginnings—discuss not only pregnancy, labor, and postnatal concerns, but also subfertility, adoption, and what many consider one of the major health problems today—teen-age pregnancies. Chapter Fourteen emphasizes the genetic ecosystem. In a time when scientists are performing previously unheard of experiments with genes, some understanding of the negotiations between the DNA and RNA is needed. Such knowledge makes genetic disease itself comprehensible and opens the door to a fuller understanding of the environmental influences on the fertilized ovum. This chapter provides that knowledge and closes with advice about genetic counseling. Chapter Fifteen discusses the health care systems in this country today. The major programs are defined and discussed, as are the shortcomings of health care in this complex society. The chapter ends with a discussion of quackery.

The book concludes with an Epilogue whose major purpose is to describe frontiers in health care. Diabetes mellitus is used as a model throughout a considerable portion of the Epilogue because it is an example of a medical problem with a past, present, and future: The ancients diagnosed it and developed treatments for it, and current research holds much hope for the future of the millions who still suffer from it.

As a nation, we have been guilty of grievous errors—of waste, of poorly conceived programs, of failures. But there are reasons also for optimism. Jean Mayer, the distinguished nutritionist and president of Tufts University, has pointed to the extraordinary success of a federal program that, within ten years, has relieved serious malnutrition in many areas of the country. A nation that has within the same period dramatically reduced the death rates from heart disease and stroke, that has ingeniously helped the blind to see, will also solve the enigmas of cancer, of pollution, and of the many other health problems that still beset us.

Thanks are due to John Leedom, M.D., Professor of Medicine at the University of Southern California School of Medicine, who critically read the entire manuscript, and to Mrs. Marion Mayne, for many years a leading public health nurse, who graciously donated many hours to this edition.

The author particularly wishes to acknowledge the contributions of all those who suggested ways in which the text might be revised and improved, including Ross O. Armstrong, Department of Health, Physical Education and Recreation, Chadron State College; Patricia Binding, Department of Health Education, Los Angeles Harbor College; Alan Briggs, Department of Health Science, Edmonds Community College; Lynne Bynum, Life Sciences Division, Monterey Peninsula College; Donald Carlucci, Department of Health Education, Los Angeles Harbor College; J. Alfred Chiscon, Department of Biological Sciences, Purdue University; Jack Criqui, Department of Health Science, Chabot College; Alan B. Davidson, Assistant Principal, Kent Meridian High School; Robert Diller, Department of Health Science, Cabrillo College; Ronald A. Fusco, Coordinator of Health Education, Queensborough Community College; V.W. Greene, School of Public Health, University of Minnesota; Donovan Horn, Department of Health and Physical Education, Mississippi State University; Michael Hosokawa, Department of Family and Community Medicine, University of Missouri; Jack Madigan, Department of Health Education, City College of San Francisco; Allen Nelson, Physical Education Department, Porterville College; Nicholas J. Pisacano, University of Kentucky Medical Center; James M. Pryde, Department of Health Sciences, American River College; Charles R. Schroeder, Department of Health, Physical Education and Recreation, Memphis State University; Henny Shepherd, Department of Health and Physical Education, Los Angeles Pierce College; Morry Storseth, Department of Health Science, Seattle Central Community College; Muriel Svec, Department of Life Science, Santa Monica College; Kenneth Swearingen, Physical Education Coordinator, Saddleback Community College: Joan Taylor, Physical Education Department, El Camino College; Jack V. Toohey, Department of Health Science, Arizona State University; Robert E. Vanni, Department of Health Sciences, Western Illinois University; C. Harold Veenker, Department of Physical Education for Men, Purdue University; Kenneth E. Veselak, Department of Health and Physical Education, Nassau Community College; Murray Vincent, School of Public Health, University of South Carolina; William E.R. Whitely, Department of Health Sciences, California State University at Los Angeles; and Verne E. Zellmer, Department of Health Sciences, American River College.

However, it is the author who must accept total responsibility for errors; corrections would be gratefully appreciated.

BENJAMIN A. KOGAN

Contents

**SPECIAL INSERT:
DISEASE AND DESTINY**

4 The Chronic Degenerative Diseases   87

5 The Emotional Life: Part I   123

HEALTH
THIRD EDITION

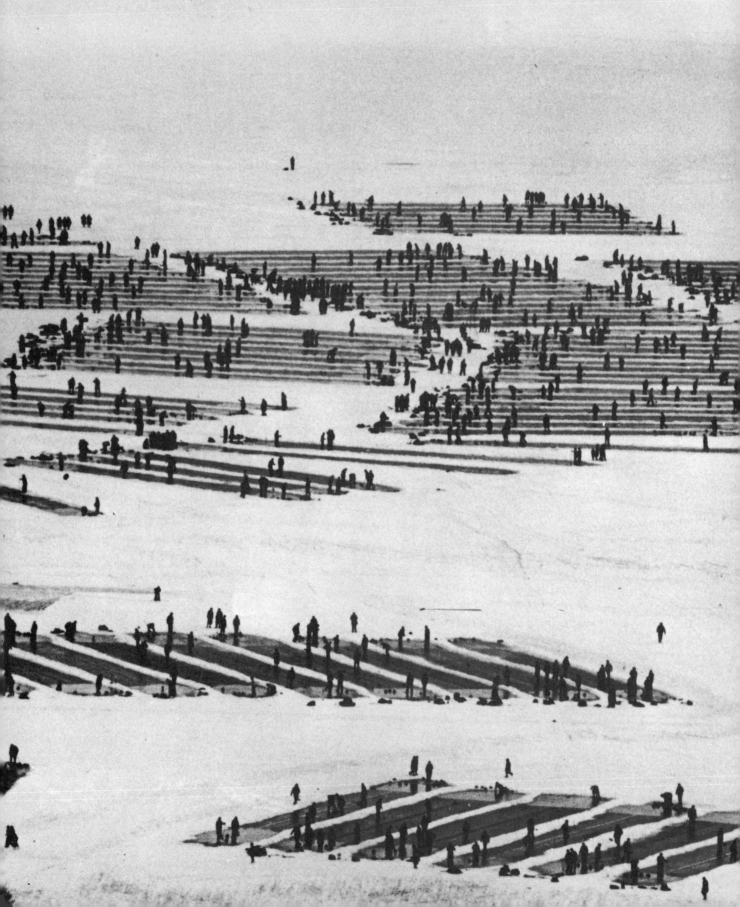

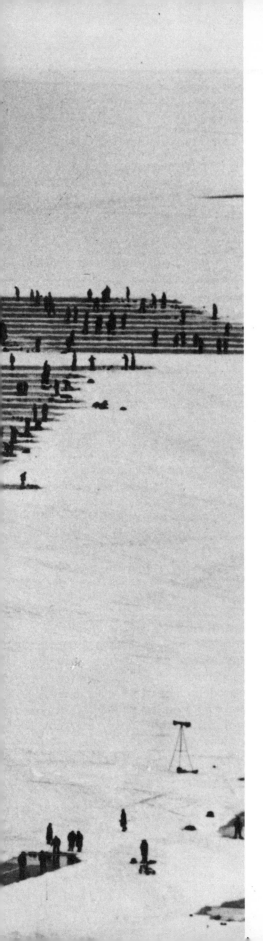

1

Health: The Individual and the Community

The Scale of Health

What is health? Is it visible—seen as a gleaming smile, for example? Not by those Asians who chew betel nuts to blacken their teeth for beauty. Or is health felt? Many people feel well yet harbor infectious illness. Perhaps a formula, something short and magical, like $E = mc^2$, could define health. But formulas such as Einstein's equation apply best not to people but to objects. Since there is no human equation, there is no health equation. Health is as complex as human beings, as variable as life, and any attempt to define health within strict limits is as idle as to seek the mind in the dissecting laboratory. In this is its endless fascination.

Any concept of health must be viewed as much with imagination as with words. Imagine, then, a scale or a ruler of as yet unmeasured length. At one end of the scale is a pole marking zero health (death); at the other end is the pole of perfect health, which as yet remains an unknown ideal. Between the poles of death and perfect health are the many gradations or degrees of health. It is along this scale that living things and people constantly move and shift directions. Nothing stays at the same place on the continuum because all of life consists of successions of changing occurrences. Consider, for example, the following series of events.

At about 6 A.M. one Sunday morning, Mr. Blue, who has been feeling below par, develops a sudden shaking chill. At 10 A.M. he calls his physician, who arrives within the hour. By that time Mr. Blue has had severe chills half a dozen times, sharp pains that knife through his right chest, and a slight cough, which produces a rust-colored material. His breathing is labored, and his oral temperature is 104° F. After examining the patient, the physician promptly hospitalizes him. From X-ray and other studies it is clear the patient has pneumonia. Mr. Blue is dangerously ill. He has been rapidly moving toward the death pole of the health scale.

But treatment is prompt and effective. The patient is given oxygen and antibiotics while fluids are dripped into his veins. Slowly, he improves. Mr. Blue moves away from death toward a safer, healthier level on the scale. He regains his strength, develops good health habits, and eventually moves further along the scale approaching perfect health.

Although life is not always as dramatic as a case of near-fatal pneumonia, something is always happening to everybody. And each person, because of his or her unique make-up, responds to things differently. Does this statement seem obvious? Actually it is neither understood nor accepted by everyone.

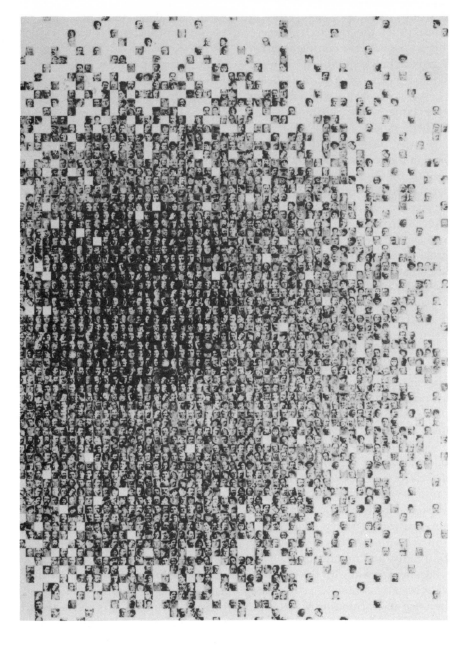

Health and the Individual

All People Are Not Created Equal—In Health

"We hold these truths to be self-evident, that all men are created equal." Written in a passion for liberty, these words still give our nation purpose in times of trial. There is only one thing wrong with them: They are not true. All people are not created equal. On the scale of health each human being is born to a particular place and pace. No two people occupy the same place nor have the same speed.

If you consider for a moment the endless hereditary variations that exist among the more than four billion people living on the earth, you can see why the idea of equal birth loses its meaning. Nobody has ever happened before. Nobody will ever happen again. One infant, born a symphony of nerve and muscle, may someday run the hundred-yard dash in nine seconds. Another, crippled, will find walking five feet an agony. One human being may be born an idiot, another a genius. Of course, individual differences are usually much less obvious than these. Nevertheless, human individuality is a fact of life, a fact made evident by the difficulty in surgically transplanting tissue from one person to another. Indeed, to achieve success in transplant operations, changes must be made in the person receiving the transplant.

Lower on the biological scale, tissue transplants are less difficult. Skin from one frog may be successfully grafted to another frog. On a still lower level, different parts of two earthworms may be grafted together as long as all the segments point in the same direction.

Viruses are at the bottom of the scale of "living things." Indeed, many experts place them in a middle position—between living creatures and nonliving things. Some years ago scientists at the California Institute of Technology performed a remarkable experiment. They placed various parts of a number of viruses of the same type into a test tube. All of these viruses were incomplete in some way. Some lacked hereditary chemicals (genes) to make heads, others had no genes for tails, still others had no "collar" genes, and so on. But by mixing these incomplete viruses together in a test tube, the researchers were able to assemble a complete virus. Compare this lack of individuality to the complexity of a human being whose tissues ordinarily will reject transplants of even his or her own mother's skin.

On the basis of individuality, then, humans clearly occupy the top position on the biological scale. Variety in people is present not only in the great variations in such obvious external features as height, eye color, and bone structure, but in internal organs as well. Studies of the human stomach, for example, have revealed a wide range of normal variations in size and shape. But what about the heart? Surely any deviation in heart structure would be unhealthy, even deadly. Nonsense. Hearts vary so much among people that careful training and experience are needed to distinguish between problems and normal variations. Since no organ of any person is exactly like that of another person, it follows that the chemical functions of these organs also vary from person to person. In humans, even the activity of body chemicals and the composition of hair, skin, bone, stomach juices, and blood differ from individual to individual.

Becoming aware of the normal, wide variations among people is a first step in learning to avoid making hasty comparisons. This lesson certainly applies to generalizations about health. Many ideas about health are really no more than observations. Eight hours of sleep may be what some people need, but many others get along beautifully on six. Some need ten. "Drink milk" is good advice for most people, but there are those who are sickened by milk; they may even be allergic to it. "I can't start the day without a lot of breakfast," one person insists.

Another finds the thought of a heavy breakfast distasteful. No one should try to force his or her personal health ideas on anyone else.

In Its Proper Place, Health Is Important

How much does one need to think about health? Imagine a man and a woman stranded on a desert island. Would their first order of business be to sit down and have a conversation about health? Not likely. They would think about their basic needs—food, shelter, and sexual expression (although not necessarily in that order). Only insofar as health furthers or frustrates the satisfaction of these needs would they have to pay much attention to it. Without doubt, health is a superb adornment to life. It certainly makes human needs more possible to satisfy. Nevertheless, until it is in jeopardy, health is of secondary, not primary, importance to most people.

But what of death? How much does one need to consider the other end of the health spectrum in the normal scheme of things? A modern wit has described death as "nature's way of telling you to slow down." The number of such wry references to death seem only to emphasize our inability to deal realistically with it. Jokes are like whistling in the dark: For many people they relieve some of the terror. But death is the natural end of life, and, as such, ordinary people usually stand in awe of it, refusing to think of it until they have no alternative. The result is that in our society, death is often hidden away within hospitals and nursing homes. When death comes, we frequently must face it alone and unprepared.

Health and Rhythm

To every thing there is a season,
And a time to every purpose under
the heaven.

These lines from the Bible's Ecclesiastes (3:2) convey the ancients' feelings about a rhythm, or beat, to life. This notion is no less valid today. In a study of biological rhythms, one researcher wrote of a Cambridge athletic team that adjusted its playing schedule according to the rate at which water accumulated in the knee joints of its star player.[1] This disability occurred regularly every nine days and lasted for two or three days. Although this is a rather extreme example, it suggests the extent to which body rhythms play a part in human adaptation to a changing environment. It is through our body rhythms that we become attuned to and get in harmony with our surroundings. This timing mechanism in the body is what some scientists refer to as the "inner biological clock." Its rhythm is built into every living cell. There is scientific reason to believe that there is also a rhythm in nature outside of the cells and body. This is sometimes called the "outer cosmic clock." The word *cosmic* is used to distinguish the whole universe from the earth alone. The outer cosmic clock is related to the relative positions of the earth, sun, and moon, as well as to all the other physical factors of the universe, such as radiation and magnetic fields.

Rhythm characterizes all life patterns, and the question of whether this rhythm is governed by the inner biological clock or by the outer cosmic clock is now the subject of scientific inquiry. That there is a relationship between the two no longer seems questionable. Consider, for example, the fiddler crab. At sunrise every day it begins to blacken. In this way it is protected from both the sun's glare and its enemies. At sunset its dark coat rapidly blanches back to a cool silvery gray. If captured and kept in a dark room, it will keep this gray color. This example illustrates how closely the lives of creatures are related to earth's cycles of day and night, which in turn depend upon cycles of the universe.

Human rhythms are no less marked than those of lower animals. There are the obvious rhythms of a beating heart, of walking, sleeping, breathing, loving. And there are the more secret rhythms of body functions. Within a twenty-four-hour day, for example, a person's temperature may vary from 1 to 1.5 degrees Fahrenheit. The "normal" temperature (about 98.6° F orally) typically is highest (reaching about 100° F) in the late afternoon or early evening. At four or five in the morning, it is normally lowest (approximately 97.6° F). Such rhythmical cycles that repeat themselves at approximately twenty-four-hour intervals are called **circadian rhythms.**

Most people who travel by jet plane over several time zones in one day will testify to the fatigue (and even illness) resulting from interference with their individually timed cycles. A woman leaves Chicago at 6 P.M. The flight takes eight hours, but she arrives in London when the English are having breakfast. For the Chicagoan it is bedtime. She may feel ill. How can she avoid this insult to her body rhythms? She can begin the trip rested, she should allow a day to adjust, and she should avoid overeating. Diplomats who travel to distant lands must deal with upset rhythms before they deal with upset international relations. Even long before the existence of jet planes people understood this. In the Declaration of Independence the authors voiced this complaint about the English king: "He has called together legislative bodies at places unusual and distant . . . for the sole purpose of fatiguing them. . . ."

Even attacks of illness seem to occur in a rhythmic cycle. Asthmatic and heart attacks, for example, seem to be most common at 4 A.M., and many epileptics tend to have a seizure always at about the same time of the day.

Some emotionally ill patients have been noted to behave very abnormally for a twenty-four-hour period, then, within a few minutes, to return to normal behavior for the next twenty-four hours, and then, again within a few moments, to return to abnormality. Such abnormal-normal changes have occurred in certain patients in cycles ranging from a few days to as long as ten years. Sometimes rhythmic emotional problems are truly extraordinary. One emotionally sick young man felt he was a male for three or four days and then felt like a female for the next three or four days. These changes in his feelings were very regular. Another case has been reported about a salesman who regularly became so depressed for twenty-four-hour periods that he could not get out of his car. He would sit in it for hours, miserable and unable to carry on his business. The rest of the time he was a fine, talkative salesman. How did he solve his problem? He simply adapted to his rhythmic cycle and made appointments only on "good" days.

The complex rhythmic individuality of human beings should caution against total reliance on average health measurements. True, averages can be very significant indicators. Health workers use such average measurements as height and weight, blood sugar content, and white blood cell counts for a variety of important purposes. But many people do not fit into averages, nor can they be forced into them. For the average population, smog tolerance levels may tell whether the smog level is safe or not. But for those with severe chronic bronchitis, a "safe" level may be dangerous. Some of these people could become ill and perhaps even die before the average tolerance to smog is reached. Those who set legal tolerances for smog levels must, then, set them low enough to protect the sick. More than a hundred years ago, the American writer Henry David Thoreau gave us some good advice about individual differences: "If a man does not keep pace with his companions, perhaps it is because he hears a different drummer. Let him step to the music which he hears, however measured or far away."

People *are* individuals, but no person nor any living creature moves along the health scale alone. Life, health, sickness, recovery, and death are related happenings, experienced and shared by all who live within a community. The community molds and, in turn, is molded by all within it.

Perhaps a good analogy is to think of people's lives as looms, on which everyone has an individually patterned fabric of good health and disease. Then, these endlessly varying fabrics, manufactured on billions of different looms, must fit together into a working harmony called humankind. And the same unified system of life exists not only between people but between people and all other forms of life. Everything that lives has a rhythm that is in tune with the individual rhythms of all that relate to it. To understand health one must understand how people relate to one another in their community and to the whole community itself. Therefore, we turn our attention next to health and the community.

Health and the Community

In this book the word **community** is used to refer to a group of people living in the same place and sharing the same rules for survival. Other forms of life may live in association with the humans in the community, and these creatures will share their own rules for survival. Thus, since they share a common organization and purpose, they are a society too. One may speak of a community or society of human beings, or dogs, or squirrels, or cells, or insects, and so on. We may begin our examination of a community by looking at the behavior of some creatures existing in a remarkably successful society. The Bible reads, "Go to the ant, thou sluggard; consider her ways, and be wise." We need not emulate ants: They are slaveholders, thieves, and inefficient workers. Yet the similarities and differences between ant and human societies are such that a comparison offers some useful lessons.

An Insect Need Not Learn

A morsel to tempt some finicky Mexican brides at their wedding break-

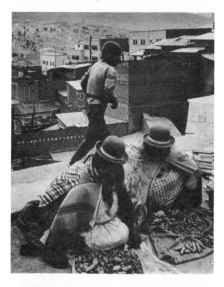

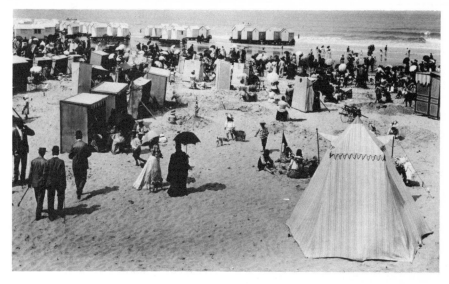

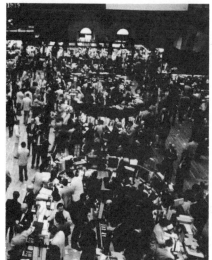

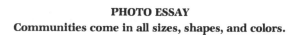

PHOTO ESSAY
Communities come in all sizes, shapes, and colors.

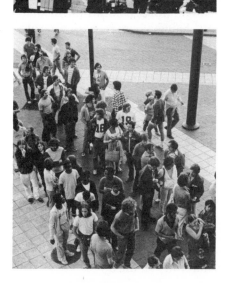

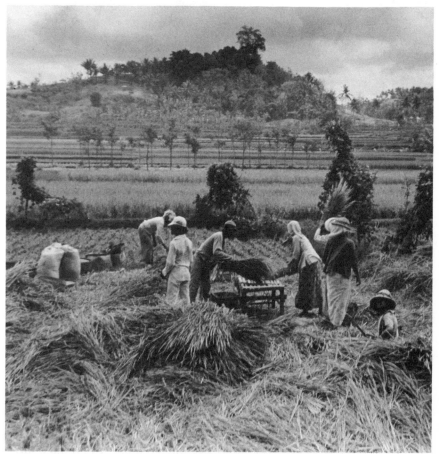

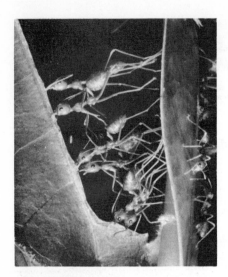

Weaving ants. These workers are busy pulling together a breach cut in the nest.

fast might well be an insect honey-ball. This delicacy is a collection of ants, swollen like tiny barrels, purposely stuffed by worker ants with honeydew. In times of short supply these "cask" ants provide food for worker ants. These living mason jars are but one of the countless clever arrangements that exist in ant communities.

Ants also maintain slaves and babysitters, keep cattle, engage in agriculture, construct cities, skyscrapers, and freeways, and have a regular system of patrols. Soldiers (undeveloped females) defend the nest from outside invasion. A stray ant that wanders into a strange nest will be attacked, but a native ant that is lost and gone for weeks will be welcomed back. There is even a "doorkeeper" ant, whose head is fashioned into a plug to close nest entrances.

The devotion shown by individual ants to the common good of the community would be hard to better. Yet "among the marvels of ant and termite societies, one thing is conspicuously absent. Nowhere is there a school for the young workers or soldiers!"[2] The ant's behavioral patterns are not learned. All these complex occurrences happen according to instinct.

People Must Learn the Rules of Community Life

The need to learn rules is one of the basic differences between life in human and ant communities. For the ant, behavior is instinctual. The ant need not learn. Without training, it becomes expert at particular tasks once it reaches a given stage of development. In contrast, the human must be trained, and only after prolonged growth and de-velopment does he or she achieve certain abilities. Consider what this difference means:

Should all the members of an ant community perish, for example, except one fertilized female, the lone survivor would be capable of rebuilding the entire social edifice in all its original complexity within the span of a few short generations. A society of humans could not similarly recover from catastrophe if all humans suddenly disappeared except one adult couple organically intact but innocent of knowledge and all other social learning. . . . it would take tedious thousands of generations to rediscover the ways and wisdom needed to run any human society now in existence. This is because humans, unlike insects, order their lives and interpersonal relations largely by means of socially acquired signals.[3]

So human beings rely primarily on learned behavior, or culture, for survival. It is this guidance, this learned behavior, *transmitted from generation to generation*, that enables people to constantly adapt to change. Insect communities do not change; human communities change constantly, and it is this change that makes progress possible.

Still another difference between human beings and lower forms of life is the length of time required for the development of independence. No other creature remains dependent on adults for as long as the human does. Insects have a brief period of immaturity followed by a relatively long period of productivity. While the young monkey busily seeks food in the supermarkets of nature, a human of the same age idly examines his or her fingers. A human being requires almost one-third of a life span to reach maturity. One reason we need so much time is that it takes this long to learn the rules of the community. Another reason is that humans have an unusually long postreproductive life span. Nature grants us extra years in which to learn the demands of our human community and even more years in which to make use of this wisdom. But, in the developmental years, people pick up problems as well as wisdom. And, in the productive years, we tend to create even more problems for ourselves—problems that can flaw our health and thus our productive energy.

So although we humans are unique in terms of our behavior, the process of learning is not without cost. The price will depend on our ability to create a balance between ourselves and our communities, and too often our inability to strike this balance costs us our health.

Health, then, helps to create communities, and communities help to create or damage health. (How the community can cause ill health will be explored in the pages that follow.)

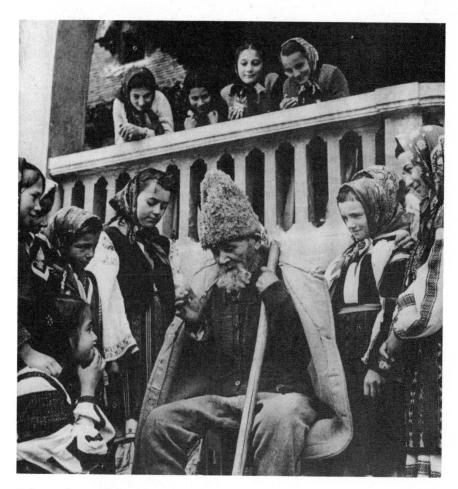

Culture: ". . . and there is wisdom in the selection of wisdom."

BERGEN EVANS

To the Human Community a Third Dimension Is Added—Culture

The human community differs from all others in one major respect. For all other life forms the community is made up of two related parts: The physical (or nonliving) and the biological (living). But human communities are complicated and enriched by a third dimension—**culture**. Culture is the sum of what people have learned *and transmitted* from generation to generation. It

is that sum that makes us different from all other life forms and that gives us our special ability to plan for and adapt to change independently of the physical or biological occurrences that may have caused the change.

Consider again the pneumonia patient discussed earlier. A biological imbalance between the cells in his lungs and a pneumonia-causing bacteria changed his state of health from good to near disaster. In an earlier time he may even have died. Fortunately, however, human culture had produced penicillin, which was able to correct the imbalance,

thus bringing about the change back into a favorable condition for the patient.

Unhappily, human culture does not always provide such positive change agents. We have, for instance, developed the technology to extract uranium from the earth. But along with the potential advantages that uranium provides comes the fact that the miners have at least three times the incidence of lung cancer as do other humans from comparable age groups. Exposed daily to the physical stimulus of radioactive uranium, a miner experiences biological changes in his lung cells—changes that produce lung cancer. Helplessly, he moves toward the death end of the health scale. But are not all people subjected to the physical stimulus of some natural radiation? Yes. And some cells are damaged while other cells die. But for most people, the total radiation dose at any one time is so small that there is time for cellular recovery and replacement, and for restoration of the balance in the cellular community that makes up the body. The uranium miner is less fortunate. The sustained and unusually high doses of radiation to which he is exposed make counterbalance impossible. His healthy cells are overwhelmed and he becomes critically ill. Eventually the miner dies.

But the imbalance set in motion by the radioactive uranium does not end here. The miner's death creates both grief and concern in his community and sets in motion a whole series of cultural processes. For instance, the miner is mourned in a certain way. His funeral strictly follows prescribed cultural rules. Finally he is buried in accordance with the customs of the community.

Beyond this, pressure may be brought to bear on government officials to enact new safety laws. Only after some time has passed since the miner's death will his community be restored to a greater degree of balance.

To what extent are people affected by imbalances within themselves and within their communities? The scientist René Dubos has written:

All living things, from men to the smallest microbe, live in association with other living things. . . . an equilibrium is established which permits the different components of biological systems to live at peace together, indeed often to help one another. Whenever the equilibrium is disturbed by any means whatever, either internal or external, one of the components of the system is favored at the expense of the other . . . and then comes about the process of disease.[4]

One of the ways in which we have learned to cope with the processes of change and imbalance is through religion.

"All living things . . . live in association with other living things."

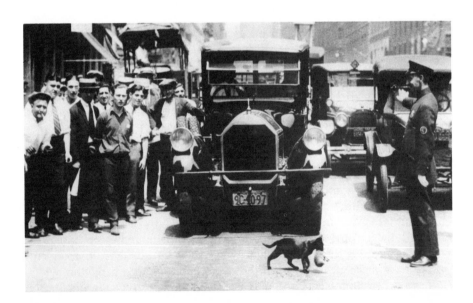

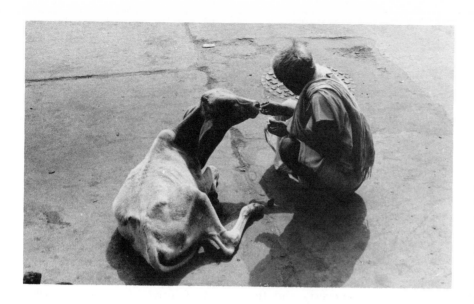

Religion and Health

For most of the world's religious people, faith has deep emotional meanings. But there is more to religion than emotion. Into its rules have often been built practical community-saving ideas—ideas that are often involved with health. The sacred cow in India is one such example. Throughout their history, Indians have endured dozens of famines. Yet the Hindu religion prohibits the killing and eating of cows. In that hungry country, cows eat ten million tons of food fit for humans yearly. To Westerners, such a situation would be intolerable.

Why do so many Indians reject beef? Is the religious belief in the sacred cow a product of stupidity, foolishness, or ignorance? No. The Hindu religion forbids the destruction of the cow on the grounds that killing is antilife and thus sinful. Yet there is a much more practical reason involved here. Without the bullock the Indian farm could not exist, and cows produce the bullocks that pull the plows. Cows, even if old and ailing, also produce lavish amounts of manure. For millions of

Indians, manure is the only source of fertilizer and fuel. In addition, it provides a usable building material. What the Indian religion has developed is a cultural balance in the community. Killing and eating the cows would indeed feed several million Indians for a short while. But the long-term result could well be agricultural disaster.

Poverty: The Mother of Disease

Those who attempt to improve the public's health are often stymied by an indifference that does not necessarily stem from attitudes about health and death. Rather, this indifference is born of poverty and bred by a sense of hopelessness. Every community health worker is witness to this tragedy; no complete health survey fails to demonstrate it.

Consider a common experience revealed by a recent survey conducted by a large West Coast health agency. The survey had been part of the preplanning activity necessary for a campaign to promote immunization against "regular"

measles (rubeola). A safe and effective vaccine was available. The year before, a similar campaign had seemed to stop an epidemic. For protection against the disease, thousands of parents had brought their children either to their family doctors or to the health department. But the new survey showed that there were still large pockets in the community containing thousands of unvaccinated children. It was certain that a high proportion of them had not had the disease. Lacking immunity by vaccination or by an earlier attack of regular measles, they were liable to contract the illness and also its serious complications.

The health workers studied a pin-studded map indicating areas of low vaccination levels. They drew circles around a few pockets in the middle-class areas, but the survey showed that relatively few children in these sections of the county were still susceptible to measles. The circles surrounding the disadvantaged areas of the community enclosed the majority of the pins. Although health department workers had provided the vaccinations free of charge, the children of the poor were the least immunized. Here was the old story of the *behavioral* or *performance gap*—the gap between the preventive health services offered and those accepted. That gap between the available benefits of modern, preventive health care and the indifference to them by a large segment of the poor is hard to bridge.

The great majority of poor people do understand the importance of health. It has been pointed out that

. . . poor people understand the relationship between their ill health and poverty. Health is one of their major concerns. Good

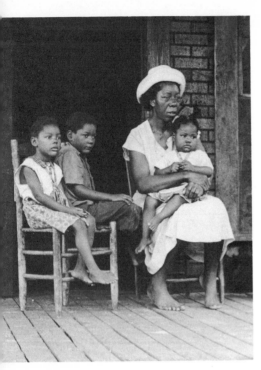

One of the many faces of the mother of poverty.

health to the poor is the lifeline to all else.[5]

Nevertheless, a great many poverty-stricken people do not take advantage of available preventive health programs. The reason is that most of these people are part of what has been called "the culture of poverty." The people in this culture do not feel a part of the major institutions of the surrounding society. Generally they have little or no effective community organizations beyond the family. They have a very brief childhood, and they often feel helpless and inferior. There is a difference between poverty and the culture of poverty. Despite their desperate circumstances, many of the poor of Africa, Asia, and South America, for example, have a sense of belonging to and participating within the larger group. Of the estimated forty to fifty million poor people in the United States, only about 20 percent live in the culture of poverty.

In the United States, those in the culture of poverty are mostly blacks, Chicanos, Puerto Ricans, American Indians, and many rural Southern whites. It is clear that the prejudice and discrimination directed toward the members of these minority groups accounts for some of their resistance to government-sponsored health services.

The active participation of minorities in all phases of health planning would, of course, improve the situation. And money is essential to relieving the economic problems, although it alone cannot eliminate prejudice or the behavioral gap. High death rates among children and pregnant women, shorter adult life expectancies, malnutrition—these are among the bitter realities of the poor that need urgent attention.

Poverty, however, is not the only cause of resistance to health programs. Sometimes it is due to senseless refusal to accept scientifically proven information. Consider the following example.

"Them Dogs Don't Vote"

In a large western city some years ago, it was unsafe for a child to play in the streets, much less to walk home from school. Rabid dogs roamed the area, biting and possibly infecting any human being who happened across their paths. A safe and effective vaccine to prevent rabies in dogs had long been available. All responsible scientific organizations supported compulsory vaccination of dogs. Yet for many years, a small, very active, and seemingly well-financed minority successfully led the fight against rabies vaccinations of dogs. The advice of public health officials, distinguished deans of medical and veterinary schools, and other leading scientific figures in the community went unheeded.

It was usually the children who paid the price of such ignorance. A child does not easily understand that a sick dog can carry death and so must be left alone. And even if a child does understand this, pity usually gains the upper hand over judgment. In that city, children had to be taught to fear dogs—sick dogs in particular. Frequently, both children and adults had to endure the fourteen to twenty-eight injections that, in those days, were needed to prevent rabies in humans. To survive rabies is very rare; the preventive vaccine was the best procedure. However, the only vaccine that could be used at that time caused paralysis about once every two thousand times it was used. The following true story illustrates the problems that resulted.

Tommy, a nine-year-old newsboy, was brought to the family physician by his mother because he had been bitten by a dog that "was acting funny—he was limping around and had a funny bark." The boy had tried to help the animal, and it had bitten him savagely on the hand. Before coming to the doctor, the mother had reported the dog bite to the health department. The doctor immediately telephoned the health department and asked the resident veterinarian about the animal. The dog had been caught. It was rabid. The bite in the child's thumb was a deep tear. The doctor washed the wound with soap and water for a long time, and then started the preventive injections against rabies.

After nine injections into the soft tissue around his navel, Tommy developed a fever, a headache, and a "'lectric like" feeling over the right ribs and arm. "See, doctor," he said, more curious than concerned, "I can't hold a pencil." The doctor saw only too well. The boy's symptoms indicated possible paralysis as a result of the treatment. He turned to the mother. "We will have to stop his treatments," he said slowly.

"But won't he get rabies?" Her voice rose. She fought to control it.

"He could. But right now, with this reaction from the vaccine, the chances of his getting rabies are not as great as the chances of a permanent paralysis. It's a matter of measuring the risks. And there is a good chance, the best chance, that nothing at all will happen and he will be all right."

"When will we know?"

The doctor paused. He had seen two cases of human rabies. Now, as he looked at the boy, he remembered them. "In about a week or two we should know pretty well.

But we can't be absolutely positive, not for some months."

After the frightened mother left with her child, the doctor telephoned a city councilman. He explained the case in detail. "Why don't you vote for rabies vaccination?" he asked. "It's even good for the dogs."

"Listen, doc," the politician said bluntly, "when we took up this rabies vaccination thing, the council chambers were swarming with dog lovers. They raised a row. These days two things bring people to a council meeting—taxes and dogs. You know how many people came to talk for vaccination? One was this run-down botany professor whose sleeves were too long for him. The other was the president of the medical society, and nobody likes him because he drives a Cadillac. Where were you? There were twenty dog lovers for every kid lover. Everybody gets what he deserves. As for them sick dogs, well, them dogs don't vote."

The doctor telephoned the mother. "I just wanted to ask you," he said, "do you remember the city council meeting on rabies vaccination last month? Were you there?"

There was a long pause. "I wasn't there," she said. "I'm getting what I deserve."

The child recovered, but his mother did not rest until, in the next year, compulsory rabies vaccination for dogs was the law in her town.

So it has been since this country began. Public health is sometimes accepted only after years of effort by an informed citizenry that is finally aroused. In Colonial America, the Reverend Cotton Mather was widely hated for his advice that people be protected against smallpox. Indeed, in 1721, a hand grenade was thrown into his house. Attached to it was this message: "Cotton Mather, you Dog, Damn you, I'll inoculate you with this, and a Pox to you."

Smallpox vaccination, rabies vaccination, water fluoridation, milk pasteurization—these and other health advances have been met with the bitter resistance of the misinformed. Though experience is usually the best teacher, too often that experience is in the form of dead and disabled human beings.

In the past pages much has been said that is relative to the environment in communities. Whether plant or animal, insect or human, all living things exist within the earthly environment. Even astronauts, who temporarily escape this planet, cannot live without the capsule of earth they take with them. Since our earthly environment is essential to life, it would do us well to learn more about it. After all, it is the only one we have. This, then, is the subject of the following section.

Ecology: A System of Environmental Checks and Balances

In northern California there are communities of giant redwoods. The trees are cathedral. Away from the choking highways, a person can observe a hurrying ant and not feel like one. The quiet is so complete that the visitor may be misled into thinking that not much is happening.

Yet, amid the seeming peace of the forest, as much is happening as in a big city. Through its roots each tree must slake its thirst and feed its outermost buds. At the tree's top each leaf must find light or die. Silently, each tree competes with every other tree for life. By living together, however, trees are better able to resist wind and water damage. A dense grove of trees, for instance, prevents fallen leaves from being blown away, and thus moisture and nutrients are maintained in the soil. About each tree, on it, and in it are numberless forms of life that also are striving for existence, competing with and yet adapting to one another.

So it is with human beings who live together in a community. People are not rooted to one place, of course, but, like the tree, we compete with the rest of life for our place in the sun. Swarming inside and outside of us, too, are countless other organisms, all competing, all adapting.

Any discussion of the environment in a community automatically involves us in a major field of science called **ecology**. This word is derived from the Greek words *oikos*, meaning "home" or "household," and *logos*, meaning "explanation." Thus the ecologist seeks to understand and explain the shared interaction between living things and their environmental household. A key word in the ecologist's vocabulary is **ecosystem**. Ecosystem refers to the systematic, orderly combination or arrangement of living organisms reacting with one another in a shared environment. One may sharply define the area of an ecosystem even to the simplest unit of ecology. For example, a single-celled bacterium thriving in the human gut has its own ecosystem. But the concept of an ecosystem may also be much wider. There are complex interrelationships between the ecosystem of one bac-

terium in an intestine and millions of other bacterial ecosystems within the same gut. Nor could anyone deny a relationship between the

The silent forest is as full of life as the noisiest highway.

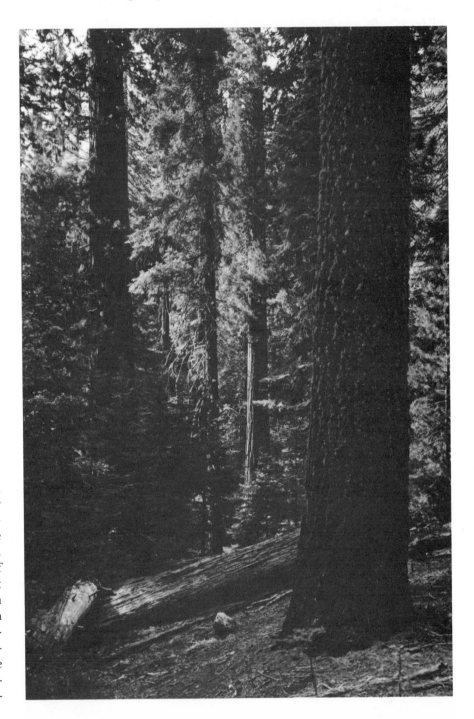

bacterial ecosystems in the gut and the ecosystems of the human hosts. So, innumerable ecosystems interrelated with one another can be distinguished. One may speak of the ecosystem of the Atlantic Ocean, or of a person swimming in it, or of a bacterium swimming in the person. You can see from these examples that ecosystems cannot be separated from one another. They are all interdependent and interrelated. Indeed, the basic chemicals that constitute the heredity material within the nucleus of every human cell are similar to those in each living cell of all plant and animal life, and these chemicals are even found outside the earth in other parts of the universe. "We are brothers of the boulders," wrote the astronomer Harlow Shapley, "cousins of the clouds." This grand concept of a unity of all creatures and things within the universe was movingly described more than half a century ago by the English poet Francis Thompson:

All things by immortal power
Near or far,
Hiddenly
To each other linked are,
That thou canst not stir a flower,
Without troubling of a star.[6]

For Balance, Ecologic Challenge Changes People

Every creature characteristic, from the opening of a flower to the opening of a hand, is determined by both heredity and environment. Formed and stored many thousands of years ago, the chemical pattern of each human being's uniquely arranged set of hereditary chemicals (**genes**) changes with the very slow speed of evolution. Genes and environment interplay to produce a creature with the best chance of meeting any particular environmental challenge. Thus people, by means of their hereditary structure, remain in balance with the ecosystems in their environment.

Can environmental stimulus alone produce rapid change? Yes. Normally, human hereditary characteristics change little, if at all, from a single generation to the next. Yet, in the years since the Second World War, one environmental change, diet, has helped produce a whole generation of larger Japanese and Israeli children. Another recent environmental change accounts for the earlier sexual maturity of today's Western teen-ager. From their parents, modern teen-agers have inherited unchanged reproductive systems. But the culture within the modern ecosystem, which is less dependent on genes, has stimulated new attitudes toward sexuality and marriage.

The characteristics of ecosystems exert even greater changes on human physical characteristics. The fair skin of northwest Europeans affords them the greatest benefit of the little ultraviolet radiation that passes through the cloudy skies of their environment. This is important because the sun's radiation is needed for the skin to make vitamin D, which is necessary for proper bone development. Thus only people with a genetic trait for fair skin were able to adapt successfully to this environment. On the other hand, the dark skin of black people, evolved in the distant past in tropical climates, was doubtless a protective adaptation to guard them against overexposure to the ultraviolet rays of the sun while still allowing them to get enough of those rays to manufacture vitamin D.*

Eskimos have short noses. Were their noses as long as those of the average desert dweller, there would surely be an epidemic of frozen

*Without enough ultraviolet radiation from the sun, rickets, a bone disease caused by too little vitamin D, is the result.

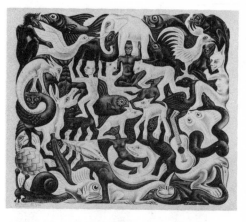

Review the definition of an ecosystem on page 16; can you see how this drawing by E.M. Escher fits the description given in the text?

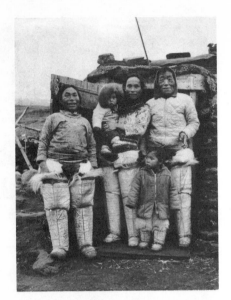

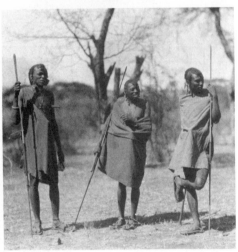

That people are molded by their environments is demonstrated by the Eskimos (top), whose squat, padded bodies, short, broad noses, and tough skin help them to survive their rigorous climate, and by the Masai of East Africa (bottom), whose tall, lean bodies are admirably suited to the hot climate of that region.

noses in the Arctic. Eskimos and the people of eastern Siberia live in what may be the coldest places in the world. They have short noses, narrow nasal passages, and flat faces. Their squat bodies are padded with fat that helps keep them warm. In the African heat, a body frame so covered with fat would be a discomfort. To the Eskimo and the Siberian, it is essential for survival. Thus do ecosystems in the environment influence human characteristics.

People Battle for Control of Their Ecosystems

We turn now to some of the life forms that present challenges to our control of the environment. Their actions spell ecological imbalance for people. Their weapon is disease.

The Staphylococcus Versus Penicillin: A World War

Staphylococcus aureus is a germ that lives in the nose and throat. It is carried by numberless people throughout the world—including those who work in hospitals. Fortunately, though, most people who carry the germ are usually unaffected by it. They and the staphylococci coexist in a state of ecological balance. Occasionally, however, the germ overcomes the resistance of its host. On these occasions, the person carrying the germ experiences such conditions as pimples, boils, or eye infections.

At one time, most staphylococci were very sensitive to penicillin. Small doses of the antibiotic destroyed vast numbers of the germs. And so physicians would saturate the germs' environment with penicillin, and most of the staphyiococci would die. There were always a few, however, that could resist the drug. The originally penicillin-resistant staphylococci did not evolve as the result of a particular change brought about by the antibiotic. Rather, they had a hereditary resistance to penicillin, which enabled them to live through the antibiotic onslaught. As the susceptible staphylococci died, the resistant ones lived. In time, they multiplied enormously. Today they threaten to infect every hospital in the world. Worse, staphylococci have come to develop resistances to antibiotics other than penicillin.

Organisms of higher species also exhibit this resistance to human attempts at control. Consider the louse.

About Lice and People

A striking advantage of being human is our ability to shape our culture in accordance with what we have learned. Insects, by contrast, do not learn. Their attempts at environmental control happen entirely by instinct, as we saw earlier in our description of the ant community. In other words, they have a community but not a culture.

About three-fourths of the insect's brain is eye. It sees much but learns nothing. An insect's sexual instincts, for example, frequently depend on its sensitivity to definite odors. Imagine the confusion of the male insect when scientists, who have been able to isolate the insect sex chemical, spray it over a given area. The poor creature is surrounded by glamorous females who are not there. One would think the frustration enough to kill him. In fact, it does. Scientists, at least in this instance, have outwitted the insect.

But in our constant war with insects for environmental control, we have not always been so victorious. The humble body louse, for example, is able to frustrate human efforts to control it. On the warm body of a human the louse gets free room, board, and transportation. It finds a temporary ecological peace. But the favor goes unreturned. In the first place, lice will make a person itch. Second, some lice carry serious, even deadly epidemic diseases, such as typhus fever. Lice are especially partial to soldiers and their clothing; however, anybody will do. It was with some relief, therefore, that during the Second World War, DDT was found to kill the body louse. For some time during and immediately after the war, soldiers and other affected persons were deloused with this agent.

Imagine the disappointment that occurred when, during the Korean War, it was found that DDT was no longer useful in killing the body louse. The foot soldier had lost a valuable chemical ally. What had happened? During the Second World War, DDT had been introduced into the louse environment. That environment became more tolerable for humans, but intolerable for many lice. Most of the exposed lice died. Most—but not all. Some lice lived. To understand why, one must remember that great numbers and varieties of lice exist. Enormous numbers of lice, with various hereditary combinations, produce tremendous numbers of offspring.

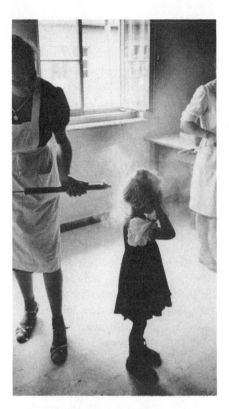

A European child being deloused with DDT. Such spraying was commonplace during and just after World War II.

These offspring contain an even greater number of hereditary combinations. A few of these hereditary combinations resulted in lice that were resistant to DDT. These DDT-resistant lice then produced offspring with hereditary combinations as resistant to DDT as their parents (some were even more resistant). In this way DDT acted as a selector of DDT-resistant lice. Since all the DDT-susceptible lice were killed, in the end only DDT-resistant lice were left. Survival of the species was dependent on adaptation to DDT. Adaptation occurred, and the species survives.

The staphylococcus and the louse are examples of some organisms that have made a biological (hereditary or genetic) adaptation

to a human-made cultural change in environmental ecosystems. To defeat the staphylococcus and the louse and to protect health, the ecology of some germs, lice, and people must undergo even further change. Today, for example, there are several new chemicals that kill staphylococci and lice. These developments are the result of ecological change resulting from human culture.

Of Rain, Potatoes, and Tuberculosis

It is more than a hundred years since the Irish potato famine, but the scars of its deep wounds can still be seen. The great famine was the result of an ecological imbalance brought about by a combination of cultural and environmental changes.

The potato, originally a wild root native to the Andes mountains, had been brought to Ireland as a new food. Along with it came a fungal parasite that had long infested the plant. But with careful farming and reasonably good weather, Irish farmers had been able to keep the fungus at bay. The Irish potato became a delicious food and a staple in the population's diet.

Then the crop failed. Why? For two basic reasons. First, by growing only the best varieties, Irish farmers had refined the potato, making it tastier but also more delicate. It could no longer resist the fungus as well as its hardy Andean ancestor could. Second, in 1845 the weather in Ireland was pitiless. Rain and fog upset the now-delicate ecological-biological balance between potato and fungus, and the potato was overwhelmed. It lay soaked, rotting. The crop was ruined, and so was Ireland.

The enormity of the calamity can hardly be imagined. More than a million people died of hunger. Others perished from scurvy (due to a lack of vitamin C), dysentery, and typhus. Insanity and blindness were common. The former was doubtless due to prolonged stress and lack of vitamins. The latter was probably caused by lack of decent nourishment.

Fearful people of Europe, then as now, looked to the New World. In desperate droves, the rural Irish, starved, disease-ridden, left Ireland for New York, Philadelphia, and Boston. There they met with other miseries. Accustomed to the gentle pace and space of the Irish farm, they were forced into the frantic congestion and speed of the cities. "The sudden and dramatic increase of tuberculosis mortality in the Philadelphia, New York and Boston areas around 1850 can be traced in large part to the Irish immigrants who settled in these cities at that time."[7]

So, because it rained excessively in Ireland in 1845, deaths from tuberculosis increased in Boston, New York, and Philadelphia in 1850. The arm of ecology is long. The physical change in the climate, resulting in a change in the biological balance between the potato and its fungal parasite, brought about vast physical, biological, and cultural imbalances affecting the health of human beings in communities thousands of miles away.

But note this: In the series of imbalances, there were counterbalances. The ecological scales were but temporarily tipped against the people. In the end, they survived. And with their help, so did the Irish potato. Why? Because human beings are able to think and to transmit their thoughts to the generations that follow. We have a culture.

People Can Use Their Learned Culture to Better Their Ecosystems, But . . .

We have seen how human knowledge, combined with cultural achievements, enables people to manipulate ecosystems to their own benefit. Another example? Not long ago large milk supplies in California were found to be polluted by a pesticide. How did this happen? Cows

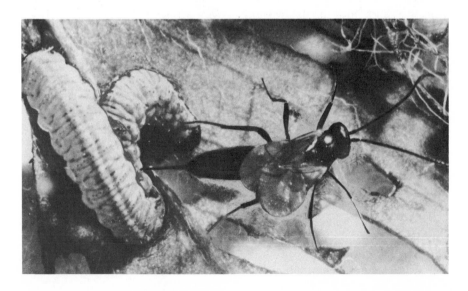

The wasp and the weevil. A natural enemy of the alfalfa weevil and a friend of the alfalfa grower, the wasp deposits its eggs within the alfalfa weevil larva, as shown here. The eggs hatch within the host, and the host then dies.

eat alfalfa. Competing for this food were hungry alfalfa weevil larvae. Wanting milk, people brought their culture to bear on the side of the cow. Alfalfa growers used a pesticide to save the cow-food crop. The weevil was eliminated, but the milk was polluted by the pesticide. Another method of destroying the weevil had to be found. Within the natural balance of the ecosystem lay the answer. It had been observed that certain wasps deposited their eggs inside the alfalfa weevil, and when these eggs hatched, the weevil larvae died. And so great numbers of wasps were deliberately let loose in the weevil's ecosystem. By this culturally inspired manipulation of the environment, the threat of the alfalfa weevil was removed without the use of dangerous pesticides.

In this way, the complex culture of scientists enters into a simple ecological picture. It is a picture of a relationship between a wasp and a weevil. Scientific skill as a part of human culture is wholly learned, taught, and transmitted from one generation to the next. But science, as much as any other aspect of culture, can harm as well as help people. It has brought us both health and disease. And although culture distinguishes us from all else that lives and lends us power over all other life, it is just this culture that in many ways has become our own worst enemy.

Summary

This first chapter has served to identify people as individuals on a health scale, as *community* members, and as a part of the earth's *ecosystem*. Alone among living creatures, people have added thought to instinct, and *culture* to inherited impulse. Human health is woven into culture. It is greatly affected not only by such basic cultural concerns as religion and money but also by the ability of human beings to manipulate their environment. While this ability is useful, it has often been a mixed blessing. Pesticides have multiplied crops, but they also present threats to human well-being. We have the knowledge to protect ourselves from serious diseases, yet in ignorance we often refuse to use that knowledge. Have we remained in healthful balance with our environment, or have we, for temporary advantage, been too careless with our ecological future? There is a line in the Bible that reads: "For the Lord thy God bringeth thee into a good land, a land of brooks of water, of fountains and depths that spring out of valleys and hills" (Deuteronomy 8:7). These words tell of a world washed pure. Have we kept the land this way? Study the next chapter for some answers.

References

1. Curt Paul Richter, *Biological Clocks in Medicine and Psychiatry* (Springfield, Ill., 1965), p. 92.
2. Theodosius Dobzhansky. *Evolution, Genetics, and Man* (New York, 1955), p. 343.
3. Benjamin D. Paul, ed., *Health, Culture, and Community* (New York, 1955), p. 461.
4. René Dubos, "The Germ Theory Revisited," quoted in Stewart Wolf and Helen Goodell, eds., *Harold G. Wolff's Stress and Disease*, 2nd ed. (Springfield, Ill., 1968), p. 190.
5. Philip R. Lee, "The Problems of the Minorities Rest Not with Them, but with the White Majority," *California's Health*, Vol. 26 (May 1969), p. 4.
6. Francis Thompson, "The Mistress of Vision." From *The Poetical Works of Francis Thompson*, edited by Wilfred Meynell (Oxford Standard Authors series; 1937).
7. René Dubos, *Mirage of Health* (Garden City, N.Y., 1961), p. 90.

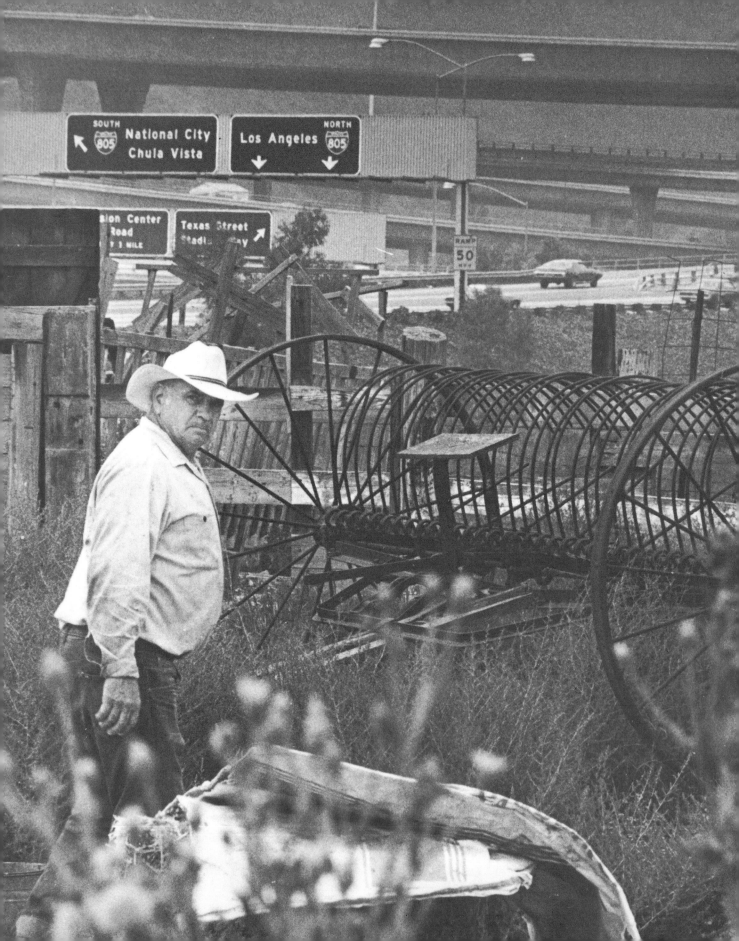

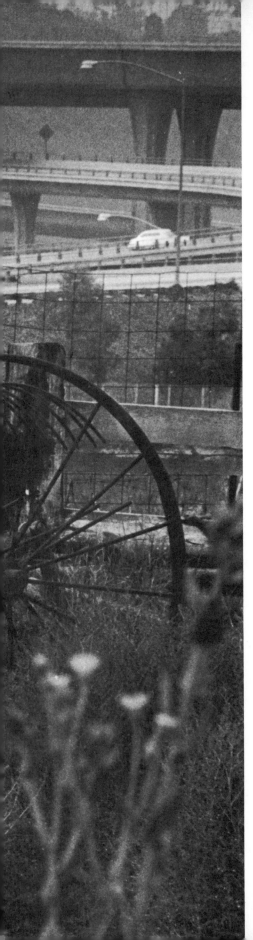

2

People Versus People

Pollution Problems

What is the use of a house if you haven't got a tolerable planet to put it on?

HENRY DAVID THOREAU (1817–1862)

To live is to pollute. This fact of life is common to all creatures, not just humans, but human pollution has begun to seriously menace the planet. And now human garbage is not limited only to the earth. Junk from satellites and spaceships orbits the globe and litters the moon. Chemical vapors may be threatening the fragile gaseous layers that surround the world and protect all earthly life from sickness and death.

Long ago far more of the earth was covered by forest than it is today. But to serve the increasing needs of a growing population, people destroyed countless trees. New growth failed to keep up with the demand for this valuable resource, and whole forest ecosystems were ruined, thereby upsetting nature's balance. At the same time, ignorance of proper farming methods caused fruitful land to be replaced with deserts. Today, *desertification* — the creation of deserts from once fertile, productive land — is still a major problem. It affects every part of the world but Europe. In 1975, the southern rim of the African Sahara Desert, the Sahel, which is poor in grazing land, suffered desertification. During the past century in the United States, New Mexico and Arizona have lost vast lush grassland to desertification.

There were other problems, too, some of which had a more direct effect on people's health and well-being. "Why should cities be erected," mourned Noah Webster, "if they are to be only the tombs of men?" Webster had good reason to be gloomy. According to the May 3, 1799, issue of the newspaper *Aurora*, Philadelphians were often "saluted with a great variety of disgusting smells . . . from filth thrown in heaps as if . . . to promote the purposes of death."[1]

The ten years or so following 1790 saw yellow fever epidemics sweeping through North American cities. In 1793 alone, more than 10 percent of the population of Philadelphia perished. A few years later New Yorkers were dying of the same disease. A few correctly guessed that there was a relationship between the "clouds of musketoes" and the sickness. Fear made the survivors try improved methods of water supply and sewage disposal. But it was not until the nineteenth century that the idea of a water-carriage system for human wastes was accepted. This separation of people from disease-carrying wastes was "the major sanitary advance over the centuries."[2]

During the early nineteenth century the underfed undergraduates at Harvard and Princeton universities often used a fork for more than eating. With it they would pin onto the undersurface of the dining table a few scraps of today's meat for tomorrow's dinner. Property rights to these leftovers were respected by all but stray dogs. At Harvard, pigs were the campus garbage disposal system. If college students turned up their noses in those days, there was good reason. Waste was usually thrown out dormitory windows. The lower floors stank and probably were reserved for freshmen and other wanderers.

Today, pollution problems have changed. We have highly sophisticated water purification and waste disposal systems, yet our relationship to our environment has not improved. Rather, it has gotten worse as the number of people on the planet has increased and their needs have multiplied.

Radiation poisoning. Accidents. Noise. Pesticides. Water pollution. Air pollution. Destruction of countless ecosystems. The growing list of environmental damage includes hundreds of species of life that are already extinct or endangered. Now our own existence is threatened. How can we remain healthy while pollution goes unchecked and uncontrolled? We cannot. We learned in the last chapter that health requires a balance between the inner functioning parts of the body and between the individual and the external environment. So our inner ecosystems must be in balance with our outer ecosystems. What has gone wrong with our outer ecosystems? What parts of the environment have been particularly endangered and, in turn, have endangered our lives?

Water Pollution

In developing and developed countries alike, water maintains life. But in affluent countries, water is also used, wastefully, to maintain *a way of life*. Nature does provide us with a constant supply of water, but it is unevenly distributed. In one country people experience a drought; in another they fight floods. To get the water that daily drips from a leaky faucet in this country, a thirsty Asian or African may need to walk a dozen miles. All peoples of the world have a stake in learning to make better use of their water re-

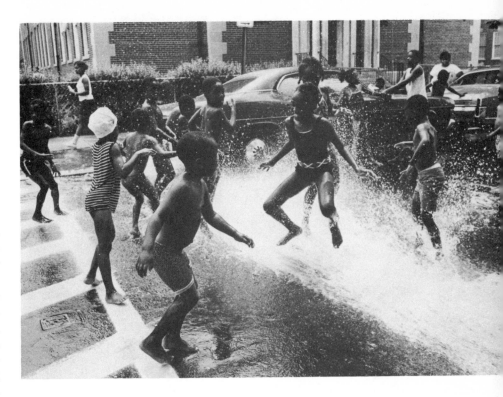

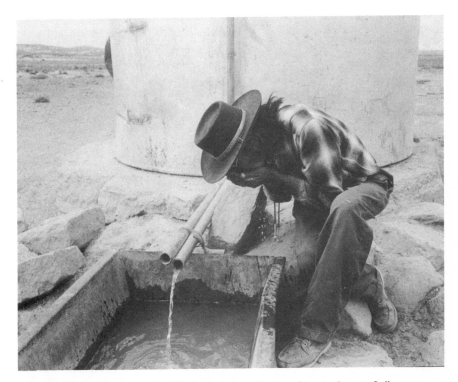

"Till taught by pain men really know not what good water's worth."

LORD BYRON

sources. And what better place is there to start than by dealing with the worldwide problem of water pollution.

PROVIDING SAFE DRINKING WATER

A safer supply of drinking water is a triumph of modern public health technology. Any water supply can be thought of as a system composed of its *source, treatment, storage,* and *distribution to consumers.* The methods of making a water supply safe for human consumption will depend to a considerable extent on its source. For example, waters from lakes and rivers are usually filtered through sand. Then chlorine is added to the water in order to neutralize the effects of otherwise dangerous microorganisms. Before delivery, some water may need special treatment for taste, odor, and softening. Not all water in this country needs filtration. If the source is protected from human and industrial waste, it may need just the added safety factor of chlorination and perhaps some further treatment to improve quality. Sometimes a community gets its water from deep wells. However, the water wells must then be built so that they cannot be contaminated by surface drainage or possible subsurface germ-laden sewage. Often, again depending on the source of the well water, chlorination is added as a safety factor. Laboratory testing of water taken at various distribution points is vital. Such care has eliminated cholera from the United States and made typhoid fever a rarity; however, there is still room for improvement. The relatively recent claim that some present methods of water chlorination result in the formation of chemicals that may cause cancer certainly

poses the need for more investigation. It should not be thought that all of this nation's water supply meets the high standards set by the federal Public Health Service. More than six thousand public water supplies serving about sixty million people fail to meet the standards set by the federal government.

For many millions of people in the developing countries safe drinking water is only a dream, while waterborne disease is a bitter reality. Almost nine million people crowd the four hundred square miles of Calcutta in India. (By way of comparison, in the four hundred square miles of Los Angeles there are less than three million people.) Millions of Calcutta residents have only unfiltered hydrant water for cleaning and drinking. Human waste runs through many streets because there is a shortage of waterborne sewage systems. To alleviate this problem, between 1971 and 1975 thirty thousand latrines (outhouse-like public toilets) were provided for more than one million people. As a result, cholera has lessened somewhat. But getting people to use the latrines, keeping them clean, and providing them for children have presented many problems in implementing the program.

TREATING HUMAN WASTE AND POLLUTANTS

The modern sewage-treatment plant is currently the best-known method we have for dealing with human waste (in which disease microorganisms breed) and pollutants. From toilet bowl, laundromat, bathtub, shower, and sink, waste leaves the home by pipes leading to main sewer lines. By these routes it reaches sewage-treatment plants. There, body waste and other pollutants are removed or reduced to simpler parts. Finally, a disinfectant, such as chlorine, is added and the now reasonably safe sewage is discharged into natural waterways. Unfortunately, even some modern cities do not use the best treatment methods, or their methods are incomplete. As a result, a major problem has developed—the vast pollution of rivers, lakes, streams, and deep wells.

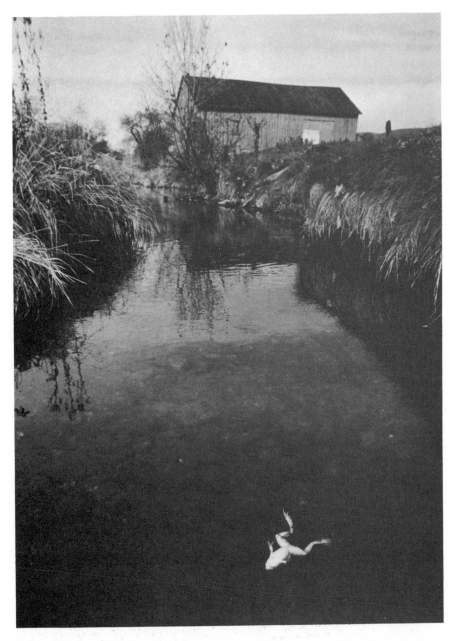

NONHUMAN WASTES

Water pollution is not the result of human waste alone. In the United States, modern hog and poultry production is centralized in factory-like operations. "A cow [for example] generates as much manure as sixteen human beings. . . . In total, farm animals produce ten times as much organic waste as the human population."[3] Disposal of such huge amounts of animal waste has become a matter of much concern, as has the problem of how to dispose of the more than 500,000 different chemicals that are regularly added to U.S. waters. Hundreds of these are believed to contaminate some drinking waters.

LEGISLATING CLEAN WATER

The efforts of an aroused citizenry have shown that the pollution of water resources by people can be reversed. In 1972 the prime minister of Canada and the president of the United States signed the Great Lakes Water Quality Agreement. This was the first pact between two nations to protect and improve a shared environmental resource. It is just these sorts of agreements that are able to save such waters as the once-dying Lake Erie.

The Safe Drinking Water Act of 1974 was an important beginning step in improving our drinking water, and other efforts to control water pollution are now being made. Not long ago, for example, Oregon's Willamette River was a vast toilet flushed by water released from federal dams. Today, it is a testimony to what can be done by people who care. Old laws were tightened; new laws passed. Now the Willamette safely serves the recreational, industrial, and agricultural needs of Oregonians. The enforcement of old laws as well as the addition of new ones, combined with better sewage-disposal methods, is also slowly reducing the pollution of the Hudson and Mississippi-Missouri rivers. But much remains to be done.

Industries and governments are studying their waste disposal processes, and they are making money doing it. For many years the Bethlehem Steel Company plant at Sparrows Point, Maryland, near Baltimore, has used the treated water wastes of the sewage of almost a million people in their productive process. This economically and ecologically responsible practice of waste-water reuse is beneficial to all—citizens and industry alike.

Poison Tanks

In Niagara Falls City they called it Love Canal. It had been built in 1894 by William Love to serve as a power source and barge route. These plans never materialized. Many years later what did materialize was an ecological horror that is now known to exist in dozens of other places in the nation.[4]

After the original plans failed, Love Canal became a swimming hole for the children in the area. Then a chemical corporation used it as an industrial landfill. Into the canal and along its banks they dumped thousands of metal drums containing chemical wastes. In 1953 the chemical company generously sold the sixteen acres to the Niagara Falls Board of Education for $1. The canal was filled in. On part of the filled-in land a school was built. The other part was sold to developers to build homes. For more than ten years the Love Canal area was an undisturbed middle-class neighborhood. But during all that time the buried drums were corroding and leaking poisons into the earth. By 1976 the chemicals had surfaced. More than eighty have been identified; some may be cancer-causers. Today it is estimated that as many as one hundred thousand drums may be stored there. Among the women in the neighborhood, the incidence of miscarriages, birth defects, and liver disease rose above

normal. About 240 families were evacuated. New York State bought the homes, and the whole site was surrounded by a chain-link fence.

But that was not all. Near another Niagara Falls city a whole baseball field swelled as chemicals seeped to its surface. It also contained the deadly drums. So did other nearby sites. Dioxin, a herb-killer, was found in some of them. Until 1970 it had been used in Vietnam. And dioxin, like DDT, accumulates in the body fat. In 1976 it was dioxin that caused people to be evacuated from Seveso, Italy, because of a plant explosion near the town (see page 40). Depending on the amount of exposure, the signs and symptoms of dioxin poisoning are a severe skin condition called chloracne and various nerve disorders. Dioxin is also thought to affect the unborn child. Some problems occur years after the initial exposures.[5]

Today we know that chemical dump sites are a national problem. Texas, Ohio, Pennsylvania, Louisiana, Michigan, Indiana, Illinois, Tennessee, West Virginia, California, New York, and New Jersey are among the states that must deal with dioxin, polychlorinated biphenyls (PCBs), cyanides, pesticides, arsenic, mercury, and a number of other chemicals, some of which are still unidentified.[6] The greatest danger is to ground-water used for drinking. About half this nation's population depends on this source for drinking water; in Florida, for example, the figure is over 90 percent. In 1979, the federal Environmental Protection Agency planned to use its authority under the Safe Drinking Water Act to strengthen regulation of all deep wells so that the amount of hazardous wastes that will pollute the drinking water will be limited.

But who is responsible for the

clean-up of this vast ecological mess? The companies? They had broken no existing law. The federal government? The enormous expense will not please Congress. The states? They too are sensitive to tax expenditures, as are the cities.[7] But the cleaning operations must be begun on known polluted sites, and the search for unknown polluted sites must be continued. Only time will tell how many people must pay more than money for this additional insult to the environment.

Solid-Waste Disposal

The story is told of the housekeeper who, when asked what she did with her garbage, replied, "Oh, I just kick it around till it gets lost." That more or less is how much of the housekeeping of this country is conducted. Every year in the United States, billions of cans and bottles and countless pounds of paper products and plastics are produced. And much of this solid waste is never really disposed of—it just gets kicked around. The trouble is it will not get lost. Moreover, getting rid of solid waste is often expensive. For example, it costs more to dispose of the Sunday edition of *The New York Times* than it does to buy it.

Most solid waste consists of food wastes and rubbish from households, institutions, and commercial establishments. Garden sweepings, soiled hospital bandages, and discarded automobiles and refrigerators are just a few other examples of the types of refuse that clog the ecosystem. Solid wastes do not usually transmit disease. True, their improper disposal breeds rats, insects, and vermin that, in turn, can spread such illnesses as plague and gastrointestinal (stomach and intestine) infections. But today's greatest

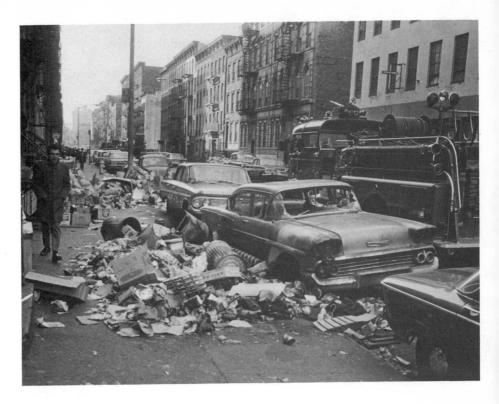

danger of improper solid-waste disposal lies in its spoliaton of the environment.

There are a variety of new ways of disposing of solid wastes. In fact, trash has become a valuable natural resource. In 1976 Congress passed the Resource Conservation and Recovery Act. Its purpose is to take advantage of our trash resources by finding ways to reuse solid wastes. This is called **recycling**. When burned in a modern incinerator, for example, some solid wastes may be reduced to an ash that can be used to surface roads. The heat of such burned solid wastes may be used to provide warmth for office buildings and swimming pools. Garbage is also used to fill land. A hill in one U.S. city is a heap of garbage covered with layers of clay, dirt, and sod. In the winter it provides fine toboggan runs.

Sanitary landfills may someday be a source of methane gas energy.

Large waste materials, such as stoves and sofas, may be passed through shredders or pounded by a hammermill and the remaining material used in the construction of new products. In Japan, where compression of waste material is a common practice, bigger bales of rubbish are sunk in the sea; smaller cubes are used for building river banks and sea walls.

In St. Louis the Union Electric Power Company turns waste into power by heating garbage to high temperatures with little or no air present to produce the energy needed to run its power-generating system. Thus a home's trash may be transformed into its bright lights. Baltimore and Milwaukee are other cities that are now using trash profitably. Even automobiles and light steel products, such as refrigerators, may be recycled by being scrapped and then made a part of steel production.

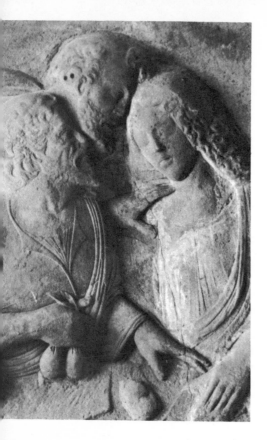

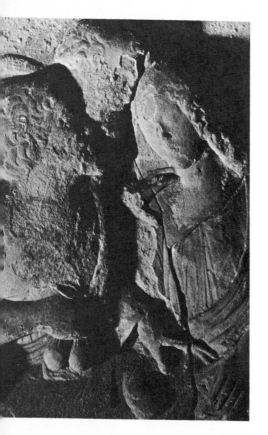

A stone sculpture in Venice, Italy. The top picture was taken in 1900, the one on the bottom in 1973. The erosion is the result of air pollution in this increasingly industrialized city.

The Dirty, Dangerous Skies

*O dark, dark, dark, amid the
   blaze of noon,
Irrecoverably dark, total Eclipse
Without all hope of day!*

JOHN MILTON, *Samson Agonistes*,
lines 80–82

An obelisk is a monument—usually a large, tapering shaft of stone. In this country, the best-known obelisk is the dulled Washington Monument in the nation's capital. Cleopatra's Needle is one of two Egyptian obelisks; however, neither is in Egypt anymore. One is in London, and the other is in New York's Central Park. Made in 1460 B.C., the latter was given to the city in 1881 as a gift from the then ruler of Egypt. But in one century, New York smog did what thirty-three centuries of Egyptian climate could not do: The ancient Egyptian carvings, once so clear, can hardly be made out today.

Some time ago a nagging question arose. If polluted air eats away stone, how does the seven- to ten-thousand quarts of polluted air each person inhales daily affect soft, delicate lung tissue? In seeking an answer to this question, first consider the source and nature of this aerial rubbish.

LONDON–TYPE SMOG

The nineteenth-century English poet Percy Bysshe Shelley wrote that "Hell is a city much like London—a populous and smoky city." What so troubled the ailing Shelley, and countless Londoners before and after him, is called **London-type smog**. The word "smog" probably originated from a 1901 scientific report blaming some 1,063 deaths in Glasgow and Edinburgh on "Smoke and Fog." London-type smog is not limited to London. It dims such industrialized communities as Detroit, New York, Philadelphia, and Chicago. It is, as will be seen, quite different from *Los Angeles-type smog*.

In both types of air pollution, however, normal cleansing of air is prevented by a phenomenon called **temperature inversion**. Ordinarily, air temperature decreases with height. For each thousand-foot rise in elevation, the air temperature drops about five degrees Fahrenheit. So, under usual conditions, the air at ground level is warmer than the air above. It is this difference in temperature that helps make possible the vertical air motion so necessary for cleansing ground-level air. But a temperature inversion reverses (inverts) this situation. (See Figure 2–1.) Because of a variety of changes in the atmosphere, a layer of warm air above traps a layer of cold air below. Thus, over the affected area there is a blanket of warm air. In London-type smog this inversion layer of warmer air usually occurs at about three or four hundred feet. In Los Angeles-type smog the warm-air blanket is higher—usually at a thousand feet or more. The lower the inversion layer, the more severe the smog. Not until the cold layer of ground air is warmed enough by the sun to break the inversion can the ground air escape and, with it, its gathered pollutants. Thus it is a temperature inversion that prevents the removal of air pollutants from the area where they originate. Since temperature inversions cannot be controlled, air pollution must be.

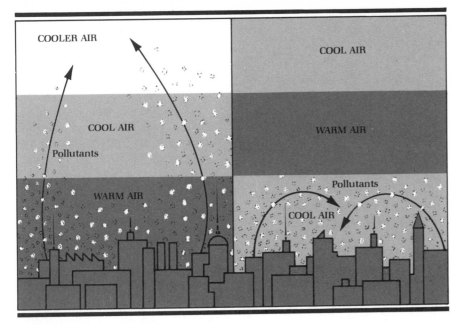

FIGURE 2–1
Normal weather conditions are shown at left. In a temperature inversion, cool air—along with pollutants—becomes trapped under a warm air mass.

London-type smog came with coal. Smoking stacks meant employment, but coal that is incompletely burned releases a harmful byproduct—sulfur dioxide (SO_2) gas. Sunlight adds oxygen to the SO_2, and sulfur trioxide (SO_3) is formed. When the sulfur trioxide combines with air moisture (or fog), the result is destructive sulfuric acid (H_2SO_4, $H_2O + SO_3 \rightarrow H_2SO_4$). Sulfuric acid is more irritating to the lungs than is sulfur dioxide, particularly if the acid is suspended in snow or in a fine mist, which is common in London. And as if this acid rain and snow were not enough, the recipe for London-type smog also includes other poisonous gases and irritating particles of soot. In the United States, the major source of London-type smog is the burning of coal, oil, and natural gas to produce electric power.

LOS ANGELES–TYPE SMOG

Los Angeles-type smog ("oxidizing" or photochemical" smog), unlike the London type, is a warm-weather irritant rarely associated with fog. It occurs in various regions of this country, where the appropriate warm-weather conditions and air pollution by automobiles and industries exist. It is therefore not surprising that this type of smog is typical of Los Angeles County, where about five million cars daily use more than eight million gallons of gasoline. And a car does not have to be running to add to smog-contributing chemicals. Fuel tank and carburetor evaporations are also part of the smog misery. Each car belches or evaporates its pollutants into the cold ground air, which is trapped beneath the warm

air by the thermal inversion. The Southern California sunshine only makes matters worse, as the ultraviolet light causes reactions between the pollutants, thus creating a poisonous pall.

THE BREATH OF DEATH

Smog worsens the illnesses of people who are already sick. And among those not already ill, smog may silently bring on the beginnings of serious sickness. Many people—particularly children and sufferers of chronic diseases of the lungs and breathing tubes (bronchi), such as asthma and emphysema—are painfully affected on especially smoggy days.

Can air pollution be linked to lung cancer? Some data seem to indicate that it can. People living in city areas have twice the incidence of lung cancer as do rural dwellers. In those areas in which coal use pollutes the air, the incidence of lung cancer is even greater. Moreover, the death rates from lung cancer of males living in areas of heavy industry in Los Angeles County were found to be unusually high. (More men than women work in heavily polluted areas, which may account for this finding.)

In November 1953, a cover of pollution blanketed New York City. Nine years later it was revealed that during that time 200 more New Yorkers died than would have been expected to die in that period. Another study showed that following a 1966 Thanksgiving weekend attack of air pollution, there were 168 "excess" deaths in New York City.

Recent years have seen a marked increase in deaths from *emphysema*, a crippling lung disease (see page 220). Some of this increase is doubtlessly due to improved diagnostic techniques, but certainly not all. Undoubtedly, a major cause of this disease is smog.

In the past quarter-century, U.S. death rates from inflammation of the breathing tubes (*bronchitis*) and *asthma* (see page 63) also have risen. The exact relationship between smog and the increases in death from these illnesses is unclear. But it is known that thousands of people died during a smog episode in London, and about a score of people were killed by an attack of smog in Donora, Pennsylvania. One fact is clear: Smog can kill.

WHAT MUST BE DONE?

Improvements in factory construction can help industrialists get rid of sulfur pollutants. Moreover, various chemical processes may not only relieve the pollution problem but, as with waste disposal processes, may become a source of income for some industries.

The major cause of air pollution, however, is the automobile, and people are now being forced to find a solution for the pollution caused by the use of gasoline as automobile fuel. It has been estimated that by the year 2025—within the lifetimes of many who are now in college— the world's petroleum resources will be almost gone. The internal combustion engine that now powers our automobiles may by then be but a memory. Experiments with other types of engines are already being carried out.

A nonpolluting new means of transportation is the recently developed automated Personal Rapid Transport (PRT) system. One type is a computer-controlled, driverless, rubber-tired minibus that carries from four to forty passengers on elevated guide rails. It has been described as a cross between an automatic elevator and a monorail. During rush hours, the minibus stops only at certain stations. At other times (as with an elevator), passengers press a call button at a station. Once aboard, they press a destination button. In 1973, a 3.2-mile, relatively pollution-free PRT system opened connecting the three campuses of West Virginia University. A somewhat similar PRT system is being built at the Dallas-Fort Worth Regional Airport. Despite an accident, San Francisco's computer-controlled subway system is attracting national attention.

AIR POLLUTION: LAWS AND ECONOMICS

Two federal laws spell out this nation's program for control of air pollution: the Air Quality Act of 1967 and the Clean Air Amendments of 1970. The federal Environmental Protection Agency has been charged with the enforcement of these clean air laws, which have established strict standards for air and automobile pollution.

It is claimed that pollution control will mean higher prices and taxes. But is it not eventually less expensive to be rid of the pollution than to keep it? Air pollution costs the people of this nation an estimated $16 billion a year. These costs vary from medical bills for those who become ill as a result of pollution to replacement of damaged materials, such as rubber used in industry.

Will pollution control result in

unemployment? Hardest hit would be small towns with only one major industry that would be forced to shut down because of the costs of pollution-control equipment. But since jobs would be created in industries that manufacture pollution-abatement equipment, the net loss of jobs in the country as a whole would be minor.

Sound Pollution: The Modern Earache

Millions of automobiles, trucks, and motorcycles roar through the streets of this nation. In and around homes, countless appliances—such as tape recorders and record players, TV sets, dishwashers, lawnmowers, garbage disposals, and food blenders—add to the national din. Above, the skies shake from the noise of jet aircraft.

Noise affects different people in various ways. The deep voice of a cello relaxes one person but distracts another. An epileptic seizure was the reaction of one Wisconsin housewife to the voices of three different radio announcers. (The successful treatment was the repeated playing of tapes of the announcers' voices until they no longer affected her.)

Noise costs money. It has been estimated that the cost to industry in terms of lost production and accidents is as high as $4 billion a year. And in this country annual compensation claims from deafness thought to be due to job noise amount to additional millions of dollars. Many companies find office soundproofing a sound investment: Typing errors drop, machine operator errors lessen, and absenteeism and employee turnover are reduced. The management of one large New York

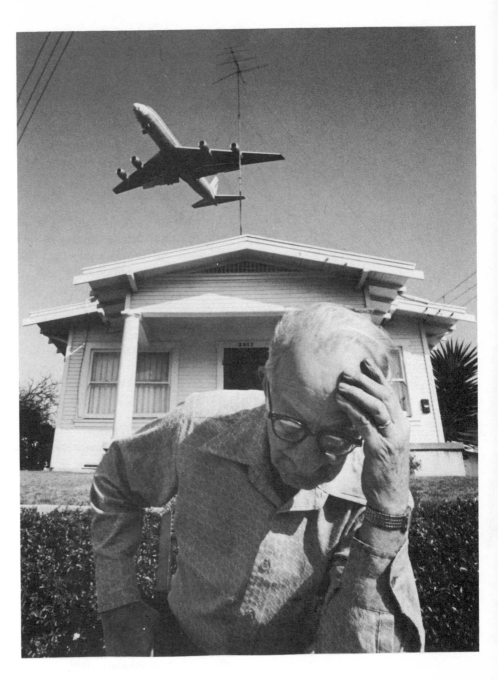

bank found a novel solution to its noise problem. Plagued by high employee turnover due to the insufferable din, the managers finally decided to hire lip-reading deaf people.

On the national level, a Noise Control Act was passed by Congress in 1972. But the basic responsibility for local noise control still rests with state and local governments. It is the responsibility of every citizen to let elected officials know of the need to reduce local noise levels.

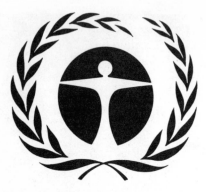

The official symbol for the United
Nations Conference on the Human
Environment, 1972.

A Worldwide Effort Against Pollution

The first global meeting on pollution was the United Nations Conference on the Human Environment held in Stockholm, Sweden, in June 1972. The conference was attended by twelve hundred delegates representing 112 nations. The African city of Nairobi, in Kenya, was selected as the permanent headquarters of the UN Environmental Agency.

Among the important results of this first international meeting was a proposal to establish a UN organization to carry out an antipollution program. Another of the 109 recommendations adopted by the conference (and later approved by the UN General Assembly) was one making nations responsible for pollution of areas outside their national boundaries.

The second meeting, called the International Conference on the Environmental Future, was held at Reykjavik, Iceland, in the spring of 1977. About 130 delegates from twenty countries attended. The intention was to bring together internationally famous ecologists to discuss global and local pollution problems. During the course of the discussion, one speaker from the United States pointed out that Reykjavik itself offers a tiny but excellent example of an "ecodisaster": the collapse of major stocks of fish brought about by British overexploitation of Icelandic fishing grounds. About this and other ecological problems, there was little optimism voiced at the conference. The experts agreed that the power to achieve an ecologically safe world lays in the hands of politicians of the Western world.

The Epidemic on Wheels

On September 13, 1899, Mr. A. W. Bliss stepped off a New York trolley and was hit by a horseless carriage. He became the world's first auto death. Since then, in this country alone, more than two million people have died in automobile accidents.

The Mathematics of Death

According to the National Safety Council, in 1978, 105,500 people died in this country as the result of accidents. Almost half of these accidents were caused by motor vehicles. Traffic accidents also account for millions of injuries a year; over 14,600 people *a day* suffer traffic injuries requiring medical attention.

In Portland, Oregon, a twenty-six-year-old woman is out for a Sunday afternoon drive with her husband and six-year-old son. She is pregnant with twins, who are due next month. The woman is a bit impatient. "I can't be comfortable with these seat belts anymore," she tells her husband, and she lets them fall unfastened. Then she turns to be certain that the child in the back seat has fastened his seat belt.

Soon they are in the country. It is a fine day. Suddenly another car comes over the hill on the wrong side of the road. They are hit head-on.

In the hospital, nine stitches repair the man's scalp. Then he is told. The child is badly shaken up, but not hurt. The wife, however, has a crush-

ing head injury. There is brain damage. The unborn twins are dead. That night the woman dies.

The woman has become one of the 51,900 who died in 1978 in auto accidents. So has the other driver, who was dead on admission to the hospital. The husband is counted with the millions who are injured. That is part of the meaning of the numbers. Not the least interesting thing about them is how uninteresting they are to so many people.

How does death occur in accidents such as this? One answer is simply mathematical. There were two crashes, not one. The first crash brought the car to a halt. But for a fraction of a second, the woman, unrestrained by a seat belt, continued traveling. In the car she continued heading for a second crash: the crash between her head and the windshield. The windshield yielded two inches, and her head collapsed two inches. Thus, after hitting the windshield, her head traveled four inches. What was the force of the blow on the woman's head? For this there is an equation:

$$G^* = \frac{\text{miles per hour}^2}{30 \times \text{stopping distance in feet}}$$

or

$$\frac{(55)^2}{30 \times \frac{1}{3}} = \frac{3{,}025}{10} = 302.5$$

The weight of that part of her upper body directly involved in the windshield blow is estimated at 20

*G is the force developed in slowing down an object, as measured in terms of the force of gravity. In this formula, 30 represents a constant number from the acceleration caused by gravity (32.2 feet per second). The 1/3 is the 2-inch yield of glass plus the 2-inch yield of the woman's head before it stopped moving against the windshield (4 inches = 1/3 foot).

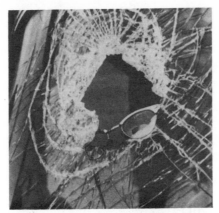
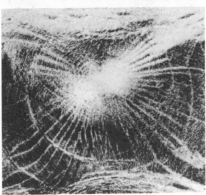

After an automobile accident, the eyeglasses of an Indianapolis woman are left dangling from the smashed windshield (top). Damage to her head was severe. A safety windshield (bottom) breaks into blunt-edged, nonlacerating granules.

percent of the weight of herself and her unborn babies (130 pounds), or 26 pounds. Multiplying 26 pounds by 302.5 G's equals 7,865 pounds —almost four tons. This was the average force with which her head impacted against the windshield.

Dangerous Drivers

For some people driving is like an accident on its way to happening. Consider the following true story. In

Pennsylvania, a motorist was killed when his car crashed into a tree. Upon examination it was found that the driver was totally blind and that an eight-year-old child had been directing his driving. Certainly this is an extreme example, but given that some states renew licenses by mail and others require an eye examination only with the first issuance of a driver's license, it may not be as rare as one might suppose.

What about drivers who are ill? Many of the drivers who have heart attacks while driving do not know they are ill until an accident happens. But there are many others whose poor health makes them accident risks, and these people should be identified and kept from driving. As for alcoholics, they, too, should be denied driving privileges until their illness is treated and under control.

Prevention of Accidents

Automobile accidents, like all other epidemics, must be considered in terms of three related factors. The *host*, or driver, has already been discussed. The two other elements are the *agent*, or automobile, and the *environment*, or roads.

AUTOMOBILES

Accidents can almost always teach us something—if we pay attention to why they happen. Had the pregnant woman in our earlier example used her seat belt, she and her unborn children might have been among the thousands of people in this country each year whose lives are saved by the use of these restraints. And those who use both lap and sash belts are even safer than those who use lap belts alone.

Unfortunately, about two-thirds of the people owning cars with seat belts do not use them, while nine out of ten ignore shoulder belts. This refusal to use safety belts cannot be attributed to the forgetfulness of the drivers, because since 1972 all cars built in this country contain a buzzer that sounds whenever the driver fails to fasten the seat belt.

In spite of the resistance of drivers to safety improvements in automobiles, research into new safety devices continues. One of the latest devices is the air bag, which inflates when a collision occurs, thus saving the car's occupants from serious injury. Though many engineering problems have been encountered, it is hoped that air bags will soon become another life-saving device required in all automobiles.

Tires are another important feature of automobile safety. The first requirement is that they be bought for their intended use. A suburban school teacher, for example, will need tires that are quite different from those required by a cross-country truck driver.

Another requirement is that the tires must be in good condition. When should a tire be replaced? Molded into the patterns of most recently manufactured tires are tread-wear bar indicators. These are solid crossbars between the grooves. When these show, it is time to replace the tire. Periodic wheel-alignment checks provide an additional assurance of safety.

Other automobile safety features now in use or planned for future use include a reshaped and padded instrument panel, collapsible steering column, shock-absorbent materials in roof areas, more securely fastened seats, rear windshield wipers and defrosters, improved seat locks, door locks with recessed handles, a

stronger wall between the trunk and the rear seat, removal of bumper projections, dual braking systems, and collapsible front and rear bumpers. Of great help in decreasing facial cuts is a new windshield (now required on all U.S.-built cars) with a plastic layer between the two panes of glass. The big side windows on two-door cars should have the same glass.

ROADS

Small highway improvements are often investments producing big dividends. By a program of "spot improvements," the County of Los Angeles has made driving safer for its millions of drivers. For example, in wet weather a section of the Hollywood Freeway was noted to be a skidding area. To combat this the pavement was regrooved. The result was almost a 90 percent reduction in accidents.

A program in which locations of consistent accidents are studied and improved has spread throughout the state. Redesigned and relocated signs and land markings, adequate roadway widening, and the construction of channeling islands are but a few of the spot improvements that in "before and after" studies have been shown to reduce accident fatalities by 53 percent and injuries by almost 25 percent. Should such programs be adopted nationwide, there could be a significant decrease in deaths and injuries due to automobile accidents.

Help for the Injured

Once an accident has occurred, how quickly does help come? The accident in which the young mother and her twins died happened in the open country, seventeen miles from a

hospital. Emergency care was not quickly available. Most rural areas have poor emergency services. In an investigation of eight hundred California accidents, it was found that 90 percent of those fatally injured in rural areas died at the crash scene within an hour of the accident. By comparison, only 37 percent of those fatally injured in urban areas were dead before they were moved by ambulance. Moreover, since rural accident victims often have to be transported twice as far as people injured in cities, more time elapses before they reach the hospital and receive treatment. And the length of time between injury and treatment is often a crucial factor in deciding the victim's fate.

Pity the Poor Pedestrian

About 20 percent of traffic deaths involve pedestrians. Of these, most are very young and very old people, who have poorer judgment and less ability to move quickly. In a pedestrian-auto collision, the pedestrian is not usually "run over." He or she is "run under." Lifted up by the car, the pedestrian's head hits the hood, roof, or windshield, or, while sprawled on the hood, the victim travels briefly along with the vehicle before being thrown to the ground. Cars without sloping hoods cause more severe head injuries than those with longer hoods, and cars with "gingerbread" projections are clearly a menace.

Motorcycle Hazards

In 1977 there were over five million motorcycles registered in the United States. Sixteen million people rode them. That same year about 440,000 motorcycle accidents killed almost four thousand young people. Most of the serious or fatal accidents involved collision with cars at intersections.

Not surprisingly, untrained and inexperienced motorcyclists are the most likely to get hurt or killed. The Motorcycle Safety Foundation in Linthicum, Maryland, has developed an excellent community course for motorcycle riders. If you drive, or expect to drive, a motor-cycle, it would make good sense to heed the warning implied in these facts and be sure you have developed adequate skills and knowledge before taking to the roads.

When gasoline became scarce in 1979, mopeds became a commonplace sight on city streets. Because their increase is so recent, there is as yet no data regarding their accident hazards. However, what is true for the motorcycle rider is just as true for the moped rider.

Dangerous Fun and Games

Some people enjoy daring death. In this country, thousands do so by racing automobiles, and many lose the race to death.

Perhaps a million others skin dive and scuba dive. Those with a history of illness, particularly if it is related to the heart or the lungs, should do neither. Some physicians would also advise people with even minor colds or only moderately high blood pressure to avoid diving. The minimum beginning age for diving should be about seventeen. Divers who are physically fit and well trained and who do not dive alone seldom are endangered. However, it is important to remember that the quality of air in the tanks is a significant aspect of skin and scuba diving. A few fly-by-night operators sell contaminated air. Local health departments are the best source of advice about where one can purchase safe air.

You do not have to dive to run a risk in the water. In 1978, over 7,000 people drowned in the United States. Statistics show that males drown more often than females, that as many as half the people in this country do not swim well enough to cope with emergencies in water, and that most drownings occur in water not specifically set aside for recreation. It is important to remember that near-drowning victims are not necessarily out of danger once they have been brought back to consciousness. Death from oxygen-shortage may still occur, which is why they should be watched in a hospital for at least twenty-four hours following the incident.

Experienced skiers know the importance of adequate ski equipment, physical conditioning, and training. The ski boots' release bindings must be properly adjusted so that when unusual stress occurs—as in a fall—the boot will easily release from the ski, preventing broken bones. Since muscles both steer and brake the skier, their condition is of great importance. Preseason exercise programs are invaluable, as are warm-up periods before starting down a hill. A tired person should not ski. Over 225,000 people are hurt every year on the ski slopes of this country. The Ski Patrol, an organization of experienced skiers devoted to first aid and rescue, should be supported by those interested in skiing, which is the most rapidly growing winter sport.

The trampoline should never be used. It has been responsible for a number of severe accidental paralyses.

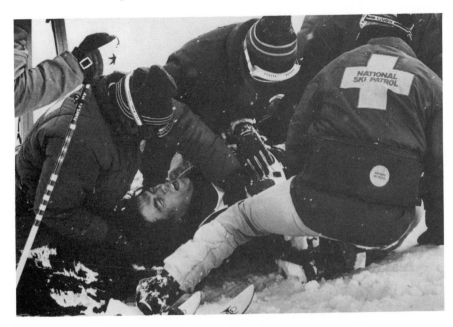

The Ski Patrol is an efficient, life-saving organization.

```
ROBERT F. KENNEDY
NEW YORK

                        United States Senate
                           WASHINGTON, D.C.

                            August 6, 1965



        Mr. Keith A. Humbert
        6440 Snowapple
        Clarkston, Michigan

        Dear Mr. Humbert:

             Thank you for letting me know your views on the control
        of firearms.

             In my judgment, regulation of the sale of firearms is
        in the national interest.  It is unfortunate that many of our
        citizens are confused and misinformed as to the effects of
        S. 1592.  This bill would give us the protection we need with-
        out unduly inconveniencing legitimate hunters, sport shooters,
        or gun clubs.  I have attached a statement I presented to the
        Senate Subcommittee on Juvenile Delinquency, setting forth my
        reasons for this belief.

             Again my thanks for your views.  I look forward to hearing
        your views on other issues in the future.

                            Sincerely,

                            Robert F. Kennedy

        Enclosure
```

"Guns Don't Kill People: People Kill People"?

These words (without the question mark) are often used by gun lobbyists in Washington. But words cannot alter the fact that every year over twenty-three thousand people in this country are killed by guns, either accidentally or in a quick rage or during acts of criminality. Millions of people own guns, and many are carried illegally.

In late 1967, Senator Robert Kennedy condemned the power lobby of the American Rifle Association. A short time later he was dead of gunshot wounds. Perhaps enough letters like the one reproduced above will someday prompt action on gun control laws in this nation.

"Be It Ever So Humble . . ."

Of the 25,000 people killed by accidents in their homes in this country during 1978, a major portion were very young (under five) or old (seventy-five or over). Falls and burns account for a high proportion of deaths from household accidents.

Falls

Fatal falls are most common among the elderly, in part because they are more likely to have spells of weakness and dizziness and in part because their bones are more brittle. Depression may be as much a cause of falling as a misplaced toy, a slippery floor, poor vision, or arthritis. An elderly person may rise in the morning feeling dreary and tired. There is no place to go. Not bothering to tie his shoelaces, he may trip going down the stairs—a fall that can cost him his life. Railings, elastic shoelaces, night lights, luminous paint around light switches, and other safety devices cannot relieve the heartache of loneliness, but they can help prevent falls by the elderly. They are also good precautions for protecting small children.

As toddlers grow, they must be protected—although not frightened—from their normal curiosity. Over a dozen young children die daily as a result of needless accidents. The crucial hours seem to be between 3 P.M. and 6 P.M., when the mother is most apt to feel that she is losing the footrace with her runabout child. A babysitter for a few hours during the extra-busy after-school hours can be a life-saving investment.

Fires

Faulty furnaces and electrical equipment, falling asleep while smoking, fireplaces without screens, matches thrown carelessly into wastebaskets, and flammable liquids are some of the most common causes of household fires. Burns are usually suffered because of clothing, bedding, or other household furnishings that are not fire-resistant. Fires can be prevented, and laws calling for the use of fire-resistant fabrics must be enforced. Wool is the most naturally fire-resistant of all fabrics. Cotton, viscose, and rayon materials burn quickly, but they can be made fire-resistant.

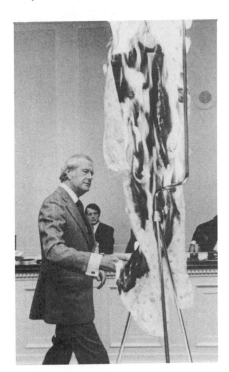

A demonstration of the dangerous inadequacy of the standards set by the Flammable Fabrics Act. A match put to a nightgown causes it to burst instantly into flames.

Glass and saran textiles resist fire. Acrylic (which is better known by the trades names Orlon, Acrilan, Creslan, and Zafron) is very flammable, but it can be combined with a flame-resistant fiber to make it safer.

Suffocation and Poisonings

Some babies suffocate on food that they regurgitate and are unable to expel. Consequently, propping up infants' bottles and leaving them to eat alone can be a dangerous practice. Plastic bags and small metal or plastic objects are hazardous to young children. The bags can fit over the child's head and cause suffocation. The small objects can fit into a toddler's mouth and clog the windpipe.

The dimming vision of the elderly is responsible for many accidents resulting from taking the wrong medication. Clear labeling of medicine bottles, adequate bathroom lighting, and diligent wearing of corrective lenses can help prevent mistakes. But most accidental poisonings happen to children. The most commonly ingested chemicals are aspirin, cleaning and polishing agents, and pesticides. These must be kept out of a child's reach in a locked cabinet. When rushing a possibly poisoned child to a physician or hospital it is important to take along the poison container. Knowing what the child took, the physician can telephone the nearest poison control center to get immediate information about the poison and its antidote. Such centers exist in all major cities.

Dangerous Substances That Help and Harm People

Pesticides and Other Chemicals

On July 10, 1976, in the small town of Seveso in northern Italy, a huge kettle of chemicals was cooking in the local chemical plant. The brew overheated, raining chemicals over hundreds of acres of agricultural grassland, trees, and houses. Among the chemicals was an extremely poisonous substance known to chemists as 2,3,7,8-tetrachlorodibenzo-p-dioxin. It is just as well to remember it as TCDD or dioxin.

The townspeople of Seveso wish that they could forget that accident, but that is impossible. Hundreds of people were forced to flee their homes because exposure to TCDD causes a severe skin disease. Only time will tell what its lasting effect will be on those who did not escape in time. And there is a possibility that environmental damage was so severe that Seveso may become a wasteland.

The disaster at Seveso is but one of a growing number of similarly alarming occurrences. In Michigan, for example, milk cows were accidentally polluted by chemical substances called PBBs (polybrominated biphenyls). In the area where their milk was sold, numerous cases of nervous system disorders were reported. A chemical called kepone has been responsible for sterility among men in California who were exposed to it, and for nervous system disease among people in Virginia and Texas.

Early in 1977, the Environmental Protection Agency banned industries from directly discharging PCBs (polychlorinated biphenyls) into U.S. waters because of their danger to the environment. And yet these chemicals were used as pesticides, which present a danger to humans. The danger is especially great because the damage these chemicals cause in people may take a long time to show itself. On June 28, 1979, the federal Food and Drug Administration lowered the legal limit of PCBs permitted in fish to less than half of what it was previously. PCBs may cause stillbirths, cancer, bone and joint abnormalities, skin rashes, and liver damage. Like other pesticides, PCBs are "fat-seeking materials" in the bodies of humans and other animals.[8]

If pesticides can harm people, why use them at all?

HOW PESTICIDES SERVE PEOPLE

For the people of the United States, pesticides have made possible a diet envied by almost everyone else on the globe. Diseases that are due to poor nutrition are less common here than they once were. Also, pesticides, intelligently used, kill the boll weevil and other insects that are destructive to important crops. However, as will be discussed shortly, there is much hope that the reliance on pesticides alone is becoming far less necessary.

Moreover, pesticides have done more than help provide a greater abundance of food and other crops. Typhus, yellow fever, the river

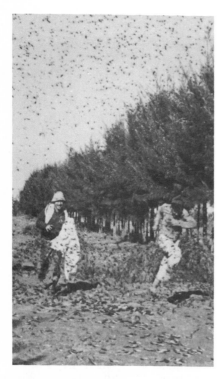

The eternal battle between humans and insects. Two farmers run from a swarm of locusts in Israel.

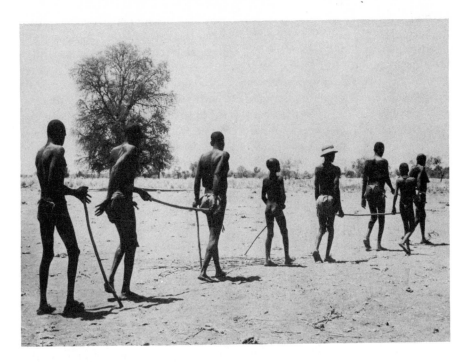

A tiny fly that transmits river-blindness has brought tragedy to many West African villages. Many people have fled, leaving behind a population in which all the adults are blind and must be cared for by their children.

blindness of Africa and Central America, and malaria are four of the insect-borne plagues that can be controlled by pesticides. In countries with extensive programs for the careful use of DDT, malaria has been brought under greater control. *Used properly*, DDT does little harm to the environment. But what of other pesticides? Has there been a trade-off between temporary advantage and disaster?

PESTICIDE PROBLEMS

Pesticides are spread by wind and water. Today they can be found in the strutting penguin of the Antarctic and the oysters of Chesapeake Bay. Some pesticides last longer than others because their components are not quickly broken down. Thus they *accumulate* in the environment. They also *concentrate* in living tissues. For example, DDT that is swallowed by small water animals will be carried up the food chain as successive predators eat their contaminated prey. Along the way the pesticide concentrates and harms fish and birds. DDT accumulated in birds causes their eggshells to be thin and thus interferes with bird reproduction.

This damage to higher life forms becomes even more senseless when one realizes that the target of these pesticides, generally insects, are capable of developing a hereditary resistance to them. In California's Imperial Valley, the unwise use of pesticide has resulted in (1) a whole new breed of insecticide-resistant pests; (2) the killing of harmless insects that once kept harmful species in check; (3) the triggering of a secondary pest invasion that brought the cotton industry in one area to the brink of ruin; (4) the destruction of tens of thousands of honeybee colonies; and (5) the resulting decline in honeybee pollination—that is, the cross-fertilization of plants that happens when honeybees carry pollen from one plant to another. This decline threatens the growth of some important food supplies. Scientists understand the pesticide problem, but what are they doing about it?

NONCHEMICAL PEST CONTROLS

Physical attractants, such as light and sound, may lure many insects to death by poison. *Chemical attractants* also offer promise. The Mediterranean fruit fly, for example, finds it hard to resist proteins from ripening fruit. Therefore, these proteins can be used to attract and poison a fruit fly. Even more irresistible to male insects are the *sex attractants*. Virgin female insects possess only tiny amounts of these chemical substances, but a little goes a long way in the insect world. Some insect sex attractants are now produced in the laboratory, and, as we saw in Chapter 1, they lure the male insect into a certain death-trap.

Scientists are also able to breed partially sterile male mosquitoes. These compete with normal males in the mating game and serve not only to reduce the present mosquito population, but—because their condition is hereditary—to reduce the future population as well. Ways to breed other hereditary defects to limit insect populations are now being researched.

Even an insect's own hormones have been turned against it. The development of most insects is controlled by hormones, so by using compounds that act like the insect's own hormones, normal development can be thwarted. Certain insect-killing viruses are also being investigated and used.

The most important development in the control of the boll weevil and other insects that destroy cotton crops is a system called Integrated Pest Mangement (IPM). Texas and Georgia cotton farmers, for example, are breeding early-maturing varieties of cotton that are vulnerable to pests for only a very short time. Certain microbes and viruses kill cotton pests; these have lessened the farmers' reliance on pesticides. Natural enemies of cotton pests, such as ants, spiders, big-eyed bugs, and others, offer a third way of controlling the boll weevil and other cotton pests. Using these methods in an integrated way has reduced reliance on pesticides by 80 percent in such states as Texas, Georgia, Arkansas, North and South Carolina, Virginia, and Mississippi. Moreover, the insects that destroy cotton pests are now able to gain the upper hand. Integrated Pest Management is surely maintaining cotton as the king of crops in the southern United States.[9]

Mercury

The element mercury is familiar as the "quicksilver" found in thermometers. It is the only metal that is liquid at room temperature. As a liquid element, mercury is not ordinarily poisonous. A person could swallow up to a pound of quicksilver without harm. So if a child swallowed just the mercury from a thermometer, there would be no reason for alarm. Nor is the mercury in dental fillings harmful.

However, there is a difference between *inorganic* and *organic mercury*. Only in unusual circumstances is it possible to be poisoned from metallic and inorganic mercury. This can happen among mercury miners who are exposed to the metal's invisible and odorless fumes for a long time. They develop dizziness and headaches, and their hands shake so badly that writing is im-

Victims of Minamata disease stand as silent reminders of the statement made by the 1972 United Nations Conference on the Human Environment: "an individual cannot be replaced."

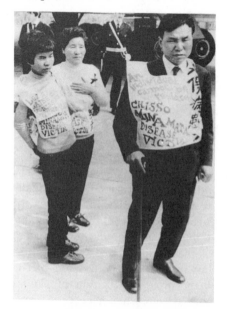

possible. In *usual* conditons of exposure, however, neither metallic nor inorganic mercury stays in the body long enough to do harm.

It is the organic chemical **methylmercury** that can be harmful because it remains in the body for longer periods of time and attacks the brain and spinal cord. It was just this compound that was responsible for a poisoning disaster in Japan some years ago. By eating fish taken from the industrially polluted waters of Minamata Bay, over two hundred people developed signs and symptoms of nervous system damage, including blindness, deafness, inability to speak, severe muscle weakness, paralysis, and mental retardation. Fifty-two people died. As a result, organic methylmercury poisoning earned the popular name of **Minamata disease**. How did this disaster happen?

In 1970 Swedish scientists reported that dumping inorganic mercury into rivers and lakes could be dangerous. Relatively harmless inorganic mercury could be changed into poisonous organic methylmercury by germs in the beds of these waters. The poisonous mercury could then leave the water bottom and pass into the bodies of fish. A certain amount of organic methylmercury in water is natural and so is its presence in fish. It becomes poisonous only when people eat large amounts of fish from waters containing very high levels of the chemical. So great was the amount of organic methylmercury in the confined waters of Minamata Bay that even the fish developed nerve-muscle disease. These fish were simply taking in organic methylmercury more rapidly than they could rid themselves of it.

There is a mistaken notion that mercury pollution has made the eating of all fish unsafe. Whether organic or inorganic, industrial mercury pollutions are limited to one area, and they tend to remain in that area. The poisoned fish of Minamata Bay cannot be compared with wide-ranging ocean fish that have lived in mercury-containing waters for millions of years. Organic mercury found in these fish is natural and not the result of pollution. For many centuries people have been eating fish that contain some natural organic mercury without harm. There is even expert opinion that tiny amounts of mercury, like other elements, may be necessary for health. Moreover, the element selenium may prevent mercury poisoning. Thus, it is not *whether* methylmercury is present in fish that is the basic factor in deciding its threat to human health, but *how much*. With these thoughts in mind, the federal Food and Drug Administration has established standards for safe levels of this chemical in foods.

Lead Poisoning: An Epidemic of Childhood

People have been digging lead out of the ground for thousands of years, and centuries of unhappy experiences have taught us to be careful with this metal. The ancient Romans added a lead compound to their wines to make them less acid. The result was a lot of lead poisoning among the ruling classes. During Colonial times in this country Benjamin Franklin warned people about lead poisoning. Yet at the turn of this century people were still surrounded by lead. It was in walls, roofing, house paint, play pens, cribs, food, toys, jugs, cosmetics—

almost everywhere. Even today, lead-containing ceramic glazes used on clay pottery produced in some countries outside the United States have caused lead poisoning and even death, because large amounts of lead are sometimes leached out of the glaze into acidic beverages or vegetables contained in improperly made ceramic pots and bowls.

Recent years have seen a growing concern about lead poisoning, or **plumbism**, in small children. Thousands of children in this nation have dangerously high levels of lead in their blood. A large number of these children have suffered permanent nervous system damage, such as mental retardation and visual disorders.

How does the lead enter the child's body? Nose-high automobile exhausts is one possibility. But a better-known source is the paint used in houses built before the 1940s. Lead-based paint tastes sweet, and unsupervised small children find flakes of lead paint to be a tasty snack. Although house paints are now nonlead-based, homes and apartments that have not been repainted with the safer paints are a hazard for approximately 120,000 children in New York City alone.

Other sources of lead poisoning are newspapers, comic books, magazines, children's books, and playing cards. Yellow, orange, and red inks are particularly hazardous. Children who habitually chew these paper products are in danger. So are the children of people who work with lead, as are children who live near smelters that emit lead.

Radiation: The Modern Janus

The ancient Romans believed in a two-faced god named Janus. Radiation has become the Janus of modern times. One of its faces is turned to a great future for humanity; the other face could be turned to the end of humankind. What is radiation? What is the source of so vast a power, a problem, and a promise?

Atoms and Their Behavior

Everything in nature is made up of *elements*. Elements are made up of *atoms*. Each atom has a central core called the *nucleus*. Within the nucleus are tiny bits of matter called *protons* and other bits called *neutrons*. Outside the nucleus and surrounding it is a whirling thin cloud composed of other bits of matter

called *electrons*. The cloud of electrons is more or less ball-shaped (see Figure 2–2). The electrons whirling in their atomic cloud decide the *chemical* behavior of an element. But within the tiny nucleus is contained a *physical* source of energy unlike anything that electrons provide. It is this energy that, unleashed, is the source of an atomic explosion.

Atoms having the same number of electrons and protons but a different number of neutrons are called *isotopes*. Many elements have more than one isotope. Some isotopes are unstable; that is, they constantly change. Why? Because their nuclei naturally break down, or decay. Energy in the form of waves or tiny bits of matter is let loose from these unstable nuclei. It

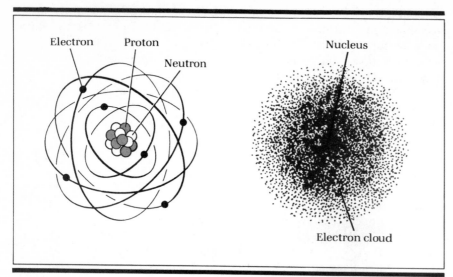

Figure 2-2
Two models of an atom: an atom of carbon 12, which has six electrons, six protons, and six neutrons (left), and a generalized model schematizing an electron cloud (right). The left diagram is highly simplified in that all the orbitals shown there are elliptical; actually, orbital shapes vary.

is this energy that can be so powerful, so full of problems and benefits. This energy is called **ionizing radiation**. The decaying isotope is a *radioactive isotope*.

How big are atoms? Well, a person who weighs 150 pounds is made up of about 6,700,000,-000,000,000,000,000,000,000 (6.7 octillion) atoms. Every time that person loses or gains one pound, about 45,000,000,000,000,000,-000,000,000 (45 septillion) atoms are lost or gained. If the person gains one pound a month, he or she has gained an average of about 17,000,000,000,000,000,000 (17 quintillion) atoms per second.

Sources of Ionizing Radiation

Ionizing radiation is a part of humanity's natural ecosystem. Radioactive materials in soil, rocks, air, food, and water, as well as in body and building materials, account for some 58 percent of radiation. From outer space comes natural radiation that bombards everything and everybody on earth. Most of this radiation is blocked from reaching earth by the atmosphere; if it were not, life would perish. Human-made sources of ionizing radiation include X-rays, some medical examination equipment, and industrial processes. These account for 41 percent of human exposure to ionizing radiation. Fallout from nuclear weapons accounts for most of the remaining 1 percent.

One Face of Janus: Human Radiation Damage

At the turn of the century, the famous French physicist Antoine Henri Becquerel discovered an important characteristic of the then newly discovered element radium. He had placed a tube of radium in his vest pocket, and before long he noticed a burn on his belly. To check Becquerel's observation, Pierre Curie (who with his wife, Marie, had discovered radium) tested radium on himself. He deliberately applied radium to his own arm. Again a burn developed. The little burn on Becquerel's belly has left its mark on humanity. This incident provided the first suggestion that radiation could cause tissue damage.

Like all other matter, human cells are made up of atoms. How can ionizing radiation damage human cellular atoms? When ionizing radiation strikes the atoms of cells, those atoms are in turn ionized. Thus, radiation upsets the chemical structure of the cell, which results in considerable cell damage. Also, poisons collect in the cell, interrupting normal cell functions.

Not only the general body tissue cells but also specialized reproductive cells (ova and spermatozoa) may be affected. The exposure of a person's entire body to too much radiation at one time can damage both body and reproductive cells. Damage to body cells may lessen the lifetime of the exposed individual. But radiation damage to reproductive cells can also harm the hereditary material within the ova or sperm, which then may affect generations yet unborn—a cruel legacy. Moreover, some scientists believe that there is no absolutely safe dose of radiation.

How much damage will excess radiation cause? This depends on the sensitivity of a person's individual cells, the kind of ionizing radiation, the radiation dose, and the length of time of exposure. Just as people vary in their sensitivity to pollen or smog, so may they differ in their sensitivity to equal doses of ionizing radiation. This is because their cells themselves differ in their sensitivity. Some cells are more sensitive to one type of ionizing radiation than another. Some ionizing radiation has a tendency to damage certain structures of the body more than others. Thus, for example, the radioactive isotopes strontium 89 and 90 will damage bone and marrow. Yet, another isotope, carbon 14, harms the whole body, including its ova and spermatozoa.

Radiation can enter a person's body in various ways. It can be ingested in foods, such as meats or dairy products, from animals that have fed on poisoned plants. It can also be inhaled with polluted air or absorbed through the skin or mucous membranes.

Spread over many years, a person's exposure to radiation may amount to a considerable total. Yet that person may show few if any bad effects, because the daily exposure has been small. The body has had time to replace or repair cells. Yet exposure during a brief time (a split second, for example) to the same total lifetime dosage may kill. Why? The immediate dose is large, and the body has no time to repair or replace damaged cells.

It was just such a tremendous dose of radiation delivered over a short time that resulted in the terrible events that followed the atomic bombing of Hiroshima and Nagasaki. Death and disfigurement from the radiation were the immediate results. But it is possible that a person who has been exposed to intense radiation for a short time will not show any ill effects for years. This tragic truth has been revealed by studies of Japanese who were ten years old or younger at the time of their exposure to the radiation of the Hiroshma and Nagasaki bombings. Among those individuals, certain cancers that appeared later occurred much more frequently than

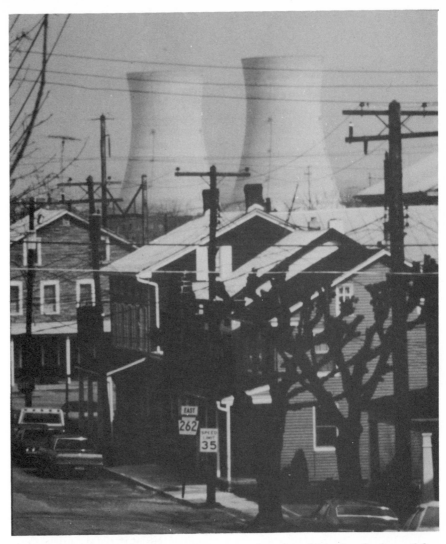

The streets of Goldsboro, Pa., a community that sits within the shadow of the cooling towers of the Three Mile Island nuclear power plant, are deserted as citizens heed warnings to stay indoors during the period of crisis.

could be expected in a normal population. So did cases of infertility and increased birth deformities in children. And to the physical problems was added severe emotional hurt.

ATOMIC ACCIDENTS HAPPEN

It was by no means the first serious accident in a U.S. nuclear power plant. The public just hadn't been

told about the others.[10] Like a failing heart, the events in the nuclear power plant on Three Mile Island near Middletown, Pennsylvania, on March 28, 1979, were apparently due to a series of valvular failures. Highly reactive elements were released into the countryside. People in the area were exposed to minute amounts of poisonous radioactive materials. How safe is a minute amount? Some physicists say that there is no safe dose of radiation.[11] A federal official estimated that the entire incident "could result in an increase of 0.1 to 0.2 cancers."[12] If that guesswork is correct, for the people who constitute that 0.1 to 0.2 increase, the increase is 100 percent. Fifteen workers were exposed to even higher levels of radiation; for the rest of their lives they will need to be monitored for cancer. The economy of the area is built around the dairy industry. Milk is the target of many of the radioactive materials that fell on the grass that is eaten by lactating cows. It will take years to know who will be affected. Some temporarily evacuated residents relieved their anxieties with signs. One read: "Gone fission." Another: "Hell, no, I won't glow."[13]

"A joke's a very serious thing," wrote the seventeenth century English poet Charles Churchill.

In 1954, a little-publicized U.S. atom-bomb-testing program (and resulting accident) brought a nightmare existence to natives of some of the Marshall Islands in the western Pacific. Forced by the atomic program from their home islands to others where food was sparse, some suffered severe malnutrition. Others, victimized by an unexpected shift of winds, were sprayed by radioactive ash. Children played in the radioactive poison. One old man rubbed it into his eyes, hoping that the "fallout from heaven" would cure his visual problem. Stillbirths, miscarriages, abnormal children, and an increase in thyroid tumors (as compared with unexposed populations) resulted. In the sea, twenty-two unlucky fishermen were exposed while fishing from their boat, *The Lucky Dragon*. The U.S. Atomic Energy Commission (now named the Energy Research and Development Administration) called this atomic test by the code name *Bravo*. But the inno-

cent natives of the affected islands, which likely will remain uninhabitable for many years, have yet to find something to applaud.

Fifteen years after the Marshall Islands incident, the worst fire in U.S. atomic energy history occurred at the Rocky Flats plant near Denver, Colorado. At this plant the element plutonium is used to make triggers for nuclear weapons. The fire did not help build public confidence in the use of atomic energy, and this plant has become one of the government's most bitterly attacked operations. The public protest is not only directed against the accident that occurred there. Over the years, a number of workers in the plant may have been overexposed to radiation. Because the state of health of workers who have left the plant has not been carefully followed, it is believed that the claims that the cancer incidence is low at Rocky Flats are not necessarily true. Moreover, some scientists believe that pollution has occurred, at various times, at levels too high for human health. Now that Denver suburbs are developing around the plant site, resident pressure to shut down the plant may increase.

RADIOACTIVE WASTE DISPOSAL

The nuclear plants themselves are not the only object of public concern. These plants produce radioactive wastes, and finding a safe way to dispose of these wastes is a growing problem. Some radioactive wastes will remain dangerous for a million years. At some storage places, liquid radioactive wastes have been found leaking out of containers into the ground. Suggested methods, such as deep-sea burial, placing them under the Antarctic Cap, or disposal in outer space, either have not been proved to be safe or are too expensive.

But getting rid of nuclear wastes is only one problem with nuclear power plants. The sale by the United States, France, and West Germany of such plants to other countries has made it possible for them to make small atom bombs from the spent fuel. Great scientists throughout the world oppose such sales, since these atomic bombs do not require the know-how of the larger bombs of a generation ago. They may easily fall into the hands of irresponsible leaders or terrorists.

THE BOMB

I beheld the earth, and, lo, it was without form, and void; and the heavens, and they had no light.

I beheld the mountains, and, lo, they trembled, and all the hills moved lightly.

I beheld, and, lo, there was no man, and all the birds of the heavens were fled.

I beheld, and, lo, the fruitful place was a wilderness, and all the cities thereof were broken down.

Thus does the biblical prophecy of Jeremiah (4:23–26) tell of a destruction that suggests the most terrible of all weapons, the atomic bomb. After scientists pressed the button of destruction at Alamogordo, New Mexico, on the chill morning of July 16, 1945, people knew they had wrought the threat of their time. For hundreds of thousands of people in Japan, the threefold body damage by the bomb—burn, blast, and radiation poisoning soon became a terrible reality.

An even more sinister aspect of atomic bombs is that they can have an effect far beyond the immediate area of explosion, as we saw from the incident in the Marshall Islands. When a nuclear bomb explodes, radioactive material is let loose into the atmosphere. This material then rains back down to earth as "fallout." Most fallout concentrates in the earth's temperate zone, within which lie the great cities of the world—London, Tokyo, New York, Moscow, Peking. And in this zone lives some 80 percent of the world's population.

Until people learn to live in peace, the control of increasingly powerful weapons will remain a problem. Both here and in Europe there has been a growing public concern about nuclear power, and the nuclear test ban is a step in the right direction. Yet we have not even learned to control nuclear power and already there is a tidier, more dangerous weapon—the neutron bomb. It will not destroy buildings. Just people. The time is growing short for human wisdom to equal human invention.

The Other Face of Janus: Radiation As a Benefactor to Humanity

If the problems of radiation hazards and the disposal of radioactive wastes can be solved, nuclear power can be converted to peaceful use on a worldwide scale. Until these problems are solved, though, public resistance will slow down the construction of nuclear power plants, preventing them from providing an unlimited source of energy for building dams, powering industry, and lighting homes.

Less trouble-plagued than the use of nuclear plants is the application of radiation to the field of medicine. Radiation has already provided new techniques for early diagnosis and treatment of some cancers. To thousands of people radiation has meant precious extra years of life. X-rays provide new ways of seeing the heart, blood, and lymphatic vessels. But X-rays are not limited to medical use; even industries have found them to be of practical value.

The machine in the photograph below is a C.A.T. Scanner. It is a diagnostic tool for detecting brain abnormalities, such as tumors. X-ray machines such as this are enormously expensive (between $200,000 and $500,000), but their benefits to medical technology in terms of saving human lives are incalculable.

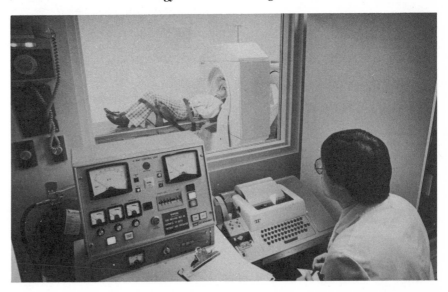

The Need for Strict Controls

In terms of human life, and in no other terms, the benefits of radiation can far outweigh the costs. Under proper conditions, diagnostic, treatment, and industrial uses of radiation are proper risks. And the risk has been reduced since better X-ray methods and machines have lessened the possibility of damage to people. Nevertheless, it must be remembered that X-ray examinations account for a large part of all exposure to human-made ionizing radiation in the United States. Steps must therefore be taken to ensure the safety of radiation equipment. Presently, there are too few inspectors to oversee all the radiation equipment used in both medicine and industry. Moreover, not enough of this nation's medical X-ray installations meet state regulations designed for human safety.

Other recent human-made radiation sources need constant watching. Microwaves, used in a variety of ways ranging from military communications to food preparation, are a type of radiation that may be harmful, especially to the eye and to the male reproductive glands, the testes. The same is true of radiation systems that are being increasingly used by industry and the military. So intense is the light energy of a laser, for example, that it can drill a hole through a diamond in moments—a process that, before lasers, took two days. Unless such systems are carefully controlled and wisely used, they could possibly cause damage that would far outweigh their beneficial uses.

The accidents in nuclear power plants and problems of nuclear waste disposal are two of the reasons that alternative sources of energy are being sought. The shortage of energy in this country is a third. Among the alternatives being studied are the sun's (solar) energy and the energy from the earth's internal heat (geothermal energy). The use of coal as an energy source is hardly new. However, depending on it as a main source of energy may upset the chemical balances within the atmosphere. This in turn may negatively affect earth's climate.

The Public Must Get Involved

President Richard Nixon signed the National Environmental Policy Act of 1969 as his first official act of the 1970s. Among the act's requirements is that any federal agency proposing a major action or project must release to the public a detailed statement of the project's impact on the environment. The **impact statement** must include a description of any harmful environmental effects and presently known ways to avoid them. The act gives the public a mighty weapon in the battle to protect the environment. Administrators of federal projects can no longer proceed without first seeking and responding to public examination. Many people dislike impact statements. They complain of paper work and delays. But ecosystems can be preserved or improved, and they are everybody's responsibility. As President Woodrow Wilson once said, "Responsibility is proportionate to opportunity."

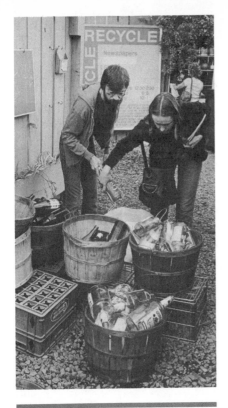

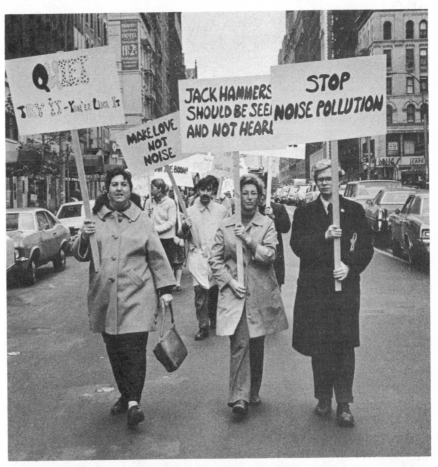

PHOTO ESSAY
We must care enough to get involved.

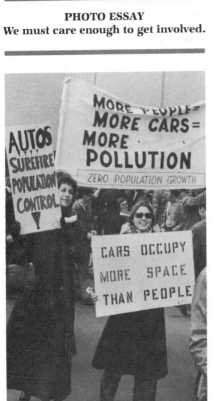

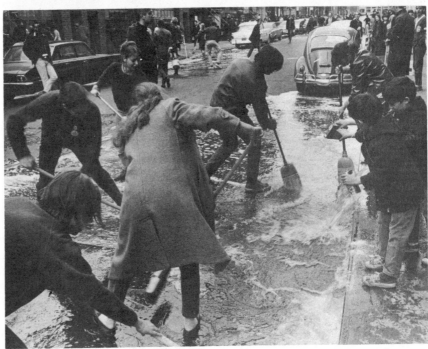

Important as they are, federal and state laws to protect the environment are not the only legal recourse available to those struggling to prevent abuse of their surroundings. Polluters use resources common to everyone, such as air and water, and may therefore be liable for the damage they cause. *Nuisance laws* give all landowners the right to use their property without unreasonable interference. *Trespass laws* prevent intentional entry into privately owned land without permission. In the case of pollution, such trespass may be hard to prove. However, one Oregon case awarded damages to a group of farmers whose crops had been damaged by fluoride gases from a nearby aluminum plant.

Active and responsible citizen participation in preventing pollution by existing legal means is spreading rapidly. In Washington, D.C., for example, the Emergency Committee on the Transportation Crisis, a group of militant citizens led by a commercial artist, has legally forced reappraisal of attempts to blight their living area. Also in the nation's capital, a young lawyer, aided by several dozen willing professional and lay volunteers, has shown what one private citizen can do for public safety and against environmental pollution. His thorough understanding and adroit use of the U.S. legal system, technology, and public opinion have been instrumental in congressional approval of the Wholesome Meat Act of 1967, the National Gas and Pipeline Safety Act of 1968, the Coal Mine Health and Safety Act of 1969, and the Occupational Health and Safety Act of 1970. His name: Ralph Nader.

Summary

We have seen that people can be their own worst enemy, creating living conditions that are hazardous both to themselves and others. While all animals pollute, the pollution of human beings seriously menaces the earth. Water is so polluted by sewage and industrial wastes that it often threatens health. Solid wastes litter the countryside. Industrial wastes and automobile exhaust released into the air, combined with a *temperature inversion*, cause health-endangering *smog*. Sound pollution not only brings about hearing problems but is also a reason for much lost working time. Recent steps taken to deal with pollution—better sewage systems, *recycling*, laws to control the source of the pollution, and environmental *impact statements*—provide hope that the problems will be successfully handled.

Risk taking and accidents lead to many deaths each year. Bad drivers and poorly maintained automobiles and roads have made automobile accidents the leading cause of accidental death. But there are many other potentially fatal activities besides driving. Skin and scuba diving, swimming, skiing, and shooting all may be dangerous unless undertaken with proper care. Without precaution, even one's own home can become a death trap. Some of the common causes of death in a household are falls, fires, suffocation, and poisoning.

Human technology has created many substances harmful to life. While pesticides can help people by controlling unwanted insects, these chemicals are often more deadly to humans and to animals that we do not wish to harm. Severe nervous-system damage can accompany *Minamata disease*—caused by organic *methylmercury*, which is released as an industrial waste—and *plumbism*—caused by lead, which was once widely found in paints. *Ionizing radiation* is perhaps the gravest threat facing life today. Not only can it have harmful immediate effects, such as burns and blindness, but it can alter hereditary material so that future generations are adversely affected.

References

1. Quoted in Nelson Manfred Blake, *Water for the Cities* (Syracuse, N.Y., 1956), p. 4.
2. Abel Wolman, "Disposal of Man's Wastes," in William L. Thomas, Jr., *Man's Role in Changing the Face of the Earth* (Chicago, 1971), p. 808
3. "Restoring the Quality of Our Environment," report of the Environmental Pollution Panel, quoted in Philip H. Abelson, "Man-Made Environmental Hazards: How Man Shapes His Environment," *American Journal of Public Health*, Vol. 58 (November 1968), p. 2046.
4. Michael H. Brown, "Love Canal, U.S.A." *The New York Times Magazine* (January 21, 1979), pp. 23ff.
5. W.A. Thomasson, "Deadly Legacy: Dioxin and the Vietnam Veteran," *The Bulletin of the Atomic Scientists*, Vol. 35 (May 1979), pp. 15–19.
6. Irene Kiefer, "Hazardous Waste," *SciQuest* (April 1979), pp. 17–22.
7. "Valley of the Drums and Other Hazardous Wastelands," *Science News*, Vol. 115 (February 3, 1979), pp. 68–69.
8. "PCB's in You and Me," *Science News*, Vol. 116 (July 7, 1979), p. 2.
9. Joan Arehart-Treichel, "Protecting King Cotton," *Science News*, Vol. 115 (April 21, 1979), pp. 266–268.
10. Lee Torrey, "Nuclear Nuggets Expose Reactor Hazards," *New Scientist*, Vol. 81 (February 1979), p. 299, referring to Robert D. Pollard, *The Nugget File*, Union of Concerned Scientists, Cambridge, Massachusetts.
11. Janet Raloff, "Radiation: Can a Little Hurt?" *Science News*, Vol. 115 (January 20, 1979), pp. 44–45; and Karl Z. Morgan, "Cancer and Low-Level Ionizing Radiation," *The Bulletin of the Atomic Scientists*, Vol. 34 (September 1978), pp. 30–40.
12. "The Three Mile Accident," quoting Harold Denton, director of the Nuclear Regulatory Commission, in *Science News*, Vol. 115 (April 7, 1979), p. 228.
13. Richard D. Lyons, "Middletown Keeps Count on Levels of Contamination," *The New York Times*, Section 4 (April 8, 1979), p. 1E.

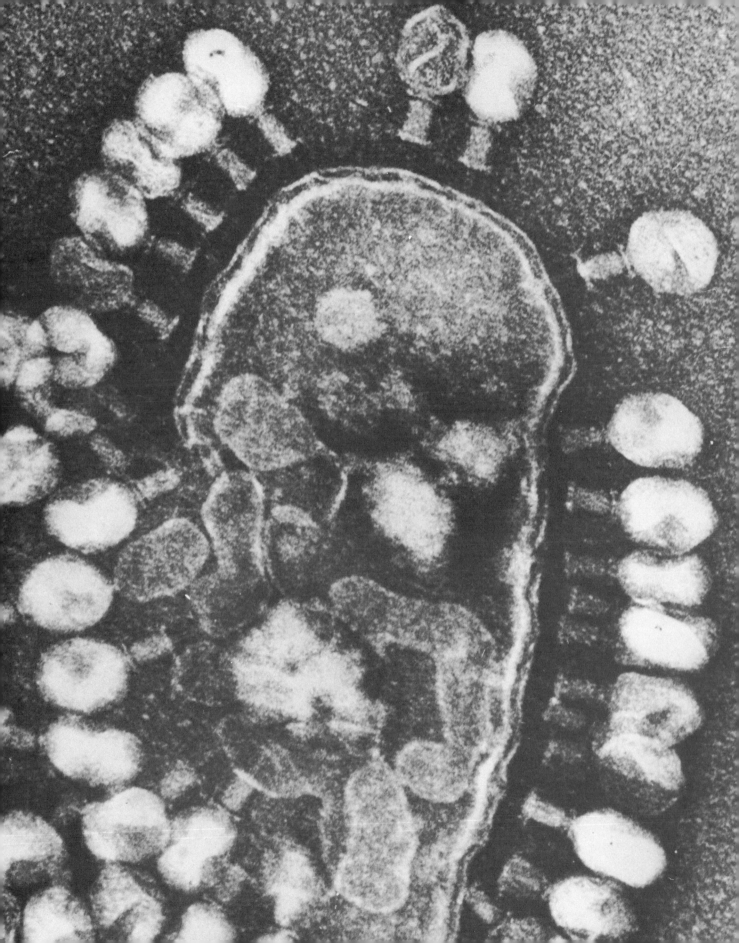

3

The Self Versus the Nonself: Communicable Disease

The "Wee" Ecosystems of van Leeuwenhoek

"Dear God," wrote Anton van Leeuwenhoek, "what marvels there are in so small a creature!" It was the autumn of 1693. The Dutch cloth merchant had made the first microscope, and with growing excitement, he explored the "wee" world of newly discovered ecosystems of living creatures. The Dutchman had made a path on which no proper signpost would be placed for almost two hundred years. For not until 1870 did Robert Koch prove that bacteria could cause disease. Then Koch, joined by other scientists (including his unfriendly rival Louis Pasteur), began a great search to identify humanity's tiniest enemies—the disease-causing **microorganisms**.

A microorganism is a living organism so small that it can be seen only through a microscope. When an organism invades the body and lives off it as a parasite, it may or may not cause disease. For disease to occur, then, there must be a causative organism (the **parasite**) invading an individual (the **host**) in an ecosystem, or **environment**, in which all act upon one another in a particular way. Some organisms are more able to cause disease than others (they have more **virulence**), and some individuals are better able than others to defend themselves against disease (they have more **resistance**). Sometimes, there may be active combat between the invading parasite and the resisting host; other times, the parasite and host might exist together in peaceful ecological balance. As discussed in Chapter 1, imbalance, as when the host loses resistance or the parasite increases in numbers or virulence, may result in disease.

An infection is said to be **contagious** or **communicable** when it can be transferred from one individual to another. Some infectious diseases are more communicable than others. For example, the microorganism causing regular measles, which is spread via droplets in the air, is much more communicable than a form of leprosy that is usually spread by skin contact. With time, an infectious disease may even lose much of its ability to be communicable. Untreated, the microorganism causing syphilitic infection may stay in the body for years, even a lifetime. Silently, it attacks the circulatory and nervous systems. But two years after the original infection, the period of active communicability is mostly over. The microorganism causing the disease does not surface to the mucous membranes to be passed on to someone else through sexual contact. It remains deep in the host's body.

Not all organisms causing disease are too small to be seen by the naked eye. Some **helminths** (parasitic worms), such as the tapeworm, can be seen without a microscope (their eggs, however, are microscopic). The helminths are the largest of the organisms that can enter the body and cause disease. Other organisms called **ectoparasites,** such as fleas, lice, and mites, may also be easily observed without microscopes. Smaller than these, and in the order of their decreasing size, other organisms that may cause infectious disease are *fungi, protozoa, bacteria, rickettsia, mycoplasma, chlamydia,* and *viruses.*

A three-inch Leeuwenhoek microscope (back view). The lens is in the small hole in the circular bulge.

The photograph on page 52 portrays a drama seen only with the aid of an electron microscope: viruses attacking a bacterium.

Varieties of Disease-Causing Agents

Helminths, the parasitic worms, are responsible for many worldwide human infections, including tapeworm, hookworm, and pinworn.

The mite that causes *scabies* ("the itch") is an example of an *ectoparasite*. It invades only the outer skin. The male of the species causing this illness is hard to see, but the female is twice as large as the male and can be seen. The female digs into the superficial skin to deposit her eggs. That causes the itching. Scabies may be spread as a result of sexual contacts.

Fungi are plants. They include the **molds** and the **yeasts**. Some of them cause human disease. Molds, for example, cause ringworm and athlete's foot. Sicknesses caused by yeastlike fungi include *valley fever*, a lung infection, *thrush*, a rare disease (usually of children) characterized by whitish spots in the mouth, as well as a more common affliction of the adult vagina.

Protozoa are one-celled, usually microscopic, animals. Among the illnesses caused by protozoa are malaria and amebic dysentery. Both diseases afflict millions throughout the world, particularly in the developing countries.

Another type of microorganism is **bacteria**. Bacteria that are rod-shaped are called **bacilli**. Bacilli cause such illnesses as tuberculosis, diphtheria, and Legionnaire's disease. (Bacilli are also responsible for the plague; see the special section "Disease and Destiny.") Spherical bacteria are the **cocci**. The gonococci (which cause gonorrhea) and the meningococci (which cause spinal meningitis) are among the best-known spherical bacteria. A preventive vaccine now exists for two kinds of meningococci. There are also *spiral-shaped* bacteria. The bacterium that causes syphilis is an example of such an organism. (Illustrations of these three types of bacteria are shown in Figure 3–1.)

Some organisms live a double life. Those bacteria causing tetanus (lockjaw), for example, have the capacity to live in a dormant state as **spores**. A spore is a highly resistant body developed by some bacilli in response to unfavorable living conditions. For years, if necessary, tetanus spores exist in an ecosystem such as soil, the dung of cows or horses, or dust. Then, when the spores come in contact with a more agreeable ecosystem—that is, one with a low oxygen supply, such as wounded tissue—they become poisonous bacteria. The bacteria multiply and release their poisons, thus causing tetanus or other serious diseases.

Mycoplasma, a genus of microorganism smaller than bacteria, can cause a form of human pneumonia, and **Chlamydia** can cause parrot fever, an eye infection called *trachoma*, and two different kinds of sexually transmitted diseases.

Rickettsia may be classified between viruses, and mycoplasma and chlamydia. They are like viruses in that they are found within cells. Unlike viruses, but like bacteria, they can be seen under an ordinary microscope. Their discoverer, Howard T. Ricketts (1871–1910), died of typhus fever, a disease caused by rickettsia.

There are some two hundred **viruses** of importance to humans. The smallest of all infectious agents, viruses cannot multiply outside a cell. But they are responsible for many human illnesses, ranging from the "cold sore" to poliomyelitis.

Because they are the most common causes of communicable disease in this country, bacteria and viruses will be the major topics of this chapter.

How Microorganisms Leave One Home and Find Another

Microorganisms have a number of ways of moving from one host to another. The material from an open sore (such as a sore of syphilis) contains the causative parasite. It may be *directly* spread from one person to another, or it may be spread *indirectly*. An example: A child with measles coughs. Within the droplets coughed out of the breathing (respiratory) system swarms the measles virus. The infected droplets are wafted about by the air currents and inhaled by susceptible people who then get measles. Or, instead of

FIGURE 3–1
Disease-causing organisms: *Mycobacterium tuberculosis*, a bacillus (left); *Neisseria gonorrhoeae*, a coccus (center); *Treponema pallidum*, a spiral-shaped microorganism (right).

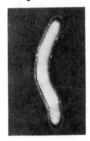
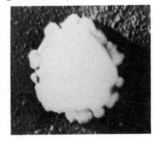
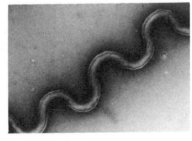

droplets in the air, other objects may act as spreading agents. Examples are handkerchiefs (contaminated, perhaps, with disease-causing streptococci and food, such as milk, in which the typhoid bacillus multiplies quickly. Insects and other tiny animals also transport disease-carrying microorganisms from place to place. A two-hundred-pound man shaking with malaria is sick because a one-celled protozoan entered his bloodstream via the bite of a female mosquito weighing 1/25,000th of an ounce.

An outbreak of communicable disease is like a mystery story.

Knowing that gonorrhea is almost always spread directly through sexual intercourse, or that an outbreak of typhoid fever is often caused by human waste that gets into and pollutes water or food, the public health detective seeks these routes to the source of the disease and to its eventual control. Once the source of the communicable disease is known, the murderous microbe can be tracked down and the linked chain of spread broken. The end of the story finds the health detective forging a new chain through which the disease is treated and further cases prevented.

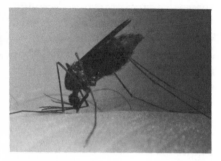

How microbes leave one home and find another. Above: An *Anopheles balabacensis*, a major transmitter of malaria in Southeast Asia. This mosquito is resting after a blood meal; note its greatly distended abdomen. Right: Blood cells containing the malaria-causing organism.

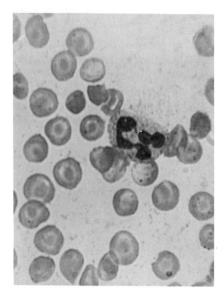

Body Resistance Against the Nonself

The human body must be able to resist foreign invaders of its tissues. A healthy body usually knows the difference between what belongs to it and in it and what doesn't. Anything that is not or should not be part of the self—that is, the foreign, nonself invaders—is quickly resisted by the body's marvelous de-

fense mechanisms. Some of these mechanisms are general and nonspecific. **General nonspecific resistance** is not directed against any particular invader. **Specific resistance** is directed against a definite, particular invader. The human body is capable of both kinds of resistance.

The Self Versus the Nonself: General Nonspecific Resistance

Foreign nonself material may be living, such as infectious microorganisms (the emphasis in this chapter), or nonliving, such as dust. Either may get inside the body through gateways called the *portals of entry.*

The *skin* and its moist continuation into the body's inner space, the *mucous membrane*, are two major portals of entry. The mucous membrane lines the body's inner cavities and openings to the outside. Together, the unbroken skin and mucous membrane are the *first line of the body's defense*. Anything breaking through them is permitted entry into deeper tissues. There are three other important portals of entry. They are the breathing (*respiratory*), *digestive*, and the combined urinary and genital, or *urogenital*, systems. Inside the body, all these systems are lined with mucous membrane.

Of these five portals of entry, the *unbroken skin* is toughest to get by and offers the best barrier to microorganisms. The entire surface layer of skin cells (those that are visible) is dead. It is constantly being replaced by new skin cells underneath that die as soon as they reach the surface. The skin's resistance to invasion is helped by the chemicals contained in its sweat and oils. But the unbroken skin is not totally resistant to foreign invaders. Other microorganisms can get by the unbroken mucous membrane (the parasite that causes syphilis is one). Like the skin, the mucous membrane also gets help to fight infection. The saliva in the mucous membrane-lined mouth contains chemicals that kill bacteria. The acid in the mucous membrane-lined stomach also kills microorganisms.

Sometimes even the membrane's structure helps, or hinders, one's resistance. For example, the mucous-membrane-lined Eustachian tube (extending from the back of the throat to the middle ear) of a child is short and straight. Infection can more easily travel from the back of a child's throat than it can from an adult's throat. Why? The adult Eustachian tube is longer and curved. Another example? Blinking eyelids constantly wipe tears across the delicate surfaces of the eyes. Without tears the eyes' surfaces would dry. Loss of resistance against infection would be only one of the problems of dry eyes. Tears also contain chemicals that kill microorganisms. And tears carry away microorganisms and other intruders, such as dust. Here too, then, mechanical and chemical actions together protect a body part—the self—from foreigners—the nonself. Such combined action against infection happens in other body parts, too. The respiratory system, as another example, works that way. It is described on pages 217–218.

Second Nonspecific Lines of Defense

What happens when invaders—bacteria, for example—get through the skin or mucous membrane and reach deeper tissues? The normal body then has two types of cells to defend itself. They are the *granulocytes* and the *macrophages.*

THE GRANULOCYTES

A **granulocyte,** a type of white blood cell, lives about ten hours. A new supply must constantly be made in the bone marrow. Granulocytes patrol the circulating blood or stick to the walls of veins and the body's smallest blood vessels, the capillaries. If no foreign microorganisms alert them to battle, they pass through the capillaries to tissue cells and die. If, however, invasion by foreign microorganisms does happen, granulocytes become combat-alert. Making their way from the blood to the bacteria in the tissue, they attack. They grab at the bacteria and try to engulf and destroy them—a process called *phagocytosis.* The bacteria fight back. They try to dodge the grabbing granulocytes. Protected by their walls, the bacteria let loose any poisons they possess. It is a bitter battle. Soon the microscopic battlefield is covered with the battered bodies of beaten bacteria and granulocytes. Surrounding tissue cells are damaged. Blood is spilled. Some cells die. Pus is formed. There is heat, redness, pain, and swelling—all signs of *inflammation.*

But granulocytes are small cells. Soon their energy is spent. They have been foot soldiers. Now they need help from heavy artillery—from bigger, stronger cells. They get it from the macrophages.

THE MACROPHAGES

From nearby supporting tissue the **macrophages** move toward the fray. The granulocytes retreat as the macrophages take over. The macrophages are also capable of phagocytosis but are far more powerful. They grab the struggling bacteria, trying to engulf them. The fight is to the death: All the bacteria must die. It takes only a short time for a dividing bacterium to become many millions. Should this happen the macrophages have lost the bat-

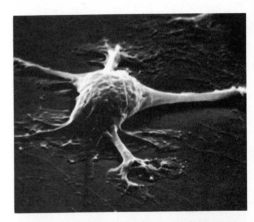

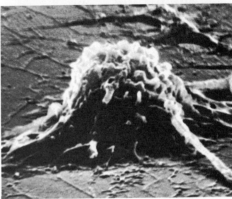

A macrophage in action. The top macrophage is dormant (× 6,000). At bottom, it has been stimulated into activity by the presence of an antigen (× 7,000).

tle, and then there is a full-scale war, involving body reserves, special weapons, and new battle plans.

What we have been describing are nonspecific and general battles with invading microorganisms. But the battles can also be as specific as a guided missile. How? By means of *antibodies*.

Specific Resistance Against Infection

Antibodies are chemical proteins that circulate in the bloodstream. They are made by *plasma cells*. But before plasma cells can make antibodies they have another job to do: They must determine the exact structure of special places on the encircling membranes of the invading microorganisms. If the invader is not a microorganism but a protein poison (toxin), they must determine the structure of a certain part of the toxin surface. These particular chosen places of the invaders are called **antigens** (or antibody generators). Then, the plasma cells manufacture the antibodies so that they fit exactly into the special chemical structure of the surface antigens. The plasma cell is like a skilled locksmith. It makes a perfect protein antibody-key to fit any antigen-lock. Once the antibody is in place, the antigen is neutralized and robbed of the ability to cause sickness. And note this: The specially shaped structure of the antigens on the membrane surface of invaders (such as bacteria) or of toxins is different from the surface structures of the membranes of body cells or of other body materials (the self). In other words, the plasma cells can recognize the difference between self and nonself antigens.

Different Kinds of Antibodies

Antibodies are special proteins. They are **immunoglobulins**. The "immuno" comes from the word *immunity*. Immunity refers to the ability of a living organism (such as a human being) to fight off infectious disease. "Globulin" refers to a group of proteins.

One kind of immunoglobulin can be found in secretions throughout the body. Should foreign fungi or bacteria invade the body, these local immunoglobulins unite with their surface antigens. This causes the invaders to stick together. For the invaders, that's not helpful. They are slowed by being clumped together with immunoglobulin hanging onto their antigen surfaces. They cannot quickly take their intended route to the deeper tissues and the bloodstream. Also they are less able to escape the ferocious attacks of granulocytes and macrophages. In this way sickness can be delayed and often avoided.

Two other kinds of immunoglobulin antibodies prowl in the blood. One kind is small enough to cross the placenta of a pregnant woman and so reach the unborn child. The newborn child then has some antibodies to temporarily resist invaders in its new worldly ecosystems. There may also be an added insurance for infants through the supply of antibodies they receive in their mother's milk.

The only problem with immunoglobulins is that they do not last long, so there is a need for artificial immunity, such as vaccines provide. (Vaccines will be discussed later in this chapter.) First it must be understood that immunoglobulin antibodies are really small jobbers. In the immune system their task is to prepare the antigen for the big

destruction, which is provided by *complement*, a third set of resistance proteins.

$C_1 \ldots C_9$: Complement

Complement is composed of nine different proteins that are manufactured in the liver. Complement refers to making something more complete. In this case, antibody immunoglobulins complement the action of the nine liver proteins. The complement proteins are named C_1, C_2, C_3, C_4, and so on until C_9. Alone they are useless. Together, and following one after the other in regular order, they are explosive. When they get together in numerical order, they can blow a hole in a cell—*any* cell. But complement cannot tell the difference between self and nonself, and so it must depend on the immunoglobulin antibodies.

When a bacterial cell invades the bloodstream, the proper immunoglobulin antibody must first fit itself onto its proper antigen. Only then can a complement fit onto the antigen-antibody surface of a microbe. Eventually all nine parts of the complement are collected in sequence (C_1 through C_9) on the antigen-antibody surface of the foreign invader. Then a hole is blasted in the wall of the invading bacterium. All this happens in a fraction of a second.

Properdin

There is a protein in the blood that is neither antibody nor fighting cell nor complement, yet it, too, is necessary to the immune system. **Properdin** combines with invading bacterial cells before they can get very far in the blood and other tissue. Like a match to a fuse, properdin activates the complement. But that doesn't happen until all other preparations for blasting the enemy have been made.

So there are many factors to human immunity against infectious diseases. Granulocytes, macrophages, immunoglobulin antibodies, complement, properdin—all make up an army of immunity. And leading this army are the cells called **lymphocytes**—the generals of the microbe fighters.

Basic Cells of Immunity: Lymphocytes

Accidentally, a hunter cuts his thumb on a dirty knife. The wound is ignored, and bacteria enter it. The thumb swells and hurts; red streaks track from the cut to the elbow. About the elbow he can feel tender lumps. These lumps are swollen *lymph nodes* (see page 94). They are swollen because lymphocytes are dividing in them, increasing in number to defend their owner, the hunter. Even when there is no infection, there are always some lymphocytes tirelessly patrolling every nook and cranny of the body.

WHERE LYMPHOCYTES ORIGINATE

With the exception of the granulocytes, the immune system originates from lymphocytes. The plasma cells that make exact antibodies and the messenger cells that bring information to the plasma cells about what exact antibodies to make both develop from lymphocytes. Granulocytes don't attack viruses, but lymphocytes do.

Unfortunately, the ability of the body to tell self from nonself sometimes can harm rather than help. For instance, a transplanted heart is a helpful foreign invader, but all the lymphocytes know is that it is foreign, and so they will attack it. Unless the lymphocytes are suppressed, the transplanted heart will be rejected.

Lymphocytes appear early in the body's development. Long before birth, as an embryo, there is a nonembryonic organ called the **yolk sac**. Within a few months, when the embryo has become a fetus, the human yolk sac withers into uselessness. But not before it has provided cells that are destined to become the lymphocytes, or *stem cells*. Fetal stem cells also originate from the fetal bone marrow and liver (see Figure 3–2).

So, long before birth, there are the architectural beginnings of the immune system. From these three fetal sources the stem cells develop further and are found as stem cells

FIGURE 3–2
The two main types of immune response, and the likely mechanisms of their generation.

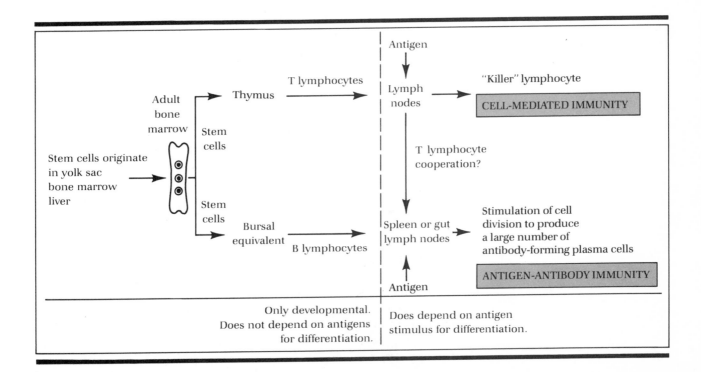

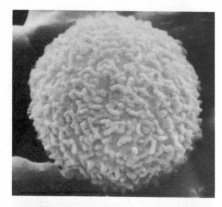

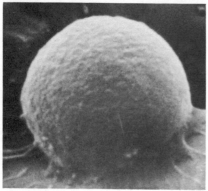

FIGURE 3–3
B lymphocytes (top) and
T lymphocytes (bottom). Many
B lymphocytes have a rougher
appearance than T lymphocytes
because they have more microvilli.

in adult bone. From the bone marrow these adult stem cells go either to (1) a gland behind the breast bone called the *thymus*, or (2) undetermined sources in the human called the *bursal equivalent*. **T lymphocytes** develop in the thymus and then go to lymph nodes where they become "killer" lymphocytes. The "bursal equivalent" cells, or **B lymphocytes**, are believed to go to the spleen or lymph nodes about the gut. There, when stimulated by a foreign antigen, they mature into plasma cells to produce antibodies (see Figure 3–3).

HOW B AND T LYMPHOCYTES WORK

Remember the hunter with the infected thumb and the resulting swollen lymph nodes. Now you can better understand what is happening. Patrolling messenger lymphocytes went into action. One of them touched the surface of the foreign invaders (bacteria) that entered the wound. It picked the antigen (antibody generator) off that surface, and then the messenger lymphocyte carried its information to the nearest lymph nodes.

Depending on the message of the antigen, the messenger lymphocyte takes its information either to B lymphocytes or to T lymphocytes. If the message is to make antibodies, many B lymphocytes are touched. The B lymphocytes then change into the antibody-making plasma cells. Countless protein antibodies pour into the blood to fit into the antigens on the surfaces of the invaders and to neutralize them. In this case the T lymphocytes simply wait.

But if the messenger lymphocyte has information that antibodies are not to be involved, then it touches the T lymphocytes. Granulocytes, macrophages, immunoglobulin antibodies, complement, and properdin all fight bacteria and fungi that do not get inside a body cell. However, viruses and certain other parasites (like the one causing malaria) do get into the body's cells. It is for these infected body cells that T lymphocytes are reserved. Prompted by the messenger lymphocytes, T lymphocytes leave the nearest lymph node on their mission to stop the spread of infection to other normal cells. The T lymphocytes unite with the sick cells. They try to kill the invading virus or other parasite. (It is the T lymphocytes that will also attack transplanted tissue cells—such as the heart transplant mentioned earlier—that have foreign antigens on their surfaces.

INTERFERON

In their fight against viral infection, T lymphocytes seem to be helped by a protein that is made in cells infected by viruses. This special protein is called **interferon**, and its function appears to be that of protecting human beings against such viral infections as influenza, some colds, chickenpox, shingles, and infectious hepatitis.

Researchers are now able to reproduce interferon in test tubes, and some exciting discoveries have recently been made about interferon. Chick interferon will not protect mouse cells; horse interferon will not protect humans; and so on. It seems, therefore, that interferon is *species specific*. Moreover, interferon is produced by various stimuli other than just viruses and by a wide variety of cells. This has stimulated extremely important research in Finland, England, Japan, France, Germany, Sweden, and the United States. And laboratories in these countries are beginning to produce some evidence that interferon can

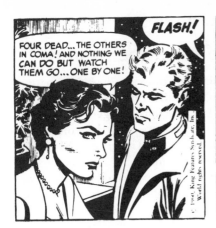

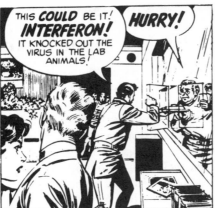

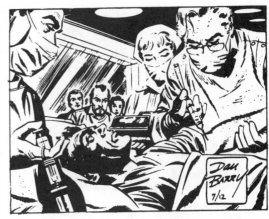

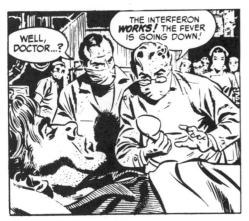

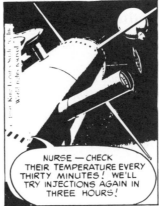

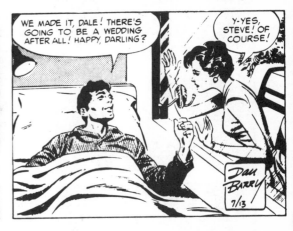

prolong the life of certain cancer patients. Will it cure cancer? Only time—and enough interferon—will tell.

The problem of obtaining enough interferon may reach a solution sooner than was hoped. Certainly one of the better present sources of interferon has been the human leukocyte (white blood cell, see page 90). But other cell sources have also been found. Moreover, since interferon is a protein, it is made up of amino acids. Scientists are trying to work out the exact structure of interferon to know the sequence of the amino acids. From this it may just be possible to discover the DNA portion that directs the production of interferon in human cells. It is already known that the gene for in-

terferon is in a certain chromosome. Is it possible that scientists will be able to splice off that part of the chromosome and insert it into a bacterial cell? Since bacteria multiply in tremendous numbers, it may be possible to produce a broth of interferon and then, eventually, to obtain pure interferon (separate from the DNA) for treatment of some cancers.

In major laboratories throughout many countries scientists are grappling with just this problem. In our own country, the American Cancer Society has organized and financed research projects in several institutions to see if interferon may be helpful in curing a wide range of malignant growths. The search is on and will continue.

The time: 1960. The place: a capsule hurtling through space. It is all very dramatic. Four of Flash Gordon's crew members lie dead. Then another falls sick. He sinks into a coma. Then still another crew member succumbs. But, in the nick of time, enter interferon! It works. The rest of the crew is saved.

Interferon is not, however, the product of cartoonist Dan Barry's imagination. It is the product of British scientists Alick Issac and Jean Lindenmann's labor. Today, twenty years later, it promises to become one of the most important lifesaving products in the history of health.

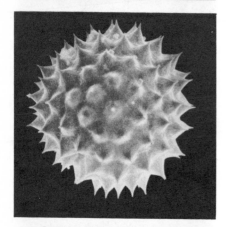

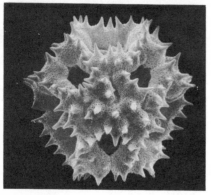

Allergens. Hibiscus (top, × 380); giant ragweed (center, × 2,380); and dandelion (bottom, × 2,340). Pollen grains, the most durable structures found in nature, are the male sex cells of flowering plants. They are encased in tough walls to protect them on their wind-carried fertilizing journeys.

Mistakes Made by the Immune System

We have seen how all parts of the immune system must work together to protect the body. But, unfortunately, the immune systems of some people do not work as efficiently as we have so far described. For these people, their own immune systems turn against them and become their enemies—actually causing, rather than stopping, disease.

The Allergic Diseases: Overacting Antibodies

Whatever turns your skin to
scum,
Or turns your blood to glue,
Why that's the what, the special
what,
*That you're allergic to.**

OGDEN NASH

A foreign substance—an antigen—that would ordinarily not harm most people gets into the body of someone who has a tendency to be allergic. This substance is called an **allergen**. The immune system overacts, making use of special immunoglobulins that the allergic person's body produces to attack the antigen.

To be allergic to a substance, a person must usually meet with it at least twice. The first time, the person gets sensitized to it—this is the time the special immunoglobulins are formed. During this first encounter the person need show no allergic symptoms. At the second meeting, however, the antigen combines with the very antibodies it had caused to be formed, and this com-

*Stanza four of "Allergy Met a Bear" from I'M A STRANGER HERE MYSELF by Ogden Nash, by permission of Little, Brown and Co. Copyright ©1936 by Ogden Nash. Originally appeared in *The New Yorker*.

bination causes a specific reaction to a specific stimulus to be changed. This change is **allergy**.

In most people the connective tissues contain *mast* cells. The mast cells are found mostly in the skin and in the mucous membrane lining of the stomach, intestines, and lungs. Their purpose is to release chemicals of protection whenever a tissue is injured. One of these chemicals consists of a group called **histamines**. Histamines act on the blood-circulatory system. They increase the flow of blood to the injured area, thereby helping the infection fighters—such as phagocytes, antibodies, and complement—get quickly to the place of injury.

In the case of allergic people, whose immune systems overreact, the mast cells have still another role. The special immunoglobulins stick to them. When ordinarily harmless foreigners wander into the body, they react with the special immunoglobulins attached to the mast cells. This causes the mast cells to let go of chemicals disagreeable to the hapless invader. And this is what causes the stuffy nose, or the hives on the skin, or the vomiting and diarrhea common to allergic reactions. The *tendency* to react this way seems to be inherited, but it is the environment that determines whether the reaction will happen at all. For it is the environment that contains antigens. If the antigen is pollen, for example, the allergic person's breathing system gets into trouble. Some foods will cause allergy; they irritate the stomach and intestines and even the skin.

How is allergy treated? First, the irritating substances must be identified so that the allergic person can try to avoid them. Sometimes moving or changing jobs helps. But many allergens cannot be avoided; dust, for instance, is everywhere. The sufferer may then undergo *desensitization*, which is a process whereby the person is made used to the allergen. First, small doses of the guilty antigen are injected. Then, over a period of many months, the doses are gradually increased and another, second, immunoglobulin to the offending allergen is formed. The manufacture of the first immunoglobulin is lessened. Also, because the second immunoglobulin combines or "binds" with the allergen, to some extent this second immunoglobulin blocks binding with the first one. At least that is the theory.

Asthma is a particularly unpleasant mixture of allergic signs and symptoms. In chronic cases, the irritated, thickened muscle fibers of the smaller breathing tubes (bronchioles) go into constricting spasms, which cause the width of these tubes to be decreased. The width is reduced even further by the tubes' swollen linings. Sometimes the bronchioles are plugged by secretions, making it easier for the sufferer to wheeze in than to wheeze out. This may cause lung tissue to become damaged. It is estimated that nine million people in this country have asthma.

There are many other common allergies. With **hay fever**, the inflammation of the mucous membrane of the nasal passages is called **allergic rhinitis**. But this is only part of the misery. Eyes itch so that tears must be wiped away. Other allergies cause skin reactions, such as **hives** or **eczema**. A drug injection or an insect sting can, within minutes, bring about a widespread antigen-antibody reaction that is violent enough to cause collapse and death. Fortunately, such a severe reaction is rare.

Rheumatoid Arthritis: The Contrary Disease

Arthritis means joint inflammation. It includes almost a hundred diseases that are all characterized by tenderness and swelling of one or more joints. In this country about twenty million people need medical care for arthritis. The major forms of arthritis are **osteoarthritis** and **rheumatoid arthritis**. Osteoarthritis is a degeneration of the joint. It is not basically an inflammation. (The stages of osteoarthritis are shown in Figure 3–4.) Almost everyone over forty has this "wear-and-tear" joint disease. Although the treatment of osteoarthritis and rheumatoid arthritis may be somewhat alike, osteoarthritis is more of a local joint disease whereas rheumatoid arthritis involves much of the body. It is a widespread inflammation, not just a local wearing-away process (see Figure 3–5).

FIGURE 3–4
A normal joint and early and late stages of osteoarthritis.

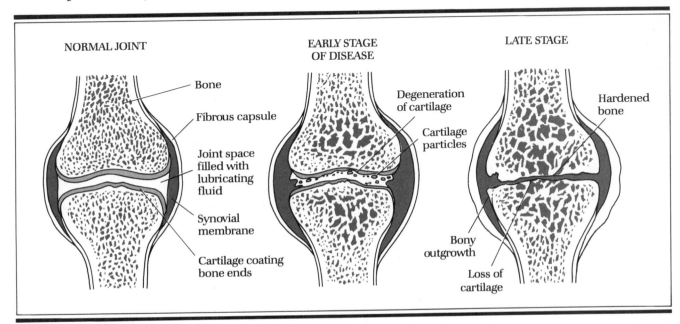

NORMAL JOINT

Bone

Fibrous capsule

Joint space filled with lubricating fluid

Synovial membrane

Cartilage coating bone ends

EARLY STAGE OF DISEASE

Degeneration of cartilage

Cartilage particles

LATE STAGE

Hardened bone

Bony outgrowth

Loss of cartilage

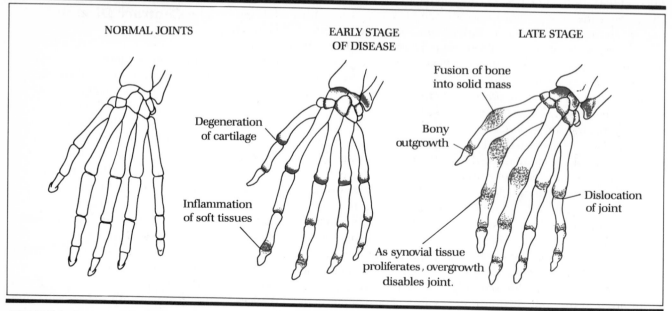

NORMAL JOINTS

EARLY STAGE OF DISEASE

Degeneration of cartilage

Inflammation of soft tissues

LATE STAGE

Fusion of bone into solid mass

Bony outgrowth

As synovial tissue proliferates, overgrowth disables joint.

Dislocation of joint

FIGURE 3–5
Surrounding the joint is a tissue called *synovium*, which keeps the joint lubricated. In rheumatoid arthritis, the synovium becomes inflamed (*synovitis*). This causes pain. As years go by the cartilage and bony joint are destroyed. The result is crippling. But in rheumatoid arthritis far more than the joints are involved. Blood vessels, bone marrow, tissues lining the heart, lungs—even the eyes—may become involved. Rheumatoid arthritis is a whole-body disease.

Although the cause of rheumatoid arthritis is not known, an interesting theory is considered valid by some specialists. They believe it to be caused by a strange antigen-antibody reaction. People who have rheumatoid arthritis have antibodies called **rheumatoid factors** in their blood. The rheumatoid-factor antibodies and the patient's other antibodies combine to form "antigen-antibody" combinations. It is the patient's own circulating antibodies that, oddly enough, act as if they were antigens. The contrary combination activates complement proteins in the joint fluid, resulting in inflammation and tissue destruction.

The most common treatment for rheumatoid arthritis is aspirin for inflammation and pain. And in recent years, surgical procedures that replace some joints (especially the hip and knee) with metal or plastic have been successfully used to treat some patients who would otherwise be crippled and bedridden.

Active Immunity Through Vaccination: Some Comments and Problems

So far our discussion has been limited to **active immunity**—that is, the process by which the body creates its own immunity. In this process, the body's *own* lymphocytes must actively develop into the plasma cells; the body's *own* plasma cells must actively make their own antibodies; and the body's *own* antibodies must actively meet the invading threat of microorganisms. So with active immunity the body does not borrow immunity; it earns it by its own active work. And like money that is earned and banked, active immunity often lasts a long time. A person achieves active immunity by being invaded by a microorganism, or possibly by developing the disease, or by being *vaccinated* against it.

A **vaccine** is a preparation given in order to cause immunity in a person (or in any animal). One type of vaccine is a suspension of whole microorganisms that are weakened but still alive. (By this suspension the microorganisms are dispersed in a fluid medium.) Such weakened microorganisms are called **attenuated**. The Sabin vaccine against poliomyelitis is made up of attenuated microorganisms. Another type of vaccine contains killed microorganisms that are still capable of causing antibodies to be made. The Salk vaccine against polio is one of these. So are most influenza vaccines. Yet another type of vaccine contains the chemically inactivated poisons that bacteria let loose in the body and that can then act as antigens. The diphtheria and tetanus (lockjaw) vaccines are examples of these. All vaccines cause the body to develop active immunity. Table 3–1 shows the immunizing agents most commonly used in the United States.

The BCG vaccine (bacillus Calmette-Guérin—named after two French bacteriologists) contains attenuated tuberculosis bacilli. The pertussis (whooping cough) vaccine is made of killed bacilli. Both the diphtheria and tetanus toxoids are made of inactivated toxin. The remaining vaccines are made of living but weakened or killed viruses. Few benefits of science have prevented as much sickness and death as have vaccines (see Table 3–2).

TABLE 3–1
Immunization Becomes More Acceptable . . .

Recommended Schedule for Active Immunization of Normal Infants and Children, with Follow-up for Adults[1]

AGE	TYPE OF IMMUNIZATION	
2 months	DTP[2]	Polio[3]
4 months	DTP	Polio
6 months	DTP	
1 year	(Tuberculin test)	
15 months	Measles, Rubella, Mumps[4]	
18 months	DTP	Polio
4 to 6 years	DTP	Polio
14 to 16 years	TD[5]	
Every 10 years thereafter	TD[6]	

[1] Schedules recommended by the American Academy of Pediatrics.
[2] Diphtheria-tetanus-pertussis (whooping cough) vaccine.
[3] Oral poliovirus vaccine.
[4] May be given as measles-rubella or measles-mumps-rubella combined vaccines.
[5] Combined tetanus-diphtheria toxoids, adult type.
[6] For contaminated wounds, a tetanus booster is needed if it has been more than five years since the last vaccination. With clean minor wounds, no booster dose should be given unless ten years have elapsed since the last one.

SOURCE: "The Vaccines Are Here. Where Are Your Children?" *Medical World News*, vol. 18 (November 14, 1977), pp. 66–68. Reprinted from MEDICAL WORLD NEWS. Copyright ©1977, McGraw-Hill, Inc.

TABLE 3–2
. . . and History Records the Changes

Reported Cases for Selected Years in the United States of Some Diseases Preventable by Immunization

YEAR	SMALL-POX	REGULAR MEASLES	POLIO-MYELITIS	DIPHTHERIA	PERTUSSIS (WHOOPING COUGH)	TETANUS (LOCKJAW)
1945	346	146,013	13,624	18,675	133,792	(Figures not available)
1950	0	319,214	33,300	5,796	120,718	486
1960	0	441,703	3,190	918	14,809	368
1970	0	47,351	28	435	4,249	148
1975	0	23,374	8	307	1,738	102
1976	0	41,126	14	128	1,010	75
1977	0	57,345	18	84	2,177	87

NOTE: In 1976 the reported cases of regular measles and poliomyelitis showed increases over 1975; and in 1977 these two diseases, as well as pertussis and tetanus, became even more common. Immunization education must be a constant effort.

SOURCE: Compiled from the U.S. Department of Health, Education, and Welfare, Public Health Services, Center for Disease Control, *Reported Morbidity and Mortality in the United States, Annual Summary*, 1976 and 1977.

Now let's consider the vaccines that are most commonly used in this country.

Vaccines Against Poliomyelitis

Unlike Salk's killed virus vaccine, Sabin's *attenuated poliomyelitis virus vaccine* contains live poliovirus that have been weakened in the laboratory. The mild poliomyelitis infection it produces is so rarely accompanied by paralysis or other symptoms that it is one of the safest of vaccines. Indeed, Salk's vaccine is no longer manufactured in the United States, though it is in Canada. The Sabin vaccine provides a more lasting immunity and, unlike the Salk vaccine, is given by mouth rather than by repeated injections.

Two Vaccines to Prevent Two Different Kinds of Measles

Two different kinds of measles, caused by distinctly different viruses, are regular measles (**rubeola**) and German measles (**rubella**). The live, attenuated, regular measles (rubeola) virus vaccine is extremely safe: It has been so weakened by laboratory procedures that it can no longer cause significant illness. It was hoped that by the early 1970s regular measles would become a rare disease. Unfortunately, partly because of the failure of parents to have their children vaccinated, this has not been the case (see Table 3–2). Apparently most people still do not realize that regular measles can be a serious, even deadly disease.

German measles, on the other hand, is a very mild disease. The major reason for the use of German measles vaccine is to prevent the occurrence of the disease during pregnancy. If a woman develops German measles during the early months of pregnancy, there is a high risk that the fetus may be born with a crippling condition called *congenital rubella syndrome* (see page 71). But the vaccine should not be given if there is a chance that the woman is pregnant, as the vaccine itself also could cause the syndrome. Because of this possibility, many physicians feel that a woman should use some reliable form of birth control for at least three months before and after vaccination for German measles. For this reason, too, it is best that women of child-bearing age be tested for their chances of getting rubella *before* being immunized against it, so that they do not get the vaccine unnecessarily. If the test for susceptibility to rubella is positive, a woman need not fear having a baby with the congenital rubella syndrome, because she is already immune.

Some people have experienced joint pains, and a few have swelling and redness of joints, after vaccination against German measles. Therefore, research is now underway for a better vaccine against this disease. A recently developed vaccine may provide immunity for a longer time than those formerly used.

The Influenza Virus Vaccine

Improved procedures have produced a new killed virus vaccine for influenza that has very few side effects. Killed influenza virus vaccines may prevent influenza for six months to a year for about 70 percent of the people who receive the immunization.

But vaccines against some viruses present a special problem because, while alive, the chemical structures of the viruses often change. Type A influenza viruses go through continuous antigenic changes; every ten or fifteen years they undergo a major change. Vaccines depend on a specific viral structure to stimulate specific antibodies, so last year's influenza vaccine may be inefficient or useless against this year's disease.

In early 1978, many people in the United States suffered epidemics of two types of influenza A. There was a vaccine for only one-fourth of the cases. Meanwhile in Russia, another type of influenza A was making people sick. In early 1978, it too had reached the United States, and no vaccine against it was available.

Influenza can be more than just an unpleasant experience for those who come down with it. Especially dangerous strains of influenza viruses can cause death among the elderly or chronically ill, especially people with heart disease, hypertension, diabetes, and tuberculosis.

SAFE OR SORRY?

Just before Christmas in 1975 Private David Lewis and the girl he was planning to marry, Peg Latham, were driving on a rural road to see his folks in Ashley Field, Massachusetts. On the way, a big pig blocked the road. Getting out of his car, David and the pig's owner got the animal to move off the road. Later, David returned to Fort Dix in New Jersey. On February 1, 1976, David had been sick for a week. He wrote Peg: "I felt a lot worse last night, like I had been hit by a truck." There was a lot of flu-like illness in the Fort at the time. Two days later David went to the dispensary but did not follow the doctor's advice. The

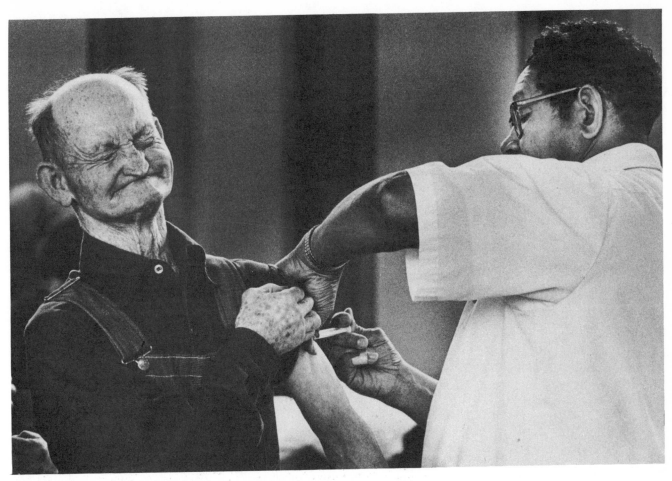

next morning, he went on a five-mile march to the rifle range. On the way back, less than a quarter mile from the Fort, David collapsed and died. The next day Peg got his letter.

An autopsy showed that David Lewis might have died of a kind of lung infection seen with swine flu. Laboratory tests strengthened the suspicion. The finding alarmed health officials. They remembered that in 1918, as World War I was ending, over twenty million people throughout the world died from a similar virus. More than half a million people in the United States alone died from influenza that year. So the health officials notified President Gerald Ford of the death at Fort Dix. There are thirty seats in the

Cabinet room, and the president asked that thirty virus advisers fill those chairs. For almost two hours the experts talked it over. There was, after all, no sure way of predicting that an epidemic would come. There was a risk of being wrong. Others feared the risk of an epidemic. The president decided. On March 24, 1976, with health heroes Jonas Salk and Albert Sabin on each side of him, President Ford appeared on television. He asked Congress for $135 million dollars to vaccinate "every man, woman, and child in the United States."

All over the country immunization committees were organized. The government assumed legal responsibility. Plans were made. Vaccine was prepared in record time, and

In 1976 a swine flu epidemic threatened the nation. Congress appropriated $135 million to immunize Americans against the virus, but the Department of Health, Education, and Welfare suspended the program after only two months when it was learned that 517 people developed a serious neurological disorder after receiving their injections. Twenty-three of those people died. Total number of swine flu cases reported: six. One of those who received an injection—and survived—was Temple Starkey (above), who also survived the great influenza epidemic of 1918.

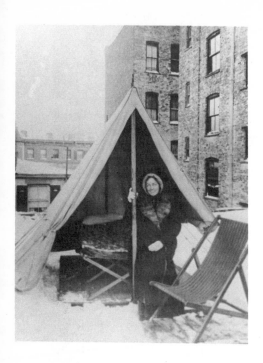

A rooftop tuberculosis sanitarium on New York's Lower East Side at the turn of the century.

clinics were opened. Then, among a small percentage of the vaccinated, a complication arose—*Landry-Guillain-Barré* syndrome. This collection of signs and symptoms adds up to a frightening paralysis. There were deaths. Moreover, the epidemic that was feared never happened.

That was the 1976 experience with the swine influenza. Should the people of the nation have had to endure the experience? One might answer with an old Belgian proverb: "Experience is the comb that Nature gives us when we are bald."

The BCG Vaccine Against Tuberculosis

The BCG vaccine is made from attenuated tuberculosis bacilli. It has found less favor in this country than abroad. Why? Because anyone receiving this vaccine who is later given the *Mantoux test*, a skin test for tuberculosis, will have a positive reaction. A positive Mantoux test may indicate either active tuberculosis or a former tuberculosis that has healed. The Mantoux test has great value in finding possible cases and suspected sources of tuberculosis, but if everyone were given the BCG vaccine, almost everyone would have a positive Mantoux test and the test would lose its detection value. Still another advantage of the Mantoux test would be lost. People whose active tuberculosis has healed and who have not received BCG will show a positive Mantoux test. Such individuals, however, have a greater chance of redeveloping active tuberculosis. These risks are much reduced by preventive treatment. But these people must be separated from those infected by BCG vaccine. Otherwise a large program of preventive treatment against tuberculosis would be impossible.

Also, tuberculosis specialists in this country have accomplished as much without widespread BCG vaccination as have specialists in other countries where such vaccination is routine practice. They control the spread of tuberculosis through use of the Mantoux test. When a person has a positive test, this is a signal that he or she has been infected by someone else. The infectious source must be sought, found, and treated. (Should the Mantoux test be negative, it may be regularly repeated.) Still, some physicians in the United States strongly recommend BCG vaccination, particularly for unusually exposed groups, such as doctors and nurses, slum residents, and people who live with a tuberculosis patient.

On Some Uses of Bacterial Poisons

When certain toxin-producing bacteria invade the body and multiply, it is not they themselves that cause sickness, but rather the poison (or toxin) they produce and let loose into the blood and body tissues. The diphtheria bacillus multiplies in the respiratory tract; the bacillus of tetanus multiplies in an oxygen-deprived wound. Locally, each produces a toxin. Carried by the blood, the diphtheria toxin may affect distant organs. With tetanus, the toxin travels along nerves to the spinal cord and a portion of the brain, thus seriously irritating the central nervous system. Fatal diphtheria often results from an affected heart, although several other factors may cause or contribute to death, such as airway obstruction or paralysis. In both cases, it is the toxin that is the antibody generator (the antigen). How can toxin-caused disease be prevented or treated?

TOXOID:
ACTIVE IMMUNITY
FROM MODIFIED
TOXIN ANTIGENS

Grow the tetanus or diphtheria bacteria in the laboratory on a rich culture medium, and they produce toxin. Filter the laboratory culture. The fluid portion passing through the filter contains the toxin. The toxin can do two things: cause sickness and even death, or cause the body to produce life-saving antibodies. How can one reduce the first effect of toxin and save the second? Treat the toxin with the chemical *formaldehyde*. The toxin antigen is modified. Its poisonous properties are destroyed. Injected into the body, however, it can stimulate the production of antibody-antitoxin. This modified toxin is now called **toxoid**. Diphtheria toxoid and tetanus toxoid can be added to killed pertussis (whooping cough) bacterial cells or to parts of these cells to produce a vaccine containing triple antigen—the *diphtheria, tetanus, and pertussis (DTP) vaccine* (Table 3–1). This is the vaccine commonly given to babies and young children. Injected, it stimulates active immunity against all three diseases.

ANTITOXIN–ANTIBODY:
BORROWED
PASSIVE IMMUNITY

Inject a small measured amount of diphtheria or tetanus toxin antigen into a horse. Each day for a period of time, slowly increase the injected dose of toxin antigen. The horse obligingly responds to the foreign toxin antigen by producing antibody-antitoxin. The horse is producing its own (active) immunity. Now bleed the horse. In the laboratory, isolate the antibody-antitoxin from the blood. The

antibody-antitoxin can be used to neutralize toxin antigen and thus render it harmless. How?

Circulating in the blood of a child desperately sick with diphtheria or tetanus, traveling via the nerves to the central nervous system, is the killing toxin antigen specific for the disease. The toxin stimulates the child's plasma cells to produce antibody-antitoxin. But the process is too slow. An emergency exists, and borrowed immunity—antibody-antitoxin—is needed immediately. Can borrowed horse antibody-antitoxin be used to neutralize the toxin antigen? Yes. When

injected into the child's vein, the horse antibody-antitoxin quickly neutralizes the child's circulating toxin antigen. And if it is used in time, the injection will save the child's life. But horse-tetanus antitoxin, once so useful, has now been replaced by a human blood product—*tetanus immune globulin* (TIG). Since it is not so foreign, it causes few of the disagreeable and often serious side effects so common with the horse product. This borrowed immunity, gotten by using another person's or an animal's antibodies, is called **passive immunity**.

Passive Immunity:
The Temporary Resistance
Provided by Borrowed Antibodies

Passive immunity, then, is borrowed immunity. Through vaccination or disease, another creature (human or other animal) must first earn active immunity—be stimulated to make actively his or her own antibodies. Then that creature is bled. From the blood the actual antibody is obtained. It has been seen that horse blood containing antibody-antitoxin can be borrowed to treat diphtheria and tetanus.

If given early enough, human antibodies, or immunoglobulins (often simply called *gamma globulin*), may be used to prevent regular measles (rubeola) and infectious hepatitis. For example, an individual susceptible to rubeola is exposed to the disease. If given within two days of the exposure, the injection of enough gamma globulin that was produced by another person will prevent the disease. A woman is exposed to a case of infectious hepatitis. She has shared the same

home and the same meals with someone who has it, and she may have contracted the virus. An injection of gamma globulin within about twenty to twenty-five days of the time of exposure may prevent her from becoming ill with infectious hepatitis.

The injected gamma globulin works by "locking into" the circulating virus antigen and making it harmless before visible sickness can occur. Within about two to six weeks, the used borrowed antibodies are mostly excreted with the urine. So borrowed immunity is like borrowed money. It lasts but a short time.

Antibodies that pass through the placenta from mother to baby are also borrowed and temporary. A newborn will lose the mother's polio antibodies in about eight weeks. The mother's measles antibodies remain with the baby for about fifteen months (or slightly less) after

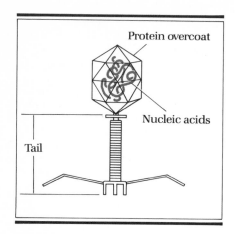

FIGURE 3-6
The structure of a virus.

birth. Children are vaccinated against both mumps and measles when they reach the age of fifteen months. Otherwise, the mother's antibodies that are still in the child will interfere with the antibody formation that would naturally take place with injected antigen (vaccine).

Viral Competitors in the Human Ecosystem

Most viruses (the smallest microorganisms) are visible only under the electron microscope. The simplest viruses are chemically composed of a tightly packed central core of nucleic acids within a protein overcoat (see Figure 3–6). It is the central core of nucleic acids (the hereditary chemicals or genes of the virus) that is responsible for causing an infection. It is the protein overcoat that determines the specificity of the virus as an antigen. In other words, the chemical *make-up* of the virus's overcoat will determine what specific disease the virus causes— whether it will cause measles, mumps, poliomyelitis, influenza, and so on. Its chemical *structure* will determine which specific antibody will be produced by the human host to fight this virus.

The central core of viral genes is of two types: RNA (ribonucleic acid) and DNA (deoxyribonucleic acid). Viruses contain either RNA or DNA, but never both. (However, cells of higher organisms, whether bacteria or people, do contain both.) Viruses also differ from one another in their *size* and *shape*. Moreover, the length of their reproductive cycles will vary, so that viral diseases will have different *incubation periods*. (This is the length of time that elapses between infection by a virus and the onset of disease symptoms.) However, all viruses are identical in one major way: They cannot multiply outside a cell. They must exist as parasites inside a cell to cause disease.

Viral Infection of an Animal Cell

When an animal cell is infected with a virus, the cell may get sick. In its sickness it can be affected in four ways and with four results: These are described below.

1 **The invading virus uses the animal cell to make more viruses.**

First, virus particles attach themselves to a cell, and then they either penetrate it (see Figure 3–7) or inject their nucleic acid into it. If the whole virus enters the cell, protein overcoat and all, the virus undergoes an "uncoating phenomenon"; that is, the protein coat opens, the virus disrobes (or is disrobed, it is not known which), and the nucleic acid molecules (the RNA or DNA) are released "naked" into the cell. If the virus just attaches itself to a cell's surface and injects its nucleic acid molecules, the protein overcoat

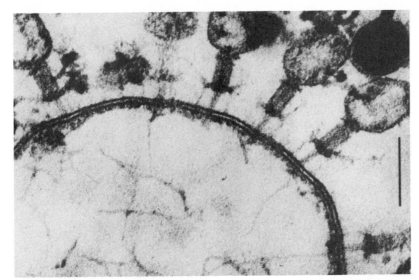

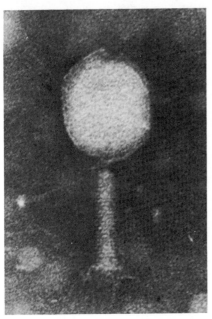

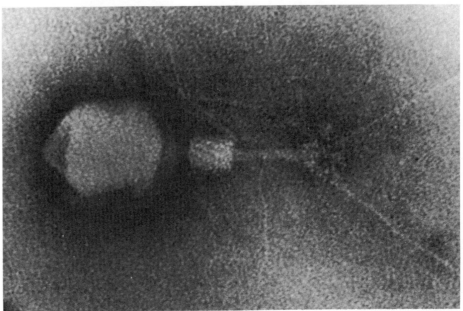

FIGURE 3-7
Left: The electron microscope reveals that each virus is bound directly to the bacterial cell wall by its short tail fibers. The tail cores have just penetrated through the bacterial wall, and dark fibers of DNA extend from the tail tips within the cell. Bottom left: An "untriggered" T2 virus (×450,000). Within its six-sided head lie coiled its genes—its infective DNA (not shown). The virus's tail is surrounded by a screw-shaped sheath. Bottom right: The virus has met with a bacterium (not shown; see the photograph on page 52). A bacterial substance caused the sheath to contract, releasing its tail fibers. The "triggered" virus (×450,000) has injected its DNA into the bacterium.

is left outside of the cell. In any event, when they are free in the cell, the viral nucleic acids containing the virus's hereditary information take over the cell's normal mechanisms. The helpless cell is forced to make more viral proteins. It is as if unwelcome visitors forced themselves into a person's home, used all the rooms, furniture, and equipment of the house, and then multiplied in such numbers that the

home fell apart. Viral infection is the supreme imposition.

2 The cell may be instructed to decrease its speed of multiplication and growth.

This is the "reverse cancer effect." During the first three or four months of pregnancy, an unborn baby can be infected by the mother's infection with the German measles (rubella) virus that passes through

the placenta. The virus takes over the hereditary, or genetic, mechanism directing an embryo's multiplying cells. The rate of cellular multiplication is slowed down, and thus fewer cells are formed. The result is *congenital rubella syndrome*, mentioned earlier. The babies are born with an inadequate number of cells; as a result, they may be blind, deaf, or retarded, or have heart and other defects.

3 Upon entering a cell, the virus may become temporarily inactive.

This is not the straightforward infection described in 1. and 2. above. This is a "slow virus infection." Chickenpox virus, for example, is usually a childhood disease. After the illness is over the virus remains *latent*, or inactive, in the cells. In a sense, then, the invading virus remains in ecological balance with the host cell. During this time there is no apparent harm to the cell. The genes of the latent virus remain in a "switched-off" state and are passed on, during cell division (*mitosis*, see page 419), from parent to daughter cells. (Exceptions are the neurons of the nervous system, which do not divide.) Often, however, if stimulated in some way, the virus can begin to multiply again. The virus migrates to the skin, the cells of which become inflamed and perhaps die. Thus, years after the chickenpox is over, the same virus may cause *shingles*. Another example of a virus that can remain latent is the common "cold sore" (*herpes simplex*), which is caused by herpesvirus 1. Still another is the genital sores caused by herpesvirus 2. Both of these herpesviruses may infect people for years, flaring up as sores (perhaps following some stress) and apparently remaining in a latent state in the cells for long periods.

4 The invading virus can cause animal cancer.

In nonhuman animals, the viral DNA or RNA captured in the cell may send messages of malignancy, meaning there is a "cancer effect." The capacity for controlled growth (previously so important a part of the normal cell's DNA or RNA func-

tion) is lost. A tumor results. As of early 1980 it had yet to be proved that viruses cause cancer in humans. Some researchers are taking the view that some human cancers are caused by the above-described (3.) latent viral infection. Inactive virus, they believe, is switched on by some stimulus, such as radiation or chemicals or perhaps another infection.

Drugs Versus Viruses

Because viruses multiply in cells, almost all known drugs are generally helpless against them. Most drugs that kill viruses kill body cells too. The problem, then, is to kill the virus without harming the cell. Bacteria do not multiply in the animal cell. They attack it from the outside. That is why drugs that are able to differentiate between bacterial and animal cells are effective against bacterial diseases. By early 1980, only a few drugs were known to be effective against human viral disease without seriously harming the human host. Scientific attacks against the virus world will probably be by a combination of vaccines and drugs. The few drugs that have proved useful against some virus infections include those for influenza A and a viral infection of the eye; a third drug is effective in one type of virus infection of the brain.

The Common Cold: The Vagrant Viruses

A cold is not, in the traditional sense, a disease. It is a collection of signs and relatively mild symptoms. Sometimes these lead to more severe symptoms and to serious disease. Signs and symptoms of a cold may be caused by a wide variety of microorganisms ranging from viruses to fungi.

An example: Suppose an unvaccinated child is invaded by the polio virus. If her resistance is adequate, she will show no symptoms. This is usual. With less resistance, she will have cold symptoms. This is occasional. Rarely, if her resistance is unusually low, she will develop paralysis or perhaps even die. All these stages are caused by the same poliovirus. At any stage her body resistance may overcome the poliovirus and then become immune to it. Later, another virus attacks. This time it may be a regular measles (rubeola) virus. Then, if her resistance is inadequate and if she is without previous vaccination, she may develop cold symptoms (respiratory symptoms usually involving the lower as well as the upper respiratory tract), a velvety rash, and, once in a thousand cases, serious brain inflammation (*measles encephalitis*). With infection, therefore, the forces of resistance are in combat with the forces of the infecting agent. The stage of condition called the cold may or may not occur, depending on the powers of the host's resistance.

With scores of other viral infections (perhaps 200 or more), similar stages occur. Influenza virus may cause no symptoms, or it may cause cold symptoms or pneumonia or even death. But viruses are not alone in causing cold symptoms. A serious bacterial disease, such as tuberculosis, may also begin with mild cold symptoms. The same may be said for some fungus diseases, such as valley fever.

The Prevention and Treatment of Colds

A cold vaccine that would include all the microorganisms that can cause

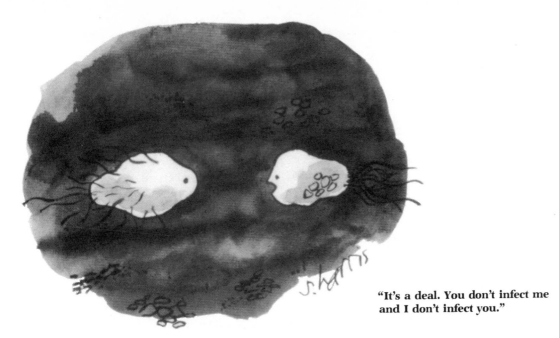

"It's a deal. You don't infect me and I don't infect you."

the signs and symptoms of a common cold may never be developed. Vaccines are, however, available for some illnesses for which a cold is introductory or in which it is a transient phase. Vaccination against measles or mumps, for example, will protect not only against these diseases, but also against the "colds" that are an early stage of them.

Penicillin is helpless against viruses. (It, and other antibiotics, can, however, often destroy secondarily invading bacteria, such as pneumonia-causing cocci. This explains their occasional use in some severe respiratory infections.) Simple aspirin will relieve aches and pains. For those who cannot tolerate aspirin, proper doses of acetaminophen will do. Alcohol, by causing nasal and throat congestion, may prolong and worsen a cold. So will cigarette smoking. To ease the symptoms and shorten the siege of an ordinary cold, one should drink enough fluids, eat what is desired, but moderately, and get extra rest. Time is a most reasonable cure for the common cold. Despite several studies, there is no conclusive evidence that vitamin C prevents or helps cure the common cold.

Viruses Affecting the Unborn

Although maternal chickenpox may end a pregnancy, there is no evidence that its virus causes malformations, as does the rubella virus discussed earlier. Children of women who develop chickenpox in the last week or two of pregnancy may be born with the disease or develop it soon after birth. This is rarely serious.

For an adult, the "cold sore" virus produces a common and usually mild infection. Fortunately, it rarely infects the unborn child. When it does, it may end the pregnancy.

Cytomegalic inclusion disease is an illness whose long name describes some of its aspects. *Cyto* (meaning "cell") and *megalic* (meaning "large" refer to the unusually large cells associated with the disease. The word *inclusion* describes certain bodies (or particles) found within those cells. In adults the disease is usually so mild that it is often not detected. But when transmitted to the fetus in the first three months of pregnancy, it often shows itself by a wide variety of malformations in the newborn child. As with German measles, children with the disease may be contagious for months after delivery. They should be isolated, particularly from pregnant women.

A relationship between mumps and birth defects has not been proved. Nor do infectious hepatitis and chickenpox have any proved effect on the unborn child. But a growing suspicion that other viruses may affect the child within the uterus indicates the need for more research in this field.

Mumps

Although during mumps infection the virus is carried by the blood to all body tissues, several particular organs most frequently show signs and produce symptoms. For instance, the parotid glands (the saliva-producing glands in front and below the ears) may swell because their ducts are blocked. But the salivary glands do not always swell, especially if the patient has not yet reached puberty. About 20 percent of all male mumps patients thirteen years of age or over develop swelling and damage as a result of inflammation of the testicle (or *orchitis*). In females, inflammation of the ovary (*oophoritis*) may occur. Since a tight capsule surrounds the sperm-forming testes, there may be testicular damage and perhaps (but rarely) sterility. This does not occur with oophoritis because no tight capsule surrounds the ovary.

Another common complication of mumps is an inflammation of the lining of the brain (*meningitis*) or of the brain itself (*encephalitis*). Ninety-nine percent of all victims of mumps meningitis recover, and almost an equal percentage show no aftereffects. Fortunately, mumps encephalitis is rare; it is much less frequent than mumps meningitis, but it is much more serious. It is fatal in about 20 percent of the cases.

Despite the usual mildness of mumps and most of its complications, many old wives' tales have been spun around the horrid effects of mumps, particularly on the testes, ovaries, and meninges. The infection is not known to directly cause impotence, although the parents' distress with an adolescent son's swollen testicles may leave the child with psychological or sexual problems. Since mumps can also cause considerable temporary discomfort and disability, the disease should be prevented by vaccination.

Infectious Mononucleosis

This is a viral disease manifested by fever, fatigue, swollen neck lymph nodes (other lymph nodes throughout the body may also be involved), and sore throat. Enlargement of the spleen and liver is common. Very occasionally the sick person may have a rash or be jaundiced. Serious complications, such as brain and heart inflammation, are rare. Some individuals may become easily fatigued for months. Recent studies suggest an association between the virus that causes infectious mononucleosis and other illnesses, but the significance of this finding is as yet unclear.

Unless helped by direct and intimate contact, the disease is not easily spread. The illness is often diagnosed in (but hardly limited to) college students. For this reason it has been variously called the "college" or "student's" or "kissing" disease.

Infectious mononucleosis usually lasts from one to three weeks. However, it can last for months. Also, the virus may remain in the throat for up to a year after infection. The

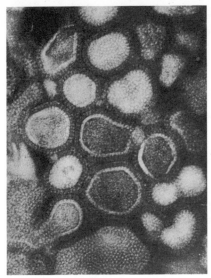

An Asian influenza virus, magnified
250,000 times.

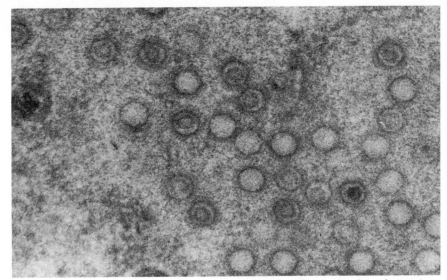

Epstein-Barr virus particles in a human lymphoblast (a developing lymphocyte).

Poliovirus particles (the clustered round objects) inside a fragment of a cell,
magnified 320,000 times.

PHOTO ESSAY
**Photographs taken through
high-powered microscopes, a
process called photomicrography,
have been an immeasurable boon to
scientific research in almost every
major field of study.**

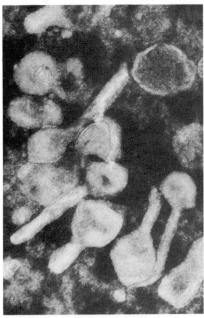

The virus that causes mouse leukemia,
magnified 150,000 times.

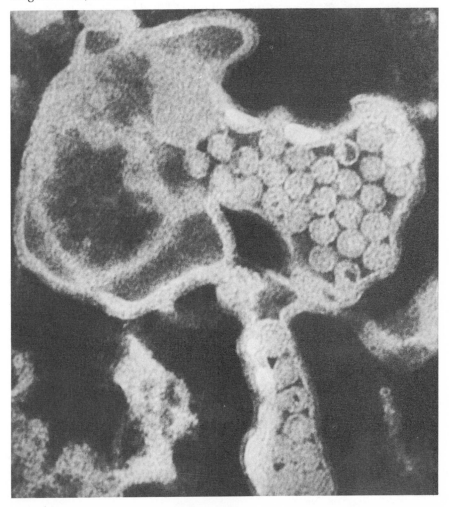

incubation period (the time between exposure to the virus and appearance of the first symptoms) is usually between two and six weeks. It is probably communicable before symptoms begin, and it may remain communicable for some time. Recovery is the rule. A vaccine to prevent this disease is presently being tested and shows promise.

Three Types of Viral Hepatitis

Most viral hepatitis (inflammation of the liver) is caused by three distinct types of infection produced by three different viruses. **Hepatitis A**, once called *infectious hepatitis*, often accompanies conditions of over-crowding, poor sanitation, and careless personal hygiene. It is easily spread by human waste (fecal) contamination of hands, food, or water. An infected individual who is careless about hand-washing after having a bowel movement may, therefore, spread the infection. **Hepatitis B**, once called *serum hepatitis*, is usually transmitted through the blood of an infected individual that enters the bloodstream of a susceptible person. This may be accomplished by transfusion of infected blood. Thus persons who have ever had hepatitis are not allowed to donate blood. Hepatitis B may also be contracted through the sharing of infected needles, syringes, or other intravenous equipment. Sharing dirty needles is common among drug abusers and people who get tattooed; thus hepatitis B is common among them too. There is also an association between hepatitis A and ear piercing. **Non-A, non-B hepatitis** has only recently been identified. (Refer to Figure 3–8.) It seems to include most of the after-transfusion hepatitis common in the United States today.

Signs and symptoms of the diseases may be very much alike. They include loss of appetite, fever, headache, nausea, weakness, muscle pain and joint stiffness, and pain in the upper right abdomen. As the diseases progress, the urine becomes dark and the stool light. With the occurrence of jaundice (yellowing of the skin), the individual may become severely depressed. The jaundice may last for about six weeks. As long as three months may be required for recovery. Chronic liver problems sometimes result from viral hepatitis. Most of the approximately fifty-five thousand hepatitis cases reported yearly in this country are of the infectious A type. Nevertheless, hepatitis B is a much more serious illness than the more common hepatitis A. This may be because people who are infected by the hepatitis B virus through medically necessary injections or transfusions are already weakened by illness or drug abuse.

There is some hope for the development of a hepatitis vaccine. Laboratory methods of identifying the hepatitis B antigen have prevented the use of infected blood that might otherwise have been used for transfusion. A test for the same purpose for the virus causing non-A, non-B hepatitis is also promising. It is possible for people to carry these virus antigens in the blood without being sick. But, again, laboratory techniques now make it possible to detect these antigens and thereby to eliminate infected would-be blood donors.

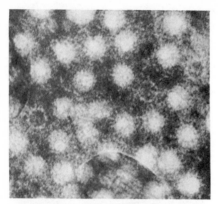
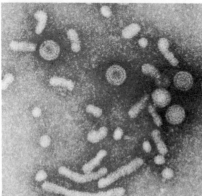
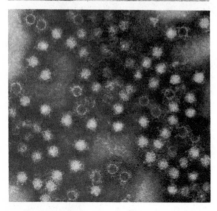

FIGURE 3–8
Electron micrograph of possible non-A, non-B hepatitis virus particles (×90,950).

Passive immunity (borrowed antibodies) by means of gamma globulin inoculation has long been available for preventing the common hepatitis A, but no active immunization has yet been discovered for this disease. However, in the case of hepatitis B there has been some progress in the development of both active (vaccine) and passive (gamma globulin) immunizations. As yet, however, there is neither active nor passive immunity for non-A, non-B hepatitis. The best tool for the prevention of all three types of hepatitis is cleanliness. Sterilization of needles, syringes, and other equipment used in blood or intravenous work is essential to the prevention of viral hepatitis of any type.

Bacterial Competitors in the Human Ecosystem

Sickness from Food Contamination

There are many microorganisms that thrive on or in foods we eat, and eating foods that are contaminated with these microorganisms can cause illness. As many as ten million cases of food-borne illnesses happen every year in this country because of these microorganisms. *Salmonella*, a large group of microorganisms that can live and grow in number in the intestinal tract, are responsible for an illness called *salmonellosis*. A continuous infecting cycle may be established because the organism can spread from animal to human, human to human, and from human to animal.

Staphylococcal food poisoning is a true poisoning. Why? Because while growing in food, the staphylococcus produces a toxin. It is the toxin, not the staphylococcus, that, upon being swallowed, causes illness. The same is true of *botulism*, which, fortunately, is rare. Botulism poison is the most deadly known. Most bacterial illness associated with food, however, does not result in death. Table 3–3 presents some basic differences between staphylococcus *intoxication* and salmonella *infection*. Information about such things as what time the symptoms began and what foods the victim ate may lead

an investigator to the cause of an outbreak of food poisoning.

The prevention of food poisoning depends to a great extent on storing or processing food at the proper temperature, as is shown in Figure 3–9. If foods are not heated at a high enough temperature for a long enough time during canning, bacillus spores may survive and later cause botulism. Leaving foods, especially milk products or those

containing milk products, unrefrigerated can also cause the food to become contaminated with harmful microorganisms.

Tetanus (Lockjaw)

The convulsions of tetanus are caused not by the bacterium itself but by the deadly toxin it manufactures. Tetanus often happens among heroin abusers, who doubtless inject

---

TABLE 3–3
Two Ingredients of Food-borne Illness: Staphylococcus and Salmonella

TYPE ORGANISM INVOLVED	MODE OF ACTION	INCUBATION PERIOD	COMMON SYMPTOMS	COMMON FOOD SOURCES	FOOD HANDLING CAUTIONS
Staphylococcus	Toxin	Under 6 hours; usually 2–4 hours	Vomiting (in almost all cases) Cramps Diarrhea No fever (temperature may be below normal)	Pastries Custards Salad dressings Sliced meats	Be scrupulous about personal hygiene (especially hand washing). Protect food from animal excreta.
Salmonella	Bacterial infection	6–48 hours; more usually, 12–24 hours	Abdominal pain Diarrhea (in almost all cases) Vomiting Fever	Poultry Raw eggs Egg products Raw milk Meats Meat Pies Fish	Clean the cutting wheel of the kitchen can opener regularly.

themselves with the tetanus organism via dirty needles, or it could be caused by the presence of the organisms or its spores in polluted heroin. In this country, tetanus still occurs with disturbing frequency (refer back to Table 3–2). But in developing countries, where immunization levels are low and sanitation is poor, tetanus is much more common. Tetanus can be transmitted from a pregnant woman to her child during delivery. This disease is responsible for many infant deaths in less developed countries. Immunization of mothers might prevent this tragedy, for tetanus toxoid is an extremely effective vaccine.

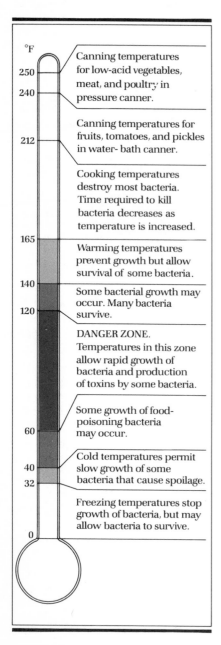

FIGURE 3–9
Temperature for control of bacteria.

The Sexually Transmitted Diseases: How Big a Problem?

There are a number of diseases that may be spread by sexual intercourse. In this country, four of the most important are **gonorrhea, syphilis, genital herpes,** and **nongonococcal urethritis** or NGU for short. (These diseases are described in the boxed insert on pages 80–81.) Three others, chancroid, lymphogranuloma venereum, and granuloma inguinale, are not common in this country.

Worldwide, about 50 million people are estimated to have infectious syphilis, and 150 million to have infectious gonorrhea—a total almost equal to the population of the United States. In the United States 287,181 cases of gonorrhea were reported in 1945. In 1977 that number was 531,558. However, in that same period, owing to the use of penicillin and other antibiotics, syphilis has declined. These drugs have also greatly reduced the incidence of babies born with syphilis and the occurrence of the late stages of the disease.

Because private physicians treat about 80 percent of all syphilis and gonorrhea (and it is believed that they also see a majority of genital herpes and nongonococcal urethritis) and report few of their infectious cases, the number of new cases of syphilis, gonorrheal infection, herpesvirus 2 infection, and nongonococcal urethritis can only be estimated. It is known, though, that by far the greatest majority of reported infectious cases of syphilis and gonorrhea in the United States are in persons between the ages of fifteen and twenty-four.

Causes

Several cultural and social changes seem to be responsible for the present epidemic of **sexually transmitted diseases.** Among these are the increasing number of sexual activities that take place with many partners; the greater availability and use of birth control devices; increased population movement; increased financial and sexual independence of women; the growing number of homosexually oriented males (many of whom, it is thought, have a higher frequency of sexual contact than do homosexually oriented women); the drug subculture; and the increased sexual permissiveness resulting from relaxation of restraints formerly imposed by religion, the family, and public opinion. Added to these is a change from public clinics as the major treatment centers of sexually transmitted diseases to private physicians, who cannot find the time or do not have adequate personnel for reporting and contact tracing. Many physicians feel that reporting a case would violate the confidence of the patient.

Still further frustrating attempts to control gonorrhea is the fact that the microbe causing this disease keeps changing. It is increasingly resistant to antibiotics, especially penicillin. And there is even one form of the gonococcus that actually produces a substance that destroys penicillin.

Three Epidemics of Sexually Transmitted Diseases among Males

Syphilis, gonorrhea, and nongonococcal urethritis are more commonly reported among males than females. Although the primary sore, or **chancre**, of syphilis does not itch and is painless, the man can usually see it. Often, however, the primary chancre of syphilis in the male may be absent or be so insignificant as to be missed. In the case of gonorrhea, the male can most often see a gonorrheal discharge, and his pain on urination may drive him to a physician. However, this is not always true. Studies of males brought to treatment for gonorrhea by contact tracing showed that although almost two-thirds had

symptoms, they had not sought treatment. Nor do all males with gonorrhea have symptoms; gonorrhea without symptoms exists in 12 to 20 percent of men examined. Not only do these symptomless men spread their disease, but as the disease progresses they risk serious complications, such as inflammation of the joints, heart, and lining of the brain and spinal cord.

Women's Special Inequality

For the woman, syphilis, gonorrhea, and nongonococcal urethritis are special risks. Her anatomy puts her at a disadvantage. The male urethra is 8 to 9 inches long, while the female urethra is only 1½ inches long. (The urethra is the canal through which urine is discharged.) Women's external genitalia are not as visible to them as male genitalia are to men. Also, the surface of the cervix (where some venereal infections may be located) and much of the vagina are without a nerve supply. A painless, invisible sore or a mild normal-like discharge can hardly give her warning of a venereal infection. The short urethra is generally not as severely involved as the male's longer one, so she does not

feel the warning signal of pain during urination. Between 70 and 90 percent of women who have gonorrhea do not know it. Nationwide this amounts to hundreds of thousands of women who have the disease and are not being treated for it. Unless found and treated, these women may remain a source of infection for months. Not until the infection has spread will pain be a sign, and by that time damage may be serious.

About 10 to 15 percent of women who have gonorrheal organisms within the opening of the cervix develop severe complications. These may be gonorrheal blood poisoning, joint and skin inflammation, and, more commonly, inflammation of one or both Fallopian tubes and ovaries. Over three-fourths of all gonorrheal arthritis occurs in women. Because joint destruction from gonorrheal arthritis can be swift, delay in treatment can be disastrous. In addition, without early treatment of gonococcal Fallopian tube infection, sterility often results. Among women, the need for surgery to cure illness due to an old gonorrheal infection is not uncommon.

About half the cases of Fallopian tube infections are thought to be gonorrheal, and such an infection can cause a pregnancy in the Fallopian tube, or an *ectopic pregnancy*, to occur. In such cases, fertilization of the egg takes place above an abscess or stricture in the infected tube. Thus, the fertilized egg often cannot pass down the tube to the uterus. Within about six weeks the tube will rupture, and this is a surgical emergency. To the danger of an ectopic pregnancy must be added this fact: Several sexually transmitted infections of the woman's internal reproductive organs lessen the entire area's resistance to invasion by other microorganisms. A

The silent epidemic. The gonococcus (left), which appears in pairs, is the bacterium that causes gonorrhea. The spirochete (right) is the corkscrew-shaped microorganism that causes syphilis.

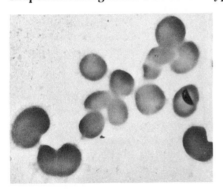
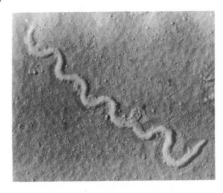

The Most Common Sexually Transmitted Diseases

(A person may have none of the symptoms but still have a sexually transmitted disease.)

Disease: Gonorrhea. *Cause: Neisseria gonorrheae, a gonococcus. Incubation period:* Within two to eight days (often less) following exposure for about 80 to 85 percent of males; two to eight days for females when symptoms occur. The *estimated* number of persons affected yearly is three million. *The disease process:* Gonorrhea is usually a local disease of the body parts affected. However, its germs may spread to involve the entire body. In the *male*, the disease most often shows itself as a burning on urination and a discharge of pus. Urination may be quite painful. Males (12 to 20 percent) may have gonorrhea without symptoms. Chronic untreated male gonorrhea often leads to involvement of other portions of the body, particularly the urinary or reproductive system. If not treated early gonorrhea may cause sterility. In about 80 percent of *females*, the early symptoms of gonorrhea are usually absent or very mild. For this reason, the infected female rarely seeks early treatment. Therefore, she unknowingly spreads the disease. Moreover, this often leads to infection of her Fallopian tubes, ovaries, and lower abdomen. The resistance of all pelvic tissue is lessened, and other organisms then complicate the picture. With these events, pain may be severe. Due to scarring and closure of the tubes, or to emergency surgery, sterility often results. Rectal infection can occur in both males and females. This occurs more commonly among men whose behavior is homosexual. In females it may occur from infectious drippings from the vagina to the anal area. Such infection is seldom recognized because its symptoms consist only of a sensation of wetness or itching around the anus. Gonorrheal arthritis is a serious disease. It is far more common among females than males. It requires emergency treatment.

Disease: Genital Herpes. (This illness was not recognized as a venereal disease until 1966.) *Cause: Herpesvirus type 2.* (Should not be confused with herpesvirus type 1, which causes infections above the waist, such as "cold sores" and "fever blisters.") *Incubation period:* Two to twenty days, average three to six days. An estimated 300,000 to 500,000 people are affected yearly. *The disease process:* The first symptom may be a slight tingling in the genital area. Then one or a group of small (sometimes itchy) blisters appears. In the *male* the blisters are on the head, the base, or the shaft of the penis. In both sexes, the blisters may be about the perineum (between the anus and the scrotum in the male; between the anus and the lower end of the vulva in the female). In the *female* the external genitalia (outer reproductive organs) and the vagina and cervix may also be ulcerated. If the cervix or vagina is involved there may be no symptoms. In both sexes ulceration of the blister-like lesions occurs, which is painful. There is also painful swelling of the lymph nodes in the groin in both sexes. The signs and symptoms last about two weeks before healing. Patients may think they are cured, but too often this is not the case. Unlike other venereal diseases, genital herpes returns repeatedly without additional sexual contact. *Other special considerations for emphasis are:* (1) Sexual intercourse should be avoided or the male should use condoms during the active phase of the disease and while it is getting better (one to three weeks). (2) Sexual partners must be examined. (3) There is a strong association between cancer of the cervix and infection with *herpesvirus 2*. Women who have herpesvirus 2 infections should have routine (at least yearly) Pap tests for cervical cancer for the rest of their lives. (4) Newborns can get the infection by contact with the mother's vagina. If the mother has herpesvirus 2 infection, she should be delivered by Caesarean section. The infection in newborns is extremely serious and often deadly. (5) Staphylococci and streptococci are among the other infectious microorganisms that are often added to the herpesvirus 2 ulcerations. Swelling occurs. Pain on urination can then be very severe. (6) Until recently there was no permanent cure, but in midsummer 1979, the *Journal of the American Medical Association* published an article announcing successful treatment with the drug 2-Deoxy-D-glucose.[1]

Disease: Nongonococcal (Nonspecific) Urethritis (NGU or NSU). *Cause:* Unknown. Several microorganisms, including *Chlamydia trachomatis*, have been implicated. *Chlamydia trachomatis* also causes a serious eye infection (*trachoma*) and is the cause of *lymphogranuloma venereum* —an uncommon venereal disease in this country but common in some developing countries. *Incubation period:* Uncertain; about 1 to 3 weeks. The estimated number of persons affected yearly is three million. *The disease process:* As with gonorrhea, nongonococcal inflammation of the urethra (*urethritis*) in the male is more extensive and, therefore, more likely to produce signs and symptoms than in the female. In the *male*, NGU begins with a scanty, watery discharge from the urethra; there is also some mild pain on urination. Also noticed is an increased frequency of urination. Some men (though not all) have a pus-like discharge, dirty gray or yellow, that will look like a gonorrheal discharge. There may be some redness and inflammation of the mucous membrane about the slit at the tip of the penis. In the *female*, the urethra and cervix become infected. The woman may experience some discomfort on urination. Some men have gonorrhea and Chlamydia infections at the same time, though they are more likely to have Chlamydia infections after they are free of gonorrhea. Frequently, other microorganisms must be sought. It is very important that the sexual partner or partners also be under medical care. True, most cases of nongonococcal urethritis clear up by themselves after six to eight weeks. However, the infections commonly return without another sexual contact. If the disease is not treated, men may develop chronic inflammation of the prostate gland. Strictures of the urethra occur occasionally. Women may develop bladder infections that are difficult to cure. If the disease is being caused by *Chlamydia trachomatis*, a child's eyes can develop a serious infection (*trachoma*) after passage through the vagina.

Disease: Syphilis. *Cause: Treponema pallidum* (a spiral-shaped bacterium). *Incubation period:* 10 to 90 days, usually twenty-one days. The estimated number of persons affected yearly is over 400,000. *The disease process:* The first sign of primary syphilis is usually a single, painless, nonitching sore called a *chancre*. It appears at the place where the germs most often enter the body—the genital area. However, chancres are often discovered elsewhere. Sometimes the chancre does not appear or is overlooked, especially in women. If it does appear, it disappears without treatment in about two weeks. In a short time, which may vary from a few weeks to six months, *secondary syphilis* signs appear. The disease is then no longer local. The entire body is infected. The initial infection involved perhaps a few thousand syphilis microorganisms. Now billions are swarming in the blood. Unchecked, the later stages of the disease can affect the body so widely that it is called "The Great Imitator" of other sicknesses. Although different people have different symptoms, the most common are lesions (an injury or other change in normal structure), which may be few or many, large or small, and which may appear on various body areas. A widespread rash is not a common lesion; frequently it is absent. If present, the rash, and the chancre that came before it, abound with the corkscrew-shaped *Treponema pallidum.* So do whitish patches in the mouth or throat. "Motheaten" or "patchy," falling-out hair, low fever, painless swelling of lymph glands, and pain in bones and joints may also be signs of secondary syphilis. While the primary and secondary signs and symptoms persist, the disease is highly contagious. Without treatment, the secondary symptoms often disappear in less than a month, although they may persist for a longer period. Since both the chancre of primary syphilis and the signs and symptoms of secondary syphilis disappear by themselves without treatment, there is a ready field for the quack. His phony treatments "cure" these signs and symptoms, but the patient is left with the destructive living microorganisms in the body. After the secondary stage, the disease enters a period of early latency. The degree of communicability associated with *early latent syphilis* depends on the reappearance of secondary skin lesions. Because of such a constant possibility, the disease is considered communicable for approximately two years following initial infection. Occasionally, the latent phase may be a year or two longer. The final stage, *noncommunicable late latent syphilis*, may eventually cause heart disease, insanity, paralysis, blindness, or death. These end results of untreated syphilis may not take place until ten to forty years after the primary infection. Often they do not occur. Too often they do.

Other Sexually Transmitted Diseases

DISEASE, CAUSE, AND INCUBATION PERIOD	SIGNS AND SYMPTOMS	COMMENTS
TRICHOMONIASIS ("Trich"); *Trichomonas vaginalis*, a *Protozoa*; incubation, 4–28 days	Frothy, odorous, greenish-yellow discharge. Genital soreness and itching. Pain on urination. Symptoms usually absent in males.	Inflammation of glands and tubes in reproductive or urinary systems. Spreads to sex partners. Can occur in the female nonsexually. *Trichomonas* may live for years in the vagina without symptoms.
MONILIASIS: *Candida albicans*, yeast, fungus; incubation varies with case.	Severe genital itching. Thick, white, odorous discharge. Disease may be triggered by pregnancy, diabetes, birth control pills, antibiotic treatment, lowered resistance.	Frequently returns. Spreads to sex partners. Oral, penile, anal infection happens in males. Most often the disease has a nonsexual basis. Causes "thrush" in babies. Can be spread to newborn babies. Early treatment of pregnant women essential.
CONDYLOMATA ACUMINATA ("Venereal Warts"); *Viral cause*; incubation, 1–3 months.	Similar to, but not the same as, common skin warts. Single or multiple growths around genital or anal regions; may be pink, indented, and moist with a cauliflower-like feel, or hard and yellow-gray.	Depending on location, may be chronic irritation and secondary infection. May obstruct passage of urine or bowel contents. Disfigurement. Recurrence. Possible spread to sex partners.
PUBIC LICE ("Crabs"); *pubic louse*; incubation, 7–9 days.	Slight to severe itching. Possible mild rash.	Spread to sex partners and nonsexually to household members. All above contacts must be treated. Can be gotten from unclean beds or toilet seats.
GENITAL SCABIES *Mite*; incubation, several days to weeks.	Severe itching. Small, reddish, elevated track or break on skin surface.	Scratching may lead to secondary infection. Spread to sex partners. May be nonsexually spread. Body and linens must be kept clean.

chronic infected condition may then develop. Although unproved, many specialists believe that nongonococcal urethritis can also cause chronic pelvic inflammatory disease (PID) just as often as does untreated gonorrhea.

For women the problem is made even worse by yet another factor. Birth control pills reduce the acidity of the vaginal ecosystem. This encourages the growth of microbes that cause gonorrhea and other diseases. Women who are taking oral contraceptives and are exposed to gonorrhea are over twice as likely to develop the disease.

Sexually Transmitted Diseases and the Unborn Child

Syphilis, gonorrhea, and herpesvirus infection may all affect the unborn child. Syphilitic infection of the unborn child can take place any time after the seventeenth week of pregnancy. Before then the syphilis germs cannot pass through the undeveloped placenta. Should a woman contract syphilis and remain untreated, she will be able to give the disease to her unborn child during the late stages of pregnancy throughout the first six to eight years of her untreated infection. Thus, although after two years the disease cannot be spread through sexual intercourse, it is in the deep tissues of the mother's body, from where it can easily be caught by the child. However, even late in pregnancy, proper treatment of the woman can prevent syphilitic infection of the unborn child. Many physicians think it wise to have blood tests for syphilis done several times during pregnancy. An infant born of a mother with untreated syphilis may show evidence of the disease at birth or shortly after.

DISEASE AND DESTINY

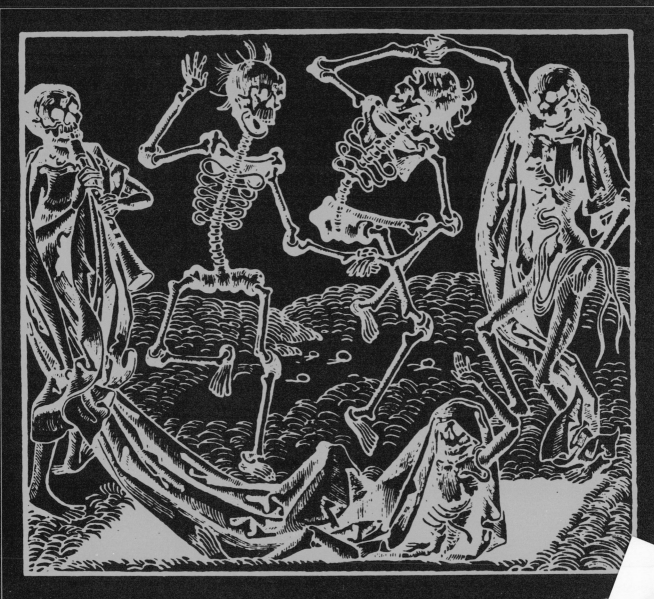

PROLOGUE

ALCIBIADES.
What is thy name?
Is man so hateful to thee.
That art thyself a man?[1]

The Dance of Death was a major artistic theme during the plagues of the Middle Ages. On the preceding page is a woodcut by Michael Wolgemuth, done in 1493, depicting the Dance of Death.

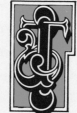

Thirteen centuries ago (in 664) the Irish kings of Ulster and Munster called a meeting of the lay and clerical leaders of their kingdoms. The problem facing them was famine. The poor earth could no longer supply the growing populations. People were starving and unable to work. What could be done?

The two kings agreed on a plan of action. Through devout prayer and a fast, a direct appeal was to be made to God. In His infinite mercy, He would surely hear and help them.

Up to this point, there was harmony at the meeting. But the content of the prayer to the Lord caused disagreement, and a debate arose. What the kings proposed to ask God for was a pestilence—a widespread, deadly infection—to kill the excess population, composed of "inferior" people. There would then be enough food for the "superior" and "worthier" survivors. As to who would be included among the survivors, there seemed to be no doubt.

One man disagreed. Would it not be more in keeping with God's way, St. Gerald suggested, to pray, not for pestilence, but for more food? Certainly such a prayer could just as easily be answered. And the chances of being heard by a compassionate God would surely be greater.

But this motion failed to carry. In opposing it, St. Fechin gained favor with the lords and most of the clergy. The earlier motion was carried, and God was implored for a plague to kill off the unwanted people.

According to the records of the Church at Mayo, however, God punished this wickedness. A pestilence did indeed visit Ulster and Munster, but it was not so choosy as some had hoped. The kings and at least one-third of the nobles who had begged the Lord for the visitation were killed by it.

This immorality tale illustrates the grotesque vanity and indifference of those who enslave others. To the Irish tyrants, sickness and death were fitting ends for their serfs. They understood that sick people can never be free. Disease makes people less resistant to slavery. Parents who see their babies die of hunger, who must prostitute their starving daughters for the family bread, who taste the dust of the land, will accept any promise, any hope. Wise leaders of modern free societies labor for the health of their people. They know that a nation's vitality can come only from its people. Today, the world is much smaller than it was in 664. The social convulsions of one nation are felt far beyond its borders. Whether in Biafra or Brazil, one sick person is the business of all people everywhere.

The philosopher George Santayana said, "Those who cannot remember the past are condemned to repeat it." That is why this special section will explore the effect of disease on past events. For the sake of continuity, one major disease has been chosen: plague. Many others could be used as examples—typhus, malaria, smallpox, leprosy, syphilis, cholera. In addition, the effect of individual illness on the course of history will be discussed, with Napoleon serving as the major subject. "God was bored with him," wrote Victor Hugo. But if any one man can be said to have brought agony to his age, it is surely he.

PLAGUE: WHAT IS IT?

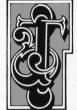

Throughout history, *Pasteurella pestis*, the *bacillus* that causes plague, has killed an estimated 150 million people. There are several types of plague, of which the two most common are the *bubonic* and the *pneumonic*. Bubonic plague is generally limited to the lymph nodes, which swell and become painful. In pneumonic plague the lungs are involved.

Plague is a sickness common to rats and other rodents, such as squirrels and chipmunks. Fleas transmit the plague bacilli from rat to rat and from rat to human. A flea takes a blood meal from an infected rodent, usually a rat. Plague bacilli get into its gut, where they multiply. In feeding on another rat or human, the infected flea vomits the bacteria into the bite. This is how the disease is passed on.

Usually, several days after being bitten by an infected flea, an infected person becomes desperately ill. A fall in blood pressure, a raging fever, and a rapid and irregular pulse are among the early signs of plague. Within hours the patient collapses and becomes delirious. With bubonic plague the pain in the neck, groin, or armpits (or all three)—where some of the body's lymph nodes are located—is unbearable. In all of these areas swellings develop rapidly. Soon these swellings, called *buboes* (from which comes the name bubonic plague), begin to abscess. The germ of bubonic plague can travel by way of the blood to other parts of the body. When the germs reach the lungs, the disease can be spread in a manner causing pneumonic plague. In pneumonic plague it is basically the breathing system that is affected. The disease is passed on through the air by tiny droplets containing the bacillus that leave the mouth of the infected person. In this way epidemics of plague can occur. Because extensive bleeding into the skin is common, often causing the skin to become a blackish-purple color, this dread disease has earned the name "Black Death."

PLAGUE IN THE MIDDLE AGES

The Middle Ages began and ended with the plague. The best known of the early medieval epidemics occurred during the reign of Emperor Justinian the Great (527–565).

The Plague of Justinian

The plague of Justinian was bubonic plague. Coming from the hinterlands of southwest Asia, it arrived in Constantinople, the capital of the Byzantine Empire, in about 532. (The Byzantine Empire in those days was the eastern part of what later became the Roman Empire.)

Lancing a bubo.

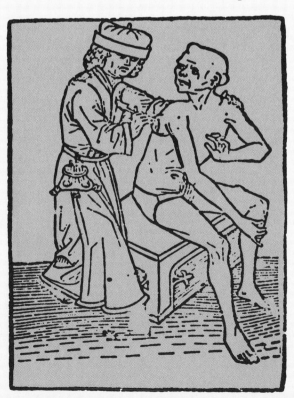

Spreading west, the plague soon assaulted all Europe. A remarkable account of the epidemic at Constantinople was left by a Byzantine historian of the time, Procopius of Caesara. Plainly, he saw disease threatening civilization. "During these times," he wrote with horror, "there was a pestilence by which the whole human race came near to being annihilated."

So accurately did Procopius describe the signs and symptoms of plague that there is little doubt as to the disease. Within a few days—at the most five—of the onset of sickness, death occurred. Soon the burial places were exhausted. The dead littered the streets. Instead of being buried, many bodies were collected and piled one on top of the other in unoccupied buildings. Inevitably, the rats infesting these buildings became infected. They carried their infection to others, and the contagion spread.

The greatest city of the Eastern Roman Empire was paralyzed. "The work of every description ceases," Procopius wrote, "all the trades were abandoned by the artisans, and all other work as well."[2] How similar this comment is to the report of a modern Peace Corps worker: "They cannot work. They cannot learn. They can't do anything but be sick and die."

In explaining a cause for the calamity, Procopius forsook scientific reasoning in favor of the blind acceptance of fate so characteristic of the Dark Ages. He wrote, "For this calamity it is quite impossible either to express in words or to conceive in thought any explanation except indeed to refer it to God."

With these words the deep night of the Dark Ages fell upon humankind.

The seventh century ushered in a new era. The plague was not the only cause of the death of the old era, but its effect on administrations, plots and plans, campaigns and countercampaigns, cannot be denied. The bacillus of plague had twisted the course of history.

The Black Death

In 1333, a drought devasted China. Famine followed, then flood. In Kingsai, at that time the capital of China, some 400,000 people drowned. Flood, famine, locusts, earthquakes—all followed one upon the other and spread across vast areas of the tormented land. Added to these sufferings was still another—plague. Starting somewhere in central Asia, the disease had spread rapidly to China and India. Finally the pestilence came to Europe. This is how.

In 1347, some Italian merchants were making their way from China back to Europe. Returning with luxury items such as furs and silks, the merchants met their ancient enemy—the Tartars. The merchants barricaded themselves in Caffa, a small fort on the Crimean Straits. There they stayed to resist the Tartar siege. Weeks passed.

One summer day, the Tartars suddenly hurled new weapons of destruction over the city walls. These weapons were the dead bodies of their own men who had died of the plague. This early attempt at bacteriological warfare was successful. The Italian merchants were terrified. Many fell sick and died. The survivors expected momentary capture, but the besieging Tartars did not attack. Hundreds of their own men were being killed by the plague. The Tartars fled, leaving the small fortress to its misery.

Those Italians who were still alive boarded four small ships and set sail for Constantinople—that great meeting place of Asia, Europe, and Africa. Along the route, they saw great ships drifting aimlessly; all on board were dead of plague. In Constantinople the merchants seeded the plague. The disease raced to Italy and then to the rest of Europe.

In the constant competition between people and their parasites, it is the plague bacillus that came closest to wiping out the human race during this fourteenth-century world-wide epidemic. Like a wind of death, the disease bereaved the world. Pope Clement VI (who escaped contagion by surrounding himself with two great fires) estimated the world loss of human life at forty-three million. The papal physicians estimated the number of dead in Europe to be between two-thirds and three-fourths of the entire population. Some thought the end of the world was at hand. Friar John Clyn, an Irish Franciscan, expecting death, left behind this touching note (1349):

So have I reduced these things to writing; and lest the writing should perish with the writer, and the work fail together with the workman, I leave parchment for continuing the work, if haply any man survive, and any of the race of Adam escape this pestilence and continue the work which I have commenced.[3]

Here the sentence trails off. The writer lived to add but two more words: "magna karistia"—great dearth. Another hand then briefly noted, "here it seems that the author died."

SOCIETAL CHANGES And so medieval Europe, terrorized by sickness, huddled under the repeated blows of the plague. As in the time of Justinian, the societal changes were tremendous. To the modern student, who sees whole populations in developing countries enslaved by disease, an understanding of these changes is essential.

First, *moral standards* were lowered. The plague had killed many policemen and judges. The courts were always closed; the process of law was stopped. Amorality became the rule. "Live today, tomorrow, death," was a way of existence. Debauchery and drunkenness were everywhere. Thievery was rampant. For a short time, stolen goods could be obtained at ridiculously low prices. But the time of low prices was short-lived. Disastrous *economic changes* followed. The surplus of goods that had accumulated as a result of plague deaths was soon gone, because the death of large numbers of people from the disease reduced the number of able hands to do the work. This shortage of labor resulted in higher prices. Diminished production and soaring prices became realities. Europe approached the brink of ruin.

The *societal character* of medieval life also changed. The newly rich who were created by the plague did not gain their wealth only from inheritance and thievery. New opportunities became legally available and were eagerly seized. Aristocratic holders of titles had died of the plague, many of them leaving no heirs. Their lands and titles were dispensed by the kings to newer favorites. But these new nobles were without tradition. "The decay in manners in the last half of the fourteenth century is an astonishing fact. The old fashioned gentility was gone; manners were uncouth, rude, brutal."[4]

In addition, there were *changes in government and the Church*. Both areas of change had evil effects on the people. Again, excess death was the cause. It had taken centuries to develop a competent governing corps with a tradition of efficiency and service. In a short time, without warning, it was gone. Positions formerly held by able men were now filled by

5

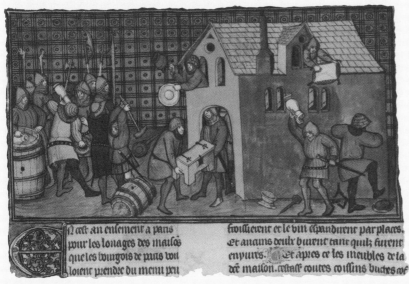

Looting during the Black Death.

incompetents and opportunists. From every quarter rose cries for reform. The Church suffered even more severely than did the government, for the people had already begun to doubt. Had not prayer failed to stop the dying? There are those who hold the view that the Black Death led to such questioning of the authority of the Church that it helped bring on the Reformation, and, indeed, the Renaissance.

Remarkable as the effects of the Black Death were on the economic, social, governmental, and religious structures, another effect was even more astonishing—insanity swept through Europe.

FLAGELLATION Whipping, as a religious activity, had been vigorously practiced by the ancient Egyptians, Romans, and Greeks. Every February 15, at the fertility festivals, the ancient Romans flogged their women. This was supposed to guard them against the inability to have children. In the eleventh century, the Church recognized flogging as a form of penance. During the Black Death of the fourteenth century, it developed into a mass mania.

Woe filled Europe. Everywhere were death and suffering. To punish people for their sins, God had sent the plague. Their only salvation lay in doing penance.

In Hungary first, then in Germany, arose the Brotherhood of the Flagellants. In long lines they wove through the cities of Europe. They were robed as if in mourning. Red crosses marked their breasts, backs, and caps. In their hands they clutched triple whips, each tied in three or four knots. In each knot were fixed points of iron.

On arriving at a chosen place of penance, the flagellants stripped off all their clothes except for a linen dress that extended from the waist to the ankles. They then lay down in a circle. The position assumed varied according to the sin. The adulterer kept his face to the ground. The murderer lay on his back. The perjurer lay on one side holding up three fingers. They were then bitterly criticized by the master. After they had lain on the ground long enough to say five prayers, they rose and were whipped. All the while they sang psalms and prayed loudly for deliverance from the plague.

So powerful did the Brotherhood of the Flagellants become that it threatened the Church. However, the core of the movement had never been wholesome. Soon, crime and degeneracy crept in. Strict action by Pope Clement and the Holy Roman Emperor, Charles IV, fought this gloomy sect. Not only had it helped spread the plague, it also played a part in spreading throughout Europe the

6

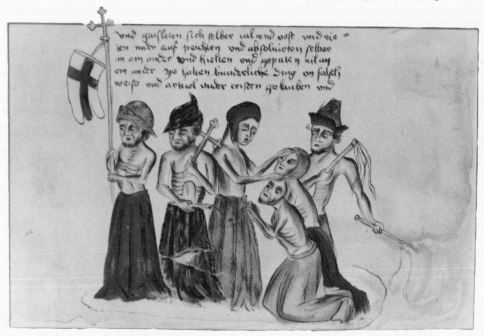

Flagellants in 1349. They often wore a cross on their hats, which earned them and their fellow penitents the name Brothers of the Cross.

plague's vicious partners—suspicion and hatred. To this day there is among some of the Indians of New Mexico a group of flagellants called the Penitentes.

THE DANCING MANIA Dancing and death have long been closely related. In primitive societies dances are often held to celebrate the death of a tribal member. Dancing was part of ancient Roman and Greek funeral rites. In his *Aeneid* Vergil, the ancient Roman poet, depicted the joy of the dance in the land of the dead. The dance of death was a favorite subject of the medieval artist.

During the height of the Black Death, a dancing mania seized parts of Europe. Particularly in Germany, and to the northwest, strange assemblages of people behaved as if possessed. Holding hands at first, they formed circles. Then they would begin to dance. They danced with wild abandon, deliriously. Finally, exhausted, they collapsed. They lay and groaned as if in agony. This was a signal for binding them in tight cloths, particularly around their waists. Apparently this relieved them. It was thought that their discomfort was due to the abdominal swelling resulting from their exertions.

Sometimes the dancing mania (called the Dance of St. John or St. Vitus) began with a convulsion—with the afflicted falling to the ground and foaming at the mouth. Suddenly springing up, they would then begin to contort wildly.

THE PERSECUTION OF THE JEWS Among the most grievous results of the Black Death was the pitiless persecution of the Jews. Since the Jews of the fourteenth and fifteenth centuries contributed many physicians to southern Europe, the maddened public suspected them of bringing about the plague. Jews were "put to the question." If they denied that they were poisoning the population, they were put to the rack. Long and detailed confessions were thus obtained. The tortured admitted, finally, that poisons from spiders and owls, some of which were colored red and black, had been provided by rabbis for the purpose of poisoning the wells. Other poison was smeared on the walls of buildings. Jews were accused of poisoning the very air. Hideous massacres took place. In Basel, Switzerland, all the Jews were enclosed in a wooden building, specially built for that purpose, and burned alive. Elsewhere, the Jews were handed over to the infuriated populace. So it was throughout Europe except in England, from which most of the Jews had already been banished.

ALAS, ALAS FOR HAMELIN! The sad legend of the Pied Piper of Hamelin was again brought to life at the time of the Black Death. The incident of the Pied Piper is thought to have occurred in 1284, a year after a violent plague epidemic. During the Black Death pandemic, over sixty years later, the story was retold again and again. Rats are associated with plague. Some droll piper may, indeed, have appeared at Hamelin long ago and offered to charm the rats away with his music. At the same time he could have taken the children of the town with him. He would come again, it was whispered, and would again steal all the children. Was it not possible that the children would be swept away on the crest of mass hysteria, even as children had joined a Children's Crusade in 1237 and had been lured away by a piper in 1284?

It was a time of mass madness, public whippings, wild dancing. It was a period of debauchery, decay, deprivation, and death. Robert Browning's wistful lines fit too innocently into those terrible times:

All the little boys and girls,
With rosy cheeks and flaxen curls,
And sparkling eyes and teeth like pearls,
Tripping and skipping, ran merrily after
The wonderful music with shouting and
    laughter.[5]

PLAGUE IN THE EARLY MODERN ERA

Let us now leave the Middle Ages and enter into the early modern era. For the plague did just this. Like all communicable disease, it knew boundaries of neither nations nor time.

Plague and the Bard of Avon

O, when mine eyes did see Olivia first,
Methought she purged the air of pestilence!

So wrote William Shakespeare in about 1602 in his play *Twelfth Night*. In the three centuries between the Black Death of the fourteenth century and the Great Plague of London of the seventeenth century, hardly a year went by that the population of some European area was not reduced by this disease. In 1592, strict measures were taken to prevent the spread of plague in London. The law read in part: "That in every howse infected, the Master, Mistris, governour, and the whole familie and residentes therin at the time of such infeccon, shall remayne continuallie without departinge out of the same, and with the doores and windowes . . . shutt."[6]

Upon such regulations Shakespeare plotted some of his play *Romeo and Juliet*. Friar Lawrence tells Juliet:

Take thou this vial, being then in bed,
And this distilled liquor drink thou off.

The drink is to render her seemingly lifeless. Later she is to waken:

In the meantime, against thou shalt awake,
Shall Romeo by my letters know our drift,
And hither shall he come, and he and I
Will watch thy waking, and that very night
Shall Romeo bear thee hence to Mantua.

But the plot goes wrong. Juliet swallows the drink, and the good Friar Lawrence gives a letter to Friar John that is to be delivered to Romeo. But the letter never reaches him because of the plague regulation. The tragedy continues:

FRIAR LAWRENCE. *This same should be the*
voice of Friar John.
Welcome from Mantua. What says Romeo?
Or if his mind be writ, give me his letter.
FRIAR JOHN. *Going to find a barefoot brother*
out,
One of our order, to associate me
Here in this city visiting the sick,

And finding him, the searchers of the town,
Suspecting that we both were in a house
Where the infectious pestilence did reign,
Sealed up the doors and would not let us
forth,
So that my speed to Mantua there was stayed.
FRIAR LAWRENCE. *Who bare my letter, then,*
to Romeo?
FRIAR JOHN. *I could not send it—here it is*
again—
Nor get a messenger to bring it thee,
So fearful were they of infection.[7]

Thus did a plague regulation prevent Romeo from knowing that the unconscious Juliet was still alive. Thinking she was dead, he killed himself.

A fifteenth-century doctor smelling a pomander (a bag of aromatic substances thought to ward off infection) while examining a dying plague patient.

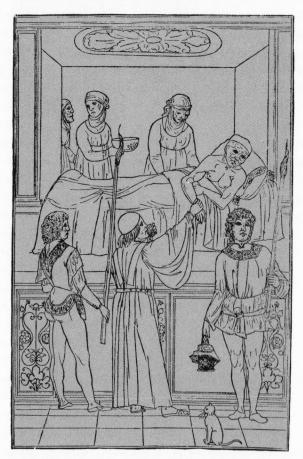

Eyam

The year 1664 had been good to the people of the ancient English village of Eyam. The passing of summer had been celebrated by the annual feast on St. Helen's Day. On that Sunday scores of visitors had been added to the usual population of about 380. There had been dancing in the alehouses. The men had toasted one another. If anyone knew of the plague raging in London, 150 miles away (which was unlikely in so remote a village), it did not dampen the enthusiasm of the celebration. The rural winds of Eyam, sheltered in the hollows of the Derbyshire hills, bore no breath of disease. That August Sunday was the last happy holiday the villagers were to know for a long time.

After the feast day, village life again became routine. It revolved around the church. The Reverend William Mompesson had recently come there, bringing his twenty-eight-year-old wife, Catherine, and their two children. The villagers respected him and liked his family.

On the third of September a box of clothes arrived in Eyam from a London tailor. It was received by a village trader, Edward Cooper. George Vicars, a servant, opened the box. Remarking on the dampness of the tailor's samples, he hung them by the fire to dry.

Three days later Vicars died in a delirium, with plague buboes swelling in his neck and groin. On September 22, Cooper's son was buried. The following day saw the funerals of Mary Thorpe and Sarah Lydall. Then two others died.

October began with two more funerals. That month twenty-two more villagers died. Like a slow stain, first apprehension, then terror spread in the village. "Pest families" were avoided on the street. The plague simmered. In November, only seven died of it. In December, nine. In January 1665, just four died. That month the villagers began to hope, but their hope was short-lived. In February, eight died; in March, six; in April, nine. In May, only three died. It was the best month in a long time and the villagers, desperate for some respite, again knew hope.

By the beginning of June, however, 74 of the 380 villagers of Eyam had died of the plague.

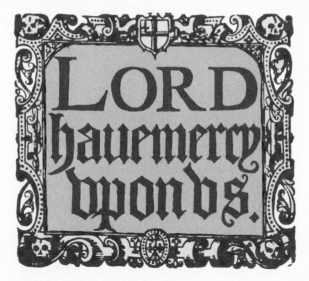

Heading from a 1636 Death Bill, a list of plague victims and health measures.

Mrs. Mompesson implored her husband to send their children to Yorkshire. Reluctantly, he agreed, but he would not leave his people, so she stayed with him.

It was in June that all the villagers began to think of flight. Some of the wealthiest had already left for other villages or the city. A few others had fled to the neighboring hills. Now the entire population wanted to run away.

At this point, the Reverend Mompesson spoke to his dwindling, stricken flock. He told them this: In their hands lay the safety of the surrounding villages. Now they surely carried the disease. Spare the others, he implored them. He promised to seek help, to remain with them.

The villagers decided to stay.

An off-limits boundary, marked by stones and hills, was drawn, encircling all the land within half a mile of the village. Beyond this, nobody from Eyam would venture. North of Eyam was a stream, which today is known as "Mompesson's Well" or "Mompesson's Brook." It was one of several places where articles were deposited for the villagers. From nearby villages people delivered provisions, placing them beside the brook and fleeing. Money for payment was left in the water in the hope of purifying it. On Mompesson's request the Earl of Devonshire also sent provisions.

Burning infected clothes during the fourteenth-century plague.

Toward the end of June, the plague grew worse. Nineteen died. Yet the living stayed on.

July was a month of indescribable suffering. Each family began to bury its own dead or to hire Marshall Howe, someone who had apparently recovered from the disease and now seemed immune. His pay consisted of the possessions of the deceased. For years after the plague, parents of Eyam quieted unruly children by threatening to send for Marshall Howe.

In July, fifty-seven were lost, and still the ordeal was not over. August was a month of utter desolation. Every thought was of death. Seventy-eight perished. One woman dug graves for her husband and six children. On the twenty-second, Catherine Mompesson died. Toward the end of that harrowing summer month, 80 percent of the village had been killed by the plague. And still they stayed.

At last, by September, the plague began to abate. Only twenty-four died that month. With the death of fifteen more in October, the plague was finished with Eyam.

Thirty-three of the original 380 villagers of Eyam were left. One of the survivors was Mompesson, who later would be ostracized by another village because he had walked among so much death.

What did the people of Eyam accomplish? Two things. First, they demonstrated rare strength of character. Second, they demonstrated the terrible price of ignorance about how diseases spread among people. By isolating themselves with their rats and fleas and bacilli, the villagers had condemned themselves. Had they all left Eyam soon after the appearance of the plague, leaving their possessions behind and submitting to isolation until the spread of the illness was no longer so likely, deaths might have been cut by 90 percent. The error was as ancient as the ignorance. Recall that during the plague of Justinian more than a thousand years before, the panic-stricken citizens of Constantinople had piled their dead in buildings and locked the doors and windows, thus guaranteeing the spread of the disease.

Even as the villagers of Eyam doomed themselves, so at the same time was London shutting up infected people in their houses, thereby spreading plague.

The Great Plague of London, 1665

O let it be enough what Thou has done,
When spotted death ran arm'd through every
*   street.*[8]

The "spotted death" about which the seventeenth-century English poet John Dryden was writing was without doubt the plague. The skin of plague victims often becomes spotted because of hemorrhages. Dryden was not the only writer of his time to write about the plague. Of the numerous descriptions of the 1665 Great Plague of London, none is more celebrated or accurate than the *Diary and Correspondence* of Samuel Pepys. Pepys sallied forth into the midst of the Great Plague of 1665, noting everything, truly touched by nothing. As his fellow Londoners suffered and died, he worried about his wig. On September 3, 1665, he notes: "And it is a wonder what will be the fashion after the plague is done, as to periwigs, for nobody will dare buy any hair for fear of infection, that it had been cut off the heads of people dead of the plague."

When Pepys first saw two or three plague houses in Drury Lane "marked with a red cross upon the doors" and a notice, "Lord have mercy upon us," he was so distressed he "was forced to buy some roll-tobacco to smell and to chaw, which took away the apprehension."

But Pepys ends his review of the tragic desolation of the plague year in his diary in a more cheerful frame of mind:

> Thus ends this year, to my great joy in this manner. I have raised my estate. . . . Pray God continue the plague's decrease! For that keeps the court away from the place of business, and so all goes to rack as to public matters, they at a distance not thinking of it.

London during the Great Plague, 1665. Fires were built in the streets; it was thought that the smoke might drive away the plague. More than a century later, such fires were built in the cities of the New World to drive off epidemics.

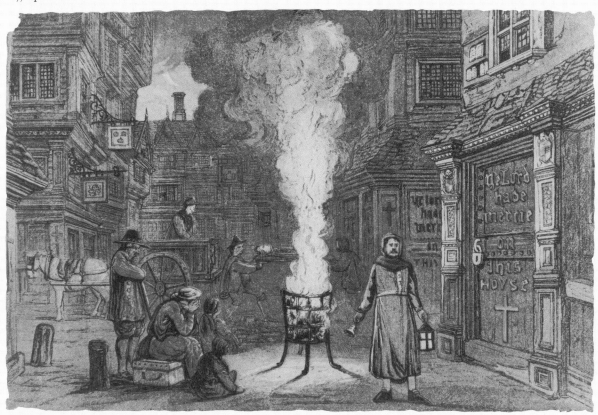

Samuel Pepys may have had a good year in 1665, but few other English people could say the same. In this, "the poor man's plague," over 100,000 Londoners lost their lives. The constant presence of death, always somehow unexpected because it was so quick, sapped the people's moral strength and drained their vitality. Trade, industry, and agriculture suffered. With the decrease in productive enterprise (which might have bolstered a flagging economy), expenditures on welfare and relief increased. Prices rose. Stores, offices, warehouses, and ships were all without workers. Because those with money feared to risk it, investment was at a low ebb. Although, as Pepys amply shows, English life continued, government administrative routines were either halted or greatly slowed. True, the social disorganizations that had accompanied the fourteenth-century plague did not now recur. The moral, political, economic, and religious convulsions of the earlier period were not characteristics of Pepy's time. Yet it is apparent that widespread sickness helped change the age and thus the course of human history.

Nonetheless, the plague was an ill wind that blew some good. From the enormous disorder came a degree of order. Dire need caused people to turn their attention to improving sanitation. Hospitals were constructed. Straw for bedding and floors (in which vermin could breed) fell into disuse. Brick replaced rotting wood for buildings. Because planners could start anew, the Great Fire of London (1666) made possible a better-organized city. Crowding was diminished. As the eighteenth century approached, the plague was gone, and London once more returned to the normal activities of living.

PLAGUE IN MORE RECENT TIMES

Up to this point, the effect of plague on the course of history has been considered in relation to the distant past.

In this century, however, one finds that the plague bacillus still abounds in India, Africa, and South America. And even the United States is still menaced. As late as 1924, the threat became reality. That year, the same plague bacillus, the same flea, the same rat that combined to produce the epidemics that killed people in Justinian's time, demoralized Europe in the fourteenth century and again in the sixteenth century, and depopulated little Eyam, were working together to kill people in Los Angeles, just as they had, around 1900, already killed in Oakland and San Francisco.

The Plague Infects Los Angeles

As certain diseases—smallpox, poliomyelitis, typhoid fever, diphtheria, and yellow fever, for example—disappear in developed countries such as the United States, increasing numbers of young physicians have only a textbook acquaintance with them. This situation is of some concern to health officers, for, despite every precaution, disease can be imported into this country. Every epidemic starts with a first case infecting an inadequately immunized person. That is why only one case of smallpox in this country would make national headlines.

In view of this limiting factor in medical education, one can hardly be critical of the physician who telephoned the communicable disease section of the County of Los Angeles General Hospital on an October day in 1924. He was puzzled and was glad to share his problem with the resident expert in communicable diseases.

On Clara Street, in the Belvedere district of Los Angeles County, he had just examined an extremely sick elderly Mexican-American woman. The patient had a high fever and a severe pain in the back and chest. A young man in the house, as well as other neighborhood people, had similar symptoms. The illness could easily be contagious. Would it not be best to hospitalize the patients and then seek a definite diagnosis? The resident agreed. Ordering an ambulance, he went along to help.

Arriving at the address, the resident found that the patient was feverish. She was coughing and crying. Lying on a couch along the wall was a young man, perhaps thirty, who also seemed to be very sick. Neither patient spoke English. A neighbor acted as interpreter.

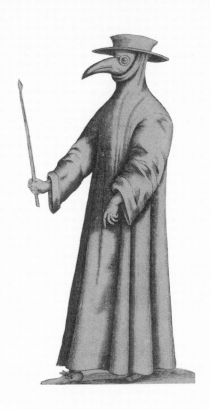

Top: *A physician as a plague fighter in Marseilles, 1720. The beak contained herbs thought to prevent infection. Bottom: Public health nurses as plague fighters in Los Angeles, 1924.*

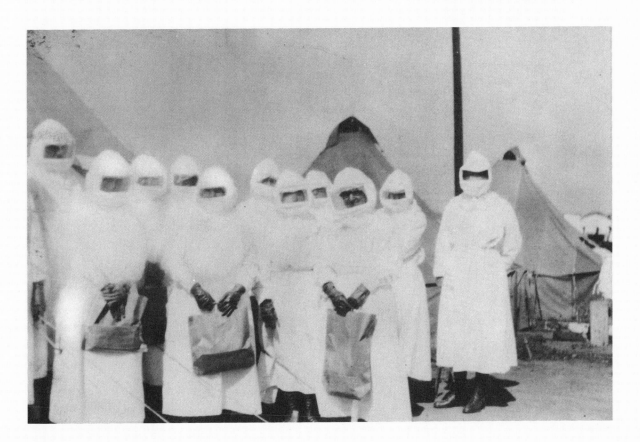

The young man had been sick all day. First he had had a pain in his chest. Within a few hours he had a backache and a fever. Now there were red spots on his chest.

The old woman had been stricken a few days before the man and in about the same manner. For two days she has been coughing. Now she was breathing heavily and coughing up blood.

As the two patients were being placed in the ambulance, the interpreter asked the hospital resident if he would be willing to look at some other people in the neighborhood who were sick in the same way. In another house, the doctor found a man in bed. He had a high fever and complained of a terrible pain in the back and chest. His young wife, in an adjoining bedroom, had similar symptoms. On a settee in the front room sat a young girl. She was holding her head in her hands. Her face was flushed, but she insisted that she was not sick. "I'm just tired," she said. "Awfully tired."

The resident made plans to immediately hospitalize this family as well. Another ambulance would soon come, he told them. He turned to leave. Again the interpreter approached him. He thought the doctor should know that not more than two weeks before the mother and father of the young man who was being taken in the ambulance had died in the hospital. They had been sick the same way as their son was now. Someone had said they had died of pneumonia. Furthermore, the interpreter continued, there were four boys in the neighborhood—relatives of these sick people—who also had this sickness. The doctor went to see the boys, and that night they, too, were brought to the hospital. On the following day six more patients were admitted. Each of the six had severe pneumonia. They spat blood. Their skins turned blue. During the first day of hospitalization three died.

An autopsy was performed on one of the patients who had died. Lung smears showed the presence of the plague bacillus. It was October 31.

On that day a nurse was admitted to the hospital. She had cared for the first patient during his few remaining hours of life in the pneumonia ward. She had plague. The next to be admitted to the hospital was the forty-eight-year-old priest who had administered the last rites to a boy ill with the plague. He was followed by one of the ambulance drivers. Of the three, only the nurse survived.

In rapid succession thirty-three people died of the plague. Of the thirty-one people who had pneumonic plague, twenty-nine died; of the six with bubonic plague, four died.

How was the plague stopped in Los Angeles? Known cases were immediately isolated in the hospital. They were seen only by those who were taking care of them. Seven blocks surrounding the Clara Street address were promptly quarantined. The entire area was roped off. Seventy-five officers were assigned to patrol its boundaries. Until the situation was under control, none of the sixteen hundred persons inside were allowed to leave the area. At one point, some of those quarantined attempted to break through the barriers. Sawed-off shotguns were provided to some of the quarantine guards. The residents stayed. To prevent gatherings of people, the theater and dance hall were closed.

In those days there was no known cure for the plague. It was dangerous work. Only after receiving special instructions, selected health department nurses and inspectors entered the area. Street clothes were not worn. "The nurse has to wear cap, mask, gloves, and gown," ordered a health officer. "Also each nurse will please wear trousers and puttees provided, and high shoes if possible." This last was to protect against contact with rats. Day after day the nurses visited homes where they knew people had been exposed to see if any of them were sick. Those who were ill were promptly hospitalized. For those who were not, other necessary help was brought. Still another precaution was taken. All undertakers were instructed not to embalm the body of any person from the plague-stricken area who had died suddenly of undetermined causes until the body had been examined by a health department physician.

Meanwhile, inside the quarantine zone and in the neighboring areas, health department workers were trying to stop the plague from spreading. A house-to-house canvass was begun. All lumber had to be elevated eighteen inches above the ground. Garbage and rubbish were collected and burned. The whole area was subjected to a general clean-up. Rats were

14

killed by the thousands. Many rats were found to be infested with fleas that were carrying the plague bacillus. A direct attack on the flea was mounted by the use of chemical sprays and lime. Since squirrels also carry plague, three men were constantly occupied in shooting squirrels found within the city limits.

To this day the County of Los Angeles Department of Health Services maintains vector control specialists. It is their job to combat the rat. Such vigilance buys freedom from plague—and from all communicable diseases.

SOME OTHER PESTILENCES

So, naturalists observe, a flea
Hath smaller fleas that on him prey;
And these have smaller still to bite 'em;
And so proceed ad infinitum.[9]

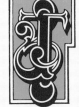his narrative has shown that one disease, plague, played a major role in the drama of human history. Soon after 1665, the disease disappeared from London. During the eighteenth century, it left Europe. It then lashed at this continent. Even today, it lurks in the wildlife of the West. In these pages, the broad review of its havoc has surely pointed to the international character of disease and its capacity to affect the course of human events. The rat that carries plague has found its way to every port. It has exerted as great an influence on history as any politician or general.

But plague is not the only pestilence that has affected human destiny. The United States was hit early by an epidemic of yellow fever. In 1793, Philadelphia, at that time the nation's capital, became literally a ghost town because of the illness. Poor advice on how to control epidemics persisted and traveled long distances. In 1665, during the Great Plague of London, the boys at Eton had been forced to smoke or be whipped. A hundred and twenty-eight years later, cigar smoking was thought by Philadelphians to prevent yellow fever. It was not until the first years of the twentieth century that Walter Reed, an Army physician, determined that the disease was carried by mosquitoes. By developing methods to control mosquito populations, Reed eliminated what was a major obstacle to construction of the Panama Canal. Today, such a defeat of epidemic disease holds great promise for the future of the world's developing nations.

In the nineteenth century, cholera demoralized armies of the Crimean War and the American Civil War. In his 1866 campaign during the Austro-Prussian War, Otto von Bismarck, the Prussian chancellor, lost more men from cholera than from war wounds. The scales of more than one war have been tipped by *typhus*—the disease of armies. Soldiers of the past were particularly prone to become victims of typhus because sanitation was poor, personal hygiene was almost impossible, and crowding was inevitable. The microbe-carrying flea or louse could easily transmit the disease from rat to man. Coming and going, Napoleon's armies in Russia were tormented by typhus. During the 1845 potato famine in Ireland, this disease added to the general misery. But perhaps the most devastating toll of human life that typhus ever took was in Russia following the Revolution of 1917. Disease has always spread with great population movements, and after the revolution, masses of Russians were on the move in search of food. Their sufferings were piteous. In some areas cannibalism was even practiced. From the starving cities

15

streamed the Mechotniki, or "sack carriers." They wandered from place to place hoping to find a crust of bread to put in their sacks. Instead they found typhus, and death. They also spread the disease. From 1917 through 1921, an estimated twenty-five million Russians developed typhus fever. Of these, three million people died.

This insert so far has dealt with the historic consequences of epidemic diseases. But what about individual health problems? Can they, too, affect the course of history?

INDIVIDUAL ILLNESS AND HISTORY

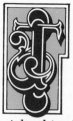

The steward and loyal follower of Joan of Arc testified that Joan never menstruated. Was this indeed true? If so, what relation might this physiological fact (a not infrequent problem in the modern physician's office) have had to her hearing voices telling her that she was to remain a virgin? And does this help account for her chasing away the women who followed the men of her armies, smiting and actually killing one with her sword? (On hearing of Joan's action King Charles is said to have asked, reasonably enough, "Would not a stick have done quite as well?") Did Henry VIII really have syphilis, and did he, indeed, give the disease to his various wives? If so, this could have been the reason that some of them had a tendency to miscarry or to have stillborn babies. Frantically Henry searched for a wife who could provide him with a male heir. When he thought that a wife had failed him, he divorced or executed her and manipulated still another marriage. His desire to divorce his first wife, Catherine of Aragon, led to his quarrel with the Church and to the establishment of the Anglican faith. Had Peter the Great perished of smallpox, in 1685, would his ambitious sister, Sophia, successfully have taken control of Russia? What effect did the emotional disorder of George III, first noted early in 1765 (and today believed to be due to a hereditary disease of body chemistry), have on the restrictive English policies toward the angered American colonies? Had Marat's inflamed skin itched less, would he have been more tolerant, and would the cruelties of the French Revolution have been eased and its bloody course changed? What effect did Robert E. Lee's diarrhea, which disabled him for two critical weeks, have on the Civil War? What would have happened to the national economy if the news had leaked out of Grover Cleveland's two highly secret operations for mouth cancer? Had Woodrow Wilson not been crippled during his last presidential years, what would the era following the First World War have been like? It has been written that his stroke was followed by episodes of paranoia. After also suffering terribly from delusions of persecution, the first U.S. Secretary of Defense, James Forrestal, committed suicide in 1949. Could this event have affected history?

But of all the aches and pains of the powerful, those of Napoleon Bonaparte most often interest footnote historians. History is a sum of events; it has many aspects of varying consequence. And the sickly Napoleon Bonaparte lends partial truth to this concept. Consider the effects of his illnesses on his Russian campaign.

NAPOLEON AT BORODINO

The Battle of Borodino was Napoleon's great opportunity to conquer Russia. Not only had a French Grande Armée been collected for the purpose, but also in the Corsican's ranks were unwilling Germans, Italians, Poles, Austrians, Swiss, and Hollanders. They wheeled through Prussia and Poland, a vast mixture of men and arms. Robbing and killing their way through Kovno, Vilna, Vitepsk, Smolensk, and Viasma, they came to Borodino, fifty miles from Moscow. Napoleon could taste victory. In all of Europe nobody had a greater appetite for it.

At Borodino, on September 5, 1812, the Russian general, Kutuzov, turned to face Bonaparte. Here he would fight it out. He waited for the onslaught. But for two days Napoleon did nothing. Why?

It has been said that Napoleon did not attack either on the fifth or sixth of September because he had a cold. The truth is, he had more than a cold. He suffered from prostate trouble; thus he could not pass urine without great pain. (Some cynics claim that Napoleon's grim expression, as he rode his white steed in Russia, may well have been caused by this factor rather than by concern for his troops.) By the time Napoleon's painful prostate eased, he had developed a sore throat and was so hoarse that he could not dictate his orders. His hand shook as he was forced to write them down.

At Borodino Napoleon failed to destroy the Russian army. Later that army returned to hound him. Some historians lay this failure to his limited ability to make decisions at Borodino. The Russian army escaped to the east. In escaping, it battered the French army with its parting shots and retreated to return at a more opportune time. Always before, Napoleon had based his success on quickly conquering a country and then living off its wealth. Had he not successfully done this in his earlier Italian, German, and Austrian invasions? Had he not taken a ragged French army and, by quick victories, rewarded them with the wealth and women of the conquered?

The Russians provided neither him nor his army with these comforts. When the French Emperor and his army entered Moscow, they found a bleak, bitter, and burning capital. Was the course of history changed because Napoleon could not pass urine? Or because he had a cold?

In his novel *War and Peace*, Tolstoy rejects the notion that Napoleon's illness affected the outcome at Borodino:

> If it had depended on Napoleon's will to fight or not to fight the Battle of Borodino, and if this or that other arrangement depended on his will, then evidently a cold affecting the manifestation of his will might have saved Russia, and consequently the valet who omitted to bring Napoleon his waterproof boots . . . would have been the savior of Russia.[10]

Tolstoy wisely goes on to emphasize the psychological state of the Napoleonic army at Borodino. "The way in which these people killed one another was not decided by Napoleon's will, but occurred independently of him, in accord with the will of hundreds of thousands of people who took part in the common action." Napoleon only thought "that it all took place by his will." True, Napoleon made the major decision in choosing to assail rather than to dislodge the Russian army. However, once that decision was made, the mood of his army was such that he could not have changed his mind under any circumstances. Men who must endure a leader's decisions may not long suffer his indecisions. Even if it were true that discomfort or sickness partly molded his decisions, sickness hardly explains the vast, overwhelming events that had brought the sensitive inflamed prostate of the French dictator to the chilled winds of Borodino.

From the Tsar, who had fled to the east, came no word of surrender. In Moscow, Napoleon awaited evidence of peace overtures. None came. He offered an armistice. It was treated with cold contempt. Moscow was a black ruin. Morale was low, and so were supplies. In the streets, the men bickered among themselves or stood silently, longing for home. A Russian winter was coming. An air of impending disaster hung over them all. There was nothing to do but get out.

On October 19, Napoleon ordered his men to

leave Moscow for home. In all of the long, sad accounts of human conflict, there is no more ghastly story than that grim retreat. Men starved and froze. Napoleon's military genius never encompassed the notion of a medical corps. He failed to understand the importance of sanitation for an army. On the way to Moscow, and in the city too, typhus had plagued Napoleon's soldiers. Now it broke out with increased severity. The loss of life was appalling. And, meanwhile, in a sort of hit and run operation, the intact armies of Tsar Alexander kept hitting him, harassing him. With Napoleon trapped in the cold vastness of Russia, time and space became the enemies of the invaders, the allies of the Russians. Disease, hunger, and cold tortured the remnants of the Napoleonic army. The living robbed the dying. There were endless desertions. Men wandered aimlessly about the countryside. Starving, they gnawed on the bones of horses and the frozen roots of plants.

Some ended up in Polish Vilna. Conditions there were unspeakable. The living stumbled over the dead and dying, who were feebly beseeching help. Gangrene was prevalent. Typhus, and now an epidemic of typhoid, were killing Russian victors and French prisoners alike.

Then the Tsar came to Vilna. To those men of Russian Poland who had sided with the invaders, he granted an amnesty. Every effort was made to relieve the agony. Hospitals were established. The remaining Napoleonic forces were well treated. It will be remembered that men of several countries served under Napoleon in Russia. The rulers of these countries sent money to help relieve the suffering. Only one man sent nothing—Napoleon.

NAPOLEON AT AUTOPSY

"Look, Doctor," said Napoleon to his physician as he came naked out of his room after an alcohol rub. "Look what lovely arms! What smooth white skin, without a single hair! What rounded breasts! Any beauty would be proud of a bosom like mine."

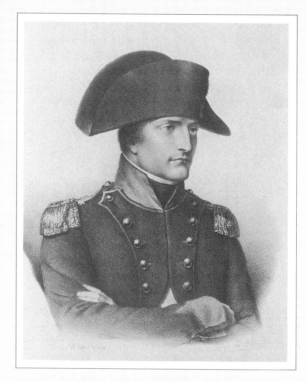

Napoleon in his early thirties, when he was First Consul of France.

Joan of Arc had heard voices inspiring her to save France. Napoleon needed no voices to inspire his belief in himself as the savior of Europe. Until he turned forty, he was remarkably successful. At that age, however, Napoleon underwent a remarkable physical change. When he should have been at his peak, he was a has-been.

As a young man, Napoleon had been thin. His eyes were piercing. He had an eager look. His movements were quick, his manner commanding. Sleep was a waste of precious time.

At forty, he was fat and slow. His eyes were dull, his expression placid. His hair, previously thick, became thin. It was curiously silken. He waddled a trifle. His body developed feminine tendencies. "He has a roundness of figure not of our sex," Count Las Casas once remarked, perhaps nervously. Napoleon began to suffer from an overwhelming need for sleep.

On Saturday, May 5, 1821, Napoleon died. On the following afternoon, at 2 P.M., seven-

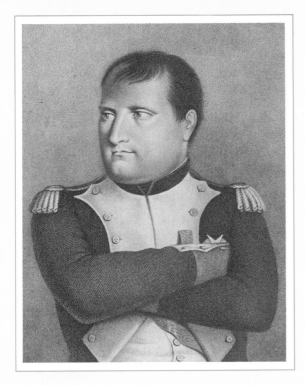

*Napoleon as Emperor, between
the ages of thirty-five and
forty-five.*

the head of George III. Antommarchi heatedly denied this final victory over Napoleon. It might be interesting to have a look.

Scientific shenanigans aside, three separate autopsy reports were made. Part of one, by the English observer Dr. Henry, is most revealing:

> The whole surface of the body was deeply covered with fat . . . the skin was . . . particularly white and delicate as were the hands and arms. Indeed the whole body was slender and effeminate. There was scarcely any hair on the body and that of the head was thin, fine and silky. The pubis much resembled the Mons Veneris in women . . . the shoulders were narrow, the hips wide . . . the penis and testicles were very small, and the whole genital system seemed to exhibit a physical cause for the absence of sexual desire and the chastity which had been stated to have characterized the Deceased.[11]

So did the colossal Corisican conqueror appear in death.

Some think that Napoleon, at about forty, had developed a disease of the hypothalamus, a small area at the base of the brain near the pituitary gland. Among its many functions is the regulation of many activities of the pituitary gland. It is thus intimately involved in growth, sexual activity, and reproduction. If Napoleon did indeed have this rather rare disease, it would surely be fair to wonder about the extent to which it affected world history. It is, however, important to indulge in such speculations only within their proper perspective.

CONCLUDING THOUGHTS

The great medical historian Sigerist has written:

> History is made by individual human beings, to be sure, and whether they are healthy or sick, sane or insane, makes a difference. Yet the place an individual holds, the power with which he is invested, and the use he is permitted to make of his power are determined by a great variety of factors, by social and economic

teen people, English and French, assembled at St. Helena for the autopsy. The dissection was performed by Dr. Antommarchi, Napoleon's personal physician. On removal of the heart and stomach, a wave of sentiment welled up in General Count Bertrand and General Montholon, members of the Emperor's staff at St. Helena. They begged for the heart. The English were not so sentimental. The heart was placed in a silver vessel. As a preservative, some spirits of wine were added. Antommarchi, who had contributed little to Napoleon's health in life, requested the cancerous stomach. By it he could prove that nobody could have successfully treated the Emperor. The stomach, however, was deposited in another vessel. Both vessels were left in the sealed coffin. In later years, there was to be some disagreement between Dr. Antommarchi and an English doctor, Rutledge, as to who sealed the vessels and, indeed, how. Rutledge claimed to have sealed the vessel containing the heart with a shilling bearing

conditions first of all, but also by hopes and fears, ambitions and frustrations and other psychological factors ... disease of an individual and even a deadly disease does not alter the course of history. A cause may collapse when the leader dies but not because of his collapse. It collapses only when the forces that carried the leader have lost their momentum. Otherwise, his death may activate the cause, as history has demonstrated more than once.[12]

Tolstoy and Sigerist agree on the relatively limited effect on history of individual sickness. Concerning past events this is reasonable. But it need not apply to the future. Neither Tolstoy nor Sigerist refers to tomorrow's risks. What can the illness of past leaders teach those who govern in this atomic age?

Leadership is an exhausting ordeal. A Washington correspondent once wrote about President Lyndon Johnson's administration:

It would be hard to overestimate the physical and nervous tension on the men at the top of this government.

They are on the go 18 hours a day, and in the President's case, often longer: endless conferences, constant testimony on Capitol Hill, a succession of tedious ceremonial dinners, pressure for more bombing, pressure for less bombing—all this, and a constant drumfire of criticism at home and abroad. The Johnson system here is based on the assumption that men can do whatever they have to do. ... It is a dubious assumption.[13]

Leaders need help and health. It is not only their responsibility but also the obligation of those they lead to make certain that they have both.

20

EPILOGUE

*There is no national science,
just as there is no national
multiplication table;
what is national is no longer science.* [14]

Malaria, smallpox, influenza, typhoid fever—these and other enemies of people have both killed them and taught them. But have they taught them enough?

> The surest safeguard against the spread of communicable disease, whether it be smallpox or Asian influenza, is control of the disease in the country of origin. In the absence of such internal control, a next safeguard is a worldwide communicable disease intelligence program geared to early detection of epidemics—and the attendant possibility of international transmissibility. [15]

This basic statement calls for a degree of international understanding more often seen in health than in other aspects of world politics. Constant vigilance is essential. Nonetheless, one cannot deny the virtual disappearance of malaria, smallpox, plague, yellow fever, cholera, and typhus from vast, formerly devastated areas. And the picture will improve. In many areas of the Western world, regular measles and poliomyelitis are disappearing. The realization by developing societies that sickness grievously impedes their development—the sure knowledge that a community riddled by malaria, for example, cannot take its place in the modern world—is a local stimulus for improvement. To those whose societies already benefit from disease control, helping to create such a stimulus in other countries is an opportunity. Those who seek a better world, who want to build bridges, not walls, between nations, must understand the absolute necessity of controlling disease. This is the fundamental proposition of this insert—a proposition whose meaning has been made abundantly clear by history.

The United States government, through the Agency for International Development, the Peace Corps, the International Health Division of the Public Health Service, the World Health Organization (WHO), and the armed services, is combining with such voluntary agencies as the Ford and Rockefeller Foundations to make an enormous health contribution to the world's developing areas. Whether it be through a technical health expert in Sierra Leone, a WHO worker in Asia, a child-health project of the Ford Foundation, or a Peace Corps worker in northern Brazil, the contribution is real and important. Moreover, the World Health Organization is promoting medical research on an international level. Such an effort promises even more than new knowledge about such health puzzles as cancer. From such international undertakings there develops a dialogue between nations that surely promotes understanding and peace between war-weary peoples. Is it too much to hope that the health worker will yet show the way to the greatest health of all—peace?

Disease knows no boundaries; this is a harsh historical experience. Even in wartime, countries have cooperated in health matters. In 1800, when France

21

and England were at war, Edward Jenner's vaccination against smallpox was being tested in England. French doctors wanted to learn about it, so special arrangements were made by the French foreign minister, Talleyrand. An English physician came to France, was treated with great regard, and vaccinated French children with English vaccine. For years, scientists have been seeking the causes of human cancers. Scientists from the United States and the Soviet Union are exchanging information for cooperative study, and they also plan to exchange personnel. On May 23, 1972, during a visit to Russia, President Richard Nixon signed a joint agreement of cooperation in the fields of medicine and public health. Projects under this agreement have begun in the areas of cancer, cardiovascular disease, environmental health, and arthritis. In September 1973, immediate exchanges of vital scientific information between scientists of the two countries were made possible by a special teletype. It was the first direct communication link between the United States and the Soviet Union since the White House–Kremlin "hot line." Is there better proof of hope for humanity?

Some time ago, a group of sixty eastern U.S. college students were asked to list the six largest (in population) cities of America. Only five included Mexico City. It is a long road from such parochialism to a sympathetic knowledge of the customs of other societies, but this kind of knowledge is being acquired. Effective international health workers no longer try to impose their own culture on others. These workers understand that other cultures have developed other ways to handle problems than those to which they are accustomed.

To assist those of the less developed world in improving their health, one must first learn to appreciate their social structures. This is one of the wise principles on which the Peace Corps is based. But there is a paradox in this. One may rightly ask: Is my world truly better? Is it really preferable to theirs? Do we not lose by heart attacks what we save by penicillin? Whose disease, whose destiny is better? Is it not best to leave them alone?

However, no longer can anyone depend on being left alone. One can only work so that each culture will gain, and not suffer, from the others. For although the scientist can distinguish innumerable ecosystems, the world is one all-inclusive ecosystem that is shared by all people.

Failing to learn this, people fail to learn anything.

REFERENCES

1. William Shakespeare, *Timon of Athens*, act 4, scene 3, lines 51–52.

2. Procopius of Caesara, *History of the Wars*, Book II, *The Persian War*, Vols. XXIII and XXIV, tr. by H.E. Dewing (New York, 1914), p. 451.

3. Friar John Clyn of the Convent of Friars Minor at Kilkenny, and Thady Dowling, Chancellor of Leighlin, edited from the manuscripts by R. Butler (Dublin, 1849), quoted in Charles Creighton, *A History of Epidemics in Britain*, Vol. 1, 2nd ed. (New York, 1965), p. 115.

4. James Westfall Thompson, "The Aftermath of the Black Death and the Aftermath of the Great War," *American Journal of Sociology*, Vol. 26 (January 1921), p. 569.

5. Robert Browning, "The Pied Piper of Hamelin," in Burton Egbert Stevenson, ed., *The Book of Verse* (New York, 1922), p. 198.

6. R.R. Simpson, *Shakespeare and Medicine* (Baltimore, 1959), p. 208.

7. William Shakespeare, *Romeo and Juliet*, act 5, scene 2, lines 2–16.

8. John Dryden, *Annus Mirabilis*, verse 267, line 1065.

9. Jonathan Swift, "On Poetry, A Rhapsody."

10. From Leo Tolstoy, *War and Peace*, in John Courno's, *A Treasury of Classic Russian Literature* (New York, 1961), p. 375.

11. James Kemble, *Napoleon Immortal: The Medical History and Private Life of Napoleon Bonaparte* (London, 1959), p. 282.

12. Henry E. Sigerist, *Civilization and Disease* (New York, 1944), pp. 127–128.

13. James Reston, "A Tired, Tense Administration," quoted in Robert E. Kantor and William G. Herron, "Paranoia and High Office," *Mental Hygiene*, Vol. 52 (October 1968), pp. 507–511.

14. From S.S. Koteliansky and Leonard Woolf, trs., *The Personal Papers of Anton Chekhov* (New York, 1948), p. 29.

15. Lenor S. Goerke, "Preface: Graduate Training for Responsibilities in International Health," in Lenor S. Goerke, ed., *Proceedings of the Los Angeles World Health Conference* (Los Angeles, 1962), pp. 2–3.

Hans Holbein the Younger (1497–1543) did forty-one woodcuts of "The Dance of Death" (1538). Reproduced on the next page are "The King," "The Doctor," "The Cardinal," and "The Husbandman."

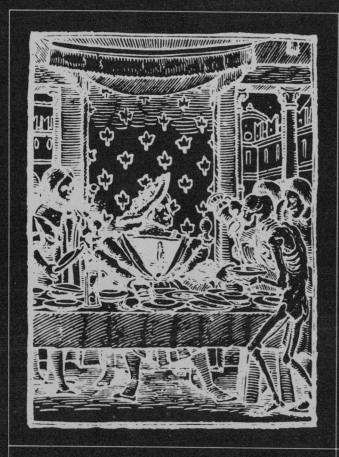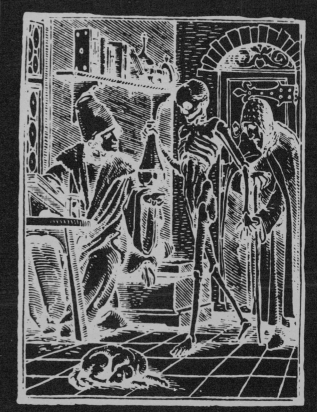

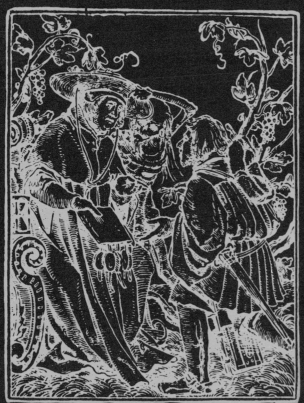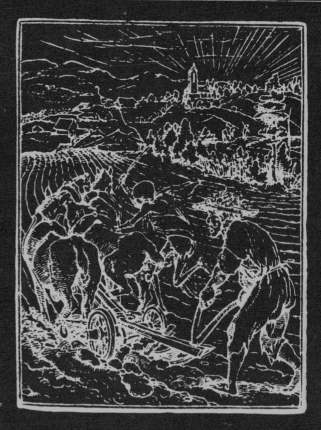

A child born of a woman with active genital herpes may get the disease while passing through the vagina. For the child this is often a calamity. So when the pregnant woman is known to have the disease, she must be delivered by way of the abdomen (**Caesarean section**). While passing through the vagina of a mother infected with gonorrhea, a child is liable to contract gonorrheal infection of the eyes. Therefore, silver nitrate drops are put in the eyes of all newborns to prevent possible blindness.

About Oral-Genital Spread of Sexually Transmitted Diseases

The oral (mouth) area is much more resistant to gonorrheal infection than to syphilitic infection. However, syphilitic infection of the mouth is more likely with "French" or "soul" kissing. This is particularly true if there is a break in the mucous membrane of the mouth. Mouth contact with infectious genital syphilitic sores is a common way of getting the disease. The primary penile chancre of syphilis teems with syphilis microorganisms as do the secondary-stage mucous patches in the mouth.

Gonococcal infection of the mucous membrane of the mouth and the tongue are occasionally seen, and a gonococcal throat inflammation (*pharyngitis*) is now quite ordinary. Gonococcal pharyngitis happens infrequently from mouth kissing or from contact between the mouth and the external female genitalia. It usually follows penile-oral contact. The gonococci that enter the body by the mouth can live best in the tonsillar area. That is because they thrive in the lymphoid tissue found in that area, even in people who have had their tonsils removed.

The person with gonococcal pharyngitis develops a sore throat a day or two after oral exposure. There may be some redness and swelling of the tonsillar area and some fever. Lymph nodes in the neck may be enlarged. Because these signs and symptoms are common with infections other than gonorrhea of the throat, there is a dangerous lack of treatment for gonorrhea. But people with gonococcal pharyngitis often develop gonorrheal signs and symptoms in other areas of the body, such as the rectum, urethra, or cervix. The gonococcal pharyngitis may be part of a picture in which there follows an invasion of the bloodstream by the gonococci, resulting in gonorrhea of the skin and the joints.

Sexually transmitted diseases can be very serious, despite one teenagers's remark that, "Aw, nowadays they're not any worse than a cold."

On Helping to Find Those Who Need Help

People who have a sexually transmitted disease almost always got it from someone. And frequently they give it to others. Infected individuals must be immediately and thoroughly treated. Follow-up visits to the doctor should not be missed.

A Brief History of Syphilis

Syphilis gives still more evidence that microbes know no borders. Two years after Columbus discovered America, Charles VIII of France (1470–1498) invaded Italy and laid siege to Naples. At that time the port city was being defended by Spaniards. Like all armies of that era, the Spanish army was accompanied by a host of harlots. Many of these women, it was thought, had been infected by sailors formerly with Columbus. If the account of the sixteenth-century anatomist Fallopius is to be believed (and it is not by everyone), the Spanish deliberately sent their debauched women to meet the French army. This unmilitary maneuver succeeded. The soldiers of the French army lost no time in meeting the harlots, from whom they caught syphilis.* Too diseased to fight, the French army retreated. In dispersing, they spread their disease throughout Europe. The Italians and Spanish called the affliction the "French disease." To the French, it was, at first, the "Neapolitan disease" and then the "Spanish sickness." The Germans named the malady the "Polish pocks." The Poles retaliated with "German pox." Bitterly remembering the Crusades, the unforgiving Turks called it the "disease of the Christians." To others, it could only be the "Persian fire." Finally, in 1530, an Italian medical man and poet, Girolamo Fracastorius, wrote of a shepherd, Syphilus, who aroused the ire of the sun god by worshiping at an altar of his king. In jealous anger, the sun god sent a plague to earth. Syphilus was its first victim. The disease was thus named, if not claimed.

*Gabriel Fallopius, *On Gallic Disease*, quoted in Herbert Silvette, *The Doctor on the Stage* (Knoxville, Tenn., 1967), p. 196.

In addition, public protection demands a thorough investigation of the source and spread of every new case. Without active contact tracing, the number of people who are venereally infected in a community grows, and thus there is a spreading sea of chronic sickness.

The venereally infected man or woman who refuses to name contacts is refusing information held, by both law and practice, to be an absolute confidence. Such people are doing no one a favor. They are personally irresponsible because they will not spare others sickness and pain. Moreover, that person may get a venereal disease again from contact with the very person who gave the illness to him or her in the first place. One recent study investigated sixty-nine venereal disease outbreaks eventually involving almost ten thousand people in twenty-eight states. "One man infected with syphilis initiated the ultimate exposure of 274 other persons resulting in 42 additional cases of infectious syphilis within a relatively short period."[2]

It pays to investigate. And to cooperate.

Summary

There are many types of *parasites* that can cause disease in human beings: *helminths, ectoparasites, fungi, protozoa, bacteria, mycoplasma, chlamydia, rickettsia,* and the *viruses.* These organisms may travel from one person to another directly, perhaps by contact with an open sore, or indirectly, as when carried by an insect.

The human *host* will resist the invasion of a parasite. *General resistance*, not directed against any particular organisms, is provided by unbroken skin, *granulocytes*, and *macrophages. Specific resistance* comes from the plasma cells, which, in response to *antigens* on the surface of the specific invaders, make *immunoglobulin antibodies.* These antibodies can neutralize the power of the foreign organisms to cause illness. There are also other body proteins—*complement* and *properdin*—that further reinforce the body's resistance.

The plasma cells that make antibodies originate as lymphocytes. Two types of lymphocytes exist: *B lymphocytes*, which become the plasma cells, and *T lymphocytes*, which unite with infected body cells to fight the invaders within those cells.

The body's immune system sometimes makes mistakes. It may overreact to a foreign substance, or *allergen*, such as dust or pollen, that enters the body and causes mast cells to release chemicals that produce the symptoms of *allergy*—*hives*, runny nose, or even *asthma*. According to one theory, the tissue destruction of *rheumatoid arthritis* results from the body's reaction to certain of its own antibodies, the *rheumatoid factors*.

Active immunity occurs when the body makes antibodies to fight the foreign invaders. This type of immunity is generally gained by being infected with the organism by chance. However, *active immunity* can be achieved through vaccination with an *attenuated*, or killed, organism that no longer has the ability to cause disease but that can stimulate the body to make antibodies against it. Although some *vaccines* have been very effective, there has been less success with influenza vaccines because the antigenic structure of the viruses is constantly changing. And the vaccine for tuberculosis, while effective, is not widely used in this country because it causes a positive Mantoux test, thus making it impossible to distinguish between those who have active tuberculosis and those who have received the vaccine.

Toxins produced by bacteria can also cause sickness. The body can gain active immunity against these toxins by immunization with *toxoid*, which is a toxin treated to destroy its poisonous properties.

Passive immunity is a temporary immunity gained from borrowed antibodies. Thus someone ill from, say, tetanus toxin or *rubeola* virus may be injected with antibodies made by another person. Babies receive some passive immunity against many diseases from their mothers before birth. This immunity protects the child against some diseases during the early months of life.

Viruses must invade living cells in order to multiply. Either the entire virus or its central core of genetic material will enter the cell and take over its normal mechanisms. However, the virus may have other effects on the cell. It may slow down (the reverse cancer effect) or speed up (the cancer effect) the cell's growth, or it may remain latent in the cell, until it is activated at some future time.

What we know as the "cold" is a collection of symptoms caused by a viral infection that, if more severe, could cause a disease such as poliomyelitis. Since so many microorganisms can cause a cold, it has been impossible to create a vaccine against it.

Virus infections can have a very adverse effect on an unborn child. If the mother contracts rubella or certain other viral diseases while pregnant, her child may be born with abnormalities.

Sickness, and occasionally death, can result from bacterial contamination of food. Salmonellosis and staphylococcal food poisoning are common food contamination illnesses.

Sexually transmitted diseases are a great problem for three major reasons: The source of infection and that person's contacts are hard to trace, diagnosis in women is difficult, and the early signs and symptoms of the diseases are often mild or disappear quickly. Gonorrhea, syphilis, genital herpes, and nongonococcal urethritis are the most common venereal diseases in the United States.

References

1. Herbert A. Blough and Robert L. Giuntoli, "Successful Treatment of Human Genital Herpes Infections with 2-Deoxy-D-glucose," *Journal of the American Medical Association*, Vol. 241 (June 29, 1979), pp. 2798–2801.
2. The Association of State and Territorial Health Officers, the American Public Health Association, the American Venereal Disease Association, and the American Social Health Association: A Joint Statement, *Today's VD Control Problems*, cited in Walter H. Smartt, "Venereal Disease," in Lenor S. Goerke et al., *Mustard's Introduction to Public Health*, 5th ed. (New York, 1968), p. 290.

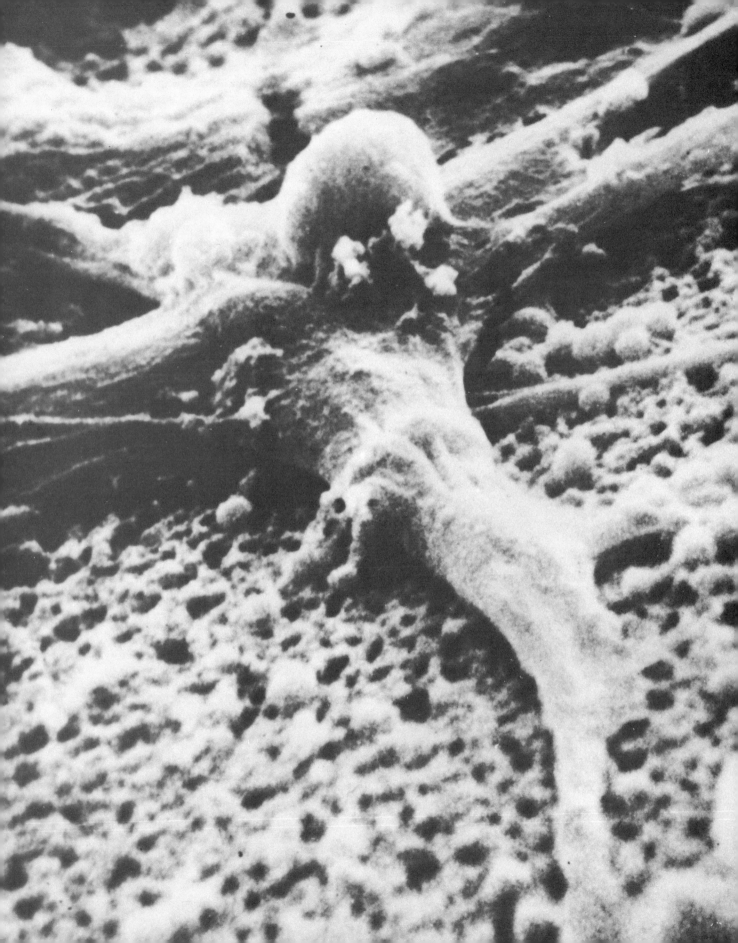

4

The Chronic Degenerative Diseases

Chronic Disease: The Price of Success?

At the turn of this century, infectious diseases were the primary health menace to this nation. Acute respiratory conditions, such as pneumonia and influenza, were the major killers. Tuberculosis, too, drained the nation's vitality. Diseases that caused diarrhea killed thousands of children. But since then a great era of public health advancement has helped change all this. Water and milk supplies have been made safe. Engineers have built systems to handle and treat infected human wastes. Food sanitation and personal hygiene have become more a way of life. True, new environmental dangers have replaced the old, but people survive to suffer them. Moreover, the constant labors of public health workers have lowered the death rates of mothers and their infants. Great numbers of children have been vaccinated against dangerous communicable diseases. Tuberculosis has been increasingly brought under control. In 1900, the average person in the United States lived barely fifty years. Today, more than twenty years have been added to this average life expectancy.

But each generation is saddled on the last. Yesterday's success often brings tomorrow's challenge. A longer life span—a mark of progress—has brought another group of basic health problems, the **chronic degenerative diseases**: "chronic" because they linger; "degenerative" because they can cause progressive destruction of tissues. As a group

---

TABLE 4–1

The Five Leading Causes of Death in the United States in 1900 and 1978 for All Ages and in 1978 for the Age Group 15–24

1900 ALL AGES	1978 ALL AGES	1978 15–24 YEARS
1. Pneumonia and influenza	1. Diseases of the heart	1. Accidents
2. Tuberculosis	2. Cancers	2. Suicide
3. Diarrhea, enteritis, and ulceration of the intestines	3. Cerebrovascular disease	3. Homicide
4. Diseases of the heart	4. Accidents	4. Cancers
5. Intracranial lesions of vascular regions	5. Influenza and pneumonia	5. Diseases of the heart

SOURCE: Data for 1900 is from an unpublished report of the National Center for Health Statistics. Data for 1978 is projected from the National Center for Health Statistics, "Final Mortality Statistics for 1977," *Monthly Vital Statistics Report*, pp. 3 and 21.

The photograph on page 86 is a cancer cell (magnified more than 3,500 times). It spreads like the roots of a tree and can invade normal tissue.

they share certain characteristics: Their causes are frequently unclear; often, they are a long time developing; usually they reduce the body's level of functioning for a long time; and, finally, their treatments are costly, because they are long term.

Chronic diseases have replaced infectious diseases as the nation's major health problem. At the turn of this century, one in seven deaths was due to heart disease or stroke. Today, in this nation, these two diseases join cancer as the three leading causes of death (see Table 4–1). And they are not limited to people who are middle-aged or elderly. Chronic illness is also a major concern of youth, among whom, as will be seen, the destructive process of a chronic disease often begins. Thus, *prevention* of chronic disease is especially important to the young.

This chapter will discuss the three major chronic diseases in the United States. First we describe the structure and functions of the circulatory system. Some of its problems, such as atherosclerosis, cardiovascular disease, coronary artery disease, and heart disease will follow. We then consider the functions and dysfunctions of the kidneys, as well as high blood pressure (hypertension), cerebrovascular disease and, finally, cancer.

The Body's Circulatory System

Two hundred years ago an autopsy was being carried out by the English physician Edward Jenner. Jenner's friend Caleb Parry recorded his words:

I was making a . . . section of the heart . . . when my knife struck something so hard and gritty, as to notch it. I well remember looking up to the ceiling which was old and crumbling, conceiving that some plaster had fallen down. But on a further scrutiny the real cause appeared; the coronaries [the blood vessels supplying the heart] were become bony canals.[1]

The man whose body Jenner examined had died of **atherosclerosis**—a build-up of fatty materials that includes bits of cells and calcium in the inner walls of the arteries.* As the atherosclerosis worsens, the calcium deposits increase. The calcium is the "hard and gritty" something that notched Jenner's surgical knife. It had made "bony canals" of once-elastic arteries.

Today, two centuries later, atherosclerosis still kills more people in this country than any other condition. To understand atherosclerosis, and other problems interfering with the circulation of the blood, one must first understand the structure of the **cardiovascular system** (heart and blood vessels) and its functions.

A sixteenth-century Persian drawing of the body's system of arteries.

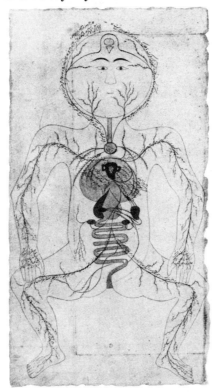

The Cardiovascular System

By means of the circulation of blood within the cardiovascular system, (1) oxygen, nutrients, hormones, and other life-giving chemicals are delivered to the cells of the body, and (2) wastes (carbon dioxide and other products) are transported from these cells to be gotten rid of at such points of elimination as the lungs, kidneys, or liver. In addition, as was seen in Chapter 3, part of the circulating blood is involved in (3) fighting infection. The circulatory system also helps (4) regulate body temperature. As the blood vessels are dilated (widened), body heat is lost; when they are narrowed, heat is kept within the body.

Consider now the blood in the vessels, then the vessels themselves, and, finally, the central organ of the cardiovascular system, the heart.

Arteriosclerosis is a general term. It refers to a condition in which the arteries thicken, harden, and become inelastic. *Athero*sclerosis is one kind of arteriosclerosis.

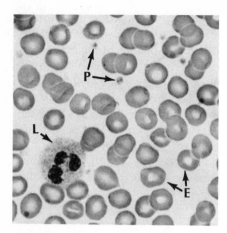

FIGURE 4–1
Human blood cells: red cells, or erythrocytes (E); white cells, or leukocytes (L); and platelets (P).

THE BLOOD: FLUID TISSUE OF TRANSPORT

The eight to nine liquid pints of blood in the body of the average human being teem with floating suspended cells. This liquid is called **plasma**. The cells suspended in the blood plasma (Figure 4–1) are as follows:

1. **Erythrocytes.** In the blood of the average adult male are some twenty-five trillion (one trillion is a million million) erythrocytes, or **red blood cells**. The average adult female's blood contains about seventeen trillion red cells. These equal 99.9 percent of the total blood cells. The average red blood cell circulates for about 120 days before it breaks apart and is replaced. During its short life it will have traveled about two hundred miles. Some 250 billion red blood cells are manufactured in the bone marrow every day.

   A complex protein called **hemoglobin** is formed in the red blood cells. The iron contained in hemoglobin gives it the ability to combine with and release both oxygen and carbon dioxide. A diet lacking iron leads to an abnormal reduction in both red blood cells and hemoglobin and results in a condition called **anemia**. Normally, there is a balance between the number of red blood cells produced and the number lost. Health depends upon this ecological balance in the blood's ecosystem. **Hemorrhage**, the loss of large quantities of blood, is one cause of anemia. This may be gradual or sudden. *A reduced production of red blood cells* due to a vita-

min B_{12} deficiency can result in *pernicious anemia*. Among the many other causes of anemia may be chemical poisons, excessive ionizing radiation, and such diseases as tuberculosis, malaria, and sickle cell anemia (page 429).

2. **Leukocytes.** Since leukocytes contain no hemoglobin to color them, they are often called **white blood cells**. Unlike red blood cells they are able to move on their own. About seventy-five billion leukocytes defend the body against various invaders, such as bacteria that cause infection. With most bacterial infections, leukocytes increase in number. This increase is called **leukocytosis**. When this happens, leukocytes attack and gobble up bacteria by a process called **phagocytosis** (see page 57). As we saw in Chapter 3, certain leukocytes, such as **lymphocytes,** are important to the immune system—the body's system of resistance to infection.

   With cancer of leukocyte-producing tissue, or *leukemia* (see page 111), white cells are overproduced. Moreover, they are usually abnormal cell types. Unlike normal leukocytes, they fight infection poorly. The enormous overproduction of leukocytes interferes with erythrocyte manufacture. Anemia results. The invading white blood cells of leukemia also overwhelm other tissues, interfering with their normal functions.

3. **Platelets.** This third type of blood cell is produced in the bone marrow. By their involvement in clotting, they help to stop bleeding. Also important to clotting are proteins called *fibrinogen* and *fibrin* (see Figure

4–2). Plasma from which fibrinogen has been separated by the process of clotting is called *serum*. Serum, then, cannot clot.

BLOOD GROUPS

Before the turn of this century, transfusion was often followed by severe reactions and even death. It was discovered that this occurred because a donor's blood was often incompatible with that of the person receiving it (the recipient). This meant that the recipient was immune to certain proteins in the donor's blood cells. As a result, the antibodies in the recipient's serum caused clumping and disintegration of the donor's red blood cells. Thus, incompatibility depends on the absence or the presence of antigens in the red blood cells and of antibodies in the serum. A person's red blood cells could contain A or B antigens, both, or neither. His serum could contain anti-A or anti-B antibodies, both, or neither. When a donor's blood, containing one or more antigens, is transfused into a recipient's blood containing incompatible antibodies, the clumping of the recipient's red blood cells that occurs is called *agglutination*. The antigens are called *agglutinogens* and the antibodies, *agglutinins*. Four main blood groups are differentiated (see Table 4–2).

A *universal donor* is a person with group O blood. Since group O red blood cells contain no A or B antigen, group O blood can usually be used for anyone.

It is sometimes used in great emergencies when blood-typing of a recipient would be too time-consuming. People with group AB blood are *universal recipients*. Since their blood contains no anti-A or anti-B antibodies, they can usually

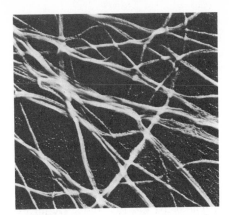

FIGURE 4–2
Fibrin strands (× 45,000).

receive any blood with relative safety.

In the United States, the frequency of group O among Caucasians is 42.2 percent; A is 39.2 percent; and B and AB are 13.5 and 5.1 percent, respectively. All the world's people have these groups among them but in different amounts. South American Indians are all group O. The Australian aborigines are half group A and half group O. So are the Eskimos. The Japanese, unlike the Caucasians, are about 11 percent group AB. All people everywhere have some O blood groups. Heredity governs the distribution of the ABO system of blood groups. The same is true of the Rh (or *Rh*esus) blood group system. (Rh is discussed on pages 431–432.) There are many other

blood group systems, but the ABO and Rh are the most significant to present medical procedures.

THE BLOOD VESSELS

Blood is carried *away from the heart to the tissues* by **arteries;** it is returned *from the tissues back to the heart* by **veins.**

Between the arterial and venous circulations are microscopic canals called **capillaries.** Some of them are so narrow that red blood cells can only pass through in single file. Between the cell walls of the capillaries are microscopic spaces. These tiny exits and entrances make it easier for delivery of the chemical needs to body cells and for the collection of wastes from the cells. These tiny spaces are the only break in the closed system of blood vessels. Fluids from the blood seep out through these breaks and make a drainage system necessary (see pages 94–96). So numerous are the capillaries that, in volume, they make up most of the cardiovascular system. The total length of the body's capillaries has been estimated to be about sixty thousand miles.

The smallest *endings* of the arteries, the **arterioles,** feed into the capillaries. The smallest *beginnings* of the veins, the **venules,** begin from capillaries (see Figure 4–3).

TABLE 4–2 The Basic ABO Blood Groups		
BLOOD GROUP	ANTIGENS (AGGLUTINOGENS) IN THE RED CELLS	ANTIBODIES (AGGLUTININS) IN THE SERUM
O	None	anti-A and anti-B
A	A	anti-B
B	B	anti-A
AB	A and B	None

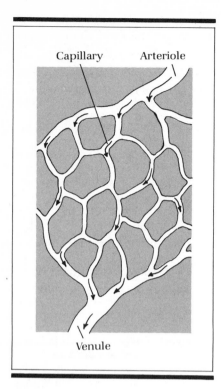

FIGURE 4–3
The relationship of arterioles, capillaries, and venules.

THE HEART AS A DOUBLE PUMP

The adult heart is fist-sized. It is mostly made up of a special muscle called the **myocardium** (from *myo*, meaning "muscle," and *cardium*, meaning "heart"). Located beneath the breastbone, the heart is in the left center of the chest. Enveloping it is a loose **pericardial sac** containing lubricating (*pericardial*) fluid.

The heart has two sides. (Refer to Figure 4–4.) They are separated by a wall, or **septum**, in which there is normally no opening. Each side has an upper chamber that receives blood, called the **atrium**. Below each receiving atrium is another chamber, the blood-pumping **ventricle**. Although each upper, receiving atrium is basically a temporary storage chamber, its walls must, and do, contract.

Each atrium is separated from the pumping ventricle below it by a one-way valve. To permit blood to flow from the receiving atrium above to the pumping ventricle below, the valve opens. To prevent blood from flowing backward, the valve closes. So, in the normal heart, one-way valves keep the blood flowing in only one direction.

Tissue cells are surrounded by wetness, and the wetness is within them too. It is through this wetness, at the cell-capillary level, that a basic chemical exchange takes place. The blood delivers oxygen, nutrients, and other needed body chemicals *to* the body cells, and it collects carbon dioxide and other wastes *from* the cells. Then, from capillaries to venules and through increasingly larger veins, the blood travels to the heart's *right atrium*. This blood that is returning to the heart is dark red because it is loaded with carbon dioxide waste. After this dark red blood fills the heart's

right atrium, the valve between the right atrium and the *right ventricle* below opens. The right atrium contracts. Blood flows from the right atrium into the right ventricle, which is the heart's first pump. The muscle of the right ventricle then contracts. Blood is pumped out of the right ventricle to the lungs through a large blood vessel. In the lungs the dark red blood rids itself of the poisonous waste carbon dioxide. It then loses its dark red color. Once the blood refreshes itself with oxygen, it becomes bright red. This bright red blood then returns from the lungs to the *left atrium* via large vessels. The left atrium fills. Then the valve between the left atrium and the left ventricle opens. The left atrium contracts, and blood pours into the *left ventricle*, which is the heart's second pump. The walls of this pumping left ventricle are the thickest of the heart. They need to be. When the walls of the left ventricle contract, they must pump freshly oxygenated blood into the great blood vessel the **aorta**. This is the beginning of a long journey. Blood containing oxygen, nutrients, and other chemicals must be carried to all of the body's cells.

THE HEART AS AN ELECTRICAL MECHANISM

The labor of the human heart is wondrous. In a seventy-year lifetime, it will beat about 2.5 billion times and pump some 600,000 tons of blood. What keeps the heart beating rhythmically? Specialized cells in the heart known as the **conducting system** are responsible for rhythmical heartbeats. Within the wall of the right atrium is the first group of such cells, called the **pacemaker**. It is also called the **sinoatrial (SA) node.** The SA node contains nerve and muscle cells and

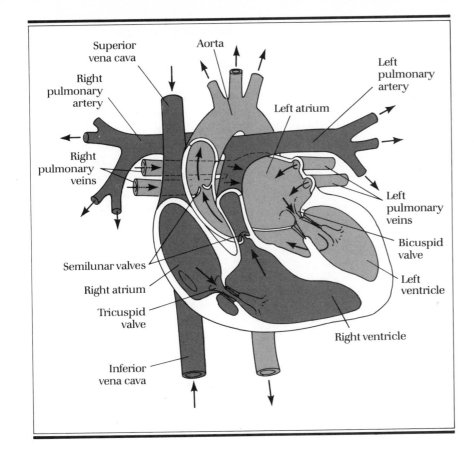

Labels on figure:
Superior vena cava
Aorta
Left pulmonary artery
Right pulmonary artery
Left atrium
Right pulmonary veins
Left pulmonary veins
Bicuspid valve
Semilunar valves
Left ventricle
Right atrium
Tricuspid valve
Right ventricle
Inferior vena cava

FIGURE 4-4
General anatomy of the heart. Blood flows from the left ventricle of the heart through the aorta. Its branches supply the head, arms, legs, and internal organs, bringing oxygen to the cells of all these parts and picking up carbon dioxide and other wastes from them. Waste-carrying veins from the lower body become the inferior vena cava, and those from the upper body become the superior vena cava. Both superior and inferior venae cavae empty into the right atrium. This completes the *systemic circulation*. In the *pulmonary* (lung) *circulation*, venous blood goes from the right atrium to the right ventricle, which pumps blood by way of the pulmonary arteries to the lungs. There carbon dioxide waste is lost, and oxygen is picked up. The oxygenated blood then travels back through the pulmonary veins to the left atrium. From here it goes to the left ventricle to be pumped into the aorta to circulate once again to the body's cells.

some fibers. The pacemaker has the remarkable ability to discharge rhythmic bursts of electrical impulses and then recharge itself about seventy times a minute. With each spreading electrical impulse, both atria contract almost at the same time. The stimulus quickly spreads to a second, similar node, which then sends electrical stimuli to the ventricles. The ventricles also contract at almost the same time. This contraction phase, during which blood is squeezed out of the heart into the lungs and systemic circulation, is called **systole**. The heart then rests and dilates. The period of relaxation and dilatation of a chamber of the heart is called the **diastole**. During diastole the chambers of the heart fill with the entering blood.

In addition to the electrical cardiac mechanism described above, the *rate* of the heartbeat can be influenced by other nerves. Some increase its rate of action; others decrease it. But only the conducting system of the heart is able to keep it beating.

BLOOD FOR THE HEART MUSCLE: CORONARY CIRCULATION

How does the heart muscle receive its own blood supply? From the blood that constantly passes through the heart? No. Only the thin innermost lining of the heart gets a little blood this way. The heart has its own blood supply. Like all other organs, arteries lead to the heart, and veins lead away from it. But the

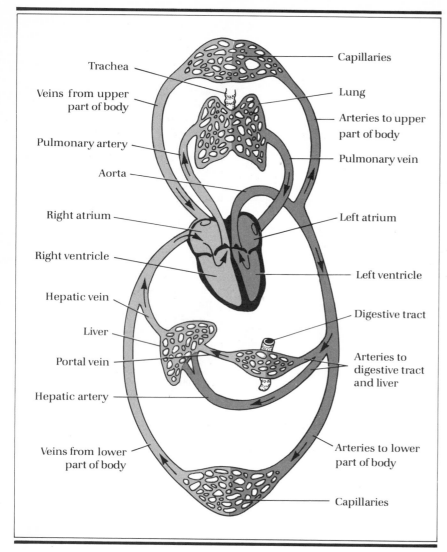

Trachea

Veins from upper part of body

Pulmonary artery

Aorta

Right atrium

Right ventricle

Hepatic vein

Liver

Portal vein

Hepatic artery

Veins from lower part of body

Capillaries

Lung

Arteries to upper part of body

Pulmonary vein

Left atrium

Left ventricle

Digestive tract

Arteries to digestive tract and liver

Arteries to lower part of body

Capillaries

FIGURE 4–5
The two circuits of blood circulation: the *pulmonary,* in which blood is pumped by the right ventricle to the lungs and back to the left atrium; and the *systemic,* in which blood is pumped by the left ventricle to the rest of the body. Oxygenated blood is shown here in darker gray.

heart receives first choice of the blood that, fresh from the lungs, is newly oxygenated (see Figure 4–5). Even before the great aorta branches off to carry blood to the head, trunk, or limbs, it gives off two branches, the **coronary arteries.** Like an inverted crown (or corona), these embrace the heart.

After supplying the heart muscle with blood, the coronary arteries grow smaller and smaller to end in a **capillary bed,** which eventually empties into venules. The venules then grow increasingly larger until finally they become veins, which discharge venous blood into the right atrium.

The Lymphatic Drainage System

Like the blood capillaries, the end vessels of the lymphatic system begin at the cellular level (see Figure 4–6). (Figure 9–3 on page 288 shows the lymphatic blood vessels in the villi of the small intestine.) Unlike the blood capillaries, the lymphatic capillaries do not act as tiny connecting canals between two larger vessels, nor do they bring the needs of life to the body cells. Their function is drainage. Originating as blind-ended, microscopic vessels, the lymphatic capillaries do not communicate with the blood capillaries, although they may mingle with them. At the level of the cells, the fluid within the lymphatic capillaries is like the fluid in the spaces outside of the cells. Within the lymphatic system, that fluid is called **lymph.** The lymphatic capillaries blend to form larger and larger vessels. Finally they empty, as two large trunks, into the large waste-returning veins near the heart. (See Figure 4–7.)

By way of the lymphatic channels, large protein molecules and fluids, which had originally left the blood to seep through blood capillaries into the spaces outside the cells, are eventually returned to the blood. In this way, a fluid balance in the body's inner ecosystems is maintained. Lymph also contains white cells, bits of dead cells, poisons, and other wastes (even bacteria) that must be kept out of the blood. This service is provided by the **lymph nodes.** Lymphatic vessels (see Figure 4–8) lead to these definite organizations of specialized lymphoid tissue. Lymph nodes are not "lymph glands," for they do not secrete anything. Before lymph reaches the blood circulation, it is filtered in the lymph nodes. Special

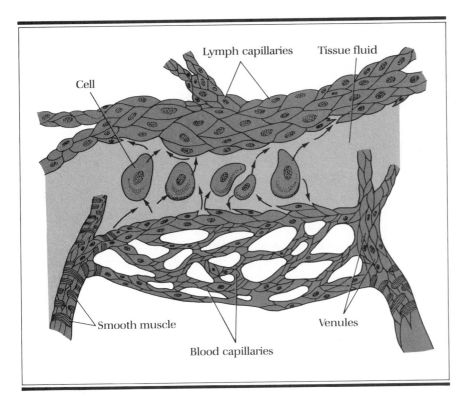

Cell

Lymph capillaries

Tissue fluid

Smooth muscle

Blood capillaries

Venules

FIGURE 4–6

Oxygen, nutrients, and other vital substances in the blood seep through the blood capillary walls into the fluid spaces surrounding the tissue cells. If there is then a higher concentration of a needed substance outside the cells than inside them, the cell membranes will admit it. Similarly, wastes traverse the cell membranes and reach the fluid spaces between the cells. The wastes may then be carried off with lymph, eventually to enter the venous blood, or they may enter venous blood by seeping directly into a blood capillary. The kidneys, liver, and lungs clear wastes from venous blood.

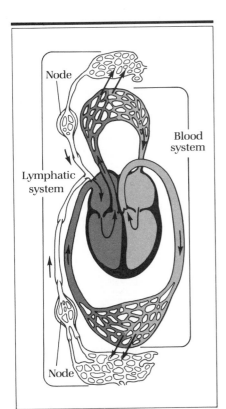

Node

Lymphatic system

Blood system

Node

FIGURE 4–7

A schematic diagram of the blood and lymphatic circulatory systems. Oxygenated blood is shown here in lighter gray.

FIGURE 4–8

Lymphangiograms—X-ray photographs of lymphatic vessels, which are made visible by injecting a radiopaque dye into them. In the normal leg (left), the lymphatics appear as thin, straight vessels. In the swollen leg (right), the lymphatics are both more numerous and widely distributed; they are also tortuous, beaded, and dilated. An obstruction to the lymph flow in the groin caused this condition.

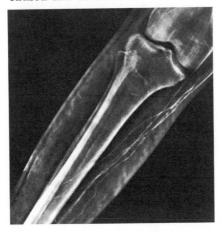

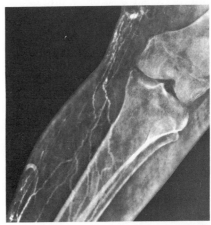

cells within the nodes digest bits of broken cells and other wastes and make them harmless. It is also in the lymph nodes that lymphocytes become the plasma cells that make antibodies (see pages 59–60 in Chapter 3).

In some parts of the body, lymph node tissue groups together to form organs. The best known of these are the **tonsils** and **adenoids**. The largest lymphoid organ, the fist-sized **spleen** (see Body Chart 9), is in front of the left kidney. The spleen filters some lymph and blood. It is, moreover, a major site for the manufacture of a clotting factor that prevents normal people from having **hemophilia,** a hereditary disease in which blood fails to clot properly. Many of the spleen's functions still are not clearly understood. Its removal, a common op-

eration, may result in a reduced resistance to infection by certain organisms. The blood-clotting factor, however, is simply taken over by other body parts, among them probably the liver.

Terms Describing the Results of Blood-flow Blockage

A local shortage of blood supply to any body part is called **ischemia** (pronounced *is-keé-mee-ah*). When either atherosclerosis (see pages 97–99) or a clot or both combine to plug an artery leading to a portion of the brain's **cerebrum,** for example, *cerebral ischemia* results. Cerebral ischemia can also be caused by a sudden contraction, or *spasm*, of the muscle layer of a cerebral artery.

A general term covering the sicknesses that result when there is not enough blood circulating to and in the cerebrum is **cerebrovascular disease,** which we will discuss later in this chapter.

When there is not enough nourishing blood supply to the heart muscle, the myocardium, **ischemic heart disease** or **cardiac ischemia** results. A lack of blood in the myocardium reduces its supply of oxygen and other life needs. The result is a pain called *angina pectoris.* The word *angina* comes from the Latin word *angere*, meaning "to strangle." *Pectoris* refers to the chest. With severe ischemic heart disease (such as occurs with complete blockage of a coronary artery or one of its branches), a portion of the heart dies from lack of blood and oxygen. Since the heart muscle

TABLE 4–3
Number of Deaths, and Death Rates per 100,000 Population, in the United States from All Causes, Major Cardiovascular Disease, Ischemic Heart Disease, and Cerebrovascular Disease 1971–1977[1]

		ALL CAUSES	MAJOR CARDIOVASCULAR DISEASE	ISCHEMIC HEART DISEASE	CEREBROVASCULAR DISEASE
1971	Deaths	1,927,542	1,017,145	674,292	209,092
	Rates	934.7	493.3	327.0	101.4
1972	Deaths	1,963,944	1,035,146	684,424	213,344
	Rates	943.2	497.1	328.7	102.5
1973	Deaths	1,973,003	1,037,492	684,066	214,313
	Rates	940.2	494.4	326.0	102.1
1974	Deaths	1,934,388	1,010,926	604,854	207,424
	Rates	915.1	478.2	314.5	98.1
1975	Deaths	1,892,879	971,047	642,719	194,038
	Rates	888.5	455.8	301.7	91.1
1976	Deaths	1,912,000	977,410	649,280	189,100
	Rates	890.8	455.4	302.5	88.1
1977	Deaths	1,898,000	960,090	637,670	182,840
	Rates	877.4	443.8	294.8	84.5
Total Deaths		13,501,756	6,135,356	4,577,305	1,491,151

1. Major cardiovascular (heart and blood vessels) disease includes both ischemic heart disease and cerebrovascular (brain and blood vessel) disease. Deaths from "all causes" refers to *all* deaths—whether due to cardiovascular disease, cancer, accidents, or any other causes—in this country for any given year.

SOURCE: National Center for Health Statistics, *Monthly Vital Statistics Report*, Provisional Statistics, Annual Summary for the United States, 1976, Vol. 25 (December 12, 1977), p. 26, and 1977, Vol. 26 (December 8, 1978), pp. 26–29.

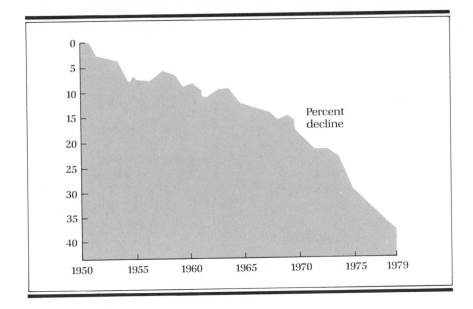

FIGURE 4-9
U.S. death rate from heart disease
(1950-1979).

is known as the *myocardium* and the portion of dead heart tissue is called an *infarct*, the term for a sudden heart attack is *acute myocardial infarction* due to ischemic heart disease. This condition, often called simply a "heart attack," is an epidemic cause of death in this country (see Table 4-3 and Figure 4-9) although recent years have seen a decline in its incidence.

Examples of how different parts of the circulatory system are related by both structure and disease can be shown by cases of increased blood pressure in the arteries, known as **hypertension**. This can result in both heart and kidney disease. Hypertension is believed to be an important factor in coronary artery blockage and heart attacks. Possibly this may be started by the damage caused by high blood pressure on the inner lining of the arteries. Hypertension can also cause heart disease when it forces the heart to beat against increased blood pressure. The heart may then enlarge and fail to work efficiently. This can result in **hypertensive heart disease**. Kidney disease can also

result in hypertension. On the other hand, hypertension can *cause* kidney disease.

In the next section we will take a look at the process of *atherosclerosis*.

Atherosclerosis: A Puzzle Only Partly Solved

A *theory* implies that (1) the thoughts about a subject may be true, and (2) the thoughts agree with some definite information, but that (3) they need further study before they can be proved true. What follows here has been filtered through present theories about the cause of atherosclerosis. When scientists find all the pieces of the puzzle of this condition, its complete picture will be revealed.

About Two Chemical Compounds and Atherosclerosis

Two of several groups of fatty substances are necessary for life. These are **cholesterol** and **triglycerides**. The amount of each that is contained in the body cells depends on

two basic factors: (1) how much of each the body cells make, and (2) how much the body gets from food. Both increase in the body when a person eats too many calories and is too fat.

Most, if not all, of the cells throughout the body, such as some in the skin and the liver, normally have the ability to make cholesterol. And one of the liver's many functions is to make triglycerides. Both substances are ordinarily found in various body tissues.

Cholesterol is needed to make up part of a cell's membrane. It also becomes a substance from which certain life-maintaining glandular chemicals are made. Triglycerides are part of the necessary chemical activity of the body. But for health and life there must be a balance of the two substances in the body's cellular ecosystems. Too little of the cholesterol or triglycerides may make cellular health and even life impossible. Too much will promote atherosclerosis. But neither triglycerides nor cholesterol travel in the blood alone. Both are carried in the blood by a group of chemicals known as **lipoproteins**. These consist of a protein combined with a **lipid** (fat). Some lipoproteins carry cholesterol; others, triglycerides; still others carry both. There are two kinds of these chemicals: low-density lipoproteins (LDLs) and high-density lipoproteins (HDLs). What role do lipoproteins have in the control of cholesterol and triglycerides? Let's take cholesterol as an example.

CHOLESTEROL CONTROL

On the surfaces of cells are molecules or combinations of molecules called **receptors**. The arrangement of the molecules on the receptors of the cell's surfaces enables cells to tell whether there are any chemicals nearby, such as gland products, drugs, or fatty substances like cholesterol-lipoprotein combinations. But the LDL receptors do more. They exert a *feedback control* on the cholesterol that is made within the cell. But what is a feedback control? Think of it this way. There must be a mechanism for controlling the amount of cholesterol made in a cell. Otherwise there would be no way of making certain that the cell would manufacture enough cholesterol to maintain its own health or that it would discontinue production before blood cholesterol levels get so high that there is an undesirable deposit of it on the arteries, resulting in atherosclerosis. In this instance, then, feedback is simply the way a cell lets

itself know that it has made enough cholesterol and should stop making more. It is the return to the cell of a part of its output of cholesterol, which is a signal to the cell to stop making more unneeded cholesterol.

It is now known that normally the LDL receptors on the surface of the cell bind the LDL-cholesterol complex to it. Then the LDL receptors transport the cholesterol into the cell. Within the cell, cholesterol acts on cellular activity to reduce cholesterol production. The LDL receptors themselves are also regulated by a feedback mechanism. When cholesterol gathers in the cell, the LDL receptors become less active. By decreasing the number of LDL receptors, normal cells can protect themselves from being overloaded with cholesterol.

Patients who suffer a hereditary absence of the normal LDL receptors on their cell surfaces have greatly elevated blood-cholesterol levels and are subject to premature heart attacks. The cells lack the important link of feedback regulation of cholesterol production. Since they do not receive the message that there is too much cholesterol in

them, they go on making more and more cholesterol and releasing it into the bloodstream. Finally this excess of the fatty substance is deposited on the walls of the arteries to begin the process of atherosclerosis.

High-density lipoproteins, the HDLs, seem to perform a more straightforward protective job than the LDLs. The HDLs simply pick up excess blood cholesterol and deliver it to the liver. From the liver the cholesterol travels by way of the gallbladder to the small intestine. From then on excretion of excess cholesterol is a matter of time. There is evidence that a decreased intake of saturated fats (see page 102) and exercise are both related to a protective, high level of HDLs. In fact, many experts believe that a high level of HDLs in the blood is a sign of protection against atherosclerosis.

Nowadays, there is a laboratory test to measure not only the amount of cholesterol and triglycerides in the blood but also the level of the protective HDLs. Such tests make it possible to identify people who have a particularly high risk of develop-

You will be meeting with the concept of feedback in other areas of study in addition to the way it works in the body. For example, when a viewer of a television program telephones a question or comment to the television station, a form of feedback occurs. Consider a more complicated example involving female body function. Hormones from the brain's hypothalamus stimulate the front lobe of the pituitary gland. The cells of this lobe produce other hormones, which in turn stimulate an ovary to release an ovum. Then, using a feedback mechanism, the ovary will send its own chemical hormonal message back to the front lobe of the pituitary gland and then on to the brain's hypothalamus signaling (or feeding back the message) that the ovum has been released from the ovary (ovulation, see pages 354–357) and that high hypothalamic hormone levels for ovulation are not now needed.

ing atherosclerosis. Once identified, measures may be possible to prevent its occurrence or progression.

The Process of Atherosclerosis

Ordinarily, the inner lining of a healthy adult artery has a glistening, smooth surface. This feature of the inner lining of the artery is important because the blood cells can then rush along to the needy cells without anything getting in their way. With atherosclerosis, this changes. As we have said, most scientists believe that cholesterol, as well as other fatty chemicals (such as triglycerides), irritate the smooth muscle cells of the inner artery linings. As if to protect themselves, the smooth muscle cells of the inner artery linings increase in number. In addition, the middle layer of the artery has many more smooth muscle cells than does the inner lining, and there is some evidence that they travel to the irritated inner artery lining. All these extra cells form a **plaque** (or patch) on the inner artery layer, as shown in Figure 4–10. Though the body is trying to protect itself, the deadly process of atherosclerosis is beginning.

The process continues as the blood cells, when passing the plaque, become stuck to it. Some of these blood cells are platelets, which help the clotting process. A clot, called a **thrombus,** forms, or organizes. As the damage to the artery lining worsens, the body does what it can to repair it. Tiny capillaries grow from nearby healthy arteries to the break (or *lesion*) in the normal arterial lining. The capillaries may rupture and bleed. The lesion worsens and becomes an ulcer. Eventually, however, the ulcer heals.

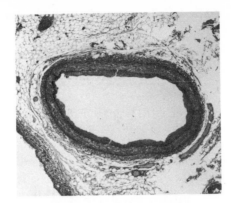

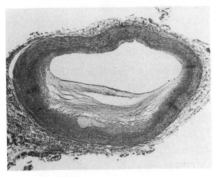

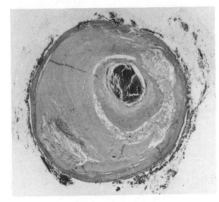

FIGURE 4–10
A normal artery (top), an artery with atherosclerotic deposits in the inner lining (center), and an artery narrowed by atherosclerotic deposits and now blocked by a blood clot, the dark inner circle (bottom).

Calcium is deposited, causing the artery to stiffen and harden. The organized clot and the hardened plaque beneath it get in the way of the passage of blood. When such an artery is cut at autopsy, an inexperienced surgeon might be forgiven

for sharing Jenner's impression of falling plaster.

The arteries of some body sites seem particularly likely to develop atherosclerosis. The atherosclerotic process tends to begin at a point where an artery branches. Figure 4–11 is a diagram showing some locations of arterial branching that are common sites of atherosclerosis. For example, note that the leg's *popliteal artery,* a continuation of the *femoral artery,* divides into branches. At the point of branching, atherosclerosis may occur and get in the way of blood circulation to the leg. Complete obstruction of the blood flow to the foot would lead to gangrene, the death of tissue cells that are without a proper blood supply.

When the average middle-aged person has a heart attack or a stroke or develops gangrene due to atherosclerosis, the damage has been a long time coming. The signs and symptoms may be agonizingly sudden, but the disease process has been brewing for many years. Few diseased conditions have so prolonged an incubation period—so long a period between the first body changes and the onset of symptoms—as does atherosclerosis. In fact, the beginnings of atherosclerosis have been found even within the arteries of small children who have died from other causes. Also, atherosclerosis was very commonly found in the arteries of U.S. soldiers killed in the Korean and Vietnam wars. How many people in the United States die from atherosclerosis? What is the tragic price of this condition? In well-to-do nations it affects people in all age groups and of both sexes. More than half the deaths in the United States are due to major cardiovascular diseases (see Table 4–3), and most of these are caused by atherosclerosis.

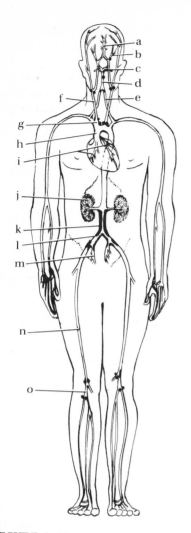

FIGURE 4-11
Common arterial sites of atherosclerosis: cerebral (a–c), basilar (d), vertebral (e), common carotid (f), innominate (g), aorta (h), coronary (i), renal (j), abdominal aorta (k), iliac (l, m), femoral (n), and popliteal (o). The dark circles indicate where obstruction is most likely to occur.

Cardiovascular Disease: Some Hard Facts and Figures

Examine still again Table 4–3. There is, of course, no point to memorizing numbers; yet several trends should be noted. *First:* From 1971 through 1977 more than six million people in this country died of cardiovascular disease. Few cities in this nation contain that number of people. As a group, the cardiovascular diseases remain the leading cause of death in the United States. *Second:* Except for 1975, 1976, and 1977, over a million people a year died of cardiovascular disease. And, for all the years shown, the table reveals that almost half the deaths in this country were caused by them. Yet there is room for optimism. Also shown in the table is this fact: In 1975 the number of cardiovascular deaths dropped below the million mark for the first time. This happened even though the population of the United States continued to increase. Although one of the cardiovascular diseases—ischemic heart disease—is still the nation's number one killer, it now causes a smaller proportion of total deaths than formerly (refer back to Figure 4–9 on page 97). Since 1967 the U.S. death rate from heart disease has been going down. This may mean a growing interest in health among our nation's citizens.

Although the statistics are encouraging, they are no reason to relax efforts against the killing cardiovascular diseases. Ischemic heart disease alone will still cost about 600,000 lives a year. And about 25 percent of the dead will not have reached their sixty-fifth birthday.

Coronary Artery Disease

Angina Pectoris: The Pain of Partial Coronary Artery Atherosclerosis

When there is atherosclerosis of a coronary artery, the signs and symptoms that the patient will experience usually depend on the degree of ischemia, or lack of blood supply to the heart. When coronary vessels are only partly blocked, the heart can still receive some blood, and the individual may experience few or no symptoms. But stress, exercise, or overeating may cause the pain called angina pectoris to appear.

Ordinarily this pain begins beneath the breastbone. It may vary from a mild sense of pressure in the chest to a viselike, crushing, even choking, pain. Sometimes it reaches to the neck or around the back. More often it travels like a nagging ache down the left arm, usually into the fourth and little fingers. Attacks of angina pectoris are a warning that a complete blockage of a coronary artery may occur. A long-term study of heart disease, begun in 1949 in Framingham, Massachusetts, revealed that some people develop an almost continuous angina pectoris. The ischemia seems to cause constant heart muscle (myocardial) pain and irritability. Frequently it kills.

Complete Coronary Artery Blockage

A coronary artery blockage may be complete when the artery is closed off by a clot, or thrombus, forming at the site of an atherosclerotic plaque, or by a plaque swollen by a hemorrhage within it. At times, a piece of a thrombus or of an atherosclerotic plaque breaks loose and travels (as an **embolus**) and goes on to plug a smaller branch of a coronary artery. Although the part of the heart bereft of blood dies, the patient may survive. In that event a blood supply develops that bypasses the dead heart muscle tissue (the myocardial infarct). At first the infarct is soft. If healing takes place, it becomes tough fibrous tissue in about six weeks. A person can have a myocardial infarct, recover, and with sensible care lead a long and active life. The Framingham study revealed another surprising fact: Some people have a myocardial infarct without ever realizing it. These are the so-called "silent coronaries."

Rhythm Disturbances

Myocardial damage may cause rhythm disturbances. What happens is that the infarct interrupts electrical pathways from the specialized pacemaking cells responsible for a regular heartbeat (see page 92). Should the ventricles beat chaotically and twitch (*fibrillate*), blood cannot be properly pumped to the

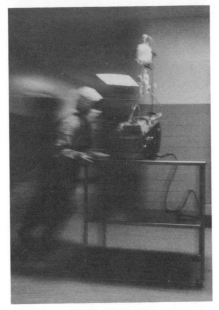

A nurse rushes to an operating room with emergency apparatus.

body. Death may occur. For those with this problem, the use of artificial pacemakers may be lifesaving.

Congestive Heart Failure Due to Coronary Artery Disease

Congestive heart failure may occur when the heart, weakened by coronary disease, loses some of its ability to pump blood. As a result, fluid of the blood backs up from the heart and gathers in the lungs or the abdomen and legs. This type of heart failure may occur immediately following a severe heart attack, or it may happen years after damage to the heart muscle. Since coronary artery disease is only one of several heart problems that can result in congestive heart failure, the latter will be discussed separately on pages 105–106.

At this point, however, we can summarize the major events that can happen when a person suffers from coronary artery disease result-

ing in myocardial ischemia. They are (1) angina pectoris; (2) coronary artery blockage (or *occlusion*) resulting in myocardial infarction; (3) loss of regular heart rhythm (*cardiac arrhythmia*); and (4) congestive heart failure, which also occurs with other heart conditions.

Heart Attack: Emergency!

The studies conducted in Framingham, Massachusetts, showed that about half the deaths from acute coronary disease in the United States occur in the first hour. Every year, more than 300,000 heart attack victims die before they reach a hospital. Emergency coronary care programs are aimed at reducing three time-consuming factors: (1) the *victim's decision time* that passes between the onset of the heart attack and the seeking of professional help; (2) the *transportation time* to a hospital's coronary care unit; and (3) the *hospital time* that passes before adequate emergency treatment is begun. Education can only partly shorten the first of these. Denial by the patient of the coronary event can result in a deadly delay. Often, a victim agrees to examination only at the insistence of someone else. Specially equipped ambulances driven by specially trained paramedical personnel help reduce the second delay. And today, 75 percent of all hospitals with one hundred beds or more have coronary care units to provide emergency help to heart attack victims.

Every study of coronary heart disease leads to a basic conclusion: The best objective is to prevent the attack. To do this, an understanding of the major concepts about atherosclerosis will help.

Plan to Live:
Know the Risks
of Atherosclerosis

Who is most likely to have an atherosclerotic artery blockage? What factors increase the risk of suffering a heart attack, a stroke, or a blood-starved leg? The exact answer cannot be complete because the exact cause is still unknown. Theories are no substitute for plain truths. Yet, long-time observation of the patterns of atherosclerosis among groups of people have given a lot of information about factors that seem to make the condition worse.

All over the world, babies a year or more old have the tell-tale *fatty streaks* of beginning atherosclerosis in their aortas. Among some peoples, usually in the developing countries, the streaks do not grow worse to damage the body's arteries seriously. Among other peoples, generally in the industrialized, wealthier countries, these fatty streaks do worsen. They often appear in the coronary arteries of college-aged people. At this age and stage there is strong evidence that the streaks will not worsen in nonhypertensive people who do exercises that improve heart and lung function (see Chapter 8), who do not smoke, and who are watchful of weight and diet. As the years go by, however, the condition may worsen in those who do not have such a program of personal health attention. Atherosclerotic plaques bulge into artery canals, obstructing what William Shakespeare called in *Hamlet* ". . . the natural gates and alleys of the body."

Just getting older must be considered still another important factor in atherosclerosis. Yet many old people have arteries that are in better condition than many young people. Why? The *four greatest risks (except age) associated with atherosclerosis are cigarette smoking, an abnormal increase in blood serum lipoproteins, high blood-sugar levels, and high blood pressure.* Sometimes these risks are greatly increased because of other diseases. People with *diabetes mellitus* tend to have increased blood-sugar levels. A person with a *poorly functioning thyroid gland* (the ductless gland straddling the windpipe) will develop high levels of blood-serum lipoproteins. Very high blood-serum lipoprotein levels are sometimes found in *members of the same family.* Members of such families may develop severe atherosclerosis as teen-agers or earlier. Why? They have a hereditary lack of the normal LDL receptors on their cell surfaces. Since there can be no feedback regulation of cholesterol in the cell (see page 98), the cells never give the message that they contain too much cholesterol. Uncontrolled, cholesterol piles up in the cell. Soon, there is an abnormal amount of cholesterol deposited on the artery walls. This type of increased atherosclerosis is more clear-cut than others. For example, there does seem to be a *family tendency* for heart attacks in people with this hereditary problem.

Being a male increases the chance of developing atherosclerosis. A myocardial infarct, for instance, is rare in women who are still menstruating. After the age of about fifty, however, some women, too, start developing high blood pressure and increased blood levels of lipoproteins. The incidence of atherosclerosis thus can increase in women after fifty. But even then, the number of heart attacks among women do not equal those among men until advanced age.

Lack of physical exercise, the stress of modern living, obesity, and a diet too high in saturated fats (those that usually solidify at room temperature) have all been added to the list of risks of developing atherosclerosis. Yet another cause is believed to be *gout,* a form of arthritis, most often of the big toe, caused by too much of a certain chemical compound in the bloodstream. Several of these conditions in the same person increase the risk of a heart attack or a stroke to a marked degree. (To test your risk of getting heart and cardiovascular disease, see the box "Risko.")

PREVENTION:
WHAT CAN BE DONE
TO DELAY THE DISEASES
OF ATHEROSCLEROSIS?

Those with inherited atherosclerosis need special medical attention. But even those with a family history of the diseases of atherosclerosis can do much to decrease their risks. A sensible program of exercise (see Chapter 8's discussion), complete avoidance of smoking, effective coping with excessive stress, and control of one's intake of calories, fats, and especially cholesterol all reduce the risk of developing artery-blocking atherosclerosis. "Taking the dying out of eating" is a meaningful phrase. People who are overweight should, with the help of their doctors, lose weight. Studies in different countries indicate that diets high in saturated fats and cholesterol increase the risk of coronary heart disease. Thus, foods high in saturated (but low in unsaturated) fats—including cheeses, butter, cream, lard, and meats, particularly pork, beef, and lamb—should be avoided. "Marbled" meats may be as streaked with fats as an atherosclerotic artery. Pretenderized meat

RISKO

The purpose of this game is to give you an estimate of your chances of suffering heart attack. The game is played by making squares which—from left to right—represent an increase in your RISK FACTORS. These are medical conditions and habits associated with an increased danger of heart attack. *Not all risk factors are measurable enough to be included in this game* (see below).

RULES: Study each RISK FACTOR and its row. Find the box applicable to you and circle the large number in it. For example, if you are 37, circle the number in the box labeled 31–40.

After checking out all the rows, add the circled numbers. This total—your score—is an estimate of your risk.

IF YOU SCORE:

6–11—Risk well below average	25–31—Risk moderate
12–17—Risk below average	32–40—Risk at a dangerous level
18–24—Risk generally average	41–62—Danger urgent. See your doctor now.

HEREDITY: Count parents, grand-parents, brothers, and sisters who have had heart attack and/or stroke.

TOBACCO SMOKING: If you inhale deeply and smoke a cigarette way down, add one to your classification. Do NOT subtract because you think you do not inhale or smoke only a half inch on a cigarette.

EXERCISE: Lower your score one point if you exercise regularly and frequently.

CHOLESTEROL OR SATURATED FAT INTAKE LEVEL: A cholesterol blood level is best. If you can't get one from your doctor, then estimate honestly the percentage of solid fats you eat. These are usually of animal origin—lard, cream, butter, and beef and lamb fat. If you eat much of this, your cholesterol level probably will be high. The U.S. average, 40%, is too high for good health.

BLOOD PRESSURE: If you have no recent reading but have passed an insurance or industrial examination chances are you are 140 or less.*

SEX: This line takes into account the fact that men have from 6 to 10 times more heart attacks than women of child bearing age.

*See page 108 for a review of blood pressure.

Because of the difficulty in measuring them, these RISK FACTORS are not included in "RISKO":

Diabetes, particularly when present for many years.

Your *Character* or *Personality*, and the *Stress* under which you live.

Vital Capacity—determined by measuring the amount of air you can take into your lungs in proportion to the size of your lungs. The less air you can breathe, the higher your risk.

Electrocardiogram—if certain abnormalities are present in the record of the electrical currents generated by your heart you have a higher risk.

Gout—is caused by a higher than normal amount of uric acid in the blood. Patients have an increased risk.

IF YOU HAVE A NUMBER OF RISK FACTORS, FOR THE SAKE OF YOUR HEALTH, ASK YOUR DOCTOR TO CHECK YOUR MEDICAL CONDITIONS AND QUIT YOUR RISK FACTOR HABITS.

NOTE: The fact that various habits or conditions may be rated similarly in this test does not mean these are of equal risk. The reaction of individual human beings to Risk Factors—as to many other things—is so varied it is impossible to draw valid conclusions for any individual.

This scale has been developed only to highlight what the Risk Factors are and what can be done about them. It is not designed to be a medical diagnosis.

		1	2	3	4	6	
AGE		10 to 20	21 to 30	31 to 40	41 to 50	51 to 60	61 to 70 and over
HEREDITY		No known history of heart disease	1 relative with cardiovascular disease Over 60	2 relatives with cardiovascular disease Over 60	1 relative with cardiovascular disease Under 60	2 relatives with cardiovascular disease Under 60	3 relatives with cardiovascular disease Under 60
WEIGHT		More than 5 lbs. below standard weight	−5 to +5 lbs. standard weight	6-20 lbs. over weight	21-35 lbs. over weight	36-50 lbs. over weight	51-65 lbs. over weight
TOBACCO SMOKING		Non-user	Cigar and/or pipe	10 cigarettes or less a day	20 cigarettes a day	30 cigarettes a day	40 cigarettes a day or more
EXERCISE		Intensive occupational and recreational exertion	Moderate occupational and recreational exertion	Sedentary work and intense recreational exertion	Sedentary occupational and moderate recreational exertion	Sedentary work and light recreational exertion	Complete lack of all exercise
CHOLES-TEROL OR FAT % IN DIET		Cholesterol below 180 mg.% Diet contains no animal or solid fats	Cholesterol 181-205 mg.% Diet contains 10% animal or solid fats	Cholesterol 206-230 mg.% Diet contains 20% animal or solid fats	Cholesterol 231-255 mg.% Diet contains 30% animal or solid fats	Cholesterol 256-280 mg.% Diet contains 40% animal or solid fats	Cholesterol 281-300 mg.% Diet contains 50% animal or solid fats
BLOOD PRESSURE		100 upper reading	120 upper reading	140 upper reading	160 upper reading	180 upper reading	200 or over upper reading
SEX		Female under 40	Female 40-50	Female over 50	Male	Stocky male	Bald stocky male

SOURCE: "Risko: A Way to Alert You to the Risks of Heart Attack," ©Michigan Heart Association. Reprinted by permission.

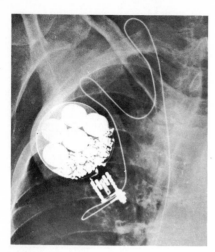

This X-ray shows an electrical pacemaker placed just under the skin of the chest. It will help to continue and control the heartbeat.

is tasty, less expensive, and more healthful. "Junk foods," such as high-fat-content hot dogs and potato chips are best abandoned. Unlike saturated ("hard") fats, polyunsaturated fats remain liquid at room temperature. Saturated fats usually come from animals. Polyunsaturated fats come from vegetable oils. Both safflower and peanut oil are high in desirable polyunsaturated fats and low in saturated fats.

Even more can be done to combat atherosclerosis. With most people high blood pressure and gout can be successfully treated. Blood-sugar levels can be controlled. Poorly functioning thyroid glands can also be handled medically.

A yet incomplete study of about two thousand schoolchildren in Muscatine, Iowa, suggests that children should have their blood pressure checked for the first time at about three years of age; weight should be controlled; and a low-fat, low-cholesterol diet is indicated for children whose cholesterol level stays high after several tests.

A personal and medically directed preventive program could have added many normal years to the life span of people now dead of atherosclerosis. Atherosclerosis is another challenge to prolonged health and to life itself.

NEW HELP FOR HEART PATIENTS

Remarkable new machines can now detect those heart muscle areas that are receiving too small a blood supply due to a blocked coronary artery. Patients are also enjoying longer lives as a result of corrective surgery, which involves a "jump" or "bypass" graft in which a vein from the patient's thigh or an internal artery of the breast is grafted to the heart muscle in order to bypass the coronary blockage to the heart and thus restore circulation. Thousands of these operations have been performed. Many are done to prevent likely heart attacks.

In this country, about one person in five thousand is kept alive by a *pacemaker*, which helps the heart to beat regularly. New advances— such as the plutonium-powered pacemaker, which has a longer life expectancy—promise to reduce the number of repeated surgeries to replace the run-down batteries of ordinary pacemakers.

Heart Conditions Not Due Basically to Atherosclerosis

Congenital Defects

With improper development of the embryo heart, nonhereditary **congenital defects** occur. Every year some forty thousand babies in this country (less than 1 percent) are born with a heart malformation. Such a heart may not be able to pump enough blood to the lungs to get oxygen. Or the heart defect may be such that it results in the mixing together of venous and arterial blood. These children may have a bluish color of the skin and mucous membrane, a condition called **cyanosis.** Such infants are termed "blue babies."

The cause of most congenital heart defects is unknown. A small percentage are due to German measles or other viral infections transmitted through the placenta during pregnancy. Fortunately, many of the more than thirty-five kinds of congenital heart defects are correctable by surgery. The heart-lung machine has been a surgical boon. By shunting the blood from the heart, it temporarily takes over the heart's blood-circulating function, as well as the function of the lungs in ridding the blood of carbon dioxide and taking on oxygen. The heart is thus "dry" and can be operated upon while the machine does the work for it and the lungs.

In recent years heart surgeons have extended the benefits of the heart-lung machine. For example, a congenital heart defect that usually kills the child during the first year of life has now been successfully treated by surgery in over 90 percent of the cases. First, the baby's body is packed in ice. Blood is then run from the baby's body through a heart-lung machine. Then the baby's blood temperature is lowered to below 18°C (64°F). At that temperature the infant's blood can be completely stopped for half an hour with little risk of brain damage. Then the tubes from the heart-lung machine are removed from the heart. This leaves the golf-ball sized heart more easily operated on than would ordinarily be the case. This chilling of newborns before heart surgery may well become a boon for newborns with other heart defects that need very early surgery.

There is concern that with some babies brain damage may result during hypothermia from the long deprivation of a normal amount of oxygen to the brain. Thus, in various treatment centers throughout the country, other techniques have been added to the hypothermia procedure that will doubtless remove this possibility.

Rheumatic Heart Disease

Rheumatic heart disease still costs about 13,500 lives yearly in this country. The disease is a secondary reaction to a specific streptococcal nose or throat infection. Like rheumatoid arthritis (see pages 63–64) and glomerulonephritis (see page 107), rheumatic heart disease occurs when the body's immune system turns upon itself. Many people get streptococcal infections. In some, however, the antibodies that are made to fight the streptococcus may also damage the lining of the kidneys, joints, and heart valves. The person, usually a child between five and fifteen years old, may have a sore throat or joint pains. He or she may just feel unwell. "Growing pains," people may say, but the problem is far more serious. A physician may need to watch the child carefully for some time.

Should the disease involve the heart valves, healing may cause one or more of the valves to scar, shrink, and thus lose their normal shape. Because of this, the leaflets of the heart valves fail to meet one another properly. After the atria contract, the valves try to close tightly but cannot. Blood leaks backward. Or a valve may fail to open completely. Blood flow to the ventricles is held back. The physician will hear significant heart murmurs. (Not all murmurs mean disease, however. Some are quite normal.)

Penicillin and other antibiotics can usually treat and prevent rheumatic fever. But one attack of rheumatic fever makes a child susceptible to another. For people who have had previous attacks, penicillin by mouth is usually given daily until at least age forty. Some specialists feel it should be given for life. This medication helps prevent future attacks. Surgical repair and replacement of valves already severely scarred by rheumatic disease are now almost commonplace.

Hypertensive Heart Disease

Hypertensive heart disease is a complication of hypertension (high blood pressure). Because the heart must beat against increased pressure, it enlarges. Hypertension also damages the inner wall of the arteries and thus promotes atherosclerosis. (Hypertension is discussed in more detail on pages 108–109.)

Metabolic and Endocrine Disorders and Heart Disease

Generally, **metabolism** refers to all the chemical reactions that constantly go on in the body. The **endocrine glands** are those that do not have ducts, such as the pituitary, thyroid, and adrenal glands (see Body Chart 15). As an example of the relationship between body chemistry and heart disease, an overactive thyroid gland, which affects metabolism, can add to the amount of stress placed upon the heart muscle.

More about Congestive Heart Failure

Any illness that causes impairment of the heart's action as a pump can result in congestive heart failure. (**Congestion** refers to the abnormal accumulation of blood or fluid in a body part.) Rheumatic fever or long-standing hypertension may, at last, by their excessive demands on the heart, seriously weaken it. A heart frittering away its energy in the wild muscular twitchings caused by a damaged conducting system will result in congestive failure. Or the heart, long ago having endured serious damage from a coronary thrombosis, will at last fail. An acute myocardial infarction may start cardiac muscle failure. So congestive heart failure is not itself a disease; rather, it is a complex combination of signs and symptoms that can result from any number of various types of heart disease.

Either or both of the two heart pumps may fail. If the left heart pump fails, the fluid of the blood backs up into the lungs. There is a "rattling" in the patient's chest. Congestion causes the patient to cough and to be short of breath. Sitting up brings a little relief. The patient seeks comfort from the support of several pillows as a backrest. Should the right pump fail, fluid backs up into the abdomen and legs. **Edema,** the gathering of too much fluid in the tissue spaces, results. Press a finger into the leg edema. For a while, the pressure point remains depressed. If both pumps fail, edema may involve much of the body.

Moreover, the kidneys cannot help. The weakened heart muscle cannot pump enough blood to them. Salt that would ordinarily leave the body with the urine is reabsorbed by the kidneys. Water is held back with the salt in the body's tissue spaces. As a result, fluid collects. Treatment may include a diet low in sodium (which is most commonly found in table salt) and the use of *diuretics*, medicines that remove sodium, and thus water, from the body by way of the kidneys.

The Kidneys Have Several Functions

Bones can break, muscles can atrophy [wither], glands can loaf, even the brain can go to sleep, without immediately endangering our survival; but should the kidneys fail to manufacture the proper kind of blood, neither bone, muscle, gland nor brain could carry on.[2]

Excretion refers to the discharge of waste products, such as urine, from the body. Every twenty minutes all the body's blood filters through the kidneys. The kidneys are not alone in their excretory functions. But the liver, lungs, and skin, important to excretion as they are, do not compare to the excretory activity of the kidneys. Yet excretion is not the only function of the kidneys. Among their other work is to control the making of chemicals that keep blood pressure at normal levels. The kidneys' chemical controls are also involved in red blood cell production. Moreover, they help to keep watch on the blood levels of drugs

and to maintain the body fluids and their contents.

Kidney Structure and the Filtration of Blood

The kidneys lie at the back of the abdomen at the level of the lower ribs. A large branch of the great aorta enters each kidney as the **renal artery.** Like all other arteries, it progressively divides to become arterioles. But these blood-filled arterioles (the **afferent arterioles**) do not, like all others, end in capillaries, which in turn become venules. Instead, each arteriole first leads into a tiny tuft of daintily coiled capillaries, a **glomerulus.**

The capillary tuft fits into the hollow of a capsule. Each functioning unit of the kidney is called a **nephron** (Figure 4–12). There are over a million nephrons in each kidney. Blood-carrying wastes enter the

capillaries of each glomerulus of every nephron. Fluid from the blood containing the waste filters through the glomerulus into the capsule. Then, the fluid containing waste travels to little collecting tubes (tubules) which eventually lead to the ureter. The ureter carries the urine from the kidney to the bladder. From the bladder the urine is finally excreted. If all the fluid leaving the capillaries was excreted as urine a person would be quickly "dried out." This does not happen because most of the fluid (minus waste) is reabsorbed in a lower part of the tubule of a nephron before reaching the ureter and bladder.

Kidney Dysfunction

Kidney disease is responsible for claiming about 100,000 lives a year in this country. Over 3,300,000 people in the United States have undiagnosed kidney disease. Some kidney diseases give immediate warning; others do not. Once kidney disease occurs, its progression must be stubbornly resisted.

Pyelonephritis is inflammation of the kidney and its pelvis. Among all age groups it is the nation's most common kidney disease. It is best treated in its early stages, because when chronic, pyelonephritis plays havoc with kidney function.

Glomerulonephritis causes most of the kidney failures in this country. It is believed that glomerulonephritis results when antigen-antibody combinations are deposited on the kidney. These combinations cause inflammation of the glomeruli. Although healing takes place, the result is scarring and destruction of kidney tissue. As far as cause is concerned, glomerulonephritis can be compared with rheumatoid arthritis and rheumatic fever. What is the antigen in glomerulonephritis? Animal studies suggest it to be a virus or a piece of a virus.

Hypertensive Kidney Disease

Diseases of the arteries that lead to the kidneys (the renal arteries) may reduce the size of their canals. Less blood flows to the kidneys, causing them to produce a chemical that causes a reaction resulting in high blood pressure. Some types of heart failure are associated with an abnormal amount of salt and water retained by the kidneys. Hypertension may be a byproduct of this.

Chronic kidney disease may result in a variety of symptoms. There may be a burning feeling upon urination, or too-frequent urination; the urine may turn a dark coffee color or appear bloody. In severe cases, swelling of body tissues occurs. Failure of

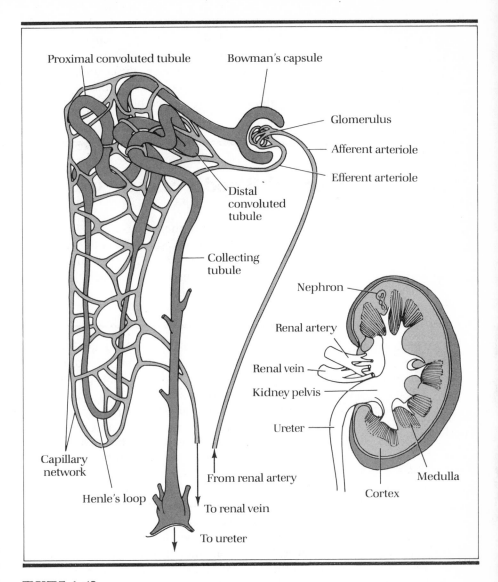

FIGURE 4–12
A nephron (left) and its relation to the kidney as a whole (right). The nephron in the illustration of the kidney has been drawn disproportionately large so as to be visible.

the kidneys to excrete wastes results in their accumulation in the blood. This is **uremia,** a most serious condition.

Modern medical techniques have prolonged the life of many kidney disease sufferers. Antibiotics fight infection. Drugs help the kidneys eliminate salt and water, thus relieving edema. **Dialysis machines** are mechanical devices that purify polluted uremic blood by filtration. A new, smaller, and less-expensive method of self-dialysis has been developed and is being tested. Kidney transplants are today quite common. A person can function with one healthy kidney.

Abnormal Blood Pressure (Arterial Hypertension)

When the smaller branches of the arteries (the arterioles) are abnormally narrow, blood cannot easily pass through them to the capillaries. Blood pressure within the arteries then increases. This high blood pressure within the arteries is *hypertension.* To overcome it, the heart must work harder. A vicious cycle begins. Artery walls toughen and lose their elasticity. The overworked heart muscle thickens. This is particularly true of the wall of the left ventricle. *Hypertensive heart disease* develops. Increased pressure of long duration may damage the kidneys and other vital organs.

For a twenty-year-old, the average **systolic pressure** — the highest blood pressure during contraction of the ventricles — is about 115 to 120 (measured in millimeters of mercury). The average **diastolic pressure** (lowest blood pressure during relaxation of the ventricles) is about 75. Exercise, tension, and excitement raise the blood pressure. So does age. Only when the blood pressure is unduly high, over a prolonged period of time, is disease likely. Many physicians consider a consistent systolic pressure of 150 questionable, and a diastolic pressure of over 90 high. Of the two, the diastolic pressure is most meaningful because it signifies the lowest constant blood pressure in the arteries. It, therefore, means more, because the high blood pressure against the arterial wall is continuous.

Partial blockage of a main kidney artery may cause hypertension. Sometimes, kidney inflammation (**nephritis**) or other kidney damage may result in high blood pressure; the exact mechanisms are unknown. By liberating adrenalin, adrenal gland (see Body Chart 15) tumors

Research conducted by the National Blood Pressure Education tion Program has illuminated four myths that are common among many of the estimated thirty-five million people in this country with high blood pressure:

1. Hypertension does not necessarily mean that a person is nervous or "high strung." Many outwardly cool, calm, and collected people have high blood pressure. Nor is it true that people undergoing treatment should take their medication only when they feel "nervous."

2. A second common fallacy is that all people with high blood pressure have symptoms. Signs and symptoms do not usually reveal themselves until there is extensive heart and blood vessel damage or even a stroke. Medicine prescribed for people with hypertension must be taken even when there are no symptoms. The purpose is to *prevent* the damage caused by high blood pressure.

3. A third common myth is the notion that a person under medical treatment for hypertension can successfully ignore the physician's advice to diet, exercise, limit salt intake, and take prescribed medication in exchange for some different, self-chosen form of treatment. Such people may well be courting disaster.

4. It is understandable for people with hypertension to hope for a *cure* for their disease. Cure is rare but *control* is common. And it is control that can save people from disability or possible death from a stroke. Thus, daily medication should not be discontinued when the blood pressure is lowered to the level set by the physician.

SOURCE: Susan W. Thompson, "To Control *Your* High Blood Pressure Doctor-Patient Communication is the Key," in "Living with High Blood Pressure, II," *The Reader's Digest,* Vol. 114 (May 1979), pp. 157–160.

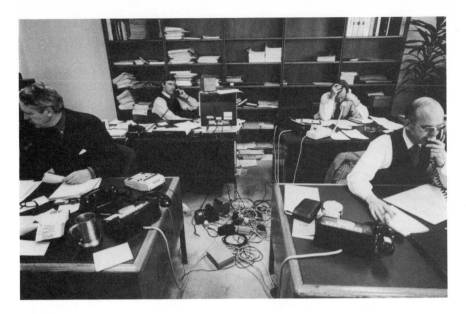

The eighteenth-century English statesman Edmund Burke wrote that incessant labor causes people to "exhaust their attention, burn out their candles, and [be] left in the dark." Today we know that overwork and high stress can also cause hypertension and other serious illness.

also may raise the blood pressure, but this is rare. Most hypertension is unrelated to any other disease, and the causes of it are unknown. In these instances, it is called **essential hypertension**—not, however, because it is necessary. "Essential" here means "self-existing" or "having no obvious, external cause."

Today's drug treatment of hypertension has produced results that were but a hope twenty years ago. Side effects from drugs have, in re-

cent years, been greatly reduced. It is important that the patient stay on the prescribed medication. Diets to reduce weight may help. Restriction of sodium (found in table salt) may lower blood pressure. For hypertensives, smoking is especially harmful since it further constricts the arteries. Attention to rest and weight, avoidance of tension, and continued use of prescribed drugs can add years to the lives of hypertensive people.

sue to die from lack of oxygen *(cerebral ischemia)*. The result is **paralysis** (loss of muscle function) and **anesthesia** (loss of feeling). Since each of the brain's cerebral hemispheres controls the opposite side of the body, right-sided paralysis indicates left cerebral involvement, and vice versa. With most people the left side of the brain is the area that controls the learning of speech. Damage to that side may deprive a person of the ability to talk. After bleeding of a cerebral artery, and the resultant clotting of the blood, there is often absorption of some of the clot. Pressure on the brain is then relieved, and some recovery is possible. However, unlike the nerve cells and distant nerve fibers (such as those in the muscles or skin), the cells and fibers of the adult central nervous system (brain and spinal cord) may not repair themselves. Some permanent damage is not uncommon.

Occasionally, a hardened and weakened small artery in the brain, under prolonged hypertension, ruptures. A small amount of blood escapes. The individual thus experiences a "little stroke"—a minor,

The Major Cerebrovascular Disease: Stroke

Although cerebrovascular disease has declined somewhat in the past several years, it is still a major threat. **Cerebrovascular accident (CVA)**, also known as *stroke*, kills almost 200,000 people a year in this country (see Table 4–3, page 96). Stroke is a group of signs and symptoms that may occur in different combinations and for a variety of reasons. A cerebral artery may burst as a result of high blood pressure, or the artery may burst be-

cause its wall has been badly weakened by atherosclerosis. Or hypertension and atherosclerosis together may cause the stroke. Bleeding occurs, and a clot on the brain develops. A stroke also occurs when a clot (thrombus) blocks a cerebral artery. A clot or a piece of an atherosclerotic plaque may travel as an embolus from another artery to block the cerebral artery or one of its branches. Such blockage of the blood flow causes some cerebral tis-

passing paralysis. It is a warning. Treatment and rest may delay a more serious stroke for many years; or one may never occur.

Severe strokes may be considered both from the aspects of prevention and of restoration of function (*rehabilitation*). Many stroke patients have no warning signs or symptoms. Weakness of one or more extremities, speech difficulties, and dizziness may be some of the warnings that a major stroke is about to occur. These warnings herald little strokes. By early treatment of little strokes, big strokes can often be prevented. Most stroke victims survive their first major attack. The patient can learn to use undamaged nerve pathways and to strengthen weak muscles. Early and intensive treatment for restoration of function can do much to return stroke victims to useful lives.

Cancer: The Lawless Cells

In a country without a government there is anarchy—no leadership, just lawlessness. No wonder the ancient Greek poet Sophocles had King Creon cry out in the great tragedy *Antigone:* "Anarchy, anarchy! Show me a greater evil!" **Cancer** is cellular anarchy. Its microscopic, greedy lawlessness is contemptuous of body government.

The basic difference between normal cells and tumor cells is that normal cells are controlled. Tumor cells are not. They are both instructed by their hereditary chemicals to divide, but, as we will see, the management of tumor cells has been taken over. Tumor cells are in ecological imbalance with the body that feeds them. Thus, they are doomed, as, too often, is their host.

Tumors Are Benign or Malignant

Tumors, as indicated above, are masses of cells resulting from uncontrolled growth. **Benign** tumors are not cancers. Of themselves, they do not kill. Only by incidentally interfering with function (for example, by obstructing the bowel) can they cause death. Benign tumors are regularly defined and have capsules limiting them. They are thus *localized:* Their surrounding capsule keeps them within bounds. As they grow, they do not penetrate tissues; they simply push against them. Surgically, they may be shelled out of their capsule, and cure results.

Malignant tumors are the cancers. By the very nature of their behavior, they can kill. Originating from the Greek word *karkinos,* meaning "crab," cancers behave like crabs. Not withheld by a capsule, they claw their way along the paths of least resistance, destroying cells in their path. Worse, cancer cells multiply faster than normal cells. And some cancer cells are believed to produce chemicals that stimulate their own blood supply and encourage their spread.

"Solid" and "Generalized" Malignant Tumors

Cancer is a disease of the cell. That is, the first event leading to a cancer is an abnormal change in a single cell. As the abnormally changed cell divides and cell division continues, the abnormal change is continued

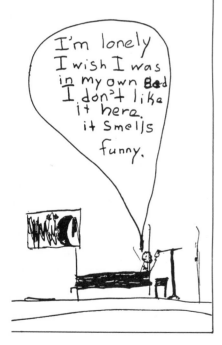

This drawing was made by Dave Martin, age 12. After therapy for a tumor, Dave is fine.

into succeeding generations of cells. The malignant cells may eventually form a mass—a "solid" tumor, or they may at once become "generalized"—widespread throughout the body. More specifically, "solid" tumors come from one source; "generalized" tumors occur all at once and at many sites. These two types are, in turn, classified according to the tissues from which they arise.

THE "SOLID" TUMORS

Carcinomas are the most common form of cancer. They arise from epithelial cells, important as a covering or lining tissue, which exists in numerous forms. Skin is composed of one kind of epithelium; when it becomes cancerous, it is designated as skin carcinoma. Other carcinomas arise from the glandular organs, such as the breast, which are composed of different epithelial tissue, as are the smooth, shiny mucous membranes such as those that line the mouth, stomach, and lungs.

Sarcomas occur less frequently. [These cancers arise] from fibrous (connective) tissue and from muscle, bone, and cartilage. Together, the carcinomas and sarcomas have been classified as "solid" tumors.[3]

"Solid" tumors—the **carcinomas** and the **sarcomas** — often **metastasize**, which means that they break loose from their original sites and travel to other body locations, near and far. Once there, the migrant cells seed new, secondary malignant growths. There are four routes by which cancers metastasize: (1) They can go directly along their paths, destroying tissue that is in their way. (2) They can, by penetrating delicate lymph-channel walls, pass through the lymph channels (see page 94) to set up secondary cancer deposits in nearby and distant lymph nodes. From these sites they might eventually reach the bloodstream via the lymphatic circulation and then endanger other organs. (3) The cancer cells may invade the veins, which are less resistant than the arteries. Following the blood circulatory routes, they can then set up secondary tumors in remote places. That is why a cigarette smoker's cancer is so often fatal. Fooled into thinking that a chronic cough is a "cigarette cough," that the pain in the chest is temporary, the smoker may not see a physician until the lung cancer has spread beyond cure. (4) Lastly, cancer cells may break off from an original location and migrate to the fibrous sacs enclosing the intestines, the lungs, or the heart. Then, after penetrating the sac, they may float in its enclosed fluid, finally settling down on an organ. They can then start a secondary cancerous growth.

THE "GENERALIZED" TUMORS

The "generalized" tumors include the **leukemias** and most of the **lymphomas**. Leukemias are cancers of the blood-forming tissues. Usually generalized from their onset, they are characterized by an uncontrolled multiplication of abnormal white cells. Lymphomas are cancers of some of the infection-fighting structures of the body, such as the lymph nodes. They may begin as a localized disease but often quickly become widespread.

The Causes of Cancer

Some specialists estimate that between 70 and 80 percent of cancer cases can be related to the environment—these include the *physical* and *chemical* causes of cancer. The two other basic categories are the *hereditary* (or *genetic*) and *viral* causes.

PHYSICAL CAUSES

Some substances emit cancer-causing radiations as they degenerate. Such radiation may produce a chemical change in the hereditary structure within a cell. The changed cell may then progress to cancer. Examples of radiation-produced cancers are the lung cancer of uranium miners, the increased leukemia rates among Hiroshima and Nagasaki survivors (the incidence of leukemia among them is five times that of the rest of the Japanese population), the increased incidence of female breast cancer (two to four times) among these same survivors, and the higher leukemia rates among X-ray workers. The sun's ultraviolet light radiation is responsible for most skin cancers (see page 116).

Many people experience the greatest exposure to the sun when they are young. Why, then, do skin cancers appear most often among older people? The answer is "time lag." This long passage of time between exposure to a cancer-causing (**carcinogenic**) agent and the appearance of a cancer is very common. It explains why many cancers occur more often among older people. It also explains why carcinogenic agents are often so difficult to identify. And, finally, it explains why so much research is being directed toward the goal of finding out which physical and chemical agents cause changes in an experimental culture of cells. Most cancer-causing chemicals produce changes in the hereditary make-up of cells. (However not all genetically

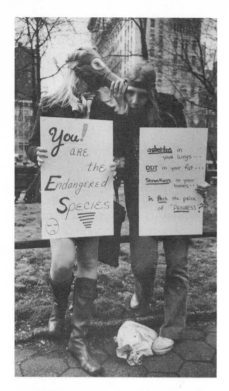

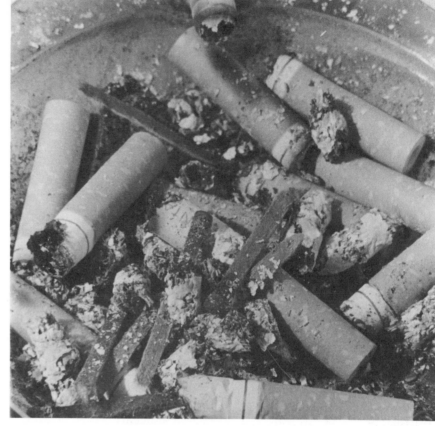

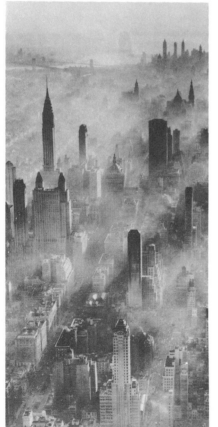

PHOTO ESSAY
Cancer-causing agents are not always as easy to identify—or to avoid—as are those found in cigarettes. They also are present in the sun's rays and in much of the air we breathe, and they contaminate many of our workplaces.

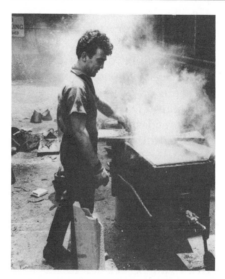

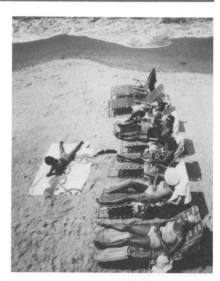

changed cells are cancerous.) An early step in such research is to find out what a certain agent does to bacterial cell-culture systems. These systems are made up of media designed specifically for the growth of certain bacteria.

CHEMICAL CAUSES

Sometimes chemicals combine with physical injuries, particularly burns, to cause cancer. In Panama, some washerwomen smoke cigarettes with the lit end inside their mouths. Among them, mouth cancers are frequent.

Today, people are virtually surrounded by possible chemical carcinogens. The air is the most notable example. Although scientists have not yet reached a final conclusion about the effect of atmospheric pollution, recent research suggests that smog may be one of the causes of cancer. Industries that use coal tar and chemicals made from it present dangers for their employees; these elements are the largest single source of occupationally induced cancers. Other likely cancer agents are the chemicals used in the rubber and cable industries. Alcohol can also be a carcinogen: Deaths from cancers of the mouth, pharynx, larynx, esophagus, and liver have been associated with heavy drinking.

HEREDITARY CAUSES

Very few cancers result from strictly hereditary or genetic causes. Those that are hereditary include an uncommon tumor of the eye's retina and one of the nervous system, each of which is determined by a specific gene. Certain cancers seem to happen more often in some families. Statistically, female relatives (particularly sisters) of breast cancer pa-

tients have two to three times the tendency to develop the disease as do other women. But the higher-risk group also includes other factors. Among these are early onset of menstruation, menstruating for more than thirty years, having done little or no breast feeding, having had few or no pregnancies, and having had some previous breast disease. So a lot of variables are involved. One could hardly suggest that a woman with one of these variables will always develop breast cancer. But several or all of them together make for a "high-risk" woman.

VIRUSES AND NONHUMAN CANCERS

In 1911, medical researcher Peyton Rous showed that chickens developed certain tumors from viruses. But little attention was paid to his work. Years later, others were able to show that a virus from a mouse produced cancers in rats, guinea pigs, hamsters, and other animals. A new research race was on. And perhaps to mark it, fifty-five years after his original work, Rous was awarded the Nobel Prize.

It is understandable that a possible solution to part of the cancer riddle is being sought by some scientists working with viruses. It has been said that cancer is a disease of the cell. And in Chapter 3 it was pointed out that viruses are obliged to multiply in living cells. Like all viruses, the viruses that can cause animal cancers consist of a protein overcoat and a core of hereditary chemicals, DNA or RNA (never both). Remember that the protein overcoat is the part of the virus that gives it specificity as an antigen—that is, that determines the disease the virus causes—and it is the core

A hero of cancer research: the guinea pig.

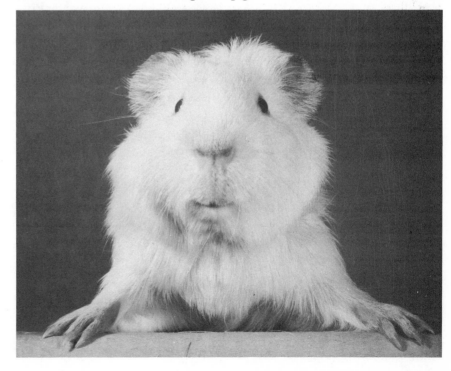

TABLE 4-4
Cancer: Estimated Casualty Figures for 1979, Warning Signals, and Safeguards[1]

SITE	ESTIMATED NEW CASES 1979	ESTIMATED DEATHS 1979	WARNING SIGNAL (IF YOU HAVE ONE, SEE YOUR DOCTOR)	SAFEGUARDS	COMMENT
Breast	107,000	35,000	Lump or thickening in the breast; unusual discharge from nipple.	Regular check-up; monthly breast self-exam.	The leading cause of cancer death in women.
Colon and Rectum	112,000	52,000	Change in bowel habits; bleeding.	Regular check-up, including digital, occult blood, and proctoscopic exams, especially after age 40.	Because of accuracy of available tests, potentially a highly curable disease.
Lung	112,000	98,000	Persistent cough; lingering respiratory ailment.	80% of lung cancer would be prevented if no one smoked cigarettes.	The leading cause of cancer death among men and rising mortality among women.
Oral (including pharynx)	24,000	9,000	Sore that does not heal; difficulty in swallowing.	Regular check-up.	Many more lives should be saved because the mouth is easily accessible to visual examination by physicians and dentists.
Skin	14,000[2]	6,000	Sore that does not heal; change in wart or mole.	Regular check-up; avoidance of over-exposure to sun.	Skin cancer is readily detected by observation and diagnosed by simple biopsy.
Uterus	53,000[3]	11,000	Unusual bleeding or discharge.	Regular check-up, including pelvic examination with pap test.	Uterine cancer mortality has declined 70% during the last 40 years with wider application of the pap test. Postmenopausal women with abnormal bleeding should be checked.
Kidney and Bladder	51,000	18,000	Urinary difficulty, bleeding—in which case consult doctor at once.	Regular check-up with urinalysis.	Protective measures for workers in high-risk industries are helping to eliminate one of the important causes of these cancers.
Larynx	10,000	3,500	Hoarseness; difficulty in swallowing.	Regular check-up, including laryngoscopy.	Readily curable if caught early.
Prostate	64,000	21,000	Urinary difficulty.	Regular check-up, including palpation.	Occurs mainly in men over 60. The disease can be detected by palpation at regular check-up.
Stomach	23,000	14,000	Indigestion.	Regular check-up.	An 80% decline in mortality in 50 years, for reasons yet unknown.
Leukemia	22,000	15,000	Leukemia is a cancer of blood-forming tissues and is characterized by the abnormal production of immature white blood cells. Acute lymphocytic leukemia strikes mainly children and is treated by drugs that have extended life from a few months to as much as ten years. Chronic leukemia strikes usually after age 25 and progresses less rapidly.		
Lymphomas	39,000	20,000	These cancers arise in the lymph system and include Hodgkin's disease and lymphosarcoma. Some patients with lymphatic cancers can lead normal lives for many years. Five-year survival rate for Hodgkin's disease increased from 25% to 54% in 20 years.		

1. All figures have been rounded to the nearest thousand.
2. The estimated new cases of nonmelanoma skin cancer are over 300,000.
3. If carcinoma in situ is included, cases total over 98,000.

SOURCE: American Cancer Society, *Cancer Facts & Figures 1979*. Incidence estimates are based on rates from National Cancer Institute SEER Program 1973–1976. Reprinted by permission of American Cancer Society, Inc.

of the hereditary chemicals that determines the actual cellular infection.

Now, consider an animal cell instead of a virus. Within the nucleus of the animal cell, there are hereditary chemicals called **chromosomes.** Chromosomes are made up of **genes,** and genes are made up of DNA. In the animal cell it is the DNA that directs the formation of RNA. Note that the core of a DNA virus contains hereditary chemicals that are basically similar to the nuclear core of ordinary animal cells. Thus some DNA viruses can enter nonhuman animal cells and compete with the cellular DNA to cause cancer. How, then, may RNA viruses cause nonhuman animal cancers? It has been discovered that a chemical complex known as *reverse transcriptase* can produce DNA from the RNA of certain viruses. Thus, DNA formed from the RNA of tumor viruses may become part of a cell's DNA.

So, in nonhuman animals, cancer-causing viruses with either DNA or RNA move into an animal cell, become a part of the cell's DNA, and then, after lying inactive for a while, are "switched on" by some stimulus to direct the cell to disaster. The stimulus may be radiation or a chemical or perhaps another virus. This taking over of the functions of the cell's DNA by viral hereditary chemicals robs the cell of its ability to direct its original destiny to make healthy cellular protein. The ability of healthy cells to stick to one another is also lost. In short, viral DNA, or viral RNA that can produce DNA, upsets all the normal life processes of the cell. In doing so the viral intruders use the cell's structures. The cellular DNA can now send only messages of malignancy. Cells made malignant divide into malignant daughter cells that carry the deadly instructions of their parent cells, including the capacity for uncontrolled growth. A cancer is born.

Are Cancers Communicable?

Some one hundred different viruses (both DNA and RNA) have been proved to cause cancer in various species of nonhuman creatures. But are these cancer viruses contagious? Studies suggest that chickens spread a leukemia virus to other chickens, and cats transmit a leukemia virus to other cats, but neither transmit their virus to humans. Do cancer viruses spread among human beings? As of early 1980, there was no evidence to show that viruses spread cancers among human beings. Moreover, no virus has yet been proved to cause human cancer. Indeed, some researchers have given up the hope of finding a virus that causes breast cancer. Yet viruses may play a role in at least some cancers. Exactly what that role might be, though, is still unknown.

The Extent of the Cancer Problem

For thirty years cancer has ranked second only to heart disease as the leading cause of death in the United States. At present rates, over fifty-five million people in this country—one person in four—will develop cancer. In early 1979 the American Cancer Society made its annual—and usually devastatingly accurate—prediction of cancer casualties (Table 4–4). In 1979 the estimated number of new cancer cases in the United States was 765,000. Figure 4–13 gives a break-down of the rate at which various kinds of cancers are expected to occur in both men and women.

There has been a startling increase in cancer among blacks. No comparable increase of cancer among whites of either gender has been noted. Why the sharp increase in cancer mortality among U.S. blacks? One reason may be increased exposure in the past twenty years to urban pollutants and industrial carcinogens. A greater degree of unemployment and less educational opportunities, resulting in delayed diagnoses, might be other reasons. As employment and educational opportunities increase for blacks in this country, more will certainly seek regular medical examinations and profit from the benefits of early diagnosis and treatment.

Information going back thirty years shows that in the first year of treatment for cancer, poor patients do not live as long as the comparatively well-to-do. This may be due, in part, to the fact that poor patients seek treatment later in the course of their disease than do wealthier patients. However, after the first year of treatment, poor, nonpaying patients do live as long as patients who can afford to pay their health-care expenses. Such information emphasizes once again the great need for better health education and for easily available health services for the poor.

Prevention and Early Detection of Cancer

Using health education techniques as a common denominator, any disease prevention program is concerned with the *prevention of its occurrence* and, failing in this, *pre-*

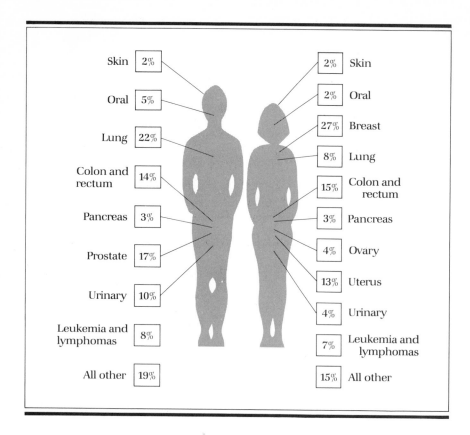

Skin	2%		2%	Skin
Oral	5%		2%	Oral
			27%	Breast
Lung	22%		8%	Lung
Colon and rectum	14%		15%	Colon and rectum
Pancreas	3%		3%	Pancreas
			4%	Ovary
Prostate	17%		13%	Uterus
Urinary	10%		4%	Urinary
Leukemia and lymphomas	8%		7%	Leukemia and lymphomas
All other	19%		15%	All other

FIGURE 4–13
1979 estimates of cancer incidence by site and sex. Not included here are nonmelanoma skin cancer and carcinoma in situ of the uterine cervix.

vention of its progression. Three basic recommendations are offered to help prevent the occurrence of cancer: (1) avoidance of those ecological factors associated with a high incidence of certain cancers; (2) removal of lesions that, although not yet malignant, may become cancers; and (3) discouragement of marriages that would produce children with a high risk of developing cancers (although, as emphasized earlier, such strictly "hereditary" cancers are very rare).

Consider a few *ecological factors.* Excessive, long-term exposure to sunlight is a major cause of *skin cancer,* especially among fair people. Although it has a 95-percent cure rate, skin cancer is the most common cancer and still causes about six thousand deaths a year in this country. It usually occurs in people over fifty. People who must spend a lot of time outdoors should consult their physicians for the most effective sunscreen preparations.

Two factors associated with a high incidence of *cancer of the uterine cervix* are unusually frequent sexual intercourse at an early age and poor hygiene of the external genitalia. Promiscuity or an early marriage may account for the first of these. Poor personal hygiene, particularly in some uncircumcised males, results in the collection under the covering penile skin fold (the *prepuce*) of a thick, creamy, ill-

smelling secretion called *smegma.* With the female it may collect around the clitoris. Smegma has been shown to cause cancer in animals. Some (but not all) cancer experts agree that women whose husbands are circumcised (and who are, therefore, able to practice more thorough personal hygiene) have a much lower incidence of cervical cancer than women whose husbands are not circumcised. A simple, painless examination of vaginal fluid, the **Papanicolaou (Pap) test** (named after its originator, Dr. George Papanicolaou), provides excellent diagnostic information about cervical cancer. The Pap test must be a routine part of a woman's physical examination.

Cigarette smoking causes *lung cancer,* which is among the least curable of all cancers. Cigarette smoking is, moreover, associated with an increased incidence of other malignancies, such as those of the mouth and urinary bladder. Cigarette smoking is killing people, and it should be condemned. But despite the widely published findings that confirm this fact, cigarette sales are higher than ever. However, the *per capita* consumption has been gradually decreasing. In 1978, for example, the number of cigarettes purchased per person per year (based on the entire U.S. population) declined to 4,000 from 4,148 in 1973. Moreover, some progress has been made in this country in manufacturing a "safer" cigarette, that is, one with less tar, nicotine, and other harmful substances.[4] By no means, however, is there yet a completely safe cigarette.

Much has been accomplished in terms of removing cancer-causing agents from industrial environments, but much remains to be done. For example, workers and other people exposed to *asbestos*

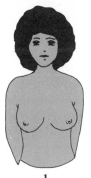 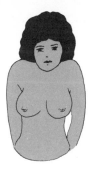 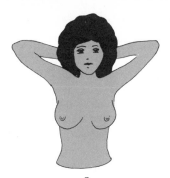 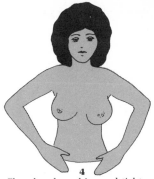

1
Stand with arms down.

2
Lean forward.

3
Raise arms overhead and press hands behind your head.

4
Place hands on hips and tighten chest and arm muscles by pressing firmly inward.

Breast Self-examination
**Follow these steps to examine your breasts regularly once a month.
This is best done after the menstrual period.**

Looking: Stand in front of a mirror with the upper body unclothed. Look for changes in the shape and size of the breast and for dimpling of the skin or "pulling in" of the nipples. Be aware, too, of any discharge from the nipples or scaling of the skin of the nipples. Abnormality in the breast may be accentuated by a change in position of the body and arms.

Feeling: Lie flat on your back with a pillow or folded towel under your shoulders and feel each breast with the opposite hand in sequence. With the hand slightly cupped, feel for lumps or any change in the texture of the breast or skin; also, note any discharge from nipples. Avoid compressing the breast between the thumb and fingers as this may give the impression of a lump which is not actually there.

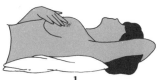 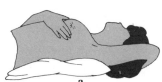 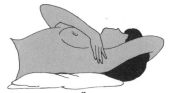 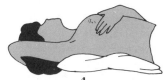

1
Place the left arm overhead. With the right hand, feel the inner half of the left breast from top to bottom and from nipple to breastbone.

2
Feel the outer half from bottom to top and from the nipple to the side of the chest.

3
Pay special attention to the area between the breast and armpit including the armpit itself.

4
Repeat this same process for the right breast using your left hand to feel.

Source: Breast Self-Examination, U.S. Department of Health, Education, and Welfare, Public Health Service, National Institutes of Health, DHEW Publication No. (NIH) 76-649.

fibers and uranium miners exposed to *ionizing radiation* have higher than average lung cancer rates.

Precancerous lesions always indicate an immediate, often lifesaving visit to the family physician. The warning signals listed in Table 4–4 may indicate not cancer, but a cellular change that may become malignant if neglected.

All women must be on constant guard against breast cancer. At the end of each menstrual period (but continuing after the menopause), self-examination of both breasts must be a regular part of every woman's life. A woman who habitually examines her breasts over the years becomes increasingly aware of subtle changes in them that otherwise might go unnoticed. The self-examination procedure is described in the accompanying boxed insert.

Since early breast cancer is usually painless, any change in the breast, particularly a lump or a thickening, merits immediate consultation with the family physician. These routine self-examinations supplement, but do not replace, periodic physical examinations by a physician. New X-ray techniques are available that can detect breast tumors that are not otherwise noticeable. One of these techniques is called *mammography.*

Mammography is a special kind of breast X-ray that has been the subject of much discussion among medical people. The claim had been made that the examination itself could cause breast cancer. Late in 1977, a conference of experts was held by the U.S. National Institutes of Health. It was decided that mammography could safely be used, along with a physical examination, in women over fifty. *Routine* mammography screening for the average woman under fifty was not indicated. Between the ages of forty and forty-nine, mammography should be used only with women who have already had a breast cancer or whose mothers or sisters have developed the disease. Between the ages of thirty-five and thirty-nine, only women who have had the disease should be screened, and women under the age of thirty-five were generally not to be given this particular test. However, the word "generally" is important. When a physician strongly feels that a patient may have a breast cancer, mammography should be used at any age.

Added to traditional X-ray for detection of tumors is a *computerized scanning* machine. This device is of special use in locating tiny tumors in the brain and in other areas of the body that are hard to see by X-ray. Some *radioactive substances* also concentrate around certain tumors and make them more visible. Cancer cells contain antigens, and some may be detected in the bloodstream by special techniques.

The major element preventing the progression of any cancer is early diagnosis. Among the most common internal cancers are those of the rectum and colon. Delay may mean death. Early diagnosis can mean cure. Using a recently improved instrument for seeing the affected area with little or no discomfort to the patient, doctors can now diagnose almost three-fourths

of these conditions early enough for successful treatment.

In the race for life, cancer always has a head start. But it need not win. "Through early diagnosis and prompt treatment of cancer, the present survival ratio could be one in two."[5]

All physicians have a high index of suspicion. They must in order to begin a time-consuming but always worthwhile investigation. If a cancer is localized, they can offer hope. If it has escaped from its origin, if there is regional involvement,

hope lessens. For example, if cancer of the breast is localized, the five-year survival rate is 85 to 90 percent, but only 40 to 45 percent of the women with regional involvement are alive at the end of five years. (Figure 4–14 plots the five-year survival rates for various cancers.)

If cancer is found during a routine physical examination in a person without signs or symptoms, the outlook for a five-year cure is brightest. Breast cancer, for example, if diagnosed before signs or symptoms appear, has as much as a 34-percent

FIGURE 4–14
Five-year cancer survival rates for selected sites (adjusted for normal life expectancy). Diagnosis before the cancer spreads is lifesaving.

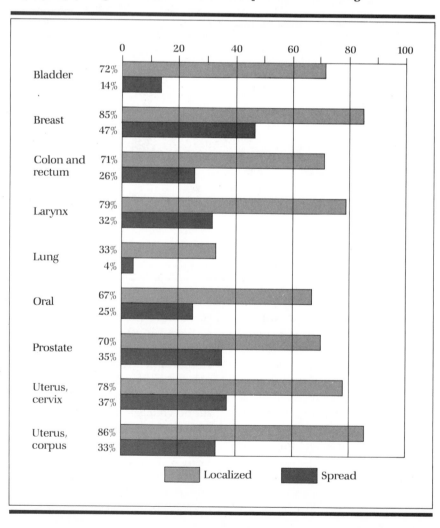

better chance of cure than if diagnosed after the appearance of signs and symptoms. Similarly improved chances for cure also apply to other cancers.

Every family doctor's office is a cancer detection center. His or her routine physical examinations for cancer save countless lives. Moreover, many communities sponsor cancer detection programs. These provide routine cancer examinations for those without symptoms. A cancer detection program, provided for all, could save approximately eighty thousand lives a year in this country.

"Many cancers run their course from 'early operable, easily removable and highly curable' to 'advanced stage . . . , inoperable and incurable' in the course of less than a year."[6] The tumor may have been present for many years, but the changes in it from curable to incurable may occur in less than one. One cannot overestimate the importance of immediate attention to early signs and symptoms, regular breast examinations, and thorough routine physical examinations.

The Treatment of Cancer

Today, cancers are treated by *surgical removal*, *radiation*, or *drugs*. Sometimes all three treatments are combined. Surgery and radiation are far more successful if the cancer is localized. The usefulness of radiation is limited because often the amount needed to destroy all the cancer cells may also destroy normal tissue. However, with some cancers radiation specialists are today achieving remarkable results. In one type of leukemia, a combination of drugs and intensive central nervous system irradiation has given years of life to many young people. **Hodgkin's disease**, a progressive and painful enlargement of lymph nodes, spleen, and other lymphoid tissue, used to be always fatal. Today, early diagnosis, irradiation, surgical removal of the spleen, and a combination of drugs have brought prolonged life, even apparent cure, to numerous victims. A combination of chemicals (**chemotherapy**) following surgery appears promising in the treatment of breast cancer.

THE IMMUNE RESPONSE AND HEAT THERAPY AS CANCER TREATMENTS: STILL EXPERIMENTAL

More than a century ago it was noted that some cancers seemed to disappear after an acute bacterial infection. Could the *immune response* be responsible? The immune response is generally considered to be any reaction involving a specific antibody response to an antigen, or a specifically changed reaction of a host's cells, following stimulation by a foreign antigen. Treatment that stimulates the immune response may one day benefit some cancer patients. Today, experience with organ transplant failures is an added dividend in the search. Recall from Chapter 3's discussion that organ transplants are foreign invaders and that they are rejected because the "killer" white blood cells (certain lymphocytes of the recipient—see page 59) attack the antigens that are on their surfaces. Thus, a person who receives a transplant must take certain drugs that depress the natural immune response. But such a patient is more prone to develop cancer, possibly because the immune response that would control a cancer has been suppressed.

It is now known that certain antigens are on the surface of cancer cells that are not present on normal cells. It is believed that the immune system can recognize these cancer antigens. Efforts to stimulate the immune response, exciting as some of them are, must still be regarded as experimental. Immunotherapy is hardly a guaranteed cure for cancer.

Heat treatment (thermotherapy) for cancer is being used in several famous clinics in this country. The heat may be generated in a variety of ways, including microwaves and ultrasound (high-power energy produced by soundlike waves above those that can be heard by people). The temperature used must be measured with extreme precision. Thermotherapy is being tried for cancers of local surface areas, various regions of the body, and even the whole body. *Patients must be referred to these clinics by a physician.* Results of thermotherapy, especially for body-surface tumors seem most promising.[7]

POSSIBILITIES FOR DETECTION, TREATMENT, AND CURE

The search for a solution will yield no single method of detection, no single treatment, no single cure for so complex a group of diseases. Despite the poor results with some cancers, the picture is by no means all gloomy. The Pap smear and better personal hygiene are together responsible for a remarkable decline in the death rate from cancer of the cervix and uterus. In forty years the death rate from uterine cancer has dropped about 65 percent. Since the 1930s the incidence of cancer of the stomach in both men and women has declined almost 70 percent. Drug treatment is now a basic factor responsible for long-term survival in at least ten types of widespread cancer occurring largely in children, adolescents, and young adults.

Various agencies of the United States government have ordered that many industrial carcinogens be banned from use. The use of some possibly cancer-causing pesticides and food additives is being sharply limited. Allowable levels of radiation exposure have been lowered. As has been stated, there is even evidence that the number of nonsmokers in the nation is increasing. If continued, this may eventually result in a decline of lung cancer.

There is still work to do—but there is also hope.

Summary

In the United States today, the *chronic degenerative diseases* are the major health problem. Among the major chronic diseases are those of the *cardiovascular system*, kidney disease, and cancer.

To understand cardiovascular disease, it is necessary to know the structure of the heart and circulatory system. Blood is a tissue composed of a liquid, called *plasma*, with millions of cells—*erythrocytes, leukocytes*, and *platelets*—suspended in it. Also in the blood are certain antigens and antibodies that determine one's blood type and the compatibility of one person's blood with another's. The blood is carried away from the heart by *arteries*, which branch into smaller *arterioles*, and eventually into *capillaries*. Through the walls of the capillaries the blood cells give up oxygen and other life-giving needs to the tissue cells and pick up carbon dioxide and other death-dealing wastes from them. Then the blood returns to the heart through the *venules* and the *veins*. The heart is a double pump made up of the *atria*, which receive blood, and the *ventricles*, which actually pump blood to the lungs and to the general body circulation. A *conducting system*, controlled by the *pacemaker*, keeps the heart's contractions in proper rhythm. Another circulatory system is the lymphatic drainage system, which returns to blood circulation those fluids that leak from the capillaries — *lymph* — and molecules of material too large to enter the capillaries, such as bits of cells. Wastes are filtered out of this *lymph* fluid by the *lymph nodes* and destroyed there.

Atherosclerosis is the major impediment to blood flow, causing blockage. It is the usual precursor of such heart conditions as cardiac and cerebral *ischemia*, coronary artery disease, and other conditions resulting from the obstruction of blood flow through the arteries. The process of atherosclerosis begins when there is an excess of *cholesterol* in the blood. (*Triglycerides* are also involved.) The low-density *lipoproteins* will carry this excess cholesterol to the arteries and deposit it there. This irritates the arterial lining, and extra smooth muscle cells of the artery migrate there to form a *lesion*. Red blood cells gather about this irritated area, and the platelets, a blood component, cause a clot to form. This *thrombus* (clot) or a piece of the atherosclerotic *plaque* can break loose and travel, as an *embolus*, to a smaller artery.

Some of the conditions that arise from blockage of a *coronary artery* are acute myocardial infarction, a pain called angina pectoris, disturbances of the heartbeat rhythm, and congestive heart failure.

In this culture atherosclerosis is an ordinary process of aging, but those who exercise, do not smoke, eat a diet low in saturated fats and cholesterol, and control high blood pressure can often successfully control this disease process.

Many heart conditions are not due basically to atherosclerosis. These include the *congenital heart defects*, rheumatic heart disease, and heart disease due to hypertension or to metabolic and endocrine disorders.

The kidneys filter wastes from the blood. The functioning unit of the kidneys is the *nephron*. Within each nephron is a *glomerulus*, or coil of capillaries, surrounded by a capsule into which fluid containing wastes passes. As this fluid moves through the tubules of the nephron, the wastes are removed from it. Then most of the fluid is reabsorbed through special tiny vessels back into the body. One type of kidney dysfunction, hypertensive kidney disease, may cause certain types of heart failure.

Cerebrovascular accidents, or strokes, which are associated with *cerebrovascular disease*, occur when a cerebral artery bursts or becomes blocked by a thrombus or embolus. *Hypertension* can occur without a known cause. Atherosclerosis can cause hypertension, and both conditions can result in a stroke. *Paralysis* and *anesthesia* are common results of a stroke, but rehabilitation to regain function is often successful.

Another major chronic disease is *cancer*, which results when cells divide uncontrollably. *Malignant* cancer *tumors* may be solid, such as the *carcinomas* and *sarcomas*, or generalized throughout the body, as with the *leukemias* and most *lymphomas*. But even solid tumors may *metastasize*, or spread throughout the body.

Cancer can be caused by environmental factors such as radiation and chemicals. There are also a few types known to be hereditary. Viruses are also suspected of having a role in the development of this group of diseases.

Cancer is a primary cause of death in the United States. But its occurrence can often be prevented by avoiding exposure to known irritants, such as sunlight (in too great amounts), cigarettes, and industrial *carcinogens* like asbestos fibers. Routine self-examination for breast cancer can lead to early detection of tumors; chances of recovery are then much greater. Many cancers can be successfully combated by the combined approach of surgical removal of the tumor, radiation, and *chemotherapy*.

References

1. Caleb Hillier Parry, *An Inquiry Into the Symptoms and Causes of the Syncope Angiosa, Commonly Called Angina Pectoris*, quoted in Henry J. Speedby, *The 20th Century and Your Heart* (London, 1960), p. 84.
2. Homer W. Smith, *From Fish to Philosopher* (Boston, 1953), p. 4.
3. *Progress Against Cancer 1969: A Report by the National Advisory Cancer Council*, National Cancer Institute, U.S. Department of Health, Education, and Welfare, pp. 52–53.
4. E. L. Wynder and D. Hoffman, "Tobacco and Health," *The New England Journal of Medicine*, Vol. 300 (April 19, 1979), p. 898.
5. CA—A Cancer Journal for Clinicians, Vol. 18 (January–February 1968), p. 13.
6. Francis D. Moore, "Hesitation and Delay as a Social Phenomenon," *New England Journal of Medicine*, Vol. 289 (July 5, 1973), p. 41.
7. David N. Leff, "Hyperthermia: Hottest News in Cancer Therapy," *Medical World News*, Vol. 20 (May 14, 1979), pp. 52ff.

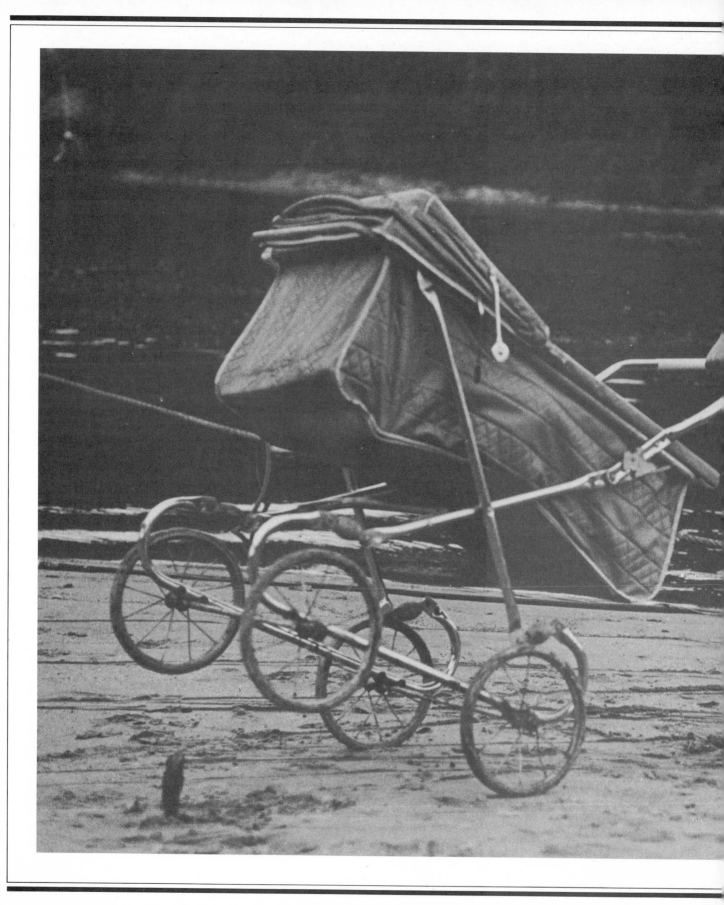

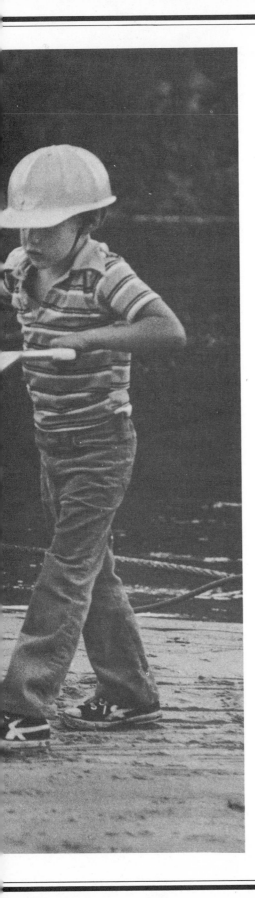

5

The Emotional Life: Part I

Personality Development

About Freud's Concepts

Maslow's Theory: A Step-by-Step Pyramid to Self-actualization

Erikson's Theory: Eight Stages of Personality Development
The Infant: Basic Trust Versus Basic Mistrust
The Toddler: Autonomy Versus Shame and Doubt
The Preschooler: Initiative Versus Guilt
The School-age Child: Industry Versus Inferiority
Adolescence: Identity Versus Role Confusion
Early Adulthood: Intimacy Versus Isolation
Middle Adulthood: Generativity Versus Stagnation
Late Adulthood: Integrity Versus Despair

Personality Disorders and Emotional Problems
The Limits of Labels
"He Who Can Simulate Sanity Will Be Sane"
An Overview of Emotional Disorders

The Nervous System: Its Functions and Chemistry
How Nerve Cells Communicate with One Another
Chemical Neurotransmitters and Emotional Disorders: The Drug Connection

Aging
Some Problems of the Aged
Some Myths about the Aged

Death: "The Birthday of Your Eternity"
The Silent Minority
Dying: A Life Process

Summary

Personality Development

And if the soul
is to know itself
it must look
into a soul:
the stranger and enemy, we've seen
*   him in the mirror.*[1]

Begin at the beginning. Begin with the birth of the baby. This time the newborn is a boy. He can suck and he can look, but not at the same time. Through eyes vacant like tiny unwashed windows, he is aware of light and dark. He can cry and perhaps raise his head a trifle. Although six months will pass before a tooth will be seen, he has an immediate sweet tooth. He dislikes bitters. He can smell, and even before he was born he could hear. Three to ten minutes after he is born, he will turn his eyes toward a sound. He can feel pressure and warmth and cold. He can cough and sneeze. For a day or two, he will eliminate a blackish-green material called *meconium* from his rectum. This matter was formed during life within the uterus, when trial secretions of his digestive glands mixed with swallowed fluid. In a few days he will eat. Most of the time his gut will be able to push the food down, but sometimes he will spit it up. It will be months before he can suck and look at the same time.

During his first day, he will pass between one-half and one and one-half ounces of urine. This amount will increase. His heart beats about 150 times a minute, and he breathes 30 to 50 times a minute. If his head was born first, as is ordinarily the case, he was probably breathing even before he was completely out of the womb. At about six weeks he can smile, and not because of a gas pain but because he knows pleasure.

If infants do not weep at birth, they are often spanked until they do. But whatever the reason for that first cry, it heralds the change from a watery to an earthly life — an evolutionary change that required millions of years. After his first crying spell, the infant sleeps. When he awakens, he cries again. No other creature can howl so mightily at such a tender age. What are the roots of his suffering? This is among the questions we seek to answer in this chapter.

Collecting stress and distress, often the child reaches adulthood only to feel like Shakespeare's Antonio in *The Merchant of Venice:*

In sooth, I know not why I am so
*   sad.*
It wearies me, you say it wearies
*   you;*
But how I caught it, found it, or
*   came by it,*
What stuff 'tis made of, whereof
*   it is born,*
I am to learn.
And such a want-wit sadness
*   makes of me*
That I have much ado to know
*   myself.*

What sadness makes Antonio feel a "want-wit"? What is the root of his anguish? In every time, in every tongue, in every lonely troubled corner on earth, this bewilderment has been uttered. Why? Before the work of Sigmund Freud there were few answers.

About Freud's Concepts

About the middle of the nineteenth century, the modern era of medicine began. Great discoveries in the natural sciences by Mendel, Darwin, Pasteur, Koch, and others formed the backdrop for the Freudian stage. Sigmund Freud began his career with significant discoveries about the anatomy of the nervous system and went on to revolutionize the investigation of human emotions. Before his death, in 1939, he had become one of the most influential thinkers in history.

Freud's concepts were fundamentally ecological. He began by calling attention to the child. He believed that within each child are basic unconscious instinctual drives that are both sexual and aggressive. But the child must develop in a world of reality, which imposes its own demands. Of these the child must grow conscious. When the unconscious demands of instinct conflict with the conscious demands of reality, the child experiences *anxiety*. This emotional state occurs when the **conscience** exerts its influence. The conscience is the unconscious

and powerful ally of reality: It sets limits on instinctual demands in accordance with the demands of reality. Thus, the child's conscious life of reality is caught between the twin pincers of powerful unconscious forces—basic instinctual drives and an altogether human conscience. From the constant coping negotiations between the developing child and the demanding environment, human personality results. With severe emotional trauma, or with serious, unresolved conflicts and crises, the child's personality development lags. The resultant adult behaves like a child. The adult personality, then, is molded by the way the child learns to cope with the stresses of childhood. "Pubescence," Freud wrote, "is an act of nature; adolescence is an act of man." In this way Freud emphasized the difference between merely growing and growing up. Moreover, Freud taught that the conflicting stresses of childhood can be modified, and therefore the patterns of behavior that are developed as reactions to conflict and stress can also be

changed. Ineffectual responses to early painful stress, which remain deeply buried in the unconscious for long periods of time, often are the cause of later emotional problems. Answers may come from uncovering, confronting, and resolving the original conflicts. This is the aim of traditional Freudian therapy.

As is true with most original thinkers, Freud had, and has, many followers, imitators, and critics. Some rejected all or parts of his theories; others emphasized one part over another. Freud, too, frequently revised his own thinking. It cannot be the purpose of this section to review all the changes and developments that resulted from Freudian beginnings. However, the work of two people, Abraham Maslow and Erik Erikson, can be taken as examples. In addition, we will explore some recent, though incomplete, studies which suggest that some chemical-biological balances may play a role in emotional health. These will be discussed later. Consider now some of the thoughts of Maslow and Erikson.

Maslow's Theory:
A Step-by-Step Pyramid to Self-actualization

Freud, whose training was in medicine, became a therapist. Maslow was trained to be a therapist. As a student of the mind his ideas about human motivation were inspiring and generous. Within all people, he theorized, was a Valhalla of good. That is, everyone possesses an inborn desire to find truth,

goodness, and beauty. In addition, humans seek to get the most out of their uniqueness as individuals, meaning that there is a desire to fulfill all possibilities, to be creative, and to come as close as possible to a human ideal. For Maslow, human needs or motives develop in a series of step-like stages leading to the top

of a pyramid (see Figure 5–1). Maslow theorized that the attainment of each successive step depended on the conquering of the step before. One starts with the basics.

The bottom step has to do with body functioning, or *physiology*. Such basic human needs as hunger, thirst, and sexuality have to be met.

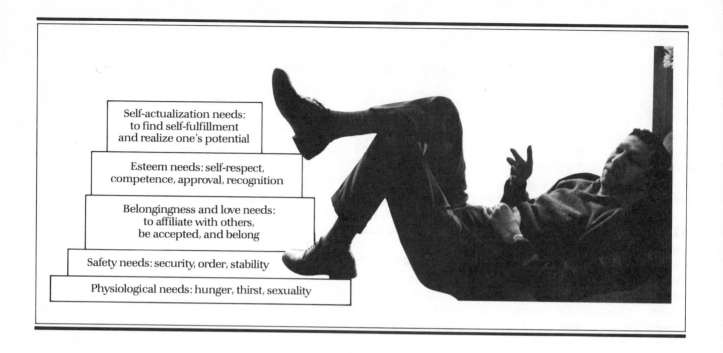

FIGURE 5–1
**Abraham Maslow and his pyramid
of needs.**

Self-actualization needs:
to find self-fulfillment
and realize one's potential

Esteem needs: self-respect,
competence, approval, recognition

Belongingness and love needs:
to affiliate with others,
be accepted, and belong

Safety needs: security, order, stability

Physiological needs: hunger, thirst, sexuality

Only then can the second step, that of *safety*, be reached. By safety Maslow meant a sense of order, of stability, and of security. These having been met, a person can then manage the third step of the pyramid of needs—a sense of *belonging* and *love*. The fourth step is the level of *self-esteem*. This has to do with the self-respect that comes with a feeling of achievement in life. The highest plateau of Maslow's pyramid of motives is that of *self-actualization*. Self-actualized individuals have made the most of their creative potential. They accept the worth of the self and the value of others, and they find living to be a rich experience. Self-actualized people are attuned to life's meanings and mysteries. They find amusement in its comedy and are not hopelessly embittered by its tragedy. They find their work meaningful and are content. They are what they could become.

Maslow was hardly blind to life's realities, however. He was no idle dreamer and was fully aware that self-actualization was a high goal. But he believed it was a goal that can be reached. He understood all the disappointments, disadvantages, and emotional privations that make the goal difficult, even unreachable, for many, if not most, people. Yet he believed that even though the final step might never be attained in totality, many people can—and do—achieve moments of self-actualization throughout the course of their lives.

To many psychologists Maslow's concepts are almost like a religion. Others consider them far too optimistic. It has been said that "the optimist proclaims that we live in the best of all possible worlds, and the pessimist fears this is true." Yet it cannot be denied that there is much food for thought in Maslow's recipe of life. Is it not a concept of hope, that the best of humankind can and will prevail? "There is," said Mark Twain, "no sadder sight than a young pessimist." To this he might well have added older people too.

Erikson's Theory:
Eight Stages of Personality Development

Among the most influential of Western psychologists who built on part of Freud's theoretical ideas is Erik Erikson. Like Freud, Erikson is aware that human behavior is created by and helps to create its own environment. His schema of personality development provides useful and sensible ideas about the flow of events through which people must live in order to reach emotional maturity.

Erikson believes that every human being's personality develops in eight stages, each of which takes place during a particular age. In each stage the individual is faced with a specific task that must be satisfactorily resolved before he or she can enter healthily into the next stage. If the task is not successfully resolved, the individual is ill-equipped to handle the task of the next stage. Future attempts to resolve tasks are hampered by the emotional impediments created by past failure. To heal these wounds to the personality, the individual needs help. Adequate help at critical times stabilizes the individual. Preparation for the next stage and the transition into it are then accomplished with a greater sense of personal competence and security. Without help, the person's inadequately resolved tasks turn into cumulative emotional scars that may result in personality disorders.

Each of Erikson's eight stages is named for the task that must be confronted. The name identifies both the desirable resolution of the task and the contrary development that takes place if the task is not resolved. The desirable resolution of

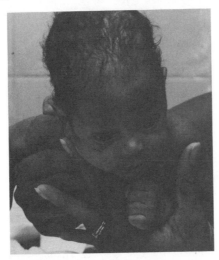

The infant: "...completely self-centered yet utterly dependent."

the task of the first of the eight stages, for example, is *basic trust*. Its contrary development is *basic mistrust*. Thus the first stage is named *basic trust versus basic mistrust*. But there are no sharp dividing lines between Erikson's stages. During the later stages the resolution (or lack of resolution) of the tasks of earlier stages continues to exert its influence.

As a result of continuous interactions with the environment during these stages, a person develops a self-identity, which Erikson calls **ego-identity.** This is central to human personality development. Human ego-identity is awareness of oneself as a distinct person with an influential past, an active present, and a controllable future. What must a person live through in a realistic world to achieve feelings of identity and competence? This is the basic question that Erikson sets out to answer.

The Infant:
Basic Trust Versus
Basic Mistrust

Infancy may be considered as the time of life between birth and about eighteen months of age. In the first year, the infant will make a decision, based on the quality of maternal care, as to whether the world is dependable and safe or filled with frustration and fear. It is not a decision reached as the result of one incident or even a few. Erikson does not mean that this stage (or any other) is like an obstacle race in which a few missteps forever doom the participant to emotional illness. Rather, the infant's decision is the product of the ripening relationship with the mother. Completely self-centered, yet utterly dependent, the child will inevitably be disappointed. No mother can always immediately meet all her baby's needs.

As a part of normal development, therefore, the child must learn to cope with a degree of frustration. The infant's ability to do this will depend on his or her overall sense of security or insecurity. If frustrations are not excessive in amount or in frequency, the child will learn that although things are not always to his or her liking, most of the time they are fine. A baby can adjust to that. Indeed, such lessons will help the child face situations that will arise as the first year is reached, particularly those that involve some degree of separation from the mother. If all that has preceded has been characterized by anxiety, the child will approach this and future problems with fear and basic mistrust. But if most of the child's experience has been characterized by basic trust, a sense of self-esteem will have been gained. That sense of self-worth will always be a necessary part of the healthy personality.

A CASE OF
SEVERE BASIC MISTRUST

What happens to a baby without an opportunity to develop a degree of basic trust? The story of Joey, the "mechanical boy,"* provides an instructive, though dramatically extreme, example. "He wanted to be rid of his unbearable humanity," his psychiatrist, Bruno Bettelheim, wrote, "to become completely automatic."

"I never knew I was pregnant," his mother said, meaning that she had already excluded Joey from her consciousness. His birth, she said, "did not make any difference." Joey's father, a rootless draftee in the wartime civilian army, was equally unready for parenthood. So, of course, are many young couples. Fortunately most such parents lose their indifference upon the baby's birth. But not Joey's parents. "I did not want to see or nurse him," his mother declared. "I had no feeling of actual dislike—I simply didn't want to take care of him." For the first three months of his life Joey "cried most of the time." A colicky baby, he was kept on a rigid four-hour feeding schedule, was not touched unless necessary, and was never cuddled or played with. The mother, preoccupied with herself, usually left Joey alone in the crib or playpen during the day. The father discharged his frustrations by punishing Joey when the child cried at night.

Joey's existence never registered with his mother. . . . When she told us about his birth and infancy, it was as if she were talking about some vague acquaintance.[2]

This parental indifference taught Joey little but basic mistrust. To be touched, to be held, to be cuddled, to be played with—none of these baby needs were met. Only mechanical devices could be relied on to satisfy Joey's greatest needs. Years later Bettelheim described his bizarre behavior:

Entering the dining room, for example, he would string an imaginary wire from his "energy source"—an imaginary electric outlet—to the table. There he "insulated" himself with paper napkins and finally plugged himself in. Only then could Joey eat, for he firmly believed that the "current" ran his ingestive apparatus. . . .

Many times a day he would turn himself on and shift noisily through a sequence of higher and higher gears until he "exploded," screaming "Crash, crash!" and hurling items from his ever-present apparatus—radio tubes, light bulbs, even motors or, lacking these, any handy breakable object. (Joey had an astonishing knack for snatching bulbs and tubes unobserved.) As soon as the object thrown had shattered, he would cease his screaming and wild jumping and retire to mute, motionless nonexistence.[3]

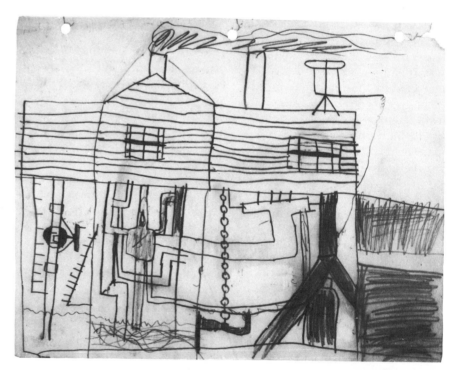

One of Joey's early drawings. Notice that the house is small and simple while the mechanical sewer system is large and complex. Joey's impersonal and rigid toilet training is reflected in his obsessive interest in sewage disposal.

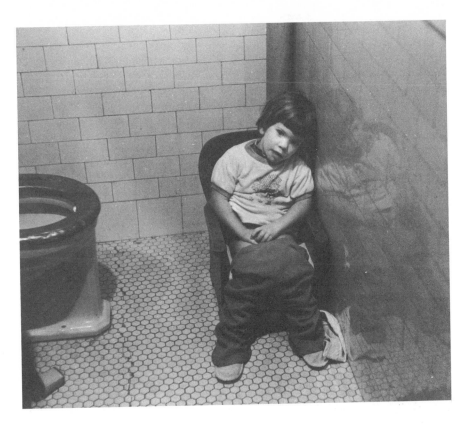

Toilet training requires patience and flexibility. This is a crucial period for a child, and parents need to be aware of the effects their attitude will have on the youngster's future development.

The Toddler: Autonomy Versus Shame and Doubt

The time of toddlerhood extends from about eighteen months to about thirty-six months of age. Autonomy is derived from a Greek word meaning "independence." This stage is marked by increasing individual muscle control. The toddler learns to consciously control the bowel and bladder. He also learns that attention can be gotten by withholding control. If a new baby enters the family and is seen as a competitor, the toddler may withhold bowel and bladder control as one method of regaining attention. The parents must learn patience. Having a rigid attitude or causing the youngster to feel shame can create lifelong emotional scars. "From a sense of *self-control without*

loss of self-esteem comes a lasting sense of autonomy and pride. From a sense of muscular and anal impotence, of loss of self-control, and of parental over-control comes a lasting sense of doubt and shame."[4]

At this stage what happened to Joey? He was toilet-trained rigidly. And the rigidity was rooted in indifference, not love:

Going to the toilet, like everything else in Joey's life, was surrounded by elaborate preventions. We had to accompany him; he had to take off all his clothes; he could only squat, not sit, on the toilet seat; he had to touch the wall with one hand, in which he also clutched frantically the vacuum tubes that powered his elimination. He was terrified lest his whole body be sucked down.

To counteract this fear we gave him a metal wastebasket in lieu of a

toilet. Eventually, when eliminating into the wastebasket, he no longer needed to take off all his clothes, nor to hold on to the wall. . . .

It was not simply that his parents had subjected him to rigid, early training. Many children are so trained. But in most cases the parents have a deep emotional investment in the child's performance. The child's response in turn makes training an occasion for interaction between them and for the building of genuine relationships. Joey's parents had no emotional investment in him. His obedience gave them no satisfaction and won him no affection or approval. As a toilet-trained child he saved his mother labor, just as household machines saved her labor. As a machine he was not loved for his performance, nor could he love himself. . . . By treating him mechanically his parents made him a machine.[5]

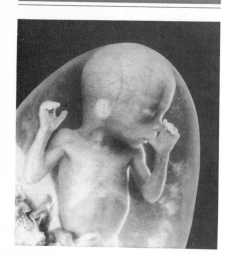

The Story of Little Suck-a-Thumb

One day, mamma said: "Conrad dear,

I must go out and leave you here.

But mind now, Conrad, what I say,

Don't suck your thumb while I'm away.

The great tall tailor always comes

To little boys that suck their thumbs;

And ere they dream what he's about,

He takes his great sharp scissors out

And cuts their thumbs clean off—and then

You know, they never grow again."

FIGURE 5–2
During the Nazi era, countless German schoolchildren memorized this poem. But thumb sucking is quite normal. Within the uterus, the unborn child may suck on a thumb; often the newborn will do so moments after birth.

The Preschooler: Initiative Versus Guilt

During the preschool years, the child, if armed with the accumulated security of the first stage and the independent body control of the second, seeks to discover more about the self. Erikson calls this stage *initiative versus guilt.*

Being firmly convinced that he is a person, the child must now find out *what* kind of person he is going to be. And here he hitches his wagon to nothing less than a star: he wants to be like his parents, who to him appear very powerful and very beautiful, although quite unreasonably dangerous.[6]

To love and be loved. What a rare and wonderful opportunity for both parents and child! Yet so many parents do not drink deeply of that precious time. It is perhaps in this stage that the crushing tragedy of Joey's indifferent parents became most poignantly apparent. For the child, needing love, can endure impatience and even passing anger. The child knows that even anger means caring. But it is indifference that is too much to bear. Is it any different with grown-ups?

The preschooler knows his or her gender and is curious about sexuality. Examination of the self and, when possible, of others is ordinary. It is learned that handling the genitals is pleasurable (Freud's "phallic phase"). A shocked, forbidding parent will convince a child that he or she is basically dirty and unworthy. A relaxed, accepting parent teaches the child a basic self-worth, and this worthiness includes the genitalia. Strongly disapproving parents at this phase create in the child a sense of guilt and a fear of punishment. Not all, but a great number of children experience the fear that their genitalia will be (with boys) or have been (with girls) cut off. (Figure 5–2 and its accompanying verse illustrate how a terrible fear can be created about an entirely normal human activity— thumb sucking. Parents need not be concerned about thumb sucking until the child is about four. Past that age, teeth may be displaced, and the family dentist should be consulted.)

Expressions of the Oedipus* complex (which is associated primarily with the work of Freud) are also likely to appear during this stage. With childhood's devastating logic, the four- or five-year-old boy reaches two conclusions. First, that his genitals cannot compare with his father's, and, second, that no matter how much he loves his mother, he cannot replace his father in her affections. Frequently, a male child may express a desire to marry his mother (Oedipus complex). The little girl may endure a similar experience (Electra complex). Mother had been her ideal; she now prefers her father. She now wants only him to put her to bed, dress her, and care for her. The mother is rejected. But the little girl still needs her mother, just as the small boy still needs his father, no matter how much he wishes to be rid of him. This will not be their last entrapment in emotional contradictions—in feelings of both love and hate. Also, as is the case with the castration complex, it

*Oedipus, in the Sophoclean tragedy *Oedipus Rex*, kills his father and marries a woman whom he later discovers to be his own mother. When he learns of the true relationship, he blinds himself. In females, the Oedipus complex is called the Electra complex. In Greek mythology, Electra is supposed to have urged her brother, Orestes, to kill their mother, Clytemnestra, who had murdered their father, Agamemnon.

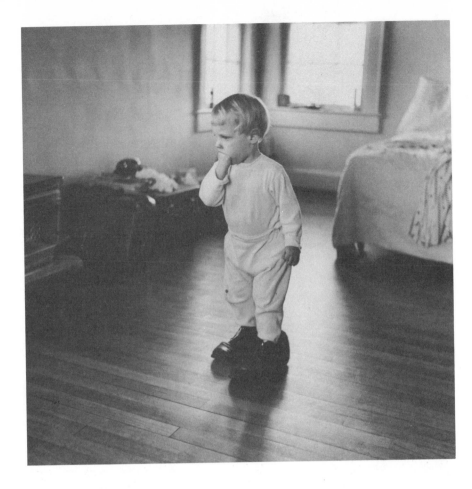

Expressions of the Oedipus complex take many forms. This little boy cannot possibly fill his father's shoes, but he must not be ridiculed for trying.

is important for the parents to know that both the Oedipus and Electra complexes may *not* occur. Moreover, when they do, neither parent nor any other individual is necessarily responsible for them.

Parental maturity and skill in handling these emotions, in preventing the humiliation of the searching child, will add to the child's sense of a worthy self. Embarrassing the child will interfere with his or her ability to conquer future crises.

The School-age Child: Industry Versus Inferiority

At the time the child enters school, the fourth stage of Erikson's scheme of personality development, called *industry versus inferiority*, has been reached.

Personality at the first stage crystallizes around the conviction "I am what I am given," and that of the second, "I am what I will." The third can be characterized by "I am what I can imagine I will be. . . ." The fourth: "I am what I learn."[7]

In an earlier chapter it was noted that because no other creature has as much to learn before self-sufficiency is possible, only human beings have such a long period of dependency. The child must learn skills, use tools, and do something satisfying for the self. Returning from school to the parents, the child will hold out the result of the day's labor. "Look," the child will say hopefully. If the work is met with appreciation, the child will attempt to do still better. If met with parental indifference, a deep sense of inadequacy and inferiority may overwhelm the child. But praise must be merited. Should the child receive praise for an effort that is obviously slipshod, respect for the person giving the praise may be lost, and the child may never learn the value of his or her truly good work.

Adolescence: Identity Versus Role Confusion

"I felt myself isolated, helpless and always shut up in myself: I do not complain of it, for I believe that my early meditations developed and strengthened my thinking powers."[8] So did Talleyrand (1754–1838), the celebrated French politician of the eighteenth century, describe his twelfth year. His was obviously a lonely adolescence. That period of life often is. Erikson terms this fifth stage *identity versus role confusion.*

Adolescence and puberty are not the same. They may start at about the same time, but in Western culture adolescence is far more prolonged than puberty. Puberty is a physical event; adolescence, a cultural event. So many changes happen during puberty that the growing person needs to become reacquainted with the self. Powerful new sexual urges may send the teen-ager soaring into confused dream worlds. These may be frightening and produce vague feelings of guilt. Added to these disturbances are the "inability to settle on an occupational identity" and "the inexorable standardization of American adolescence."[9] Erikson has further described this stage in the following manner:

There is a "natural" period of uprootedness in human life: adolescence. Like a trapeze artist, the young person in the middle of vigorous emotion must let go of his safe hold on childhood and reach out for a firm grasp on adulthood, dependent for a breathless interval on his training, his luck, and the reliability of the "receiving and confirming" adults.[10]

Anna Freud, daughter of Sigmund Freud has written of this stage of life with eloquent understanding:

[Adolescents are] excessively egoistic, regarding themselves as the center of the universe and the

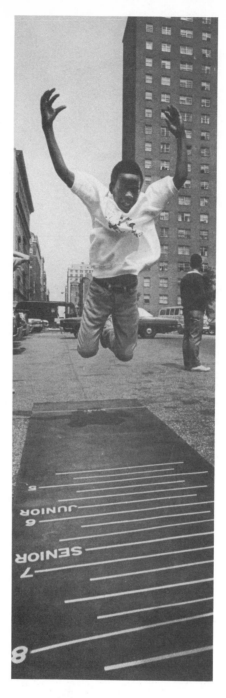

sole object of interest, and yet at no time in later life are they capable of so much self-sacrifice and devotion. They form the most passionate love-relations, only to break them off as abruptly as they began them. On the one hand they throw themselves enthusiastically into the life of the community and, on the other, they

have an overpowering longing for *solitude.* They oscillate between blind submission to some self-chosen leader and defiant rebellion against any and every authority. They are selfish and materially minded and at the same time full of lofty idealism. They are aesthetic but will suddenly plunge into instinctual indulgence of the most primitive character. At times their behavior to other people is rough and inconsiderate, yet they themselves are extremely touchy. Their moods veer between light-hearted optimism and the blackest pessimism. Sometimes they will work with indefatigable enthusiasm and, at other times, they are sluggish and apathetic.[11]

Without reasonably satisfactory resolutions in the previous four stages—without basic trust, for example—adolescence can indeed be a trial. Not identity, but identity diffusion (or role confusion) may result. In this culture such confusion is common. Temporary identity may be found by some in a gang or clique. With others, self-identity seems endlessly slow in coming. From elders, the adolescent hears apprehensive criticism. Parents have been known to say, "Grow up. Stop hanging around the public square and wandering up and down the street. Go to school. Night and day you torture me. Night and day you waste your time having fun."[12] These words were translated from a clay tablet four thousand years old. Apparently, the confusion of adolescence is no new phenomenon peculiar to modern society.

Yet despite the fact that an unresolved crisis at this stage is often a cause of severe emotional disturbance, in the case of Joey adolescence (and years of treatment) produced an opposite effect.

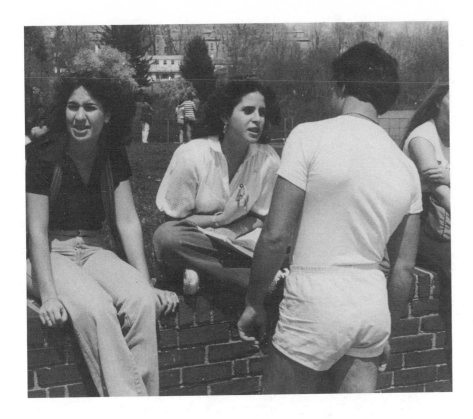

When Joey was 12, [wrote Bettelheim] he made a float for our Memorial Day parade. It carried the slogan: 'Feelings are more important than anything under the sun.' Feelings, Joey had learned, are what make for humanity; their absence, for a mechanical existence. With this knowledge Joey entered the human condition.[13]

As a small child Joey had tried to kill himself. With help, and, approaching the effervescence of adolescence, Joey began to heal.

Early Adulthood: Intimacy Versus Isolation

The first of Erikson's three stages of adulthood is called *intimacy versus isolation*. Childhood is over, and if the previous tasks have been met successfully, self-identity is established. Now the task is to seek and commit oneself to mature mutual relationships of love and friendship as well as to one's work.

> *Henceforth I ask not good-fortune,*
> *I myself am good-fortune,*
> *Henceforth I whimper no more,*
> *postpone no more, need*
> *nothing. . . .*
> *Strong and content I travel the*
> *open road.*
> WALT WHITMAN (1819–1892)
> *"Song of the Open Road,"* lines 4–7

Intimacy—a state of deep and lasting caring for others—includes the need to share experiences and may also include sexuality. It is during this stage that many people marry and form lifetime intimate friendships. Failure to commit oneself to others and to work in early adulthood results in isolation, and thus in an inability to cope adequately with the two remaining stages.

Middle Adulthood: Generativity Versus Stagnation

For many people, these middle years of adulthood are the most creative and productive period of life. The mature person understands that taking can be a way of giving, but that there is a difference between taking and exploiting. *Generativity* may include parental pride, a desire to create and guide the next generation, and a need to give pleasure to, and enrich, oneself and others. A sense of impoverishment or *stagnation* may come from the feeling that one has not accomplished earlier goals or that one's work is not satisfying or important. Generativity happens at about age forty; it is the beginning of the time of greatest possible service to others and to society.

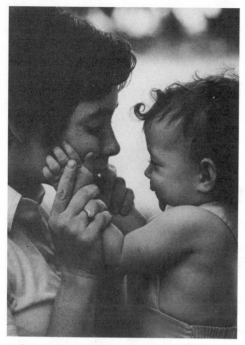

Infancy: Basic trust versus basic mistrust.

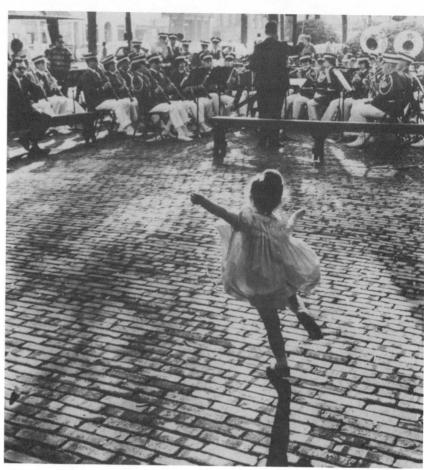

The preschooler: Initiative versus guilt.

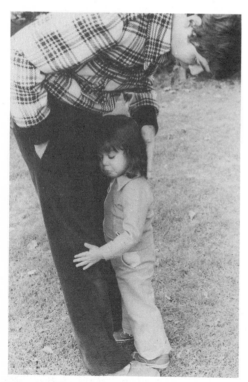

The toddler: Autonomy versus shame and doubt.

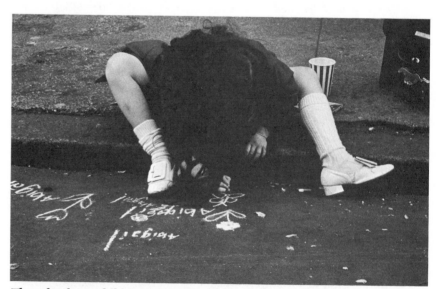

The school-age child: Industry versus inferiority.
"Learning is not child's play." ARISTOTLE

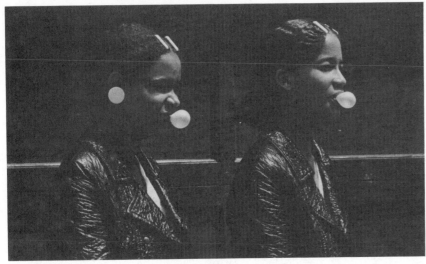

Adolescence: Identity versus role confusion.
"...the inexorable standardization of American adolescence."

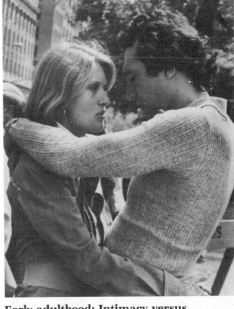

Early adulthood: Intimacy versus isolation.

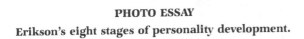

PHOTO ESSAY
Erikson's eight stages of personality development.

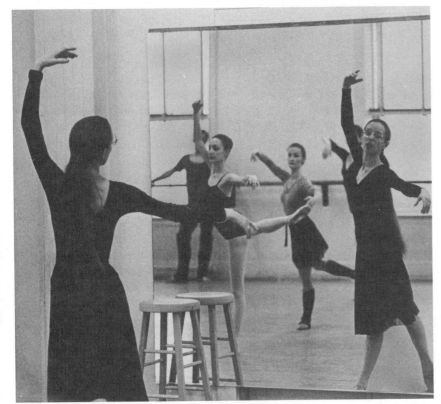

Middle adulthood: Generativity versus stagnation.

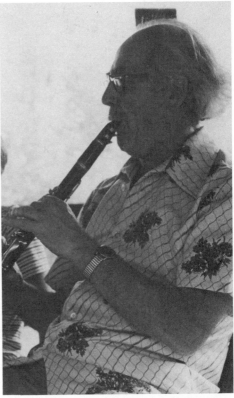

Late adulthood: Integrity versus despair.

Late Adulthood: Integrity Versus Despair

The first Earl of Balfour (1840–1930) was a gentle man and a gentleman. His had been a good and exciting life in the service of his country. His last words were, "This is going to be a great experience."

An originator and leader, Balfour met life with courage and verve. He even died with anticipation. This final stage produced a sense of *integrity*—there was no *despair* of opportunities missed or disgust by past failures.

Thus Erikson unfolds the processes of the development of the human personality. Note the importance he places on self-esteem, in the same way that for Maslow it was the basic stepping stone to self-actualization. And notice the difference between self-esteem as described by these two important thinkers and a self-centered "ego trip." The former is an absolutely necessary part of emotional health whereas the latter can lead only to a loss of faith and a sense of meaninglessness.

Most people pass through Erikson's stages without too much trouble, gaining the emotional strength to function more effectively. But at various times during their personality development, some people need help. How much help they need will depend on the extent of their problems—it may range from a few quiet conversations with a wise friend to long-term psychotherapy. The most important thing is that people know that help is available.

Albert Einstein once said that "every kind of peaceful cooperation among men is primarily based on mutual trust and only secondarily on institutions such as courts of justice and police." Without the basic trust of infancy there cannot be the mutual trust of adulthood. Surely it is difficult to see how the self-actualization that Maslow speaks of can be reached without the trust and integrity that is described by Erikson. For both personality theorists, life at its fullest begins and ends with trust and faith in others. Thus the circle is complete.

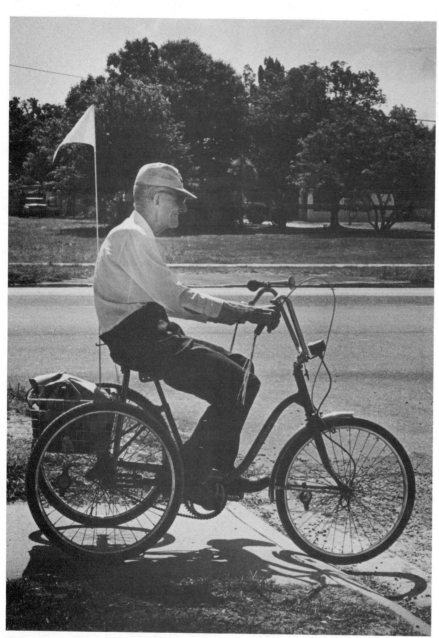

"Give me a young man in whom there is something of the old, and an old man with something of the young: guided so, a man may grow old in body, but never in mind." CICERO

Personality Disorders and Emotional Problems

Emotionally healthy people are able to meet the stresses of life realistically and to choose appropriate methods of solving problems. They have a realistic sense of their own worth and interact constructively with others. They are able to find satisfaction in efficiently performing their work. Since they adapt well in their environment and perceive it realistically, they function well on the health scale. They are able to give and take love without using it as a weapon. Emotionally healthy people behave, for the most part, in ways that are socially and culturally acceptable. It should be noted that this does not mean that well-adjusted people do not or should not question that which is unhealthy about society. There are always social ills that must be questioned and constructive alternatives that need to be proposed and taken.

Nonetheless, behavior is appraised as "normal" according to the degree to which it conforms with what most people do in the context of a particular time and place. For an example of what is meant by *degree of conformity*, consider the differences between three men working on an assembly line in an automobile factory. One comes to work every day dressed in a formal suit and tie; the second consistently wears jeans or workpants and a clean shirt or pullover sweater; and the third almost invariably shows up in bathing trunks and no shoes. None of the three styles of dress is, *in itself*, an indication of emotional disturbance: Each is appropriate to a particular time and

place. But when judged *in context*, the attire of the first and third men takes on added significance and may be seen as a sign of possible emotional disturbance. Only the second man dresses in a manner that is most appropriate for that setting.

Time is another factor in determining normality. Shrieking adolescent girls in the seventeenth century were often thought to be possessed by the devil. Today, comparable behavior at a rock concert draws little attention. *Locale* is still another context for normality. In Java, for instance, it is acceptable for two people who are arguing in public to punctuate their anger with the added insult of shedding their clothes. If this were done on a street in the United States, psychiatric investigation might well be suggested.

If the concept of "normal behavior" varies according to degree, time, and place, how can *normality* be defined? Today, many specialists who diagnose and treat emotional problems accept Freud's concept that the ability to work and to love without undue emotional impediments is measure enough of normality.

The Limits of Labels

Given the broad definition of normality as stated above, it is with reservations that we introduce here even a limited classification of emotional disorders. There are many such classifications, and they are convenient for discussing disorders.

However, they should not be used to pigeon-hole either people or their problems. Indeed, many specialists in the field of emotional health tend to dispense with the labels or classifications altogether, preferring instead to discuss *adjustive* and *maladjustive* behavior in broad, uncategorized terms. As the noted psychiatrist Karl Menninger said:

> We label mental diseases the way little girls label their dolls. And one little girl's *Helen* is not like another little girl's *Helen*. In the same way, Dr. A's "schizophrenia" is different from Dr. B's "schizophrenia." And as long as we think of mental illness as a horrible monster with a name like schizophrenia, we won't be able to prevent it.[14]

"He Who Can Simulate Sanity Will Be Sane"[15]

Menninger's concept is surely supported by an experiment designed several years ago by a Stanford psychiatrist. Eight volunteers (three women and five men), without significant psychiatric histories, presented themselves for admission to psychiatric hospitals. Among the volunteers were three psychologists, a pediatrician, a psychiatrist, a painter, and a housewife. All complained of a single phony symptom: They said they heard hollow voices. In eleven out of twelve tries, the volunteers were admitted with a diagnosis of schizophrenia. They were discharged between one and seven weeks later; the discharge diagnosis was schizophrenia in remission. The twelfth volunteer was both admitted and discharged as having a manic-depressive psychosis.[16] In the hospital, the pseudopatients behaved normally and cooperated fully. The other patients were much more perceptive than the staff. In three of the hospitalizations, 35 of a total of 118 patients expressed their suspicions, saying, for example, "You're not crazy. You're a journalist or professor. You're checking up on the hospital."[17]

The experiment was then modified in the following manner: Staffs at various teaching hospitals were advised of the results of the earlier experiment and informed that a pseudopatient would soon come seeking admission to their hospitals. Of 193 patients who sought admission, 41 were alleged to be the pseudopatients by at least one staff member. In fact, during the entire period in question, no pseudopatients presented themselves to any of the hospitals.[18]

These experiments raise disturbing questions about the labeling of emotional disorders (particularly schizophrenia), the diagnostic ability of some hospital personnel, the unwillingness to reassess patients in an institutional setting, and the extent to which hospital staff make diagnoses on the basis of what they *expect* to find. Another problem (and possible solution) of labeling concerns neurosis; it is discussed in the accompanying boxed insert.

Yet despite the inaccuracy of labels, physicians continue to find them useful, and it is estimated that on any given day approximately two million people are disabled by emotional illness in this country. From 7 to 12 percent of school-age children and young adults need professional help for severe emotional problems.

No More Neuroses— Psychiatry Has Retired Them

In recent years, more and more attention has been given to the problems of labeling and what to do about them. One proposed way to eliminate the vagueness associated with the term neurosis *is described below. The next several years should clarify the workability of this proposal.*

Neurosis is going the way of the vapors as a medical condition. After the American Psychiatric Association formally approves and issues the third edition of its *Diagnostic and Statistical Manual of Mental Disorders* at the end of next year, the word "neurosis" may still be found in medical dictionaries but not in its members' diagnostic vocabularies.

. . . The idea, says task-force chairman Robert L. Spitzer, is to name them for their symptoms rather than Freud's arguable assumption of their root cause. In Freudian theory, all neuroses are caused by intrapsychic conflicts, such as a patient's unresolved conflict concerning his mother. Also, the term has become so broad that it no longer has a precise meaning, says Dr. Spitzer, chief of biometric research at the New York State Psychiatric Institute in New York City.

The proposed new terminology is precise. The old depressive neuroses . . . include four subgroups: major depressive disorder, chronic depressive disorder, adjustment disorder with depressed mood, and atypical depressive disorder. . . .

APA's council on research and development met here for three days last month to hear arguments for and against the changes. Dr. Leo Madow, president of the American Psychoanalytic Association, was concerned that Freudian concepts of mental illness were being downgraded by the redefinition. This was perfectly all right with some members who felt the term "neurosis" was too closely linked with psychoanalysis, anyway. Others said they feared adverse information used to support a patient's assignment to a category could be misused or publicly revealed by insurers. . . .

Dr. William A. Frosch, vice chairman of psychiatry at Cornell University in New York City and a member of the APA task force, points out that some of the new narrow diagnostic criteria may be based on wrong guesses. He is worried that both the good and bad will be "cast in concrete."

The *Washington Post* has editorially bemoaned the "cultural loss" of the term "neurotic." It asserted that "neurosis" and "neurotic" call up "an implicit act of forgiveness and understanding," whereas "to excuse so-and-so by citing his disorder—the specific category of his disorder, to boot—is like excusing a car for faulty brakelining. Not only can the defect be repaired—it damn well ought to be, and quick. The burden of adjustment would sit squarely on the disorderee."

But with all its real and facetious difficulties, the change is a major advance, Dr. Frosch maintains.

Furthermore, about 10 percent of the population will, at some point in their lives, suffer serious emotional illness.

An Overview of Emotional Disorders

A Classification of Emotional Disorders

A. Psychotic disorders
  1. Organic causes: Characterized by lesions (an abnormal or harmful change in structure) in the brain.
  2. Functional disorders: No demonstrable lesion in the brain.
      a. Schizophrenia
      b. Manic-depressive psychoses
      c. Paranoia

B. Neurotic disorders
  1. Psychoneuroses (neuroses)
      a. Anxiety and depression
      b. Phobia
      c. Obsessive-compulsive reaction
      d. Hysteria
      e. Traumatic neuroses
  2. Psychosomatic disorders

C. Character disorders
  Examples include criminal behavior and the psychopathic personality.

D. Emotional disorders with possible chemical causes

Psychotic disorders (**psychoses**) are more severe than neurotic disorders. The individual displaying *psychotic* behavior has lost much contact with reality. The *neurotic* person, on the other hand, is still able to view his or her emotional problems with some degree of objectivity and to make some attempt to cope with them. A neurotic, one observer remarked, is a person who builds a castle in the air. A psychotic is the person who lives in it. And a psychiatrist is the one who collects the rent. Social divergence, rather than emotional symptoms, is the main characteristic of a person with a *character disorder*. For this reason, character disorders are categorized separately. In addition, research strongly suggests the need for another category of emotional disorders. Recent discoveries in the field of brain chemistry indicate that certain chemicals manufactured in the brain play a role in one's emotional life. Therefore, later in this chapter the nervous system and the link between chemistry and behavior will be discussed.

THE PSYCHOTIC DISORDERS

ORGANIC LESIONS   Brain tumors, severe head injuries, and serious infections, such as far-advanced untreated syphilis, commonly result in psychoses. Also, the psychotic behavior of **senile dementia** is now seen more frequently as greater numbers of people live to be quite old. This latter form of psychosis is due to deterioration of aged brain cells; advanced arteriosclerosis, resulting in prolonged lessening of blood-carrying oxygen to the brain, may be partly causative.

FUNCTIONAL DISORDERS   As the experiment with pseudopatients suggested, psychotic behavior is not so easily recognizable as is generally thought. Some people are obviously deranged. Among these are people suffering from the extreme forms of *mania* and the more dramatic types of *schizophrenia* (both these disorders will be discussed below). However, many people whose behavior is occasionally psychotic ordinarily appear quite normal. Suddenly, without warning or cause, they may go berserk. And just as suddenly, they may return for a time to normal behavior. People suffering *manic-depressive* states, for example, usually experience a temporary period of ordinary behavior between a "high" jubilant mood and a "low" dejected mood. With this disorder it is as if the disturbed individual's moods swing like a pendulum from one extreme to the other, with clear-minded intervals.

In the United States, **schizophrenia** is the most common of all the psychoses, accounting for about 25 to 30 percent of all first admissions to the hospitals for the emotionally disturbed. Today, about half the beds in those hospitals are occupied by patients diagnosed as schizophrenic. It has been estimated that 2 percent of the U.S. population will have an episode of schizophrenia at some time in their lives. In disadvantaged areas, such as urban slums, the prediction rises to 6 percent. But it is not poverty as such that is the direct cause of the disorder. Poor nutrition, inadequate medical care, the stress of growing up in a disordered family—these can combine to contribute to schizophrenia.

A great deal of recent research has focused on schizophrenia. The electrical brain waves of the schizophrenic may differ from those of nonschizophrenic people. Some investigators now consider schizophrenia to be related to an imbalance of body chemistry and function (see page 147). There are studies, which have pointed to a tendency for the condition to run in families, that suggest a hereditary aspect to certain forms of schizophrenia. The relative importance of the influence of the environment on the incidence of schizophrenia needs further study.

Because of its predominance in the sixteen-to-thirty age group, schizophrenia has been called the "psychosis of youth." The very young (six to seven years), the middle-aged, and the elderly are not, however, exempt.

People diagnosed as schizophrenic do not usually (as is popularly supposed) split totally from reality into a world of their own. Nor do they generally have sudden character changes of the Dr. Jekyll and Mr. Hyde variety. Unless the person whose behavior is schizophrenic is in a totally disorganized state, he or she does have some sense of common reality. What is happening to such an individual is that certain aspects of the environment or some experiences have no basis in reality.

Schizophrenia is a good example of the limitation of labels mentioned earlier in this section. It is not a single disease, with a determined set of symptoms, a known cause, and a single treatment. Indeed, two people diagnosed as schizophrenic may demonstrate entirely different symptoms. Nor does any known single pattern of interaction between an individual and the environment inevitably lead to schizophrenic behavior. People react to different stresses individually. The time in a person's life at which the stress occurs may be as important as the nature of the stress. For example, an emotional experience with which an individual could cope at age six might be overwhelming to him at age three.

A wide variety of sign and symptom combinations occur and may be observed in the same person. The individual whose behavior is schizophrenic may experience abnormal perceptions of reality, such as hallucinations, delusions, or both. **Hallucinations** are perceptions without real external stimuli; **delusions** are beliefs that do not actually exist. Hallucinations may fill the world of the schizophrenic in one or all areas of perception. Thus the person displaying schizophrenic behavior may experience hallucinations that are auditory (relating to the sense of hearing), visual (sight), tactile (touch), olfactory (smell), or gustatory (taste). Delusions that torment the person suffering from schizophrenia are also manifested in various ways. For example, a woman may be utterly convinced that someone intends to harm her (delusions of persecution), or a man may be convinced that he is some famous and powerful person, like Napoleon. One woman suffering an auditory hallucination as well as a delusion of persecution accused her dentist of installing a tiny transmitter in the cavity of a molar. By means of this transmitter she received constant threatening coded messages, not only from foreign powers but also from other planets.

Perhaps the most pitiful characteristics of many people whose behavior is schizophrenic is their feeling of utter loneliness and their profound sense of isolation. Confused by misperceptions, bedeviled by hallucinations and delusions, the schizophrenic is often alone in a sea of fear, and it is this very loneliness that compounds the inner terror. At times, the schizophrenic may remain motionless for hours, totally withdrawn from the environment. Another person, similarly afflicted (or the same one at a different time), moves about constantly, incoherent, wide-awake, watchful, sometimes giggling or babbling senselessly.

Next to schizophrenia, the **manic-depressive psychoses** are the most common (afflicting 10 to 15 percent of those whose behavior is psychotic). There is, of course, an enormous difference between the occasional "blue mood" to which all normal people are susceptible and this condition. The onset of manic-depressive psychosis usually occurs between the ages of thirty and fifty, and women are more commonly afflicted than men. Classically, the manic-depressive reaction is seen as elation (*manic phase*) followed by deep despondence (*depressive phase*). An attack may consist of elation alone or of depression alone, or of alternating elation and depression. A **manic reaction** may be set off by a chance remark or even a mild witticism. There then follows an excessive response with a tendency to irrationality. The **depressive reaction** is marked by retardation of both thought and activity. The patient maintains an air of general hopelessness.

Except in exceedingly severe cases, the manic-depressive suffers no lasting intellectual impairment. Even without treatment, recovery is common. The manic phase ordinarily lasts about three months; the depressive phase lasts about three times as long. There is a tendency for the symptoms to return; about three-fourths of these patients have one or more recurrences.

Today, the classic picture is rare owing to the use of mood-altering drugs. Depression can vary from normally mild and temporary to abnormally severe and chronic. It is commonly associated with anxiety. Therefore, along with anxiety, depression is more thoroughly discussed in the next chapter.

Paranoia may be manifested by

delusions of grandeur or of persecution. Paranoid patients might believe themselves to be Christ or Joan of Arc. Persecutions that such individuals feel are generally accompanied by a tendency to seek ulterior motives in the behavior of others. Such was the case of a woman who received the annual prize in law school as the student who had shown the greatest scholastic improvement. Upon graduation, she sued the school for damages. She alleged that the real motive of the faculty, in giving her the prize, was to show the world that in her work was the greatest room for improvement. In this way the faculty was demonstrating that she was not as fit as her associates to be a lawyer.[19]

THE NEUROTIC DISORDERS

Every normal individual experiences some neurotic symptoms. These symptoms, resulting from ordinary stress and inner conflict, do not interfere with effective functioning in society. Thus, a person who has neurotic symptoms does not necessarily have a **neurotic disorder,** or **neurosis.** Whether a neurotic disorder actually exists depends on the degree of involvement of the personality. Neurotic symptoms, arising from an unresolved inner conflict of needs, may take command of the personality for a prolonged time. Effective functioning becomes difficult, even impossible. It is then that a neurotic disorder exists and professional help is indicated. (On page 176 is a self-test to help you determine whether your symptoms are severe enough to merit help. If your answers are inconclusive, help should be sought, if only to remove your doubt.) Unlike most people with psychotic behavior, neurotic individuals do not lose contact with the reality of their environment. Although limited, sometimes severely, the neurotic person is generally able to carry on usual functions.

PSYCHONEUROSES **Anxiety** and **depressive states** are among the most common forms of **psychoneuroses.** Everyone shows symptoms of anxiety or depression sometimes, but the neurotic's anxiety or depression is chronic and severe, and the person is helpless to handle it effectively. Tension is constant; the person feels severe stress almost all the time. Unbearably acute attacks of anxiety, such as an overwhelming sense of approaching doom, may punctuate the chronic condition. The neurotic may suffer a variety of disagreeable emotional and physical symptoms, such as a deep sense of guilt, excessive sweating, and heart palpitations. Anxiety and depressive states are the most common form of neurosis among young people. Both are so basic to the human experience and such common emotional problems that they constitute a major portion of human emotional illness.

A **phobia** is a persistent fear of an object or situation that is not really dangerous or that has been blown out of all proportion to the actual danger. Examples are a fear of open spaces, a fear of enclosed places, a fear of high places, and a fear of the dark—a phobia common to children and some adults.

Obsessive-compulsive reactions occur with people who feel compelled to think about something that they do not want to think about (obsessive thoughts) or who are compelled to do some act that they do not want to do (compulsive acts). Among the more common compulsive reactions is excessive hand washing. For example, an individual who masturbates may respond to this behavior with abnormal disgust

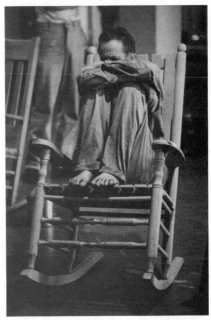

Assuming the position of a fetus, this catatonic patient has retreated into a lonely womb in which he is isolated from the world around him.

The Man with Ten Personalities

Terror stalked the Ohio State University campus last year. Between August and October, four female students were abducted, forced to cash a check or use a bank card to obtain money, then driven to a rural area and raped. Acting on a mysterious phone tip and mugshot identification by one victim, police in Columbus arrested William Milligan, 23. At first the suspect seemed like a classic young offender: physically abused as a child, cashiered from the Navy after one month, constantly in trouble with employers and police. That familiar portrait changed suddenly during a psychological exam. When a woman psychologist addressed Milligan as "Billy," he replied, "Billy's asleep. I'm David." It was the first strong clue that Milligan suffered from a rare and dangerous disorder: true multiple personality.

Psychiatrist George T. Harding Jr. was called in on the case, along with Cornelia B. Wilbur, the psychoanalyst who melded the 16 personalities of a patient known as Sybil, later the subject of a book and television play. With Wilbur's aid, Harding came to a startling conclusion: Milligan had fractured his psyche into ten "people," eight male and two female, ranging from Christene, a vulnerable three-year-old, to Arthur, 22, a rational, controlled planner who speaks with a British accent and tries to repair the damage done by the other personalities.

According to the psychiatrist, Milligan's personalities use different voice patterns and facial expressions, test at varying I.Q. levels, and turn out different kinds of artwork. Ragen, 23, who speaks with a Slavic accent, is "almost devoid of concern for others." Danny and Christopher are decent, quiet teen-agers, but Tommy, 16, who initiated the enlistment in the Navy, is depressed and has many schizoid characteristics.

SOURCE: "The Man with Ten Personalities," *TIME*, October 23, 1978, p. 102. Reprinted by permission from TIME, The Weekly News Magazine; Copyright Time Inc. 1978.

Most surprising of all, for reasons the psychiatrists cannot explain, the personality that committed the rapes is a woman, Adelena, 19, whom Milligan says is a lesbian. Allen, 18, is a sociable, talented artist and the only personality who smokes. David, 9, a frightened and abused child, may have made the call leading to Milligan's arrest. The police number was found on a pad next to Milligan's phone. Billy, 23, is the core personality—guilty, suicidal and "asleep" for most of the past seven years. When Wilbur first summoned up Billy, Milligan jumped off his chair and said, "Every time I come to, I'm in some kind of trouble. I wish I were dead."

Milligan's multiple personality, like others, is a desperate attempt to handle conflicting emotions by parceling them out to different "people" and is associated with a severely warped childhood. The illegitimate son of two Florida entertainers, Milligan was three when his father committed suicide. His stepfather physically abused his mother and sodomized young Milligan, threatening to bury him alive if he told. As a teen-ager in Ohio, Milligan fell into trances and walked the streets in a daze. He was incarcerated twice, once for rape, once for robbery, and failed at every job he had.

While nearly everyone agrees that Milligan is seriously ill, there is some doubt about whether to bring him to trial. Earlier this month, Harding reported to the court that Milligan's personalities had fused to the point where he was competent to stand trial, and Judge Jay C. Flowers set a December trial date. Last week, however, Milligan came apart again. His Ragen personality emerged and handed Public Defender Gary Schweickart a picture of a rag doll with a noose around its neck, hanging in front of a cracked mirror. Three days later, Arthur was in control, questioning the attorney closely about what had happened and how the other personalities could be protected. Said Schweickart: "The stress of jail and confinement was too much." Psychiatrist Wilbur thinks the prognosis for Milligan is doubtful. So does Milligan. His Tommy personality turned out this poem: *I am sorry I took your time/ I am the poem that doesn't rhyme/ So just turn back the page/ I'll waste away/ I'll waste away.*

Coping with a severely warped childhood by fracturing into "people" and parceling out the conflicting emotions.

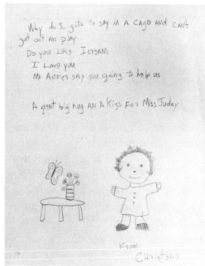

Drawing by Christene personality, age 3.

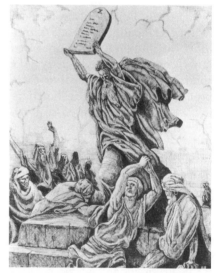

Sketch of Moses by core personality, Billy.

or an unreasonable sense of uncleanliness. These thoughts may then lead to repeated and compulsive hand washing. Compulsive individuals are aware of the absurdity of their thought processes or actions but seem helpless to control them.

Hysteria is another psychoneurotic disorder. It is divided into two categories. With **conversion reactions,** patients exhibit the same symptoms as those that indicate an organic disorder. Characteristic symptoms include paralysis of the legs; loss of sight, hearing, or speech; insensitivity to pain; and tics. In the other form of hysteria, known as **dissociative reactions,** there is a virtual temporary takeover of the individual's personality to the extent that the person no longer controls his or her own behavior. **Amnesia,** a loss of memory, and *sleepwalking* are two common examples. A third type of dissociative reaction—one that is quite rare—is **multiple personality,** which was chronicled in the popular books *The Three Faces of Eve* and *Sybil.* In this instance, two or more entirely different personalities are found in the same person. (The boxed insert, opposite, describes an interesting, and bizarre, case of multiple personality.)

Traumatic neuroses occur as a result of extreme stress. A severe automobile accident may, for example, precipitate a traumatic neurosis. But by no means does stress always result in a traumatic neurosis. Some feel that constant activity was the reason for the low incidence of reported neuroses among English, German, and Japanese civilians exposed to bombings during the Second World War. They were too busy to have emotional problems.

Those who study war neuroses usually distinguish between *combat*

exhaustion and *combat neuroses.* The neurotic combatant is frequently described as a jumpy, chain-smoking, trembling man. On the other hand, the soldier suffering from combat exhaustion may fall asleep in the middle of a roaring battle. Some soldiers may be more likely to develop chronic war neuroses than others. A soldier who has been raised in a rigid environment, for example, is more inclined to suffer from combat neuroses.

PSYCHOSOMATIC DISORDERS

When the seventeenth-century Englishman John Donne observed that "the body makes the minde," he was not reversing the ancient Roman, Ovid. "Diseases of the mind impair the powers of the body," wrote the latter. Both poets understood that mutual reactions between mind and body profoundly affect health. The expressions "as white as a sheet" or "hot under the collar" take due note of the skin as a mirror of people's emotions. Whether a person blushes or has goose flesh, anxiety is being expressed in a physical way. Why? Because the temporary release of tension via a physical reaction is easier to bear than an attempt to contain the tension.

The term *psychosomatic* originates from the Greek words *psyche,* meaning "mind" and *soma,* meaning "body." **Psychosomatic disorders** originate in the mind and are manifested in bodily symptoms. Emotional stimuli are referred by the brain to body organs, resulting in effects ranging from goose flesh to headaches. Though these symptoms have no actual physical cause, they are nevertheless very real. For example, no condition is seen more frequently by the physician than tension headache. It is caused by sustained muscle contraction about the head and neck. In en-

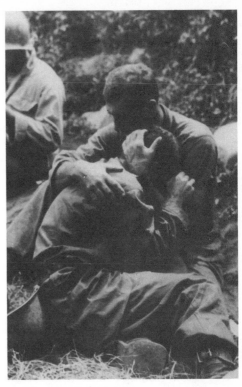

Combat stress in Korea.
"O brother man! fold to thy heart thy brother." JOHN GREENLEAF WHITTIER

during stress, such as cramming for an examination or driving in heavy traffic, the neck muscles contract in positions of maximum alertness. In several patients a physician was able to produce migraine headaches by discussing with them some of their guilt-producing life situations. Helping these patients understand the reasons for their reactions reduced the number and severity of their headaches.[20]

Asthma can be precipitated by some substances, such as dust or feathers, to which the individual is sensitive (allergic). But emotional tension may also start an attack. Or both an allergic reaction and emotional tension may be involved and overlap to affect the respiratory system in this manner.

The eye may be involved in similar reactions. A case reported by Karl Menninger concerns a twenty-four-year-old woman with prolonged disabling eye problems. These had started shortly after the death of her brother in the war. Jealous of him, she had wished him dead. Also, to see if he was really different from her, she had once peeped at him. "The guilt, therefore, was associated not only with the envy of the brother but with the peeping."[21] In such cases psychotherapy can be remarkably helpful.

The effects of the emotions on the body's organs are both numerous and common, and patients with psychosomatic illnesses are hardly rare.

CHARACTER DISORDERS

The identification of a person as someone who has a **character disorder** is not a moral judgment. This is a scientific term used to classify some emotionally disturbed people. The variation in degree of these problems is considerable. One indi-vidual may merely be a neurotic nuisance. Another constantly breaks the law. In this latter group are the **psychopathic personalities.** These individuals are utterly irresponsible. This disorder is characterized by a lack of conscience. Although psychopaths know the difference between right and wrong, they are psychologically unable to care about the difference. Preoccupied with the immediate gratification of their own needs, they are oblivious to the needs of others. They are untroubled by a sense of guilt and suffer little or no anxiety. Not necessarily lacking intelligence, they are frequently charming. But they feel no love for anyone. Friends, family, minister, and psychiatrist are unable to reach them. Their disorder may result from the absence of an affectionate relationship with an adult during childhood. The antisocial psychopath may reveal bitterness over this deprivation of love.

A habitual criminal of a generation ago, Johnny Rocco, was not a foundling, but, perhaps worse, he felt like one. These lines from the Anglo-Saxon folk epic poem *Beowulf* can aptly be applied to him:

> *From a friendless foundling,*
> *feeble and wretched,*
> *He grew to a terror as time*
> *brought change.*

Rocco suffered his way into crime because of a hostile mother. About his mother's reaction to his brother Davie's death he wrote, "When Davie died, she said she wished it was me instead." He added, pitifully, "Money I stole I would never give to my mother."[22] As a boy, he would only give her money he honestly earned selling the magazine *True Confessions.*

There is still one category of personality disorders to discuss—those that have their roots in body chemistry. But before we discuss these disorders, we need to have some understanding of the human nervous system.

The Nervous System: Its Functions and Chemistry

The nervous system is made up of two basic parts. First, there is the **central nervous system**, consisting of the brain and spinal cord. Second, there is the far-flung **peripheral nervous system,** which leads to and from the brain and spinal cord. In this way peripheral nerves connect all the body's parts with the central nervous system to influence the skin or muscles or lungs or inner ear or a powerful gland. By means of their nervous systems people sense their ecosystems, relate to them, and interact with all within them. The nervous system is the connecting messenger between the body's inner space and outer space.

A mother leans to her baby. Lightly she strokes the child's cheek, tickling it. The child's pleasure is intense. No less gently, a stranger tickles the child. The reaction: fear. The tickler must be a familiar person. To enjoy the caress, the infant must associate it with a giver of pleasure, must know that the tickler means to give pleasure, not pain, must sense

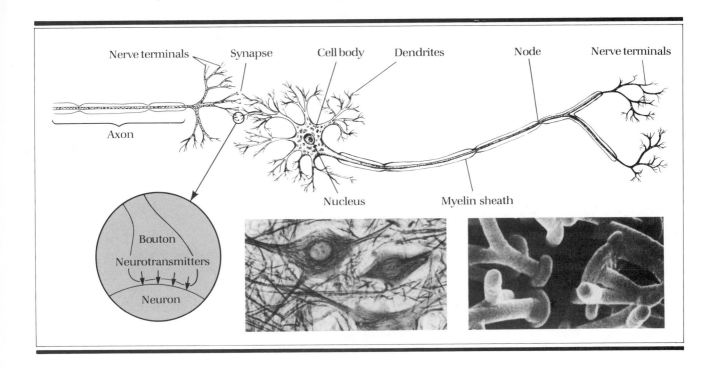

Labels in figure: Nerve terminals, Synapse, Cell body, Dendrites, Node, Nerve terminals, Axon, Bouton, Neurotransmitters, Neuron, Nucleus, Myelin sheath

FIGURE 5–3
A neuron, and its synapse with another neuron. Photograph inserts: A motor nerve cell (left), nerve fibers and synaptic knobs (right). Both photographs are highly magnified.

the difference between being tickled pink and tickled to death. So the tickle is much more than a pressure stimulus to the receptor cells in the skin. Higher brain cells are also involved. There is an *emotional* reaction. How does a simple stimulus like a tickle reach the brain, become sorted out in that citadel of the mind, and become translated into an emotion? By means of the basic working unit of the nervous system, the **neuron** (see Figure 5–3).

Although there are many billions of neurons that coordinate the human body, the structure of one is typical of them all. Like other cells, the neuron's **cell body** contains a nucleus and other structures. But unlike other cells, the neuron's cellu-

lar material extends at each end into nerve fibers. It is these fine, thread-like extensions of the cell bodies that transmit information from one part of the nervous system to another. A bundle of thousands of nerve fibers make up a nerve. At one end of the cell body the nerve fiber extensions are the many-twigged **dendrites.** They pick up sensory impulses (like a tickle) and transmit them *toward* the cell bodies. From the other pole of the cell body extends the longer, single **axon**, which carries impulses *away from* the cell bodies. Most (but not all) axons are sheathed in a whitish substance called **myelin,** which makes the neuron more effective. The destruction of this myelin sheath results in a disease called **multiple sclerosis.** *Nodes* are constrictions of the myelin sheath at regular intervals. They act as relay stations to improve the conduction of a nerve impulse. The axon ends in many branching filaments called *nerve terminals.* However, the myelin

sheath disappears just before these branches occur.

How Nerve Cells Communicate with One Another

What happens when a stimulus—such as a tickle—is received by a sensory nerve terminal? At that point the energy of the stimulus is converted into an electrical impulse in the nerve. The electrical impulse then travels along the nerve fiber, causing a small but measurable current—a **nerve impulse.** The impulse is usually transmitted in one direction—from the dendrites of one neuron, through its cell body, along the axon, to the dendrites or cell body of a second neuron or to a muscle or gland.

When considering the process of nerve-impulse transmission, it is well to keep in mind the following facts:

1. Neurons vary enormously in length. Remarkably, a single neuron may extend from the tip of the finger to the spinal cord. Or, in the brain, a single neuron may be but a microscopic fraction of an inch in length.

2. Neurons do not have simple one-to-one relationships with one another. For example, the axons of many hundreds of neurons may make connections with the dendrites and cell body of one other single neuron. How many connections between *all* the neurons in, for example, the human cerebrum (the brain's wrinkled covering of gray matter) can occur? There are an estimated ten to twelve billion neurons in the human brain. If one were to merely write out the *number* of connections made between neurons in just the covering gray matter of the human brain, one would fill up about two thousand pages of a book this size!

3. The place where the nerve terminals of one axon meet the dendrites or the cell body of a second neuron is called a **synapse**. (See Figure 5–3.) A synapse is a tiny gap or space. Each axon ends in a tiny knob called a **bouton**. An electrical nerve impulse travels along the length of the axons until it reaches the boutons. The nerve impulse then causes the boutons to release special chemicals known as **neurotransmitters**. When these chemical neurotransmitters cross the synapse, they start an electrical impulse in the next neuron. Thus, it is by way of the chemical neurotransmitters at the synapses that nerve cells communicate with one another.

Chemical Neurotransmitters and Emotional Disorders: The Drug Connection

During the past twenty years scientists have studied the brain with increasing excitement. One fact they have learned is that certain cells of the brain act as a gland, producing a variety of chemical **hormones**. These are proteins called **peptides**. Some of these hormones control the influential pituitary gland, which hangs by a stalk from the brain's base. (Refer to Body Charts 8 and 15.) This means that the environment outside the body, which stimulates the nervous system, can, via the nervous system, influence hormonal activity inside the body (see pages 156–157). Another fact that is now known is that some brain cells produce neurotransmitters called **endorphins** that have an opium-like effect on the body. The same is true of the pituitary gland. Dr. Chon Hao Li of the University of California has discovered a pituitary product named beta-endorphin. It is many times stronger than morphine. Further research into these chemicals promises a better understanding of opium dependency (see pages 197–198). Indeed, when beta-endorphin is given to morphine and heroin abusers, the desire for any more narcotics is lost. Probably this is because the beta-endorphin blocks the narcotic receptor sites in the brain. Third, there is increasing evidence that chemical neurotransmitters at the synaptic junctions may greatly affect emotional moods. In this respect there has been much attention paid to manic-depressive illness. Present research suggests that a balance of two brain chemicals are important in maintaining normal emotional balance. Too much of one chemical may be a cause of the mania; too little of the other may cause deep depression. The possibility that some cases of schizophrenia may be influenced by the brain's neurotransmitters is also being considered. Supporting these possibilities are studies that indicate a hereditary factor in both schizophrenia and manic-depressive illness. Why? The protein peptides—the neurotransmitters—are made by the cell's hereditary material.

The treatment of schizophrenia with drugs still leaves much to be desired. Nevertheless, many such patients have been discharged from mental hospitals, and there is considerable opinion that this has been done prematurely (see pages 198–199). However, there has been better success with the drug treatment of the manic-depressive psychoses. Electroconvulsive therapy (ECT) is also successfully used in moderate to severe depressive states. When ECT is used *judiciously in selected cases*, there is little evidence that it causes permanent harm. There are also patients who have permanent electrodes implanted in their brains. By pressing a button, they can reduce otherwise uncontrollable pain and prevent severe epileptic attacks.

Aging

Older people know that death is not distant; however, many of them do not waste time thinking of that future. Instead, they want a chance to be involved with the present—to be able to determine and to realize the rich possibilities of every remaining day. This attitude of immediacy perhaps can best be summed up by

Like Lord Balfour, the long life of U.S. Supreme Court Justice Oliver Wendell Holmes, Jr. (1841–1935) described a complete circle. He had spoken with a veteran of the American Revolution. He fought in the Civil War. He campaigned for civil rights. And at the age of sixty-one he was appointed a justice of the Supreme Court. There, for almost thirty years he fought for an interpretation of the law that would meet the changing needs of the people. Too often, though, his eloquent attempts to make the law a living instrument were met with a majority opposition that was stuck in the glue of the dead past; he became known as "the great dissenter." However, as he grew older he saw his concepts prevail, and his ninetieth birthday was a national celebration. This was the birthday message he read to the nation:

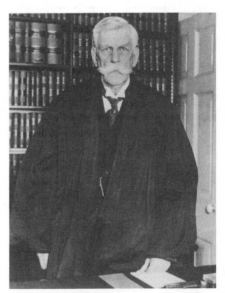

In this symposium my part is only to sit in silence.

To express one's feelings as the end draws near is too intimate a task.

But I may mention one thought that comes to me as a listener-in. The riders in a race do not stop short when they reach the goal. There is a little finishing canter before coming to a standstill. There is time to hear the kind voice of friends and to say to one's self: "The work is done."

But just as one says that, the answer comes: "The race is over, but the work never is done while the power to work remains."

The canter that brings you to a standstill need not be only coming to rest. It cannot be while you still live. For to live is to function. That is all there is to living.

And so I end with a line from a Latin poet who uttered the message more than fifteen hundred years ago: "Death plucks my ears and says, Live—I am coming."

SOURCE: Oliver Wendell Holmes, Jr., a radio talk on the occasion of a national celebration of his ninetieth birthday, quoted in Max Lerner, ed., *The Mind and Faith of Justice Holmes* (Boston: Little, Brown and Company, 1943), p. 451.

Oliver Wendell Holmes, Jr.

TABLE 5–1
Male Deaths per 100 Female Deaths by Age Groups in the United States, 1977

AGE	MALE DEATHS PER 100 FEMALE DEATHS
Under 1	136.28
1–4	148.13
5–14	195.55
15–24	298.05
25–34	243.85
35–44	177.59
45–54	175.04
55–59	173.30
60–64	173.94
65–69	161.40
70–74	143.04
75–79	113.90
80–84	84.0
85 and over	58.14

NOTE: These data do not cover deaths of U.S. civilians or members of the armed forces that occurred outside the United States.

SOURCE: *Monthly Vital Statistics Report*, Provisional Statistics, Annual Summary for the United States, 1977, DHEW Publication No. (PHS) 79-1120, Vol. 26 (December 7, 1978), p. 25.

TABLE 5–2
Life Expectancy at Birth and at Age 18 for U.S. Females and Males for 1976

	REMAINING YEARS OF LIFE	TOTAL YEARS OF LIFE
Life expectancy of females born in 1976		76.7
Life expectancy of males born in 1976		69.0
Life expectancy of females 18 years of age in 1976	60.2	78.2
Life expectancy of males 18 years of age in 1976	52.9	70.9

SOURCE: *Vital Statistics of the U.S., 1976*, Vol. II, Section V, "Life Tables," p. 12.

the words of an old Vermont farmer. Asked whether he had lived in his village all his life he replied, "Not yit."

Some Problems of the Aged

In this country a man retiring at sixty-five has about a fifty–fifty chance of living twelve more years. In 1979 more than 10 percent of the population was sixty-five years old or older, and that number continues to grow.

In fact, the fastest growing age group in the United States is the seventy-five and over population. Tables 5–1 and 5–2 reveal that women live longer than men. Combine this fact with the tendency of men to marry younger women and the result is an older population in which there are far more older women than men and many more widows than widowers.

Poverty is the constant companion of millions of the nation's aged. Although the elderly make up 10 percent of the nation's population, they constitute 20 percent of the nation's poor. An elderly person is twice as likely to be poor as is a young one; yet older people get sick and need expensive health care more often than do the young. Medicare pays less than half the costs of such care.

Can people over sixty-five find jobs? If they can, the U.S. government and industry do little to encourage them. Social security checks are reduced if a recipient earns too much. Retirement is mandatory, or at least encouraged, in many public and private industries. To many employers a lifetime of experience means little. Paychecks are reserved for younger workers.

With retirement, many older people are at a loss for what to do with their time. Compounding their boredom and frustration is the fact that they must watch helplessly as friends and loved ones die. It is no wonder that among the aged, depression is common. Statistics show that suicide is most common among men in their eighties.

These are but some of the handicaps that best the aged. What are the chances for change? They are good. The aged constitute the greatest proportion of registered voters, and they vote more regularly than the members of any other age group. Moreover, because the elderly age group is growing, its voice in determining laws that affect the well-being of older citizens can no longer be ignored. That this is so is evidenced by the 1978 federal legislation that, with few exceptions, pushed the retirement age up from sixty-five to seventy. And federal employees as well as workers in California have no age-related requirements (also with few exceptions). Other states are considering similar laws.

Dispelling Some Common Myths about the Aged

1 Most aged people are too feeble to get around by themselves and must be put away in institutions.

The facts are that over 80 percent of the aged people in this country get around without help and that 95 percent of them live within the community. Inactivity withers the will to live. Society must further encourage and provide physical, intellectual, and social activities for older people.

2 There is no sexual expression among senior citizens.

To lose desirability without losing desire is a cruel blow for most people. In this youth-oriented society the aged shuffle by, unnoticed, untouched, and thus often cruelly deprived of two basic human needs: to be noticed and touched. The old man who ventures to pat the head of a child may be regarded with suspicion, even with hidden horror. In this respect the elderly woman has the advantage; it is considered quite natural for her to cuddle and pet children. Aged males constitute less than 10 percent of adult child molesters. Yet contempt of the "dirty old man" runs deep in this society.

Few old people can satisfy their needs as did the great Indian leader, Mahatma Gandhi. Throughout his life he had punished himself (and some of those who were close to him) for what he considered his lust. In his old age he still felt sexual needs, but he found a way to forgive them in himself. He took to being cradled by middle-aged women and—as rumor had it—by young women too.

Gandhi's friends, disquieted over the fact that these women were sometimes naked, protested to the Mahatma. These protestations, however, were of no avail. Rather than quit this practice of being held by naked women, Gandhi publicly proclaimed that it provided him with a good test of his own ability to suppress arousal.[23]

To test one's own abilities is a healthy sign at any age.

Despite the taboos in this culture against sexual expression among the aged, such expression exists and, happily, to a considerable extent.

William Masters and Virginia Johnson have emphasized that the "two basic needs for regularity of sexual expression in 70 to 80 year old women...[are] a reasonably good state of general health and an interesting and interested partner."[24] The same is true of the aging male.

3 Most disabilities of the old cannot be prevented or helped.

Like the other myths, this one demands a definition. What is old? Sixty-five? That was set as the proper time for old-age insurance in Germany almost a century ago by Otto von Bismarck (after he had precipitated two wars and helped lay the groundwork for a third). But, after all, health measures have improved enormously in the past century. And new research holds even more promise for the aged. "If we could completely eliminate deaths after age 65 from the number one killer of older persons, major cardiovascular renal-disease, life expectancy at age 65 would jump from 15 years to 25 years."[25] To this the often neglected element of *preventive* medicine must be added. The seeds of a healthy old age must be planted in the young so as to prevent early death from such diseases as lung cancer and atherosclerosis.

Finally, not all older people are the same. There are old sixty-year-olds and young eighty-year-olds. An eighty-year-old square dancer once visited his physician because of a sore left knee. After a thorough examination, the doctor explained that the sore left knee was just a normal part of growing old. "If it's so normal," asked the old gentleman, "why is my right knee fine? It's just as old as the left!"

Death: "The Birthday of Your Eternity"*

People think of death in different ways. The nineteenth century U.S. poet Emily Dickinson wrote:

> Because I could not stop for
> Death—
> He kindly stopped for me—
> The Carriage held but just
> Ourselves—
> And Immortality.[26]

In these lines death is neither a process nor an event. Death is a living being who apparently drives a carriage (or has a chauffeur) and goes about picking up people. Martin Luther King, Jr., also characterized death as a personality when he wrote, "I shall die, but that is all that I shall do for Death."

Perhaps endowing death with human characteristics is one way of making it seem less mysterious. But however one chooses to see death, it seems clear that people's attitudes toward it generally reflect their attitudes toward life. There is no mistaking the stereotyped "Hollywood" attitude toward life in this advertisement that ran some years ago in *The Los Angeles Times:* "FOR SALE—Vault in Forest Lawn. Across from famous movie star. Owner moving east."

The Silent Minority

About two million people (or roughly one percent of the population) of this country die every year. They join the many billions of people who have died throughout the ages. The dead are a vast silent majority. The dying are a silent minority. And like many members of disadvantaged minority groups, they often suffer intensely. Until recently, few spoke out for their rights as human beings. Yet the incurably ill must be helped and treated.

Many of the dying have outlived those who were once dear to them, and so they have few—if any—loved ones around to make their last journey less lonely. Even when this is not the case, dying people often sense that they distress, even frighten, family members and may thus discourage those who genuinely want to help. The dying are not wrong in thinking that people turn away from death. For most people—especially the young—death is something of which they do not want to be reminded. Death, they want to believe, can happen only to someone else. So in the hospital or the nursing home the dying are shunted to a room at the end of the hall, or even to special areas secluded from visitors and other patients. In this way, death—both for the living and the dying—remains in the shadows, apart from the process of life.

What can be done to ease the pain of approaching death in a way that confronts dying as a reality of life?

Often the family can do much to keep the dying person involved with day-to-day living. For example, has a grandchild a new tooth? The dying grandparent should be among the first to know. Did Willie scrape his knee? Is Sheilah taking swimming lessons? Let the dying share the arithmetic of the lives of those they love. Dying people should be allowed to remain at home as long as possible. When they can no longer leave the hospital or nursing home, members of the family should be encouraged to participate as much as possible in the routines of the hospital.

First in England, and now in this country, *hospices* instead of hospitals have become the final home for many dying people. There the terminally ill are given pain-killing drugs before pain occurs. Thus relieved of pain as much as possible, the dying patient and the family are better able to confront and deal with the realities of impending death. There is a National Hospice Organization in New Haven, Connecticut. And in Brooklyn, New York, Tucson, Arizona, and Branford, Connecticut, there are operating hospices. More are being organized. Berkeley, California, has developed a telephone hotline for dying people. Called the Shanti Project (in Sanskrit, *shanti* means "inner peace"), it is a needed and growing service. Volunteer callers are matched to dying clients (who may be at home or in a hospital) according to age, religion, and experience with a similar disease. Since medical advances have not only lengthened the life span but also the dying period, such emotional support offered by hospices and by Berkeley's volunteer group are of increasing importance.

Prevention or lessening of lonely desolation is the most important service the living can perform for the dying. They can help by caring to the very end. And in their caring, in their goodbyes, the living will also be performing a service for themselves—the acceptance of death as a natural end to life.

---

*Death was referred to in this way by Seneca, the ancient Roman writer, almost two thousand years ago.

Dying: A Life Process

For many years, one of the most dedicated students of dying has been Dr. Elisabeth Kübler-Ross of Chicago. An early discovery she made was that dying patients are willing, even eager, to discuss their situation and their feelings about it. They need honesty and frankness from the beginning of a serious illness. And, generally, they want to be told that there is always some hope and want to know that they will not be deserted. Kübler-Ross has identified five stages of dying:

1 Denial.

"No," the patient wants to believe "it is not me. It is somebody else who is dying." In this first stage, a very human defense mechanism takes over to buffer the shock. Some patients may not want to discuss the illness at all; others assume the doctor has made a mistake or is simply incompetent.

2 Anger.

"Why me?" the patient then asks. At this stage, the person is no longer able to avoid the reality of the situation. Anger and resentment are directed against everyone who is alive and well—but especially against those who are close to the patient, such as hospital staff and family. Friends and relatives need to exercise a great deal of patience and understanding during this period.

3 Bargaining.

In the third stage the patient admits that death is approaching. Now, however, there is the wish to *bargain*, to make "deals," usually with God, typically involving promises to dedicate his or her talents and services to the good of humanity in exchange for a few more days, weeks, or months of life. Loved ones can help the patient in this stage by encouraging any type of discussion of death. This eases tension and opens the way for conversations about the realities of the situation.

4 Depression.

When the patient finally acknowledges that death is inevitable, he or she passes into a period of *depression*. There is deep mourning over the losses that have occurred and those that are yet to come. The person may weep or stare unseeing at an empty wall. Depression is a natural and healthy response and should not be discouraged. Mourning over the loss of one's life and all that is loved on earth helps prepare the dying person for the final stage of the process—acceptance.

5 Acceptance.

Although not necessarily happy, the dying person is finally no longer bitter or afraid. In this last stage the patient needs the companionship of loved ones. They need not speak; just the knowledge that someone is there who cares is enough. Acceptance is often characterized by a lack of feelings on the part of the dying person. Some have described this stage as a return to infancy, where little is expected and there is a passive acceptance of whatever is happening. During this final stage, loved ones often need more help than the patient.

"In the last analysis," wisely wrote the late United Nations secretary-general Dag Hammarskjöld, "it is our conception of death which decides our answers to all the questions that life puts to us."

Summary

Freud ushered in the modern era of the investigation of human emotions. He believed that human personality results from the attempts of powerful unconscious forces—basic instinctual drives and a human *conscience*—to cope with reality. Childhood conflicts may cause personality development to lag, and the adult may need help to resolve these emotional conflicts.

Two theorists whose work grew out of Freud's are Abraham Maslow and Erik Erikson. Maslow believed that human needs develop in a series of stages (a pyramid) to the highest stage of self-actualization. Erikson has envisioned eight stages of personality development, during which a person develops an ego-identity. Both theorists felt that failure to accomplish one stage may retard progress to the next, resulting in emotional problems. These can be severe, as was evidenced by the case of Joey, the "mechanical boy." That cure is possible is evidenced by the same case.

Any discussion of personality disorders and emotional problems must take into account a person's culture and its concept of normality. And then one must be careful of the assignment of labels to those who are believed to be maladjusted. The harm that can be done by labeling was proved in experiments with pseudopatients who sought admittance to psychiatric hospitals. With these cautions and limitations in mind, one can consider classifications of emotional disorders.

Those persons with psychotic disorders have lost much contact with reality. A psychosis may be either organic in origin, caused perhaps by a brain tumor or advanced syphilis, or functional. The functional psychoses are *schizophrenia*, characterized by *delusions* and *hallucinations*; *manic-depressive psychosis*, in which the patient alternates between elation and despondency; and *paranoia*, which is distinguished by delusions of persecution.

Next are the *neurotic disorders*, which do not necessarily keep an individual from functioning effectively in society. The *psychoneuroses* include *anxiety or depressive states*, *phobias*, *obsessive-compulsive reactions*, *hysterias*, and *traumatic neuroses*. The *psychosomatic disorders* originate in the mind but are manifested in bodily symptoms.

The *character disorders* cover a wide variety of emotional disturbances. At the extreme of this grouping are the *psychopathic personalities*, the habitual criminals who are totally lacking in conscience.

The final classification of emotional disorders, those that have a possible chemical cause, cannot be discussed without an understanding of the nervous system. The *peripheral nervous system* connects the entire body to the *central nervous system*, which consists of the brain and spinal cord. The basic unit of the nervous system is the *neuron*. Nerve impulses travel from a neuron's *dendrites*, through its *cell body*, then along its *axon*. At the nerve terminals of the axon is a *synapse*, or gap. The *nerve impulse* stimulates *boutons* at the *nerve terminals* to release a chemical *neurotransmitter* that causes the nerve impulse to begin in the dendrites of the next neuron. Study of the nervous system has led to findings that some emotional disorders may have chemical causes. Thus, neurotransmitters may affect mood, and manic-depressive illness may be caused by an imbalance between two brain chemicals.

Aging is an emotional experience that is common to all humanity. In the United States, where the elderly are often shut away and forgotten, aging can become an emotional crisis that too often ends in suicide. The elderly face loneliness, forced retirement, poverty, poor medical care, and misunderstanding. But recent legislation has extended the legal retirement age, and it is hoped that this will be but a first step toward making the aged an integral part of society.

Death is probably the most difficult life experience that humans must face. Living, they try to forget the end that ultimately awaits us all; dying, they often find themselves completely alone, abandoned by those who try to avoid death as they themselves once did. Extensive research by Elisabeth Kübler-Ross and others has provided a deeper understanding of the needs of the terminally ill and has helped family and friends to deal with their loss in an emotionally constructive way.

References

1. George Seferis, from "Mythistorema," in *Collected Poems 1924–1955*, p. 9. Translated, edited, and introduced by Edmund Keeley and Philip Sherrard. Copyright © 1967 by Princeton University Press. Reprinted by permission of Princeton University Press.
2. Bruno Bettelheim, "Joey: A 'Mechanical Boy,'" *Scientific American*, Vol. 200 (March 1959), p. 118.
3. Ibid., p. 117.
4. Erik H. Erikson, "Growth and Crises of the Healthy Personality," in Clyde Kluckhohn, Henry A. Murray, and David Schneider, eds., *Personality in Nature, Society, and Culture* (New York, 1953), p. 199.
5. Bettelheim, "Joey: A 'Mechanical Boy,'" pp. 122 and 124.
6. Erikson, "Growth and Crises of the Healthy Personality," p. 205.
7. Ibid., p. 211.
8. From *Memoirs of the Prince of Talleyrand*, quoted in Saul K. Padover, ed., *Confessions and Self-Portraits* (New York, 1957), p. 152.
9. Erikson, "Growth and Crises of the Healthy Personality," p. 218.
10. Erik H. Erikson, "Identity and Uprootedness in Our Time," in H.M. Ruitenbeek, ed., *Varieties of Modern Social Theory* (New York, 1963), pp. 55–68.
11. Anna Freud, *The Ego and the Mechanisms of Defense* (London, 1948), cited in Rudolf Ekstein, "Psychotic Adolescents and Their Quest for Goals," in Charlotte Bühler and Fred Massarik, *The Course of Human Life* (New York, 1968), p. 202.
12. From Samuel Noah Kramer, *Everyday Life in Bible Times*, quoted in Jerome Beatty, Jr., "Trade Winds," *Saturday Review* (March 16, 1968), p. 18.
13. Bettelheim, "Joey: A 'Mechanical Boy,'" p. 127.
14. "A Conversation with Karl Menninger and Mary Harrington Hall on the Psychology of Vengeance," *Psychology Today*, Vol. 2 (February 1969), p. 63.
15. Quoted from Ovid (43 B.C.–18 A.D.).
16. "12 Admissions of Mental Error," *Medical World News*, Vol. 14 (February 9, 1973), pp. 17–19.
17. "Being Sane in Unsane Places," *Science News*, Vol. 103 (January 20, 1973), p. 38.
18. *Science*, Vol. 179 (January 19, 1973), pp. 250–258.
19. Arthur P. Noyes and Lawrence C. Kolb, *Modern Clinical Psychiatry*, 6th ed. (Philadelphia, 1963), p. 370.
20. R. M. Marcussen and H. G. Wolff, "A Formulation of the Dynamics of the Migraine Attack," cited in *Harold G. Wolff's Stress and Disease*, 2nd ed., rev. and ed. by Stewart Wolf and Helen Goodell (Springfield Ill., 1968), p. 47.
21. Karl Menninger, *Man Against Himself* (New York, 1938), p. 368.
22. From Jean Evans, *Three Men*, quoted in Edward A. Strecker and Vincent T. Lathbury, *Their Mothers' Daughters* (Philadelphia, 1956), pp. 179–180.
23. Stanley J. Pacion, "Gandhi's Struggle with Sexuality," *Medical Aspects of Human Sexuality*, Vol. 5 (January 1971), p. 89.
24. William H. Masters and Virginia E. Johnson, *Human Sexual Inadequacy* (Boston, 1970), p. 350.
25. Harry A. Brotman, "The Fastest Growing Minority: The Aging," *American Journal of Public Health*, Vol. 64 (March 1974), p. 250.
26. From "Because I could not stop for Death" by Emily Dickinson. Reprinted by permission of the publishers and the Trustees of Amherst College from THE POEMS OF EMILY DICKINSON, edited by Thomas H. Johnson, Cambridge, Mass.: The Belknap Press of Harvard University Press, Copyright © 1951, 1955 by the President and Fellows of Harvard College.

6

The Emotional Life: Part II

Stress

For the sorcerer [witch doctor] has, as an essential part of the ritual performance, not merely to point the bone dart at his victim, but with an intense expression of fury and hatred he has to thrust it in the air, turn it and twist it as if to bore it in the wound, then pull it back with a sudden jerk. Thus, not only is the act of violence, or stabbing, reproduced, but the passion of violence has to be enacted.[1]

So did one researcher of human societies once describe the ritual of "bone pointing" by a witch doctor in a western Pacific island. (Notice in the description that the bone dart does not actually touch the victim; the act is purely symbolic.) The victim was a man who had broken some basic rule of the tribe. His punishment: death. To be read out of the living, to be damned, to be considered already dead by one's own people meant death. Terrified by his belief in the absolute powers of magic, unable to escape these beliefs, utterly alone because of loss of support of his kin, excommunicated by the very people with whom he had once shared food, shelter, and safety, the tragic figure could not endure his lonely anxiety and depression. Sinking from trembling anxiety to choking terror to tormented collapse, and finally to total resignation, the "boned" man lay on the ground silently awaiting death. Toward nightfall, members of the community who had forsaken him, returned. But they brought him no help, no word of comfort. They uttered over his still body the prayers of the dead. Then, for the last time, he was abandoned. Soon he was dead. What killed him? Stress.

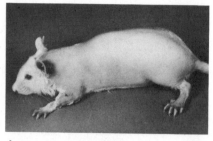

A

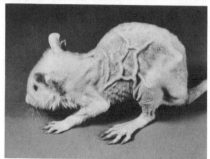

B

FIGURE 6–1
Stress and aging. There is some evidence that the changes that occur with aging are hastened by extreme stress. Both rats shown here came from the same litter. Rat A was fed a diet containing chemicals that produced stress in the animal and thus speeded up aging. However, included in its diet was another chemical that neutralized the "aging chemicals." Rat B was fed a diet containing only the aging chemicals. Although both rats are actually two months old, Rat A is young and vigorous. Rat B seems long past retirement age.

Stress as a Universal Experience

Stress, of course, is not limited to less developed cultures, nor is its effect usually so extreme. What, then, is stress? It is the body's reaction to any demand made of it, ranging anywhere from enjoying the music of a favorite orchestra to confronting a robber on a dark street. So it is not stress as such that is dangerous. It is the *kind* of stress, and the way a person *copes* with stress that decides whether health will be harmed or even life endangered.

At times everybody experiences harmful degrees of stress. Breathing often quickens. The throat tightens. The heart beats too quickly. The scalp may tingle. The stomach sours. Muscles knot. The head aches. People have common phrases for these experiences: "It makes my skin crawl," somebody may say, or "My heart was in my mouth," or "It turns my stomach," and so on. If harmful stress continues for too long a time for an individual unable to cope with it, sleep, digestion, and appetite may all become problems. Or, when a person overreacts, stress may result in raids on the refrigerator in the middle of the night. Stress may also lead to self-destructive behaviors, such as an excessive use of alcohol or other drugs. Unrelieved excessive stress can also lead to anxiety, to depression, to destruction of relationships with other people, to aging (see Figure 6–1), and, as has been seen, to death.

The General Adaptation Syndrome (G.A.S.)

Prolonged or severe stress shows itself by a set of signs and symptoms, a nondiscrete **syndrome**. This particular condition was identified as the **General Adaptation Syndrome** (**G.A.S.**) by Dr. Hans Selye, a pioneer in stress studies. Many physicians believe that the stages are not distinct, and that not all persons go through all the stages, which are as follows:

1. First there is *alarm.* The alarm stage itself produces three responses. (a) One is *stomach ulcers* that may bleed. It should be noted that stress-caused ulcers are quite different from the chronic stomach ulcers of which you may have heard. (b) A second part of the alarm stage is *enlargement of the adrenal glands,* one of which sits on top of each kidney. Chemical hormones are released from the adrenal glands into the blood. Among these hormones is *adrenalin.* It is adrenalin that increases the heart and breathing rates, blood pressure, and flow of blood to the muscles. Adrenalin is a protective hormone; it makes possible the "fight or flight" response to danger that one can observe most clearly in lower animals. Humans, on the other hand, have become so socialized into their patterns of behavior that "fight or flight" has too often been replaced by "sit and stew." This may relieve a person of the need to look for a new job, but it does not relieve stress. Furthermore, accumulated stress may impair one's ability to work effectively. (c) A third part of the alarm stage, which has been observed in animal experiments, is *shrinkage of the thymus gland* (located beneath the breast bone) *and the lymph nodes* (see page 94). The thymus gland and the lymph nodes are involved in fighting infection, which may explain why stressed people tend to be more prone to infections.

2. The second stage of the General Adaptation Syndrome is *resistance.* This is the ability to func-

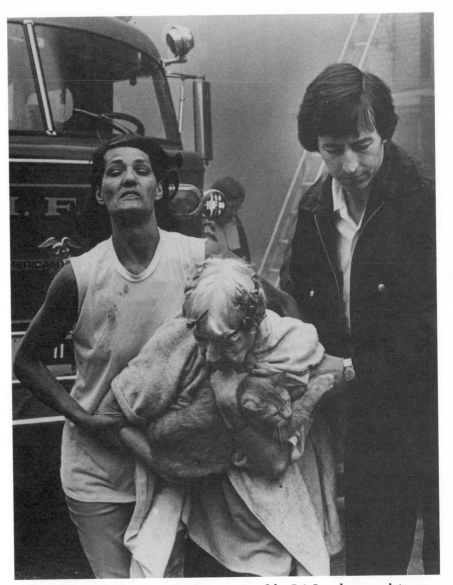

In this scene of severe stress, the three stages of the G.A.S.—alarm, resistance, and exhaustion—are almost visible on the faces of those involved.

tion despite stress. The changes that happened during the alarm stage seem to disappear. Like the release of the hormone adrenalin, the resistance stage also seems protective. It may continue until the stress stops. Should the stress continue, however, the individual loses the advantages that accompany the fight or flight response and resistance. The person then becomes over-

whelmed and utterly exhausted by the stress.

3. *Exhaustion,* then, is the third stage of the G.A.S. During the exhaustion stage many of the physical signs and symptoms of alarm reappear. Now, however, they may be devastating. Unless the stress is relieved or stopped, sickness, and perhaps even death, occurs.

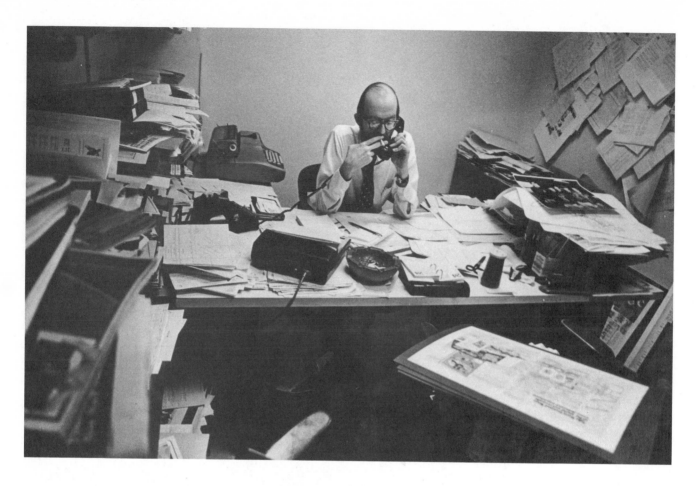

For Different People Stress Has Different Meanings

Is it possible that there might be a life situation that presents little or no real stress to anyone? The job is satisfying. The hours are regular. The boss is agreeable. The pay is good. For some, such a job is a joy. But will it bring stressless peace to all people? No. A person who strives to achieve will suffer stress because of the *absence* of challenging stress. So, stress must be individualized. It can be either good or bad for a person's health. Is it possible for a person to find some kind of average stress level that will do the most good and the least harm? To a degree, and within the limits of pres-

ent knowledge, it is. But, as has been emphasized, one must remember that people are not the same. With many people, for example, stress is the *result*, not the *cause*, of poor adjustment. Poor adaptation can lead to anxiety and depression. These, in turn, may affect the ability to respond to stress. So stress is not a simple cause-and-effect phenomenon. It may cause, or be caused by, anxiety and depression. Each person needs to find his or her own least harmful and most beneficial stress levels.

The Social Readjustment Rating Scale

The greatest cause of stress is change. Nobody can avoid change.

Six hundred years before Christ, the Greek thinker Heraclitus made this clear by saying that "There is nothing permanent except change." Twenty-five centuries later the U.S. writer Alvin Toffler wrote that people have "... a limited capacity for change. When this capacity is overwhelmed, the consequence is future shock."[2] What can be done to cope with change and to endure future shock?

The Social Readjustment Rating Scale (Table 6–1), developed by Dr. Thomas H. Holmes and his associates, begins to suggest one way. The scale lists forty-three common life events. The events are ranked in the order of their tendency to cause stress and, therefore, illness. Whether the events benefit or harm a person does not determine the risk of the illness resulting from them. It is the *event per se* that is decisive. If too many events happen within a single year, the chances of illness occurring within the next two years increase.

Referring to Table 6–1, consider this (extreme) example: In January, Marsha inherits a lot of money (38 points) because of the sudden death of her husband (100 points), and she therefore retires from her job (45 points). She remarries ten months later (50 points). Expecting to further improve her new life situation, she accepts a fine new job offer (36 points). A decrease in church activities (19 points) and an increase in social activities (18 points) result from her marriage and from the desire to further brighten her life. But in less than a one-year period Marsha has endured 306 points of change—some happy, some unhappy. Because she has gone through so much change in such a short amount of time, she has greatly increased her chances of becoming ill in the near future.

TABLE 6–1
The Social Readjustment Rating Scale

LIFE EVENT	MEAN VALUE
1. Death of spouse	100
2. Divorce	73
3. Marital separation	65
4. Jail term	63
5. Death of close family member	63
6. Personal injury or illness	53
7. Marriage	50
8. Fired at work	47
9. Marital reconciliation	45
10. Retirement	45
11. Change in health of family member	44
12. Pregnancy	40
13. Sex difficulties	39
14. Gain of new family member	39
15. Business readjustment	39
16. Change in financial state	38
17. Death of close friend	37
18. Change to different line of work	36
19. Change in number of arguments with spouse	35
20. Mortgage over $10,000	31
21. Foreclosure of mortgage or loan	30
22. Change in responsibilities at work	29
23. Son or daughter leaving home	29
24. Trouble with in-laws	29
25. Outstanding personal achievement	28
26. Wife begin or stop work	26
27. Begin or end school	26
28. Change in living conditions	25
29. Revision of personal habits	24
30. Trouble with boss	23
31. Change in work hours or conditions	20
32. Change in residence	20
33. Change in schools	20
34. Change in recreation	19
35. Change in church activities	19
36. Change in social activities	18
37. Mortgage or loan less than $10,000	17
38. Change in sleeping habits	16
39. Change in number of family get-togethers	15
40. Change in eating habits	15
41. Vacation	13
42. Christmas	12
43. Minor violations of the law	11

SOURCE: Reprinted with permission from *Journal of Psychosomatic Research*, Vol. 11, T. H. Holmes and R. H Rahe, "The Social Readjustment Rating Scale," Copyright © 1967, Pergamon Press, Ltd. See this article for complete wording of the items.

While she had no control over some of the events that brought about this change, she did have control over others. For instance, she would have experienced less stress if she had not remarried as soon as she did or if she had stayed at her original job.

Note that stress travels with a person. A stressful problem at home may be carried to, and thus affect, one's working and/or social life. Stress is then added to stress until the unhappy person breaks down physically, emotionally, or both—depending on his or her vulnerability. Moreover, the frequency of occurrence of some of the life events varies with such factors as age, marital status, education, culture, gender, socioeconomic status, past experience, and other factors. For example, the death of a spouse does not happen to single people; a change of living conditions on retirement does not happen to prisoners; college students do not often go to jail.

Dr. Holmes' scale presents variables that call for caution in application,[3] and it should be used with these limitations in mind. Nevertheless, for some people it can offer some insights into the amounts of stress they are under, thus encouraging them to think about ways to cope with it successfully. How?

Ways to Avoid Stress-Related Illness

1 Knowing the amount of stress that accompanies specific life events, one may plan to avoid or postpone certain actions.

For example, a marriage might be postponed for a few months if a close relative dies suddenly, or plans to change one's job probably ought not to coincide with plans to buy a new house. It is often better to prevent some life crises by intelligent planning than to try and cope with too many of them at one time.

2 Stress may be relieved by recreational exercise.

Some excellent types of recreational exercise are tennis, jogging, and swimming. As discussed in Chapter 8, exercise should be a regular part of every person's life.

3 Relaxation training is a way of learning to relieve stress by reducing stimuli as much as possible.

Different researchers have developed various programs for relaxation training. In general, such programs offer step-by-step exercises that are practical and effective and that can be done at home. Instructions can be memorized through practice, or they can be recorded on tape to be played back during the exercise period. Most relaxation training consists of four basic elements: (1) Extreme tensing and then relaxing of muscle groups makes the individual more aware of tension and relaxation. Most people, for example, do not realize how often the brow is tensely furrowed, the jaw muscles clamped shut, and the teeth tightly clenched. Deliberately causing these muscles to tense and then relieving them is part of the relaxation process. (2) Deep breathing; (3) repeating in one's mind a word or phrase that has a calming effect, such as "relax"; and

(4) visualizing a pleasant scene during relaxation exercises may all be helpful.

One method of relaxation training is as follows: Sit comfortably in a quiet, darkened room. Close your eyes. Take several deep breaths, hold them, and breathe out slowly. In this way relaxation is begun. Holding your breath or taking a series of slow deep breaths increases the amount of carbon dioxide in the blood. A mild sedative effect is achieved.

The next step is to first tense muscles and then relax them. Concentrate on the calm that results when the muscles relax. Deep breathing should be continued. With each exhalation a word or phrase should be repeated in your mind. It can be a word or phrase of your own choice that signifies relaxation. People who practice Transcendental Meditation (to which the present process is very similar) refer to this word as their "mantra." Visualization of a peaceful atmosphere is the final step. It may be a long-forgotten path in a quiet woods or the surf of a deserted beach. There are people who devote half an hour a day to this training procedure.

4 Another way of dealing with stress is assertiveness training.

It is based on an honest, open attempt at a *considerate* exchange of feelings between people. Notice the emphasis on the word considerate. Assertiveness is not hurtful aggression, nor is it "telling someone off," even though it is a sharing of feelings. One of the needed skills of life is learning to make one's feelings clear without being cruel or destructive. One cannot expect to be understood without first being

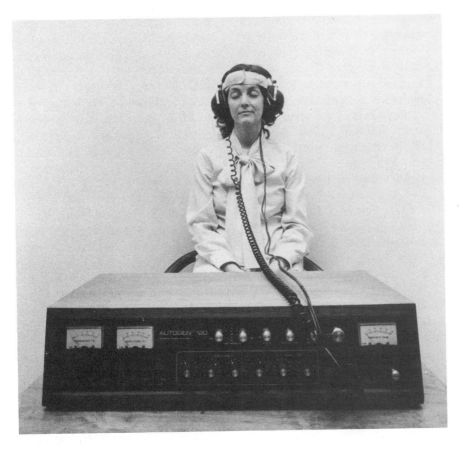

In this biofeedback technique, the subject is made aware of her own brain waves, which are monitored by an electroencephalographic machine. Here the device is being used to achieve a meditational state of mind.

understanding. Much tension can be relieved through an honest and nonhurtful exchange of feelings. Such sharing is not a new idea. Over three and a half centuries ago the English scholar Robert Burton wrote in *The Anatomy of Melancholy:*

> . . . the best way for ease is to impart our misery to some friend, not to smother it up in our own breast; for grief concealed strangles the soul; but when as we shall but impart it to some discreet, trusty, loving friend, it is instantly removed.

Today, assertiveness training is often a part of group therapy. A well-trained and sensitive group leader is essential. A poorly trained, insensitive leader can do great harm to already troubled people.

5 Still another method of relaxation is biofeedback.

This more expensive method involves the use of machinery that monitors the results of some body action, such as muscle tension, on a continuous basis. The information is fed back to the individual as a signal. In this way the person may learn to control the particular body function being monitored. Biofeedback is still somewhat experimental, and it should be practiced only by people who are proved professionally competent. Medical associations, appropriate university departments, mental health departments, private physicians, clinical psychologists, and psychiatric social workers and nurses are good sources for information about biofeedback practitioners.

Coping with Personal Change: A Creative Process

> *The ability to react to stress emotionally, to come apart, and then to pull oneself together again is the heart of the creative process—a process that requires calling upon important inner resources as they are needed.[4]*

In this chapter it has been noted that change is the most common cause of stress. And in the last chapter it was seen that the changes of physical and emotional growth are often accompanied by some stress. But even as personality development causes stress, so does stress demand growth of the personality. Psychiatrist Frederic Flach adds insight to the process when he writes that stress may result in a demand for creativity. In this sense stress becomes an opportunity to mature. True, life is beset with change. But, within limits, people can make practical creative choices and thus often turn personal defeat into personal victory.

Flach contends that when reacting to stress one passes through three stages.[5] First, there is the *impact*. A broken love affair or a job that is lost are two common examples. This is followed by *functional imbalance* within the person, who then tends to fall apart. Falling apart emotionally is a necessary response to stress and requisite to the third, or *healing*, phase, during which the person goes through the process of restoring emotional balance.

Flach lists four principles of creative thought that can help people make wiser choices in dealing with changing and stressful situations.

1. **Defer judgment.** Impulsive action robs the individual of the chance to obtain more information, to choose, to let go of old notions, and to consider new ideas.

2. **Quantity leads to quality.** This is tied to the first principle. The more ideas that one can entertain, the more choosing one can do. There are unconscious sources of creativity. Let them come to the fore.

3. **Redefine the problem.** Looking at all aspects of the stressful situation and expressing it in different ways stimulate creative problem solving. For example, James is considering getting married. It is a major change guaranteed to cause some stress. He must think creatively, asking such questions as these: What do I expect of marriage? Have my expectations changed recently? Why? How well do I expect to handle not being single? What about the marriage's effect on others? What would happen if I decided not to get married? The answers to these and similar questions can help make James's decision easier and also clarify, and possibly reduce, the potential stress.

4. **Distancing.** Being too near a problem may stifle ideas about its solution. Getting away from it for a while makes room for new creative ideas to be considered.[6]

Some extremely stressful situations will require the help of a trained therapist or counselor, such as a psychiatrist, clinical psychologist, or psychiatric social worker. Many people often recognize the need for help but do not actually seek it. Actively obtaining professional advice when it is needed is in itself a creative act of self-help.

Even when changes are not all clustered together into too many at once, it may still be a good idea to try to avoid some or to find a better approach to dealing with them. Some changes and stresses may be worth enduring to achieve a long-term purpose. And if some of them are not, what other choices are available? It is always advisable to consider alternatives before acting. *Realistic* knowledge that alternatives to a stressful situation exist in itself helps relieve stress and enables one to avoid needless surprises that often cause a sinking feeling of helplessness. Research has shown that helplessness may be a learned response to stressful situations. In other words, some people over the years come to believe that their actions can make no difference in creating pleasure or reducing pain; eventually they convince themselves that they are "born losers." This belief, among others, easily spawns the twin troubles of stress—anxiety and depression. Consider them now.

Anxiety

What is **anxiety**? It is a feeling of apprehension or uneasiness related to something that is about to happen. As a term it is more closely associated with worry than with fear. What is the difference between fear and anxiety? Fear is caused by an immediate situation. One is fearful of something or somebody specific and present. However, anxiety may be quite vague, and it is always associated with concern about the future.

People have a reservoir of anxieties—most have been conquered, but others are either half-remembered or deeply buried in the subconscious. The first strange face, the initial separation from the mother, the first day at school—these childhood anxieties are added to the countless anxiety-associated strivings, defeats, and victories that are part of living.

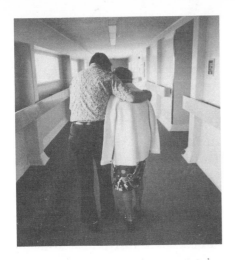

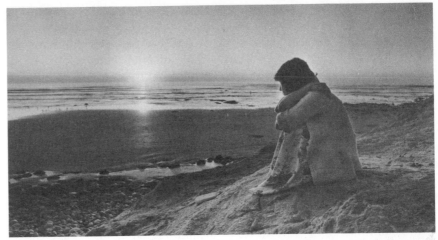

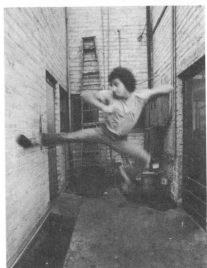

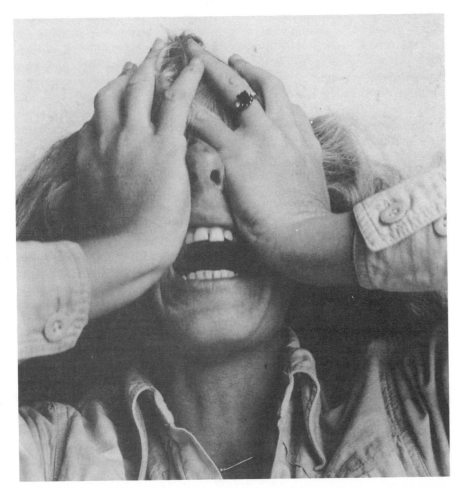

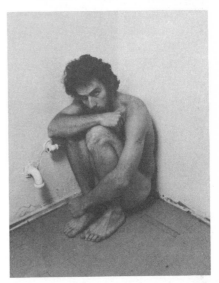

How Anxiety Is Expressed

Anxiety has the power to move the whole of one's emotional life. Its more severe signs and symptoms are only too recognizable: the dry throat, the quavering whisper, and, in extremes of anxious terror, the stifled scream. Less dramatic (but just as distressing and more common) signs of anxiety are restlessness, cold sweat, palpitating heart, muscular tension in the back of the neck, chest pain, and a hopeless, helpless sense of impending disaster. However, people differ in their reactions to similar situations. For one person a financial setback does not mean lasting ruin. Anxiety is used profitably. Work achieves recovery. Another person becomes so anxious by the possibility of a relatively minor loss that action to recovery seems impossible. Still another person is made anxious by a spot on his or her clothes. Yet when someone asked Albert Einstein why he was so indifferent to his clothes, the great physicist merely answered, "It would be a pity if the wrapping proved better than the meat."

Anxiety may be contagious. Observe a line of small children waiting to be immunized. Approaching the needle, a child begins to cry. One by one, many of the others will also cry. And who has not at some time been made anxious by a sweating, nail-biting classmate during an exam? Moderate, controlled anxiety causes the student to study more than usual. The student passes. Anxiety has been a motivating friend. Had the student been so anxious as to be unable to concentrate, anxiety would have been a foe. If the student had failed the exam, he or she might have experienced some passing depression but, one hopes, would have gained some determination to do better the next time. It is

contagious anxiety that tyrants use to control people. But it is also contagious anxiety that encourages humankind to combat tyranny.

One Cause of Modern Anxiety: Rapid Achievement Overtakes Human Wisdom

Along with increased knowledge comes an increase in the number of anxieties besetting people in modern society. "It has been determined that a weekday copy of *The New York Times* has as much to read as the educated individual in sixteenth-century Europe absorbed during his lifetime."[7] Moreover, the content of this reading material offers a comparable increase in anxiety-provoking stimuli: Murder, rape, highway accidents, and wars are served up in the daily newspaper along with one's breakfast. People are anxious because they are unable to control not only what they know, but also what they are about to know. Nuclear power, pollution, inflation, and unemployment are real threats that have given people every reason to feel insecure.

Yet it is not science and social problems alone that people fear; people also fear people. Why? Because we do not know each other. Our knowledge of ourselves and our ability to communicate with others has not kept pace with technological discoveries. We can communicate with astronauts on the moon, but not always with people across the table. Today, the failure to establish genuine human contact not only disturbs personal relationships but has the potential to disturb, and destroy, the entire human population. Human knowledge has outstripped wisdom.

So, worldwide anxieties are an unavoidable part of these times. There are perhaps few of us who can do much to control the fate of humanity, but by understanding the sources of personal conflict and anxiety there is much we can control closer to home.

Childhood Anxiety

If there is anything that we wish to change in the child, we should first examine it and see whether it is not something that could better be changed in ourselves.

CARL JUNG (1875–1961)

Long before birth, the fetus's first heartbeat pumps not the mother's blood, but the fetus's own blood, which is independently produced. Thousands of such independent steps—from rolling over in the crib to walking to going off to college—mark the child's progress away from the mother. But it is a long and frustrating journey. Prolonged dependency gives the child the time needed to learn the behavior expected by the culture. But this extensive period of dependency can also produce frustration, stress, depression, insecurity, hate, guilt, and anxiety.

The childhood struggle for freedom takes place in an atmosphere of both love and hate. Children love their world and all in it when it gratifies them, and they hate it when it frustrates them. Parents are loved when they give comfort, hated when they exert control. This love-hate feeling, which is carried into later years, is a major source of stress and anxiety. And the frustrations of dependency continue, as hostility, into adulthood. The parent loves the child; the parent hates the child. The adult loves the mate; the adult hates the mate. This emotional paradox is universal and not peculiar to modern people. Twenty centuries ago the Roman lyric poet Catullus wrote these perplexed lines:

At once I love and hate
You ask why this should be,
I know not, 'tis my fate
A fate of Agony![8]

Adults who understand that it is common and natural for feelings to contradict one another will be less stressed, depressed, and anxious by the experience. But children cannot realize this, and often they suffer a great deal of guilt and anxiety over what they consider "bad" or "evil" feelings. The loving parent can help by understanding and by explaining that it is all right to have such feelings. But should help not come, the child will struggle on alone, still seeking independence but hampered by confusion and anxiety. Should the parent impede the child in the normal quest for independence, the child will retaliate with hate and suffer guilt and anxiety because of this.

During each stage of personality development, any normal child is bound to collect problems. Usually the child learns from them, and they do not become serious emotional traumas. But traumatized or not, the child will continue to seek competence and independence. Should the heart form imperfectly and leak, it will, nonetheless, beat as long as possible. Should a child's oral needs be thwarted too often, those needs may well crop up in later life and the adult may cope with them by constant emotional overeating. But, to repeat, the child will develop

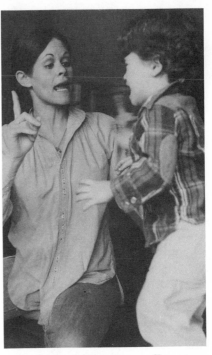

A mother's scolding is usually not an expression of hatred for the child, but usually the child—at least temporarily—hates his mother when she scolds him.

nonetheless. Well equipped or not, the child will seek competence and independence. This, then, the wise parent will accept.

Striving for independence, the developing child needs to understand discipline, not continuously suffer from it. The more the child clearly comprehends what the parents expect, and why, the less discipline will be needed and the less the child will suffer when discipline is necessary. The mother who literally screams her emotional responses to a child's behavior is more successful, at least in this respect, than the parent who is sanctimoniously silent and is seen as being mysterious. Mysterious parents frighten their children. There is room for mystery in love of God or in love between the sexes. There is no room for it in parent-child love. A child who never really knows how a parent feels has problems with discipline.

One day, a little girl pulls the pots and pans from the cupboard. She is kissed and told she is cute. The next day, repeating the same performance, she turns happily to her mother. But her mother is in a different mood, and the child is scolded and spanked. The little girl is hurt, not corrected. One day the father answers his little girl's proposal of marriage with "Sure, honey, aren't you my best girl?" (a lying answer to an honest question). The next week, the little girl repeats her proposal. It is met with cold indifference or even with harsh hostility (adding injury to error).

Children are not miniature adults. They do not spring fully formed into adulthood. They develop gradually. So do their anxieties. Children need constancy, not confusion. That is why they love peek-a-boo games and why they never tire of hearing the same bedtime story. They know what will happen; they can count on it. Discipline of children works best when it arises from constant love, not intermittent hate. And the cruelly overdisciplined child may develop a costly belief—that violence works. Violence breeds violence. Child-beaters almost always have one thing in common: They were themselves heartlessly beaten as children. So the sins of the parents are indeed often visited upon the children.

Parents often have more influence on their children than they realize.

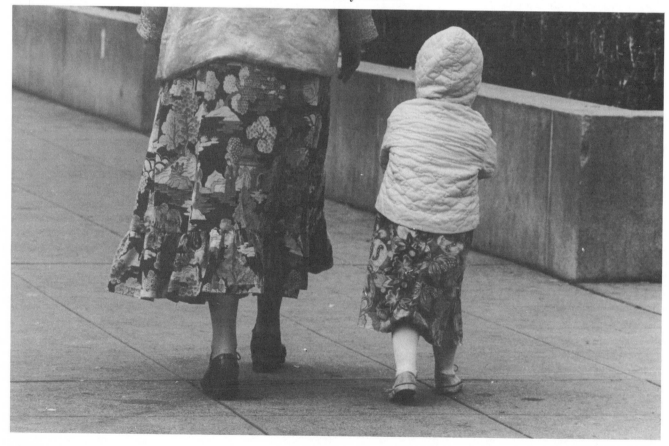

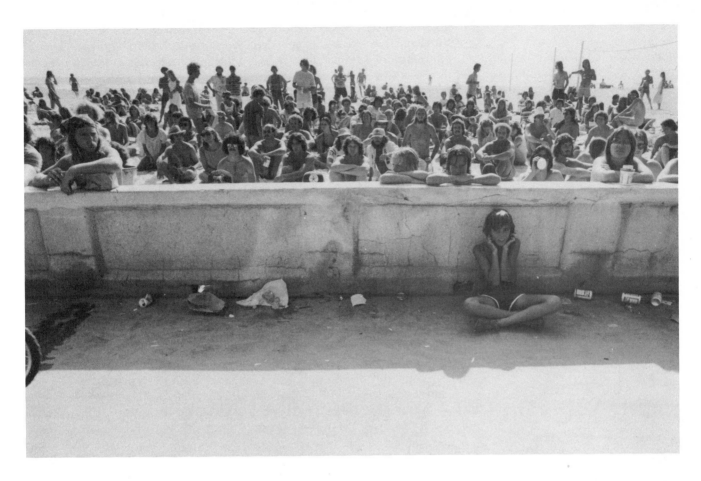

Teenage-age Anxiety

Each youth sustains within his
   breast
A vague and infinite unrest.
He goes about in still alarm,
With shrouded future at his arm,
With longings that can find no
   tongue.
I see him thus, for I am young.[9]

Today's teen-age culture is largely a phenomenon of wealthy societies. True, a great many teen-agers do not have much money, and they must shoulder the responsibilities of an adult—possibly prematurely. Nonetheless, a significant share of this nation's economy depends on this powerfully monied leisure class. Without the money teen-agers spend on movies, records, cosmetics, clothes, cigarettes, and second-hand cars, a good portion of the economy would be sorely shaken. Madison Avenue flatters, cajoles, and caters to teen-agers; adults criticize them; and along all the remnant Main Streets of the nation, grown-ups at home, school, and church collectively wag a reproving finger at them—wondering how long it will take them to straighten out. By "straighten out," the adults mean, of course, to be more like themselves.

The adult desire for self-perpetuation is natural. The Indian poet Tagore wrote that "we must not forget that life is here to express the eternal in us."[10] But if children are truly to meet the parental need for the eternal, and if they are to develop the deepest purpose of their

Who has not, at times, felt alone in the world? Among teen-agers this feeling can be particularly overwhelming.

lives, their lives must have purpose. In the past, teen-agers made a definite financial contribution to their families. This is generally no longer expected of them. It is not completely true that teen-agers today have a different set of values than adults. Like their elders they simply buy the pleasures they can afford. And many teen-agers just imitate the adults they know. They are out for the bigger, the better, and—that ultimate measure of having made it—the most. And like their parents, the pursuit of "things" has not made them happier or less anxious.

The same matters trouble today's teen-agers that used to nag their parents. Who am I? What am I? What will become of me? "Be yourself, Debbie," one kindly parent advised her adolescent. "How can I," came her answer, "until I find out who I am?" And hers is not the best age for waiting. Only too keenly does the teen-ager understand the penetrating remark made by one cowboy, "I ain't what I ought to be, I ain't what I'm going to be, but I ain't what I was."[11] How can teen-agers find themselves? How can they avoid the confusion that Erikson has spoken of as "self-diffusion"?

The answers cannot be found in the mirror. The startling changes taking place in teen-agers' bodies hardly afford reassurance that life will remain constant and predictable. And their new and overwhelming emotions often provoke only fatigue and worry. With the sharp and cruel insight that comes with their age, teen-agers are quick to see the glaring faults of their elders and of society in general. It would be surprising if they were *not* filled with anxiety.

The fortunate adolescent will meet an adult who can listen and who faces both adolescent and adult problems squarely. Such an adult will have learned that love means knowing and being known by another person. Such an adult will help prepare the young person for the dignity of adult intimacy. But finding such an adult is not easy.

WHERE CAN A PERSON FIND A PERSON?

Today's youth has a communication problem. The young person needs to talk to an older person who sees the past and the present, but not through worn-out spectacles. An older person can help a younger one handle the knowns of the past and the unknowns of the future.

As never before, an overwhelming confusion of rapid changes besets the modern student. Nevertheless, yesterday's answers do not always fit today's questions. What is right? What is wrong? Tomorrow is unpredictable, uncontrollable, undependable, so why make any plans? All this and more must be talked over with somebody. Yet every place is a crowd. Where can a person find a person to talk to? At home? For some, home is too far away. For others, there is nobody home. Still others have no home. In the church? Too often one goes to church out of habit, not because one really wants to go. Teachers? Some teachers look like listeners, but there is often a long line there. The search for a willing adult ear often ends in forlorn failure.

Adults today must hear and heed these words of the ancient Greek thinker Socrates: "Citizens of Athens, why is it that you turn and scrape every stone to gather wealth and neglect your children to whom, one day, you must relinquish it all?"

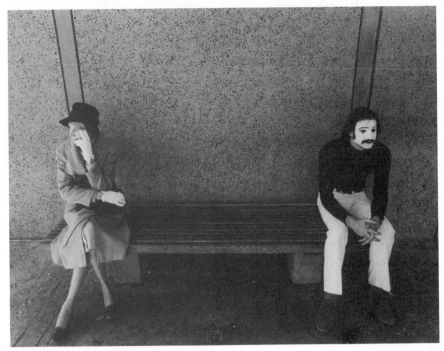

Where can a person find a person?

Parenting and Anxiety

A confused young mother presented her dilemma to her family physician this way: "It's my fault," she said, "I should have breast-fed my baby." Suddenly she was angry. "But I wanted to go back to work—I didn't want to be tied down for months, and I never liked it anyway. Then I read an article in this magazine." She held up a popular family journal. "Is it really that unnatural not to breast-feed your baby? You told me to forget about it. But a friend of mine read that unless you breast-feed your baby, there is something wrong with you. Is that somebody's idea of a joke? I don't understand all the mixed advice I'm getting. Everybody says something different."

Some women want to breast-feed their babies. That is good. They enjoy it and do it easily. Others, who are just as normal, do not enjoy breast-feeding or do not want the responsibility that breast-feeding demands. These women should not breast-feed their babies. An angry or guilty mother, resentfully holding her child to her breast, will do that child no good. It is the total experience of dining, of human comfort and tenderness, that is essential to the baby in this stage, which Erikson calls basic trust versus mistrust (refer back to pages 127–128).

The young woman described above is an example of how young parents can be victimized by an endless barrage of conflicting advice. Don't pick up Billie when he screams. Pick up Billie when he screams. Exclude Susie from the bedroom; what if she does feel left out? Don't exclude Susie from the bedroom; she'll feel left out. Never take Willie's hands away from his penis; if you do, he'll masturbate in public. Always divert Willie when he's doing his exploring; if you don't, he'll masturbate in public. And so on, endlessly. The result is needlessly confused parents, doubtful of every action, suspicious of their own ability to love, convinced of their inadequacy, and suffering from anxiety and guilt.

The relation between infant and mother is a ballet, in which each partner responds to the steps of the other.[12]

The infant feels hunger. Hunger hurts. There is threat, stress, anxiety. The child cries and is fed. Tension and anxiety are relieved. But sometimes the child cries, and the breast (or bottle) does not come. The child can do nothing but cry more. The hurt is more. Stress

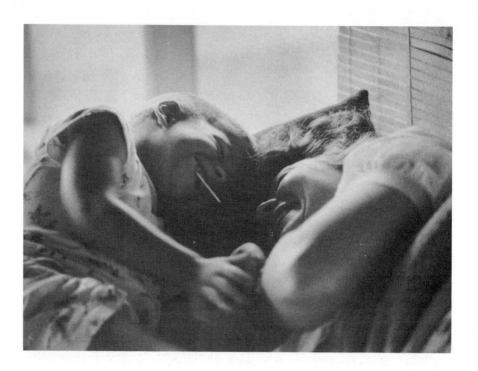

grows, and so does anxiety. Too much frustration will teach the child that the most important person cannot be counted upon. The child loses basic trust.

It can be seen, then, that parents must develop too. As the Friedmans have noted,[13] parents pass through stages related to the stages of their child's development (see Table 6–2). Parents and children develop together, experiencing singular, yet interwoven problems. And, like their children, parents in the throes of one stage may still be occupied with unsolved problems of a past stage.

In the first stage, the parents try to learn how to interpret such cues as howling. What is the baby trying to tell them? The child is dry, fed, fondled. No diaper pin pierces the bottom. Why, then, does the child weep? Is it still another gas bubble? Or is it because the bed was accidentally moved six inches from the window and the usual shaft of bright light is missed? The infant

in this stage loves only the self. Moreover, parental love is given without conditions: It is free.[14]

In the second stage, the infant who did little but lie around and sleep and cry is suddenly a toddler and getting into everything. It is as if the child cannot find time to do everything possible. And the parents find that they have no time to do anything but try to keep up with the child. The toddler is confronted with the fact that love is no longer unconditional; it must, through many small and seemingly big demands and commands, be earned. Love has a price.[15] Finally the third stage of parental development— separation—is reached.

The pain of separation is not limited to children. The sight of the child going off alone on the school bus or walking alone through the door of the nursery or kindergarten class is not one that many mothers or fathers soon forget. Nor is the fourth stage, characterized by the child's new-found independence,

any easier for the parents. Their child's "declaration of independence," may cause hurt and anger. It is almost as difficult for the rejected parents to remember that they are still desperately needed as it is for them to understand the rejection. The fifth stage of parental personality development is marked by an opportunity for the parents to rebuild their lives, now with themselves more in mind.

Parental development begins with the parents' own childhood. Parents need help, and many come to realize that their children are trying to give that help. This effort, in turn, helps the children understand their parents and grow with them. The combined effort is mutually beneficial.

THE CHILD'S DEVELOPMENT: WHOSE RESPONSIBILITY?

Parents have become the scapegoats of modern times. "Look at

TABLE 6-2
Child and Parent Development

STAGE ONE: INFANT
Approximate age: first 18 months

Parent Development: Learning the cues.

Parental Task: To interpret infant needs.

Child Development:
- Erikson: Trust.
- Spock: Physically helpless; emotionally agreeable.

Ogden Nash: *Many an infant that screams like a calliope*
Could be soothed by a little attention to its diope.

STAGE TWO: TODDLER
Approximate age: 18–36 months

Parent Development: Learning to accept growth and development.

Parental Task: To accept some loss of control while maintaining necessary limits.

Child Development:
- Erikson: Autonomy.
- Spock: A sense of his own individuality and will power; vacillates between dependence and independence.

Ogden Nash: *The trouble with a kitten is*
THAT
Eventually it becomes a
CAT.

STAGE THREE: PRESCHOOLER
Approximate age: 3–6 years

Parent Development: Learning to separate.

Parental Task: To allow independent development while modeling necessary standards.

Child Development:
- Erikson: Initiative.
- Spock: Imitation through admiration; learns about friends.

Ogden Nash: *But joy in heaping measure comes*
To children whose parents are under their thumbs.

STAGE FOUR: SCHOOL-AGER
Approximate age: 6–12 years

Parent Development: Learning to accept rejection without deserting [the child].

Parental Task: To be there when needed without intruding unnecessarily.

Child Development:
- Erikson: Industry.
- Spock: Fitting into outside group; independence of parents and standards; developing conscience; need to control and make moral judgments.

Ogden Nash: *Children aren't happy with nothing to ignore*
And that's what parents were created for.

STAGE FIVE: TEEN-AGER
Approximate age: 13–19 years

Parent Development: Learning to build a new life [in the context of changing family relationships].

Parental Task: To adjust to changing family roles and relationships during and after the teen-ager's struggle to establish an identity.

Child Development:
- Erikson: Identity.
- Spock: Peer orientation; [development of] reality sense by reality testing, with [parental] inhibition fostering idealism.

Ogden Nash: *O adolescence....*
I'd like to be present, I must confess,
When thine own adolescents adolesce.

SOURCE: Alma S. Friedman and David Belais Friedman, "Parenting: A Developmental Process," *Pediatric Annals*, Vol. 6 (September 1977), pp. 10–22. Reprinted by permission from the authors and Insight Publishing Co., Inc. "Pediatric Reflection," copyright 1931 by Ogden Nash; "The Kitten," copyright 1940 by Ogden Nash; last stanza of "A Child's Guide to Parents," copyright 1936 by Ogden Nash; "The Parent," copyright 1933 by Ogden Nash; and an excerpt from "Tarkington, Thou Should'st Be Living in This Hour," copyright 1947 by Ogden Nash (originally appeared in *The New Yorker*), in *Verses from 1929 On* by Ogden Nash, by permission of Little, Brown and Co.

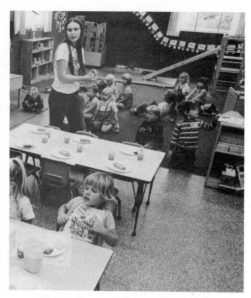

Properly staffed and adequately funded day-care facilities are a boon to parents and children alike. Even when the mother does not work, many parents are choosing the alternative of day-care centers for the enriching preschool experiences they provide.

how badly you raised me" is the accusation and excuse of many emotionally distressed young people. The parents' sense of guilt is deep. But "the fact is that children, too, possess freedom of choice. It appears at an early age and develops with the intelligence and other capacities of the youthful personality. Children, then, share the responsibility for their behavior and emerging characters with their parents, relatives, teachers and friends."[16]

And freedom of choice is a durable freedom that may remain when all other freedoms are gone. Psychiatrist Viktor Frankl writes:

We who have lived in concentration camps can remember the men who walked through the huts comforting others, giving away their last piece of bread. They may have been few in number, but they offer sufficient proof *that everything can be taken from a man but one thing: the last of the human freedoms—to choose one's attitude in any given circumstances, to choose one's own way.*[17]

True, parents need improving, but the child must share in the responsibility for his or her own development. Such responsibility is an opportunity as well as an obligation, for it allows the child to help not only himself, but also his parents.

THE WORKING MOTHER

The life of the average mother today is not like that of her grandmother or even her mother. Today's average mother will live well past the age of seventy-five. She will have borne less than three children by the age of twenty-seven, and she will have raised them before she is fifty. Production of basic services outside the home (education, recreation, food), combined with labor-saving devices, add perhaps as much as ten more years to her life and help make child raising less than a full-time occupation. Even a woman who manages to keep busy at home throughout all the child-bearing years can count on only about fifteen to twenty years of being occupied with this task. What is more, some 80 percent of married women become widows—many at a young age. Widows and divorced women often find themselves having to compete with new college graduates for jobs in the marketplace. Younger women often are given preferential treatment.

These facts do not contribute to the modern woman's desire to consider the home a full-time, lifetime occupation. Child rearing is now a temporary and often part-time job. Indeed, during the period 1950–1975, 16.2 million women entered the labor force in the United States compared with only 9.6 million men. Moreover, the success of women in industry testifies to their growing acceptance in the formerly male-dominated business world. Over half of all U.S. mothers of school-age children now have careers outside the home. And one-sixth of the nation's children live in single-parent families, usually headed by a working mother.

Although millions of mothers work outside the home because of financial necessity, the past ten years have seen a dramatic increase in the number of mothers who choose to work because they want to. For these women, housework and child rearing are not adequately fulfilling occupations. They want an identity outside of the home and enjoy the independence that comes with earning their own income.

The major problem that working

mothers face—whether they are single parents or not—is finding responsible and affordable day care for their children. It is in this area that society must take greater responsibility. There is seriously inadequate government support for the working mother and father. Work shifts are not arranged so that one parent will always be home. Also, day-care centers are expensive; often they are distant. In many areas zoning laws prohibit them. Government-assisted day-care centers that are conveniently located and properly staffed should be made an intrinsic part of the economy.

Depression

"The black dog" was Winston Churchill's name for the depressions that hounded him throughout his long life. A century earlier, another statesman had described his depression this way: "If what I feel were equally distributed to the whole human family, there would not be one cheerful face on earth." The year was 1841, and the speaker was Abraham Lincoln. Lincoln's deep depressions, worsened by dreams in which he viewed his own coffin, added much to the despair of his marriage. Even in the few portraits that show him smiling, his eyes betray an ever-present sadness.

Like Churchill and Lincoln and many of the world's greatest writers, musicians, and painters, depressed people can lead highly productive lives. But these are the exception. Ordinarily, depression is characterized by apathy and a lack of productivity.

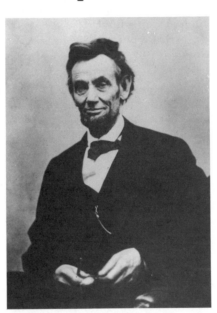

Throughout the years of his presidency Lincoln suffered from the misery of chronic depression. Carefully, he saved a file of some eighty letters marked "Assassination."

Extent and Degrees of Depression

Every year at least eight million people in this country visit their physicians because of depression. For about 250,000 of those seeking help, depression is so severe that hospitalization for treatment is necessary—sometimes to prevent suicide. Nevertheless, depression is not necessarily abnormal, serious, or long-lasting.

There are three categories of depression. (1) *Mild depression*, or sadness, is normal and happens to most people every once in a while. The episodes are usually brief, depending on the specific situation and on the individual personality, and the depression cures itself with time. Often, talking over problems with a sympathetic listener is all that is needed for recovery from temporary sadness, pessimistic feelings, and/or discouragement. (2) *Moderate depression* slows the person down markedly in both thought and action. There is a tendency to blame oneself for all sorts of evils, and minor problems are seen as disasters. Often the person begins to doubt the worth of living, and thoughts of suicide begin to pervade the consciousness. (3) *Severe depression* shows itself by the person's complete withdrawal and lack of response to anyone or anything. Both moderate and severe depressions need professional treatment.

Note that whether mild, moderate, or severe, depression is not a feeling by itself. Usually it is accompanied by some other emotion, such as anger or anxiety. For example, a student becomes mildly depressed and also angry at himself or with his teacher after failing an examination. Anxiety that he may fail the course will overlay the depression. But the student does not cease to function because of all this. He understands the source of his feelings and begins to take some positive action to correct the situation—namely, he studies harder and pays better attention to class lectures. Eventually his good work is rewarded with better grades, and the depression and anxiety disappear.

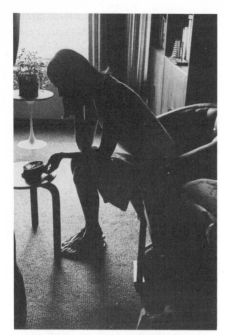

"I know not why it should be that I am so sad; there is a fairy tale of olden days that I cannot get out of my head."

HEINRICH HEINE

There Is Always a Cause for Depression

Oftentimes people feel depressed "for no reason." There is a generalized feeling of indifference toward almost everything, and no specific situation seems to be responsible for causing sadness or anxiety. Nevertheless, there is always a cause. It is just that the person cannot recognize it. Usually such depressions disappear by themselves, but if they persist for weeks or months, professional help needs to be sought to help unearth the reason and to find ways of successfully dealing with the problem. (The boxed insert on page 176 is meant to give you some idea of whether you are in need of professional help.)

Agitation: A Signal for Professional Help

It may happen that a whole range of emotions, including severe depression, anxiety, anger, guilt, and resentment, is experienced simultaneously. Such a severe combination may create a brew of **agitation**. Symptoms of agitation include wringing the hands in anguish, pacing back and forth, crying uncontrollably, feelings of frantic despair, and rejection of any help. Agitation signals illness with severe depression. Just as depression and anxiety have an effect on other people, so does agitation. And it should be noted that severe depression, such that requires professional help, need not be marked by agitation. Indeed, as mentioned earlier, withdrawal may be the most noticeable sign of severe depression.

Temperament and Depression

An important feature of the personality that is often overlooked and just as often misunderstood is **temperament**—the attitude one takes toward life and its happenings, both good and bad. Parents, for example, will notice that children are very different in their temperaments. One will make his or her way through life cheerfully, not too much disturbed by the winds of ill-fortune. Another child will tremble like a leaf and be depressed with every breeze of bad news. The first child may be appreciated more than the second child, and the latter may not receive enough of the much-needed love and caring. Why? The first child is probably more likely to be agreeable and to make the parent feel successful. The second child, shaken, often moody, may make the misunderstanding parent feel like a failure at parenting.

Loss: The Major Cause of Depression

Human beings suffer keener and more frequent periods of depression than do other creatures because we have a greater imagination and a larger number of love objects. But depression among lower animals is not uncommon. A cow that has lost its calf can be heard bellowing all night; a dog whose master or mistress has left may lie down and die. By the same token, the loss of a loved pet will cause depression in its owner. Indeed, the death of a pet may cause a deeper depression than the loss of a great deal of money. It is not *what* is lost that determines the extent of depression; it is the *degree of attachment* one has for the lost object.

Coping with Mild Depression

Things Not to Do for Others

1. Don't refuse any attempt made to solicit your help. Saying things like "It's your problem" may be truthful, but unnecessary and cruel. If you wish to avoid excessive involvement with the person, you can still help merely by listening sympathetically without too much comment.
2. Don't suggest that dreadful consequences await the depressed person unless he or she "snaps out of it." Such admonitions, even if made with the best intentions, can only increase the depression by adding another cause for worry.
3. Don't be a "know it all." Even mild depression can have complex origins, so be cautious about giving advice based on superficial knowledge of the problem. Don't tell the depressed person what to do.
4. Don't minimize the person's feelings. Saying "It's nothing, don't worry about it," or words to that effect, can make the person feel that he or she is misunderstood or that no one cares, which only increases the depression.
5. On the other hand, don't try to "push" the person into cheerfulness. It won't work, and furthermore it may cause the person to feel belittled.
6. Don't hesitate to suggest the name of someone who could be of help. This might be a mutually trusted teacher, a good friend, or a professional counselor.

Things to Do to Help Yourself

1. The first step toward conquering depression is to understand what is causing it. If there is no apparent reason—a loss, a need that is unfulfilled, trouble at home or at work—analyze yourself thoughtfully and honestly to become aware of things that trouble you. Close examination of such annoyances generally uncovers larger problems.
2. Anger at oneself is often at the root of depression. Mental or written lists of things that can be done to correct or ease the situation are helpful for turning anger into constructive action. The popular idea that the expression of anger is always therapeutic is open to question. Such expressions may bring both guilt and resentment. There are times when it may be best to vent one's fury on a tennis ball.
3. Depression is very common during and around major holidays. If possible, make plans to spend these occasions with family or friends. If you must be alone, arrange some special treat for yourself and keep busy with things you enjoy doing.
4. Try to exercise regularly. Feeling tired is one sign of depression, and frequently the tiredness is emotional, not physical. Exercise takes your mind off your troubles and relieves tension. However, avoid the stimulation of exercise before bedtime.
5. Occupy yourself with other people. Be involved with them. At first, this may be difficult, but in time genuine interest will return. Caring about others' problems and welfare helps put your own troubles in a more realistic perspective.
6. Avoid depressive situations. If a particular relationship offers more grief than joy, discontinue it. If certain music, movies, restaurants, or other things or places make you feel sad, try to avoid contact with them. Short- and long-range plans should include the possibility of change if it turns out that they increase, rather than decrease, your unhappiness.
7. Talk things over with trusted and helpful relatives and friends. However, this can be overdone. Also, try not to let your anger offend people who want to help you. Family relationships and friendships are often jeopardized by the unusual unpleasantness of the depressed person. Choose your confidants carefully, and treat them well.
8. If your own efforts and those of family or friends fail to help, seek guidance from an objective professional counselor with whom you are comfortable. Psychiatrists, psychologists, psychiatric social workers, religious leaders—any of these people may be helpful. It is difficult to tailor the needs of all individuals into one prescription for a cure for mild depression. In this, professional help may be especially necessary. Remember: Recognizing that you need professional help and then actively getting it is the first sensible step to recovery.

Do *You* Need Psychotherapy?

If you're like most people, your life inevitably has its ups and downs. You may even have wondered if you need psychotherapy. How do you decide? What are the differences between normal ups and downs and the kinds of emotional problems that call for therapy?

Psychiatrists and psychologists say it's time to consider help when you feel so bad you can't function; when your problems start interfering with your daily life, your job, your marriage. "When this situation arises," says Dr. Thomas A. Williams, chairman of the department of psychiatry and behavioral sciences at Eastern Virginia Medical School, "the next question is: for how long? If it has been going on a couple months or more, you probably could use some help."

But don't think you have an emotional problem just because you have *occasionally* felt or acted like this, especially if there's been a crisis—a death, divorce, loss of a job—that would upset anyone. With the person who could really use psychotherapy, these feelings occur frequently, usually over a period of months, and often for no apparent reason. Do you fall into this category? The following 20 questions should help you decide.

1. In new situations, such as a job interview, or a party where there are many strangers, are you afraid things will go badly for you?
a. All or most of the time. b. Frequently. c. Occasionally. d. Rarely or never.

2. When asked to do something you don't want to do, such as babysit for friends, or work late, can you say no when you really want to?
a. All or most of the time. b. Frequently. c. Occasionally. d. Rarely or never.

3. Do you ever completely lose your temper and realize afterward that you got much angrier than the situation deserved? For example, your spouse has been stuck in traffic and comes home late for dinner.
a. All or most of the time. b. Frequently. c. Occasionally. d. Rarely or never.

4. When you're with friends, can you get them to listen if you have a suggestion—like picking a restaurant or a movie?
a. All or most of the time. b. Frequently. c. Occasionally. d. Rarely or never.

5. Do you have a lot of difficulty making decisions—selecting a new coat, say, or deciding how to spend a weekend?
a. All or most of the time. b. Frequently. c. Occasionally. d. Rarely or never.

6. Do you hesitate to become involved in group activities? For example, do you find yourself standing alone at parties?
a. All or most of the time. b. Frequently. c. Occasionally. d. Rarely or never.

7. Do you seek approval or encouragement for things you do all the time, such as daily office tasks or preparing a meal for your family?
a. All or most of the time. b. Frequently. c. Occasionally. d. Rarely or never.

8. Can you express your displeasure when people take advantage of you—push ahead of you in line, for example?
a. All or most of the time. b. Frequently. c. Occasionally. d. Rarely or never.

9. Do you feel satisfied with your closest relationships?
a. All or most of the time. b. Frequently. c. Occasionally. d. Rarely or never.

10. Would you take a drink or tranquilizer to give you confidence before a job interview or a party?
a. All or most of the time. b. Frequently. c. Occasionally. d. Rarely or never.

11. Are you bothered by habits, such as smoking or overeating, that you are unable to control?
a. All or most of the time. b. Frequently. c. Occasionally. d. Rarely or never.

12. Do you have fears—as of flying, or of small places—that you are unable to control or that keep you from doing what you want?
a. All or most of the time. b. Frequently. c. Occasionally. d. Rarely or never.

13. When you leave the house, do you have to go back to make sure the door is locked, stove off, etc.?
a. All or most of the time. b. Frequently. c. Occasionally. d. Rarely or never.

14. How often is sex unsatisfactory for you or your mate?
a. All or most of the time. b. Frequently. c. Occasionally. d. Rarely or never.

15. Does it take you more than an hour to go to sleep, or do you wake up more than an hour earlier than you want to?
a. All or most of the time. b. Frequently. c. Occasionally. d. Rarely or never.

16. Have you lost weight recently without a medical reason or a diet?
a. Very little, if any. b. More than 5 pounds. c. More than 10 pounds. d. More than 15 pounds.

17. Are you very concerned with cleanliness or contamination of yourself or objects you might touch?
a. All or most of the time. b. Frequently. c. Occasionally. d. Rarely or never.

18. Do you think the future is hopeless, or do you ever think of hurting yourself or committing suicide?
a. All or most of the time. b. Frequently. c. Occasionally. d. Rarely or never.

19. Do you ever see, hear or feel things that nobody else is aware of?
a. All or most of the time. b. Frequently. c. Occasionally. d. Rarely or never.

20. Do you think you have superior powers or that other people are using superior powers against you?
a. All or most of the time. b. Frequently. c. Occasionally. d. Rarely or never.

What Your Answers Mean

First of all, this is *not* a test involving right and wrong responses. We all lose our temper now and then over something trivial; we all occasionally feel dissatisfied with our closest relationships. In normal circumstances, however, the well-adjusted person will usually give the following answers:

1.	c or d	11.	c or d
2.	a or b	12.	c or d
3.	c or d	13.	c or d
4.	a, b or c	14.	c or d
5.	c or d	15.	c or d
6.	c or d	16.	a or b
7.	c or d	17.	c or d
8.	a or b	18.	d
9.	a or b	19.	d
10.	c or d	20.	d

Questions 1 to 10 evaluate how well you express your feelings and how much self-confidence you have. If many of your answers differ from the ones indicated above, it simply means you have problems expressing feelings or aren't very sure of yourself. If you want to change some of these feelings or behavior, psychotherapy would probably help you.

Questions 11 to 14 involve behavior that usually accompanies an emotional problem. If many of your answers differ from the ones listed, and if you think your problems are interfering with your daily life, it might be a good idea to see a professional and get an opinion.

Questions 15 to 20 deal with behavior patterns that could be important early-warning signs of a serious emotional problem. If some or many of your answers differ from the ones given here, you should get a professional opinion right away. If therapy is needed, it will be easier if you don't delay.

SOURCE: Lee Fowler, "Do *You* Need Psychotherapy?" Reprinted from May 19, 1978 issue of Family Circle Magazine. © 1978 THE FAMILY CIRCLE, INC.

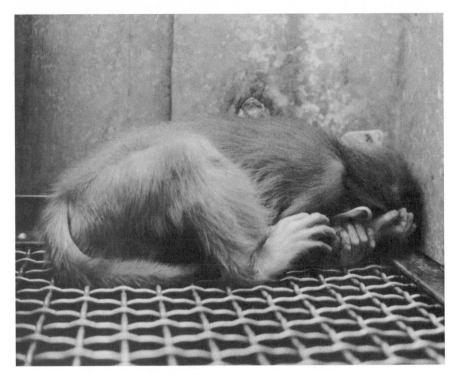

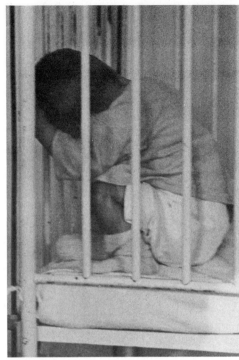

Laboratory monkeys raised without mothering grieve piteously. At times they clasp their heads in their arms and rock. Some pinch the same patch of skin hundreds of times daily or develop grief-stricken mannerisms. Others fail to mate successfully. Anxiety and depression have been induced in laboratory animals by exposing them daily to stimuli similar to that which would cause those reactions in humans.

Loss comes in many forms; it is not just about death. Loss of territory will cause depression in both humans and lower animals. Dogs and cats often mourn for weeks or months when a rival "takes over" the neighborhood. And it may well be that one of the reasons for the rising incidence of depression in this country is that so many people are constantly on the move. Ordinarily, people are not eager to move far from familiar territories. College freshmen leaving home for the first time often suffer the same sort of

depression as do families who have transferred to new locations for business reasons. It takes time to become adjusted to new people, a new bed—a new territory. Thus, the combined loss of group and territory may intensify normal depression.

Loss of self-esteem is also a basic cause for depression. Thus, all of the following people are likely to suffer depression: a frequently punished child; someone who has an automobile accident after thirty prideful years of accident-free driving; a person who is demoted or fired from a long-held job; an individual who is promoted to a job beyond his or her wants, needs, or capabilities; a divorced person, and the children who are going through the divorce; someone whose love goes unreturned; a prisoner—or one who feels imprisoned. This list could go on and on; these are but a few examples of people in situations that cause a loss of self-esteem.

Abandoned and placed in an institution, the child shown above turned his back on the world. Rejected, he rejects. The depression, immobility, and withdrawal of many children suffering maternal and other deprivations may be worsened by insomnia, loss of appetite, loss of weight, and other grave manifestations.

Like the child, the baby monkey shown at left was denied normal contact with his mother and peers. Overwhelmed by his sense of abandonment, he shuts out the world.

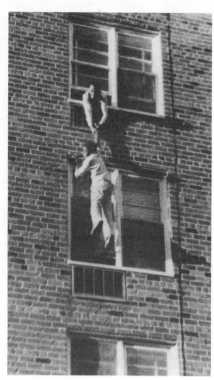

A cry for attention—answered.

People also take longer than lower animals to get over depression. We relive and brood over past losses and worry about those that might come. A depressed dog or cat, on the other hand, is depressed only as long as the unhappy situation lasts.

A Cry for Help

Often the test of courage is not to die but to live.

CONTE VITTORIO ALFIERI
(1749–1803)

He who has a why to live can bear almost any how.

FREDERICH NIETZCHE
(1844–1900)

Officially, about twenty-five thousand people in the United States (some four thousand between the ages of fifteen and twenty-four) are reported to kill themselves every year. Yet experts in the field of suicide—*suicidologists*—do not accept the U.S. government estimate. Why? First, many coroners do not call killing accidents or other death-causing mishaps suicides when, in truth, they very likely are. Indeed, studies of single-auto accidents strongly suggest that many are suicides. Moreover, this culture condemns suicide. And because it is taboo, relatives often try to hide the fact that it has happened. But suicidologists make up for this serious underreporting. The rule is to multiply the officially reported number by three to give a total that is one-third of the total *attempts* at suicide. Thus, a more realistic estimate is that about seventy-five thousand people a year commit and about a quarter of a million people a year attempt to commit suicide. Compared with the 1960s, the suicide rate among young people

has almost doubled. And while it is true that the rate of suicide among older people is also increasing, the *rate of increase* in the number of suicides among the young is greater, particularly among males between fifteen and twenty-four years of age. In the past twenty years the suicide rate in this age group has increased over 250 percent.

WHY SUICIDE?

The reasons for suicide are multiple and complex. Among the most common reasons are the following:

1. It is a crushing experience to graduate from high school or college and find that the effort has not been enough to earn a job. Unemployment among young whites is high; among young blacks it is double that of the whites. The result is a sense of hopelessness.

2. Many young people are not nearly so happy as older people think they are. It is healthy to want to do "one's own thing," to "cut the apron strings" and strike out on one's own seeking complete independence. But to do so requires strength to cope and wisdom. One cannot totally and suddenly sever oneself from accustomed moorings and go off into the world almost completely alone. Everyone needs to feel a sense of belonging: Its absence is a common cause of depression and suicide. In one tragic case, a student was dead in his room for eighteen days before he was found. Nobody seemed to know or care that he was missing.

3. A third cause of suicide among the young is a troubled, changing

family. The unwanted growing person receives little love and finds it hard to accept the pitifully small amount that is offered. Living in such a family, the young person, according to suicidologist Dr. Herbert Hendin, develops a protective emotional numbness and deadness. Yet even that sorry state has a certain security to it. But if there is nothing to replace it, the wish to die eventually replaces the numbness and deadness that was a way of life while maturing.

4. Many people develop a sense of meaninglessness to life. Risk taking—whether by taking drugs or racing cars and motorcycles—is often symptomatic of such feelings. Few high-school or college students do not know that cigarettes cause lung cancer. Yet cigarettes are their (and their parents') favorite drug. Alcohol abuse is common. And suicide is dozens of times more common among alcoholics than it is among nonalcoholics. Drug abuse surely must be considered, among some people, a roundabout, slow way of committing suicide. It may, at first, be a way of saying to someone, "Listen to me!" It may end when nobody can listen anymore.

5. Another cause of suicide is pressure to achieve. In many highly industrialized societies, such as ours, there seems to be one four-letter word that is forbidden the young—*fail.* This adds to stress, and if failure should occur—or even if it is only *thought* to have occurred—the success-oriented youth loses his or her sense of self-worth. Ironically, it is often brilliant students who worry most about failure.

Helping By Knowing the Facts

1. Listen for warnings. Over 75 percent of people who kill themselves have talked about it seriously. "I wish I were dead" is a cry for help. Suicide threats must not be ignored. People who commit suicide do not often do it on an impulse. They give many clues over a period of time, hoping someone will understand and help them.

2. Look for warnings. Hopelessness, helplessness, depression, isolation, withdrawing from people—all are signs to watch for. So are sudden changes in behavior.

3. People often commit suicide just when they appear to others to be getting over their depression. Do not be misled by seeming improvement. Most people who kill themselves do so within three months after appearing to be over a suicidal crisis. Share your concern about someone's suicidal signals with others, such as parents, friends, counselors, and teachers. Signals that indicate a possible suicide attempt should not be kept secret. Break the confidence. It may save a life.

4. "People have a right to kill themselves." But the fact is that most people who are saved from suicide are grateful later. What if they had not been helped? People do have a right to live, and if they can be helped to do so, then that help must be given.

5. When a suicidal crisis is over will other crises follow continuously? It is not likely. People are not often suicidal forever. Once helped over a suicidal depression, most people go on to lead normal, productive lives.

6. "Rich people don't kill themselves. Only poor people do." False. All kinds of people in society commit suicide.

7. "People who attempt or commit suicide are those who suffer from chronic emotional disturbances." Not necessarily. A temporary emotional disturbance plus a sense of helplessness and hopelessness can trigger a suicide attempt.

8. The tendency to commit suicide has nothing to do with heredity.

9. Never leave a suicidal person alone. Stay until help arrives.

10. Professional help for a potential suicide victim is essential. The counseling of a psychiatrist, psychologist, psychiatric social worker, or psychiatric nurse is invaluable during a suicidal crisis. After the crisis is passed, help should be continued. Sometimes more than one professional is needed—one for the suicidal person and others for close family members, such as parents.

6. Karl Menninger, like the great Sigmund Freud before him, considers suicide a form of murder. The murderer and murdered live within a single person. Freud saw this as a hate-love feeling of the child toward the parent. Unable to harm the parent, the child punishes that which is seen in the self as being like the hated parent.

7. Others kill themselves because "it is so romantic." This is a holdover of a view of death fashionable in the eighteenth and nineteenth centuries and popularized in many novels and movies. The great composer Frederic Chopin (1810–1849) is a case in point. Mortally sick with tuberculosis, he nevertheless gave concert after concert, hemorrhaging delicately on the keyboards of Europe. People flocked to his concerts, moved by his pale elegance. But as he grew weaker and could barely press down the keys there were inelegant complaints that he could not be heard. Much has been written of his romantic love affair with the celebrated novelist George Sand. But her unromantic reference to him as "my dear corpse" is not often mentioned. Chopin's suicidal concertizing did raise money for his native Poland, but it could not last. His music did. What a pity he did not live to write more! So it is with those who fantasize that death will at last bring appreciation or love or a reunion with a loved one who is dead. So far as anyone knows, suicide only brings death. And to those left behind, the feeling is generally anything but appreciation. Certainly there is no reunion.

They Found a Home in the Army

In this closing section of the chapter, a true story is told that summarizes much of the preceding discussions of human development and emotional disorders. But most important, perhaps, is that it emphasizes the human need for values and order. The narrative begins with an extraordinary staff meeting at a famous eastern hospital.

That meeting would be long remembered. Looking back, nobody could have foretold all that would happen. Present this time had been almost all the staff of the adolescent ward of Jacobi Hospital in the Bronx. At best their job was never easy: that of helping some two dozen eight- to eighteen-year-olds with serious emotional problems. Some had already attempted suicide. Because routine was often a welcome ally, any suggested change was carefully examined. So the decision to abandon nurses' and aides' uniforms in favor of street clothes was not made casually. Almost the whole meeting had been given over to the new proposal. Many staff insecurities had surfaced: anxiety about losing status, job identification, lines of authority, control over patients and one another. At last it had been agreed to try the no-uniform policy for three months.

At a second meeting the young patients were told of the plan. Like the staff, the children were anxious, but their reasons were different. Impostors would come to care for them, or nobody would. If the uniforms left, so would the nurses. One small boy, a possible runaway, cried, "The nurses will escape!" Gently, the basic reason for the change was explained: The atmosphere would be more relaxed, and patients would feel more comfortable.

There followed a seemingly uneventful period that lasted six days. Then the adolescent army appeared. It was complete with insignia of rank proclaimed in Magic Marker on pajamas. All was military. An eleven-year-old girl was corps bugler. Around her neck was a carved wooden instrument. Four of the older boys were officers. As allies, they were no longer afraid of one another. There were privates, corporals, and others. The disturbed daughter of an army colonel, a pretty and flirtatious girl of sixteen, served as general of this children's army. Accustomed to command, she merely adapted her power to a military format. Armaments (wooden guns) had been manufactured in the occupational therapy shop.

> [The army] appeared to meet every patient's most acutely felt needs and to solve each one's currently most distressing problems. Depressions lifted. Rivalries waned. Aggression became so bound up in the organization that no one appeared frightened of his own or his fellows' impulses. Individual sexual conflicts were so ingeniously ... incorporated into the matrix of military roles ... that they went unnoticed.... Never were the lines of authority clearer. Never had the dependent and infantile felt better cared for, or the fearful more protected, or the rejected more valued. No one was

lonely. Everyone had a vital role and an unmistakable identity. No invading impostors were to be feared. Anyone who craved structure found all he could use. Ambiguities ceased. The vanished uniforms had been restored, as if to demonstrate their value and function to anyone who had not yet gotten the message.... The only hitch was that this marvel of a device left out the staff.[18]

And the staff did not accept this lightly.

> Despite its formidable accomplishments the insurgent army was greeted by the now un-uniformed staff ... with distinct displeasure, with dismay and consternation. It was a revolution. The tables were turned.... Considering how little the army did that was actually disruptive, the near pandemonium that ensued among the staff bears testimony to the extent of their own emotional involvement.[19]

What actually happened? To both the sick children and some of the staff members responsible for their care, a change in clothing that was an emblem of their institution, authority, codes, or values was threatening. However, the staff members were free to leave the ward. Their anxieties could be relieved. The disturbed children had no such advantages. Yet they too had sought to adjust. They had met the threat to themselves with a threat to others. A usual reaction. A not unusual result.

The children's army reflected in miniature a well-known human reaction. For whole nations do no less than did these emotionally sick youngsters. Whether the threat is real or imagined matters little.

Temporarily, at least, martial law establishes authority, security, purpose, and direction. But the formation of the children's army excluded the possibility of treatment and cure. It was the order of the desert, not of hope. This the sick children could not see. And it is this that today's mature young student sees only too well. He needs hope within order. Clearly, the student understands that "the art of progress is to preserve order amid change and to preserve change amid order."[20]

But the student also sees that, too often, nations are like sick children. Why? Why are nations like armed camps? In a biology class the student learns that even animals that are instinctively hostile to one another can learn to live peacefully together. In an English class one is told of Stephen Crane, the great war novelist who wrote that "the essence of life is war." Bewildered, searching, the student turns to the writings of more than a generation ago. In the lyric prose of Thomas Wolfe, one of the celebrated spokesmen of those days, the student reads this:

> With a tender smile of love for his dear self, he saw himself wearing the eagles of a colonel on his gallant young shoulders. . . . For the first time he saw the romantic charm of mutilation. . . . He longed for that subtle distinction, that air of having lived and suffered that could only be attained by a wooden leg, a rebuilt nose, or the seared scar of a bullet across his temple.[21]

Modern students, reading this, begin to reject the past. They feel a part of a "new race" well described by Ralph Waldo Emerson a century ago:

There is a universal resistance to ties and ligaments once supposed essential to civilized society. The new race is stiff, heady, and rebellious; they are fanatics in freedom; they hate tolls, taxes, turnpikes, banks, hierarchies, governors, yea, almost laws.

So some students reject the past. All of it. To them, no past values fit the present scheme of things. And since the past is gone, there is no future. What matters is the present.

People need not be retarded by the past nor be worshipful of it. But they do need to understand it. Then they might see, for example, the need for both peace and national defense. The past helps to teach what is solid earth and what is shifting sand. As the well-known naturalist Loren Eiseley has written:

> The lessons of the past have been found to be a reasonably secure instruction for proceeding against the unknown future. To hurl oneself recklessly, without method, upon a future that we ourselves have complicated is a sheer nihilistic rejection of all that history . . . can teach us.[22]

So one cannot disregard past institutions, codes, and values. It does not matter whether their symbol is a nurse's uniform, a wedding ring, or a sergeant's stripes. It does matter how a human need for order is met. Institutions, codes, and values need constant, careful reappraisal. Some need changing. Others need to be discarded and, to avoid chaos, replaced by other institutions, codes, and values. In itself, mere rejection of a value is not a value. And people cannot do without values.

This much, at least, the emotionally disturbed children in the Jacobi adolescent ward understood.

Summary

Stress is the universal reaction of the human body to any demand made upon it. Prolonged or severe stress brings on the *General Adaptation Syndrome (G.A.S.)*, which has three stages—alarm, resistance, and exhaustion. If the last stage is reached without relief from the stress, sickness or even death may result. Stress can hasten the process of aging.

Change, whether beneficial or harmful, is the major cause of stress. The University of Washington Stress Test measures stress by a ranking of life changes. One of the best ways of preventing stress is to avoid undergoing too many life changes at once. Recreational exercise, relaxation techniques, assertiveness training, and biofeedback are all useful methods for reducing stress. One psychiatrist, Frederic Flach, feels that stress, properly dealt with, can be a creative process that can provide a person with the opportunity to mature.

Anxiety is a vague feeling of apprehension or uneasiness that, unlike fear, is concerned with something that *might* happen. It can be communicated from one person to another. People exhibit their anxieties by a variety of signs and symptoms, including restlessness and muscular tension. One of the primary reasons for modern anxiety is the tremendous increase in technology, which has not been accompanied by advances in interpersonal communication.

Childhood anxiety is a natural outgrowth of the conflict between the need for discipline and a child's struggle for independence. The child best copes with these anxieties if he or she is dealt with in a loving and consistent manner.

The primary causes of teen-age anxiety are the prolonged period of adolescence (during which teen-agers are seldom able to make productive contributions to society) and the overwhelming emotional and physical changes they undergo at this time. The teen-ager facing such anxiety can be greatly helped by an understanding adult who can support the teen-ager's search for self-identity and a sense of purpose.

Having total responsibility for a child's life and development is a cause of anxiety to parents. A parent must grow along with the child and accept the child's gradually attained independence. A child will eventually share the responsibility for his or her own growth. Parents, especially working mothers, should not be overwhelmed with guilt if they are unwilling to sacrifice their lives totally for their children.

Depression is a common emotional condition generally characterized by apathy and a lack of productivity. Though a mild depression may go away by itself, a moderate or severe condition may persist and require professional help. Severe depressions may be marked by *agitation.* By the very fact of their *temperament,* some people are more prone to depression than others.

The major cause of depression is loss. The extent of feeling will depend on the degree of attachment to the lost object. The sense of loss does not only accompany death. Loss of territory and self-esteem can also precipitate episodes of depression.

Guidelines have been suggested for dealing with depression, whether it be your own or a friend's. But one thing is certain: This emotional state must not be ignored, since in its severer forms it can lead to suicide.

Besides depression, suicide can have many causes—a sense of meaninglessness to life, a troubled family situation, the romanticizing of death, and others. Knowing the facts about suicide can help one to recognize the warning signs of suicide and to help another person through this emotional crisis.

The story of the emotionally disturbed children of Jacobi Hospital emphasizes the points of this chapter. Faced with a change that they viewed as a threat, the children formed their own society, complete with its own uniforms, values, and authority. Anxiety was reduced by the substitution of a sense of belonging, security, and meaning. Individuals will vary in their reactions to situations that provoke stress, anxiety, or depression. They will, however, have a good basis for dealing with their emotions if they understand, as did the children of Jacobi Hospital, that they cannot do without the values that provide the sense of belonging and purpose human beings so desperately need.

References

1. Bronislaw Malinowski, *Magic, Science and Religion* (Garden City, N.Y., 1955), p. 71.
2. Alvin Toffler, *Future Shock* (New York, 1971), p. 342.
3. Minoru Masuda and Thomas H. Holmes, "Life Events: Perceptions and Frequencies," *Psychosomatic Medicine*, Vol. 40 (May 1978), pp. 236–261.
4. Frederic F. Flach, *Choices: Coping Creatively with Personal Change* (Philadelphia and New York, 1977). This is a big little book that is highly recommended. It says much that is wise in little space.
5. Ibid., pp. 26–27.
6. Ibid., pp. 139–141.
7. William Baker, president of Bell Laboratories, quoted in W. R. Kleinfield, "Ma Bell's Great Dream Machine," *The New York Times*, Section 3 (May 28, 1978), p. 1.
8. "Ode LXXXV," quoted from *Catullus*, tr. into English verse by T. Hart-Davies (London, 1879), p. 122.
9. An Oklahoma high-school boy, quoted in Evelyn Millis Duvall, *Family Development*, 2nd ed. (Philadelphia, 1962), p. 297. Reprinted by permission of Harper & Row, Publishers, Inc.
10. Rabindranath Tagore, "The World of Personality," in Clark E. Moustakas, ed., *The Self* (New York, 1956), p. 82.
11. Erik H. Erikson, *Childhood and Society* (New York, 1950), p. 219.
12. Jerome Kagan, "The Child: His Struggle for Identity," *Saturday Review* (December 7, 1968), p. 80.
13. Alma S. Friedman and David Belais Friedman, "Parenting and Child Behavior," *Pediatric Annals*, Vol. 6 (September 1977).
14. Dorothy V. Whipple, *Dynamics of Development: Euthenic Pediatrics* (New York, 1966), p. 420.
15. Ibid., p. 423.
16. Corliss Lamont, *Freedom of Choice Affirmed* (New York, 1967), p. 32.

17. Viktor E. Frankl, *Man's Search for Meaning* (New York, 1959), p. 112.

18. The incident at the Adolescent and Latency In-Patient Service of Jacobi Hospital, Bronx, Municipal Hospital Center, New York City, is described in a paper by Donald J. Marcuse, "The 'Army' Incident: The Psychology of Uniforms and Their Abolition on an Adolescent Ward," *Psychiatry: A Journal for the Study of Interpersonal Processes*, Vol. 30 (November 1967), p. 362.

19. Ibid., p. 364.

20. Alfred North Whitehead, quoted in *Saturday Review* (March 2, 1968), p. 19.

21. Thomas Wolfe, *Look Homeward, Angel* (New York, 1929), p. 533.

22. Loren Eiseley, *The Unexpected Universe*, quoted in *Science*, Vol. 165 (July 11, 1969), p. 129.

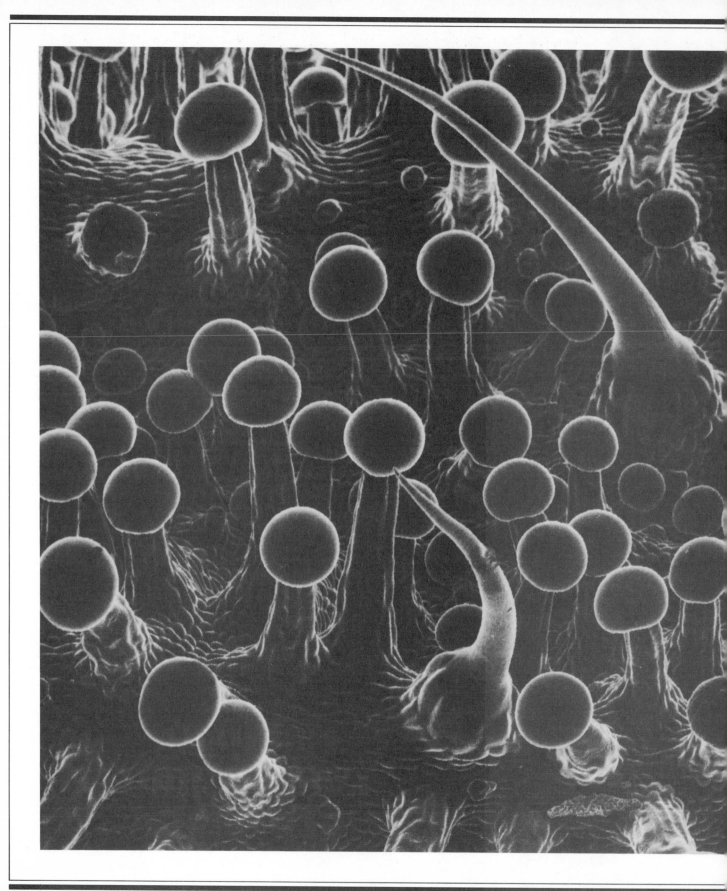

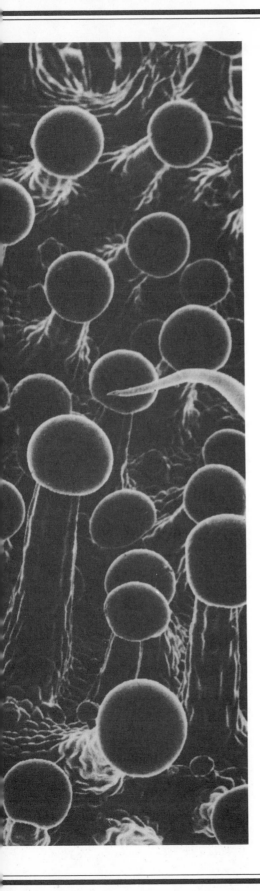

Drugs: Escape into Captivity

Some years ago a professor in Riverside, California, concocted a brew made from nightshade plant and took a large dose of it. His wife became so alarmed by the bizarre behavior that followed that she called the family physician. In a nearby hospital, a barred-window cell was found for the befuddled professor. There he had to be tied hand and foot, spread-eagle, to the bedposts. From this secured vantage point he could clearly watch the goings-on in his tiny cell. Part of the account of his experience, which he later published, reads as follows:

The vent in my cell was located just above the door. To my amazement it began to fill up like a small football stadium with tiered rows of my former students. They were wearing brightly colored berets and horn-rimmed colored glasses. Each had a bottle of coke and a bag of popcorn. They single filed into the bleachers, finally filling it to capacity. Now they sat very rigid without appearing to notice my presence. However, when I turned my head as if to look at some other area of the room the scene suddenly became highly animated. As they guzzled their cokes and stuffed popcorn into their mouths they pointed their fingers at me and laughed. Whenever I focused my eyes on their antics, they suddenly froze and took no notice of me. It is of interest to note that I recognized every face in the group and that I had given each and every one of them the D or F grade in beginning Biology.[1]

The photograph on page 186 is a marijuana leaf (*Cannabis sativa*) magnified 450 times.

Then, there was Margaret Thompson who took snuff, as did other London ladies of her day. She died on April 2, 1776, leaving a will that has caused her to be long remembered:

I, Margaret Thompson . . . being in sane mind . . . desire that all my handkerchiefs that I may have unwashed at the time of my decease . . . be put . . . at the bottom of my coffin, which I desire may be large enough for that purpose, together with a quantity of the best Scotch snuff . . . as will cover my deceased body.[2]

She was not the only one who wanted to take her vice with her. Some years ago in Camembert, France, a man obeyed his wife's wish by preserving her in the town's best brandy cider before burial. In her memory, he composed this touching rhyme:

Here lies my wife. Her dying wish:
"I think it would be dandy
To be preserved, when comes the end,
Like a ripe plum in brandy."[3]

What is buried in some graves is surprising. What is on some of the stones marking them is no less startling. Consider this memorial found in a churchyard in Burlington, Massachusetts:

Here lies the body of Susan Lowder
Who burst while drinking a Sedlitz Powder.
Called from this world to her heavenly rest,
She should have waited till it effervesced. 1798[4]

The California professor perhaps took nightshade so as to publish (though he almost perished instead). Mrs. Thompson snuffed for pleasure. The French lady left these earthly premises as she wished — stewing in her brandy. And poor Susan Lowder probably never revealed why she took a powder.

Why Drugs?

People have found a variety of purposes for a variety of drugs. Many have deep attachments to them. Several of the substances that produce dependence will be considered in this chapter, as will the reasons why people become attached to them. It is well to remember, however, that the effects of a drug often vary from individual to individual, and from time to time with the same individual. And the picture is further complicated by the fact that, whether legally or illegally, many people often take several drugs at one time, sometimes with harmful results (see Figure 7–1).

There is no single answer to the question of why people take drugs. Poverty, pleasure, the pressure of friends, the desire to be rebellious, television advertising, availability, excessive prescribing by physicians, tensions, stress, disillusionment— all have been blamed. To these must be added the overriding fact that some drugs mean vast money profits for criminals of several continents.

Those who buy drugs from street sellers invite deception. For example, tests performed on confiscated samples of street drugs, as well as drugs peddled at some rock concerts, revealed that the animal tranquilizer phencyclidine (PCP) (see page 210) was sometimes substituted for THC

(tetrahydrocannabinol), the most active ingredient of marijuana. PCP is used with caution by veterinarians, for in large doses the drug can cause an animal to convulse. In humans PCP can be extremely dangerous— even deadly. Mexican marijuana may contain anything from cow dung to the herb-killer paraquat (page 217). The person who buys street drugs often gets more than was bargained for.

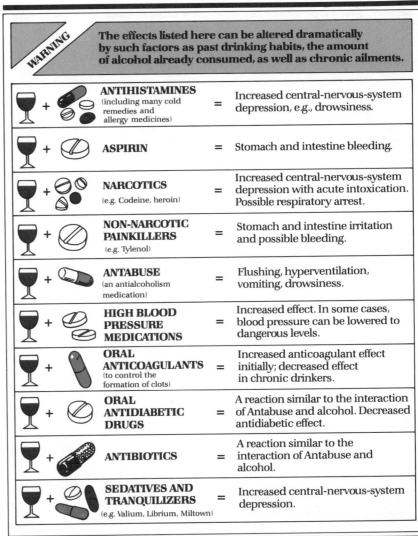

**FIGURE 7–1
Dangerous mixes of
alcohol and drugs.**

Terms and Classifications

The World Health Organization Expert Committee on Drugs has recommended substitution of the term **drug dependence** for both "drug addiction" and "drug habituation." "Drug dependence is a state of psychic or physical dependence, or both, on a drug, arising in a person following administration of that drug on a periodic or continuous basis."[5] How does the committee define **drug abuse**? Certainly the general public has reason to be confused about the term. Drug abuse may be said to be a "persistent or sporadic [occasional] excessive drug use inconsistent with or unrelated to acceptable medical practice."[6]

A variety of chemical substances affect the central nervous system of people, thereby causing a psychological (psychic) dependence. Other drugs also provoke a physical dependence. This latter type of dependence is evidenced by **withdrawal symptoms** (called the *abstinence syndrome*) when the effects of the drug are interrupted. A physically dependent drug abuser will suffer withdrawal symptoms when (1) the

---

TABLE 7–1
Some Characteristics of Certain Types of Drugs That Induce Dependence

TYPE OF DRUG DEPENDENCE[1]	BASIC ACTION	PSYCHOLOGICAL (PSYCHIC) DEPENDENCE	PHYSICAL DEPENDENCE	WITHDRAWAL SYMPTOMS (ABSTINENCE SYNDROME)	DEVELOPMENT OF TOLERANCE
Morphine and morphinelike drugs	Depressant	Yes, strong	Yes, develops early	Severe, but rarely life-threatening	Yes
Barbiturate-alcohol	Depressant	Yes	Yes	Severe, even life-threatening	Yes, but only partial for alcohol
Cocaine[2]	Stimulant	Yes, strong	Possible	No	No
Cannabis (marijuana, hashish, hashish oil)	Depressant[3]	Yes, moderate	Undecided	Minimal with some people	Yes, possible
Amphetamine	Stimulant	Yes	Possible	Possible	Yes
Hallucinogen (LSD)	Stimulant	Yes	No	None	Yes, rapid
Nicotine	Stimulant or depressant	Yes, strong	Yes	Yes	Yes
Caffeine	Stimulant	Yes, mild	No	Minimal	Yes, slight

1. Khat is not included here because the chewing of its leaves (which produces an amphetaminelike drug effect) is not yet a problem in this country.
2. Cocaine use in this country is increasing (see pages 211–212).
3. Since the WHO Expert Committee classified cannabis as a stimulant in 1965, further research has suggested that, like alcohol, it ordinarily acts as a depressant. Others consider it a stimulant of the hallucinogen (but not LSD) type; still others feel that it is too unique a drug and defies present methods of classification.

drug of dependence is abruptly withheld or (2) when another drug is given that nullifies the effects of the one on which there is dependence.

Experience with the more severe evidences of withdrawal provides the drug abuser with good reason to fear it. A delirium may occur, which is often characterized by *hallucinations* (hearing strange voices and seeing alarming things that are nonexistent) and *delusions* (unreasoning, false beliefs). These symptoms, combined with body-shaking tremors, nausea, and vomiting, cause intense suffering. Some experts suggest that drugs that produce the abstinence syndrome—such as alcohol, barbiturates, and morphinelike drugs—interfere with the "dream sleep" that occurs during the last third of the night and that is associated with rapid eye movements (REMs). Abrupt withdrawal of such drugs, they theorize, results in a sudden and overwhelmingly chaotic return of the dream sleep, and this "brain quake" then brings about the delirium of sudden withdrawal.

Many drugs that produce dependence, both psychological and physical, also produce **tolerance,** which means that increasingly larger doses of the drug must be used to achieve the effect obtained with the beginning doses. Sometimes, tolerance to a drug may become so great that the abuser regularly takes doses that would be lethal to anyone else. Also, tolerance to one drug can result in tolerance to a similar one, as is the case with heroin and morphine.

This phenomenon is called **cross-tolerance.**

The World Health Organization Expert Committee has described seven different types of drug dependence according to the patterns of their action and the responses they bring about.[7] These types are:

1. morphine type
2. barbiturate-alcohol type
3. cocaine type
4. cannabis (marijuana) type
5. amphetamine type
6. khat type
7. hallucinogen (LSD) type

Table 7–1 indicates some of the basic criteria by which part of this classification was made. In addition, it includes nicotine- and caffeine-type dependence.

Depressants

THE JUNKIES

*When they are
in the street
they pass it
along to each
other but when
they see the
police they would
just stand still
and be beat
so pity ful
that they want
to cry.*

MARIE FORD, 12 years old*

Basically, **depressants,** such as opiates, barbiturates, and alcohol, act on the central nervous system by

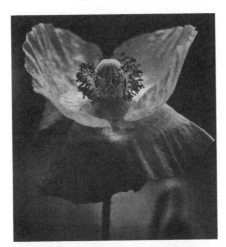

The opium poppy: bearer of both relief and suffering for millions of people throughout the world.

reducing psychic and motor stimuli. Abusers of these drugs often are unable to function either physically or mentally. Thus they are physically

or emotionally incapacitated. Senses are deadened, and abusers exist on the foggy border between consciousness and unconsciousness, drifting in and out of a troubled sleep. Frequent losses of consciousness limit the amount of the drug that can be taken. Antisocial behavior, such as stealing, is rooted in the need to secure more drugs.

The Morphine Type of Drug Dependence: The Opiates

Throughout the ages, writers have woven images of the poppy into their plots. It is a good device. For humankind, the poppy has powerful and exotic meanings. The sleep-producing plant *Papaver somniferum*, the opium poppy, flowers

25 Years of Rock Casualties

Between 1954 and January 1979, the majority of the rock musicians listed below died of drug overdose, premature chronic disease, or unusual accidents. The unique pressures and demands that accompany rapid success and the easy availability of drugs undoubtedly contribute to the high death rate among this population group.

1979

DONNY HATHAWAY. Fell or jumped from his hotel room. Age 33.

SID VICIOUS (Sex Pistols). Drug overdose, 21.

1978

SANDY DENNY (Fairport Convention). Accidental fall at home, 31.

TERRY KATH (Chicago). Accidental self-inflicted gunshot, 31.

KEITH MOON (The Who). Drug overdose, 32.

1977

MARC BOLAN (T. Rex). Auto accident, 29.

LYNYRD SKYNYRD (Ronnie Van Zant, Steve Gaines, Cassie Gaines). Plane crash. In their late 20s.

ELVIS PRESLEY. Heart ailment, 42.

WILLIAM POWELL (The O'Jays). Natural causes.

1976

FLORENCE BALLARD (The Supremes). Cardiac arrest (medication/alcohol-related), 27.

FREDDIE KING. Blood clot, ulcers, 42.

PAUL KOSSOFF (Free). Heart ailment, 27.

PHIL OCHS. Suicide, 35.

PHIL REED (Flo & Eddie). Fall from hotel room, 25.

1975

TOMMY BOLIN (Deep Purple). Drug overdose, 25.

TIM BUCKLEY. Drug overdose, 28.

PETE HAM (Badfinger). Suicide, 27.

AL JACKSON (Booker T. & the MGs). Shot by intruder in his home, 40.

1974

NICK DRAKE. Drug overdose, 26.

CASS ELLIOTT (The Mamas and the Papas). Choked on sandwich, 30.

ROBBIE MC INTOSH (Average White Band). Accidental drug overdose, 28.

1973

JIM CROCE. Plane crash, 31.

BOBBY DARIN. Heart ailment, 37.

RON (PIGPEN) MC KERNAN (The Grateful Dead). Liver disease, stomach hemorrhage, 26.

GRAM PARSONS. Drug overdose, 26.

CLARENCE WHITE (The Byrds). Hit by a car, 29.

1972

LES HARVEY (Stone the Crows). Electrocuted by microphone during show.

CLYDE MC PHATTER. Heart attack, 41.

BERRY OAKLEY (Allman Brothers). Motorcycle accident, 24.

DANNY WHITTEN (Crazy Horse). Drug overdose.

1971

DUANE ALLMAN (The Allman Brothers). Motorcycle accident, 24.

KING CURTIS. Stabbed, 36.

JIM MORRISON (The Doors). Heart attack, 27.

GENE VINCENT. Ulcer, 36.

1970

JIMI HENDRIX. Barbiturate intoxication, 27.

JANIS JOPLIN. Drug overdose, 27.

TAMMI TERRELL. Brain damage, 24.

ALAN WILSON (Canned Heat). Accidental drug poisoning, 27.

1969

BRIAN JONES (The Rolling Stones). Drug-related drowning (coroner's verdict: "Misadventure"), 27.

1968

LITTLE WILLIE JOHN. Pneumonia in Washington State Penitentiary, 30.

FRANKIE LYMON. Drug overdose, 26.

1967

OTIS REDDING. Plane crash, 26.

1966

RICHARD FARINA. Motorcycle accident, 29.

BOBBY FULLER (Bobby Fuller Four). Asphyxiation from automobile fumes, 22.

1964

JOHNNY BURNETTE. Boating accident, 29.

SAM COOKE. Shot by a motel manager, 29.

1960

JESSE BELVIN. Auto accident, 26.

EDDIE COCHRAN. Auto accident, 21.

1959

BUDDY HOLLY. Plane crash, 22.

J. P. RICHARDSON (THE BIG BOPPER). Plane crash, 23.

RITCHIE VALENS. Plane crash, 17.

1958

CHUCK WILLIS. Illness, following surgery, 30.

1954

JOHNNY ACE. Self-inflicted gunshot wound playing Russian roulette, 25.

SOURCE: *Los Angeles Times*, Calendar section (February 25, 1979), p. 78. Copyright, 1979, Los Angeles Times. Reprinted by permission.

into beautiful white, red, and purple petals. But the poppy's milky juice oozes not from its delicate petals but from its unopened seed capsules. For centuries, the use of the drugs derived from this juice has freed people of pain. Their abuse has imprisoned many others.

The air-dried juice from the unripe capsule of the opium poppy, then, is **opium**. The principal active ingredient of opium is **morphine**. Another weaker ingredient of opium is **codeine**. Opium and heroin (which is derived from morphine) are termed the **morphinelike drugs** and are generally classified as **narcotics.**

The risk of dependence on morphine is as great as are its pain-killing properties. Heating morphine with acetic acid (acetylation) produces the more potent drug heroin. Codeine is commonly used in cough medicines, and many would-be drug abusers start with this substance. There are artificially produced (synthetic) compounds that are not directly obtained from the opium poppy but that have effects like those of morphine. These laboratory-produced morphinelike chemicals include *dilaudid*, *Demerol*, *methadone*, and *Darvon*. Darvon has been marketed for over twenty years, and over twenty billion doses have been prescribed. Except for the barbiturates, it causes more accidental (overdose) and suicide deaths than any other drug. Because of its unique properties, which are described later in the chapter, methadone is used in the treatment of heroin abusers.

EFFECTS AND ABUSE

The depressant actions of the morphinelike compounds include *analgesia* (relief of pain), *sedation* (freedom from anxiety, muscular relaxation), *hypnosis* (drowsiness and stupor), and *euphoria* (a sense of well-being and contentment). The chronic opiate user, moreover, loses interest in sexual expression.

Morphinelike drugs can chain people in two ways. The first way is by their creation of a physical dependence, which occurs with repeated but increasingly larger doses of the drug. Eventually, if the dependent abuser is without the drug for about twelve hours, he or she begins to experience withdrawal. The second chain is forged by the body's ability to adapt to the drug (tolerance). Because tolerance requires increasing quantities of the drug to produce the desired effects and to avoid the intense discomforts of withdrawal, the degree of dependence also increases. And the greater the dependence becomes, the more the tolerance is increased. A vicious cycle of entrapment results.

It is not only a fear of withdrawal that enslaves the abuser of morphinelike drugs. It is also a fear of life. The word "narcotic" is derived from the Greek *narkotikos*, meaning "a benumbing." Emotional numbness is what the narcotic abuser seeks. Uninvolvement is the goal. Hovering on the border of withdrawn sleep, the abuser does not—indeed, cannot—confront and deal with life's problems. Obtaining more of the drug is the only reality, the only problem.

"Nodding out" on heroin. For temporary escape into oblivion, heroin abusers sacrifice their body and soul.

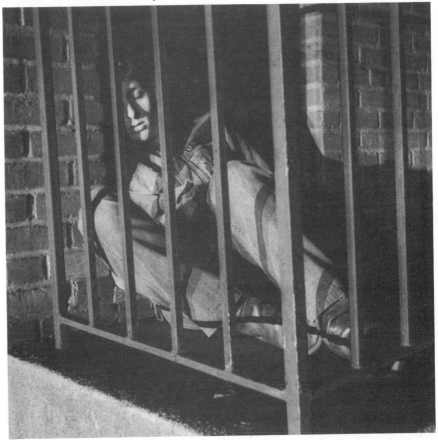

But other problems are unavoidable. Abusers of morphinelike drugs have no way of being certain how much active drug is contained in the substance being shot into their veins, and overdose is always a possibility—although this is more a problem for beginning abusers than for long-time abusers. More common is the likelihood of becoming infected by unclean needles and syringes. A liver infection called *hepatitis B* (page 76) is a serious illness among heroin abusers; it often results in death. Death also may be caused by reactions to impurities in the drugs such as quinine. Also responsible for many so-called heroin deaths is the interaction between the injected heroin and other drugs in the body. In addition, a wide variety of microbes (among them the one causing tetanus) and other contaminants (found on dirty needles and in syringes, and in the drugs themselves) often cause dangerous infections that can result in death.

Heroin abuse can also cause an absence of menstruation (*amenorrhea*; see page 360) and menstrual irregularity. This also occurs with methadone. With methadone, however, the menstrual difficulties often disappear or improve in about a year, which is not the case with heroin. Ninety percent of women on methadone maintenance treatment (see pages 195–196) return to their normal menstrual cycles within three years. Both heroin and methadone alter menstruation by affecting the hypothalamus, that part of the brain that controls the release of pituitary gland hormones affecting ovulation, menstruation, and other functions.

EXTENT OF HEROIN ABUSE

It is estimated that there are almost half a million heroin abusers in this country. Most people who are dependent on morphinelike drugs live in large cities and resort to crime in order to sustain their drug needs. Usually, it is only through stealing, prostitution, and drug dealing that they can obtain the large amounts of money they need. (Preoccupation with the drug normally prevents the abuser from holding down a job.) Dependence on a drug can become an impossibly expensive problem, costing as much as $125 or more daily. Often, to control this expense, abusers will voluntarily commit themselves to treatment centers, undergo withdrawal, and then return to lesser doses of the drug. But tolerance and dependence quickly develop again, and soon the user is back where he or she was before the treatment.

TREATMENT

There are various methods of treatment for dependency on drugs of the morphine type. Which treatment is used will depend on the nature of the patient, for there is no "typical" drug-dependent person. During treatment, the patient with morphine-type dependence should work toward the combined goals of (1) abstaining from the drug, (2) coming to grips with life's demands, (3) getting help for medical and psychiatric problems, and (4) becoming socially rehabilitated. Of course, the first step in this treatment procedure must be withdrawal from the drug—a process known as **detoxification**. Withdrawal, or detoxification, typically is accompanied by medical treatment, but sometimes it is not.

"Cold turkey" refers to detoxification without medical treatment. It can be a cruel experience, and most physicians do not approve of it.

After six to eight hours without the drug or any treatment whatsoever, the heroin dependent begins to suffer the agonies of withdrawal. "I've got superflu, man," the dependent may say. The sufferer's nose runs and eyes water. Twelve to fourteen hours after the last dose of the drug the person may fall into a fitful sleep, often called "yen." Upon awakening, the "superflu" is worse. Muscles twitch. Yawning, sneezing, vomiting, and diarrhea may be uncontrollable. One moment there is a shaking chill, the next moment a burning fever. Sometimes an orgasm will occur. The skin, crawling with gooseflesh, resembles that of a plucked turkey, which may account for the expression "cold turkey." Bones ache and muscles hurt, and the legs often make jerky kicking movements. Worst of all, there is a consuming craving for the drug.

The symptoms peak between thirty-six and forty-eight hours following the last dose of the drug, and they persist at this intensity for about seventy-two hours. But unless the person is very old, or very ill from some other disease, heroin withdrawal is not lethal. Over a period of five to ten days the symptoms gradually abate. Slowly the physical dependence on the drug diminishes, but the psychological dependence lingers on—sometimes for the rest of the patient's life.

Another detoxification procedure involves abrupt withdrawal accompanied by supportive treatment. The supportive therapy may include daily group "rap" sessions and a variety of nonnarcotic drugs that lessen the withdrawal symptoms. However, when carried out in a nonhospital environment, this form of detoxification usually fails.

Still a third method used for heroin dependence is gradual withdrawal plus the substitution for

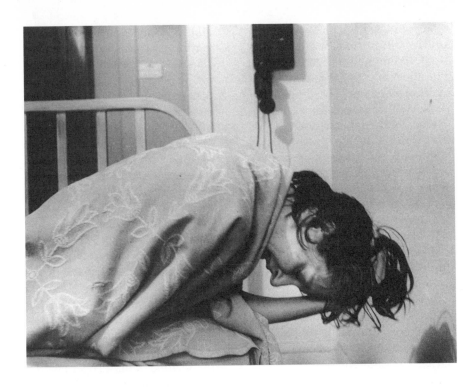

Withdrawal: an agonizing ordeal.

heroin of daily diminishing doses of *methadone*. Methadone is a synthetic narcotic that is taken orally. In treatment clinics it is usually dissolved and given in orange juice. During withdrawal, such symptoms as muscle cramps, vomiting, and diarrhea are treated as they occur. When the patient is drug-free and feeling better, rehabilitation is attempted. But methadone detoxification alone is not an effective long-term cure for the great majority of heroin dependents.

METHADONE MAINTENANCE

Methadone detoxification should not be confused with *methadone maintenance*. With methadone detoxification the heroin is replaced by methadone, which in turn is gradually withdrawn over a number of days. With methadone maintenance, on the other hand, the methadone is continued indefinitely.

Like heroin, methadone causes

severe dependency. What, then, are its advantages?

1. The effects of methadone last from twenty-four to forty-eight hours, whereas the effects of heroin last only for four or five hours.

2. Patients taking oral methadone in a clinic setting every day obtain the drug free and do not have to commit crimes to buy it, nor are they exposed to the risks of impure drugs, infected needles, and dirty syringes.

3. Those who are on methadone do not ordinarily entice others into heroin abuse.

4. With their heroin need controlled, and their intellectual and physical capacities essentially unimpaired (the "high" experienced with methadone is less than with heroin), methadone patients can become productive members of society. It is essential, however, that the methadone maintenance

program include intensive rehabilitation therapy that is tailored to the individual patient. Without it, the patient is likely to return to heroin, which provides the escape from life he or she is seeking.

There is considerable controversy over methadone maintenance programs. Because methadone maintenance involves switching patients from one narcotic to another, the treatment has been decried as immoral. However, nobody questions

the legitimacy of providing insulin for diabetics, antipsychotic agents for schizophrenics, antiseizure medication for epileptics and a variety of other medicaments to other chronically ill people. . . . Even that ancient and useful device, the crutch, is not debased by calling it *"merely a crutch"* when it permits a person to ambulate who otherwise could not do so.[8]

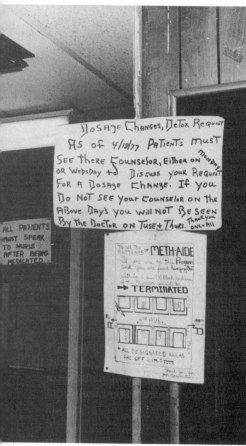

A neighborhood methadone treatment center.

Methadone maintenance hardly answers all the treatment problems of all heroin abusers. For example, with most adolescent patients, it is recommended that a program of detoxification, psychotherapy, and intensive vocational rehabilitation be tried first. Although this approach has had some success, it has resulted in dishearteningly few permanent cures. With the adolescent, the risks of sickness and death from detoxification are great, and too, it is very expensive. For these reasons methadone maintenance of some adolescents is considered worthwhile by some experts.

As of late 1979 methadone treatment programs for heroin dependents were not considered successful. Less than 10 percent of the nation's estimated heroin dependents were in such programs, and the dropout rate was over 60 percent. Why?

1. Some physicians associated with the methadone programs attribute the failure to the countless rules and regulations that must be followed. Because they deal with patients on an individual basis, they find it hard to adjust to generalized rules that dictate who, how, and when to treat, and what and when laboratory tests must be made. On the other hand, there are those who are convinced that the nature of the program makes such regulations necessary.
2. Lack of money has resulted in reduced staff, services, and programs. An actual dose of methadone is inexpensive. But the long-term cost of doctors, nurses, social workers, clerical staff, guards, and other personnel, as well as office space and rehabilitative services, is enormous.

Half a billion dollars a year, for example, is hardly enough to handle the national problems adequately.

3. Some patients claim methadone causes constipation, impotence, and decreased ability to urinate (heroin intake results in at least as many complications, without the benefit of medical care). Moreover, many methadone patients use other drugs. These, together with methadone, can be dangerous.
4. Methadone maintenance requires daily visits to a clinic, which presents many difficulties for most patients. A new, longer-lasting drug, LAAM (levo-alpha acetylmethadol), is now being tested with the hope that it will replace methadone. This drug may cut down the number of weekly clinic visits to three.
5. Other contributing factors to the failure of methadone programs include politics, organized crime, lack of consistent policies, and long waiting lists for treatment. Meanwhile, hundreds of thousands of heroin dependents go without help.

OTHER TYPES OF TREATMENT
Residential self-help centers in which no drugs are used can be an effective treatment for heroin dependence for some people. Synanon, founded in Santa Monica, California, was the first of such treatment programs. Daytop Lodge and Daytop Village, both in New York, now offer similar programs. However, not all applicants are admitted, and not every resident can abide with the rigid rules and harsh realities of these centers. The extremely supportive environment and emphasis on community life, while effective in keeping members away from

drugs, tend to create an equally powerful dependence on the community itself. There is some evidence that many residents in these programs cannot integrate back into society without returning to drugs.

Narcotics Anonymous and Teen Challenge are two other types of volunteer programs that work to help individuals with drug problems, as does Exodus House. Federal narcotic treatment centers in this country include the Public Health Service hospitals at Lexington, Kentucky, and Fort Worth, Texas. But again, despite active therapy designed to help the patient deal with life conflicts, studies of released patients show a disappointingly high rate of return to drug dependence. In both federal and California institutions the patients are detoxified and must remain until there is hope that they are cured. Unfortunately, that hope has shown itself to be small. It seems that it is much easier to get willing patients off drugs than it is to keep them off. Except for physician-patients, relapse rates are as high as 90 percent. The fact that less than 10 percent of physicians return to morphinelike drugs (usually Demerol) may well indicate the importance of having "something to go back to."

The Brain Makes Its Own Morphinelike Drugs

Scientists have long realized that the membrane surrounding each body cell does more than merely hold the cell together. The cell's membrane also acts as a sentry—permitting entry of substances the cell needs, and trying to keep out what the cell does not need. Only recently, however, has the notion of *specific receptor sites* on the cell membrane been developed. Specific receptor sites are definite chemical arrangements of molecules on the cell membrane. Many substances in the blood cannot get into a cell unless they can first fit chemically into their own definite reactor sites (refer back to the discussion of antigen-antibody combinations in Chapter 3). They are then able to be "bound" to those specific receptor sites.

This discovery has led to some interesting notions about the manufacture of morphinelike drugs in the brain cells. For instance, a person who is unconscious from an overdose of heroin is brought into a clinic. Naloxone (an antidote for narcotics) is injected into the person to counteract the effects of heroin. The unconscious person quickly becomes conscious and goes into withdrawal symptoms. How does naloxone accomplish this task? The brain has receptor sites for morphinelike drugs (including heroin), and naloxone fits into those sites, locking out the heroin. The obvious question is why should the brain have such receptor sites in the first place? After all, morphinelike drugs are not naturally a part of the brain's chemistry.

There could be only one answer: The brain must indeed make its own morphinelike drugs. Subsequent research proved this theory to be true. The first of these brain-made morphinelike substances that were found were small molecules called *enkephalins*. They are made up of five or six amino acids, which are the chemical building blocks of proteins. Then morphinelike substances of many amino acids were discovered. These larger enkephalins are called *endorphins*.

Enkephalins and endorphins are found in those parts of the brain (called the *limbic system*) that are concerned with pain and emotions. They are also stored in the pituitary gland and in the blood and spinal fluid. They may also be located along nerve pathways leading to the brain that inform people of pain.

With these discoveries scientists stand at the threshold of a whole new understanding of the nervous system. Numerous questions must be asked and answered. Does acupuncture cause the pituitary gland to release endorphins? Does this explain why acupuncture works? There is some evidence that this is possible. Is there a hereditary inability to produce endorphins? If so, would this explain why some people are more likely than others to become dependent on morphinelike drugs? Does the brain's ability to make its own morphinelike drugs explain the action of methadone? That is, does methadone, like naloxone, lock out heroin from the receptor sites for other morphinelike drugs?

There have been some cases reported of badly wounded soldiers who rejected shots of morphine before undergoing emergency surgery. Is it possible they refused morphine because their brains were releasing their own powerful pain-killing endorphins? Others have a very low tolerance for pain. Is this because their brains are unable (hereditarily) to produce enough endorphins to help them? Can morphinelike dependency somehow be explained in terms of receptor sites having been affected by repeated injections of heroin? Now that it is known that the brain produces its own powerful pain killers, can this knowledge be used in some way to treat narcotic drug dependency? Can endorphins someday be used in the treatment of emotional disorders?

Abnormally high levels of endorphins have been found in people with acute schizophrenic and manic psychoses. Using large doses of naloxone, hallucinations have been lessened in some schizophrenic patients for a brief time. Does naloxone block endorphin action? Is the brain's endorphin production involved with psychoses?[9] It has long been known that the hypothalamus of the brain is the body's thermostat, and it is known that a certain endorphin helps the body adjust to heat. Does this endorphin do the same with pain?[10]

Heywood Brown, a famed journalist of another generation, once wrote, "For truth there is no deadline." So it is with endorphins. It will take time and work to learn how endorphins can help people. But few scientific discoveries in recent years hold as much promise.

The Barbiturate-Alcohol Type of Drug Dependence

SEDATIVES: BARBITURATES AND TRANQUILIZERS

Barbiturates, which are derived from barbituric acid, are synthetic drugs that, like morphinelike drugs, are depressants of the central nervous system. They are classified as *sedatives-hypnotics* because they relieve anxiety and produce euphoria and drowsiness. Among the most common sedatives are the short-acting Seconal and Nembutal and the longer-acting Phenobarbital. Recently, a host of *nonbarbiturate* sedatives have been developed, among them Quaalude. (Because of its increasing abuse, Quaalude is discussed separately on page 199.)

"Tranquilizers" is a word that is not clearly understood by many people. It is best to consider **tranquilizers** as follows:

1. *Minor tranquilizers, or antianxiety drugs.* Examples are Dalmane, Valium, Librium, and Miltown (also known by the trade name Equanil). Valium and Dalmane are among a class of compounds known as the benzodiazepine drugs.
2. *Major tranquilizers, or neuroleptic drugs.* Neuroleptic drugs are useful in the treatment of psychoses; they are thus also called antipsychotic drugs. There are three major types of neuroleptic drugs:

   A. Phenothiazines, such as Thorazine and Mellaril
   B. Butyrophenones, such as Haldol
   C. Thioxanthenes, such as Navane

Unlike the minor tranquilizers, the antipsychotic major tranquilizers are used in the treatment of serious psychiatric illnesses, such as schizophrenia. They are, however, unfortunately associated in some patients with a serious nervous system disorder called *tardive dyskinesia.* The minor tranquilizers or

Every year, millions of barbiturates and the minor tranquilizers are used as sleeping pills. Despite this, little is known about how the pills act or what causes sleeplessness. It is evident that the effectiveness of most such pills begins to drop after seven nights. Yet most prescriptions are for thirty or more pills. It is estimated that some two million people may take the pills every night for a period of over two months.

It used to be thought that the barbiturates were riskier than the new, more frequently prescribed benzodiazepines, such as Valium, Dalmane, and Librium. But the benzodiazepines are just as risky and, in some respects, more so. Dalmane, for example, now accounts for over half the total prescribed sleeping pills. Dalmane causes dependence, as do Valium and Librium, although the degree of dependence may not be as great as it is with the barbiturates. People who use Dalmane on consecutive nights may have a gradually increasing amount of the drug in their bodies. By the seventh night, the accumulated dose may be four to six times greater than the amount present in their systems after the first night's dose. Moreover, it is claimed that Dalmane is effective for at least twenty-eight consecutive nights. This claim is based on studies with only ten people. Considering the millions of people taking Dalmane, this hardly seems an appropriate scientific conclusion. It is also claimed that Dalmane does not interfere with REM (rapid eye movement) sleep as much as do the barbiturates. This is not proved. What is more, both Dalmane and the barbiturates can be lethal when taken with alcohol.

The Food and Drug Administration (FDA) has been criticized because it is responsible for insisting on adequate prescription information. Sadly enough, it is the elderly who are most affected. They now receive about 40 percent of the sleeping pill prescriptions. Yet the insomnia of older people is a natural part of aging.

Physicians have been urged to prescribe less sleeping pills, and patients should take less of them. Losing sleep now and then is not life-threatening.[11]

benzodiazepine drugs do *not* result in tardive dyskinesia. Many people have been discharged from hospitals for the emotionally ill while being treated with a major tranquilizer only to unpredictably develop the grotesque mannerisms of tardive dyskinesia that are due to loss of muscular control, particularly of the face, tongue, jaws, and extremities. Of all the sedatives, Valium and the barbiturates are the most widely used and abused.

As will be seen, chronic barbiturate abusers walk on the edge of death. Every year barbiturates kill more than thirty-five hundred people in this country. Many of these deaths probably are suicides. As with the morphinelike drugs, prolonged and excessive use of barbiturates causes not only profound psychological and physical dependence but also rapid tolerance. Long-time barbiturate abusers may take between ten and twenty pills or capsules every day. They are not hard to get. Counting refills, millions of physicians' prescriptions for sedatives are filled every year in the nation's drug stores. And they are also available illegally. The U.S. consumption of barbiturates is about a million pounds per year, or about 4.5 billion average doses.

Acute barbiturate poisoning may, at first, make an individual seem sociable. But moodiness and depression soon replace the cheerfulness. There is some staggering. The speech slurs. The abuser seems to suffer an inner confused agony. Finally, all sensation is lost in a coma. Without attention, death occurs.

This is not the only way to die of barbiturate poisoning. To avoid a sleepless night, a barbiturate abuser may take one or two pills at bedtime. Awakening an hour or two later, the mind in a cloud of cotton, the individual takes two more pills. Again, sleep comes. A deeply disturbed person may awaken repeatedly, each time more confused, each time gulping down more barbiturates. The average killing dose of barbiturates is only about fifteen times the average treatment dose. With the respiratory and cardiovascular systems depressed, this individual, too, eventually may not awaken. Combined with alcohol, there is an even greater danger. Since both alcohol and barbiturates are depressants, one adds to the action of the other, and the combined effect is far greater than their cumulative individual effects. Worse, tolerance to alcohol produces increased tolerance to barbiturates, and vice versa (cross-tolerance). Often people are found dead with amounts of barbiturates and alcohol in their blood that, had either been taken without the other, would not have been fatal.

Withdrawal from barbiturates without careful treatment is very dangerous. During the first six to eight hours, the patient may seem improved. Then there occurs trembling, anxiety, headache, and vomiting, which in turn give way to grave threats to life. Delirium and psychoses occur, and the patient may die during a convulsion. The danger of convulsions may persist for the first week of withdrawal or even longer. Thus, withdrawal from barbiturates should take place in a hospital; it is generally much more dangerous than withdrawal from heroin. A patient undergoing withdrawal from barbiturates may require as long as six weeks of watchful care. The temporary substitution of long-acting for short-acting barbiturates has been found to make the withdrawal period far less dangerous. Psychotherapy to examine and treat the cause of the dependence is essential.

METHAQUALONE ABUSE

"Luding out" is a street term referring to the sedative-hypnotic effects of a depressant drug called methaqualone (Quaalude). Both physical and psychological dependency on methaqualone occur, and withdrawal symptoms may include delirium and life-threatening convulsions. Combined with another depressant, such as alcohol, methaqualone can be particularly hazardous. Methaqualone is mistakenly believed by some to stimulate sexual desire. Like alcohol and other drugs, it may appear to do this by lowering the sexual inhibitions of some people. But also like alcohol, increasing doses actually diminish the sexual function. Methaqualone is not necessary for medical purposes, and has a high potential for abuse. Most physicians believe that its use should be discouraged.

ALCOHOL

First the man takes a drink,
Then the drink takes a drink,
Then the drink takes the man!
A JAPANESE PROVERB

Forty centuries ago, a famous Babylonian code provided careful regulations for the sale of beer. In about 1500 B.C., an ancient Egyptian book of etiquette warned: "Make not thyself helpless in drinking in the beer shop . . . thy companions . . . will say, 'Outside with this drunkard.' "[12] Alcohol seems to have been a problem even at the ancient Greek athletic events. The Greek stadium at Delphi still has a sign, dating from about 5 B.C., forbidding wine in the stadium.

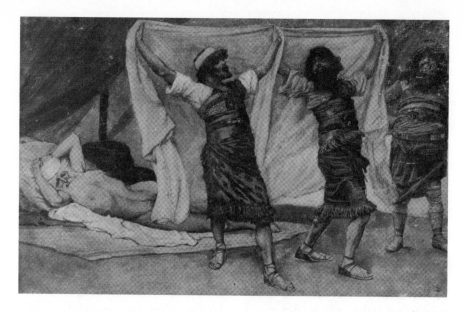

Noah's drunkenness. "And Shem and Japheth took a garment, and laid it upon both their shoulders, and went backward and covered the nakedness of their father." (Genesis, 9:23.)

Nor is the Bible short of references to alcohol. As soon as he left the ark, Noah built an altar; then he planted a vineyard and got drunk. That his drunkenness was a bad example for his sons is, however, made abundantly clear. Moderate use of alcohol was permitted among the Jews—wine "cheereth God and man" the Old Testament states—and was even part of religious ceremonies, but to be intoxicated was considered a disgrace. Self-control was the rigid rule.

The early Romans also avoided intoxication. Nevertheless, as the fall of the Roman Empire approached, widespread drunkenness accompanied promiscuity. Both Roman debauchery and Hebrew restraint profoundly influenced the early Christians. Those desiring to be known as followers of Christ were instructed, "Be not drunk with wine." However, the use of wine was not completely forbidden, as Paul's advice to Timothy makes clear: "But use a little wine for thy stomach's sake and thine often infirmities." Today, almost all of the world's major religions strongly support temperance.

It is known that many primitive peoples drank partly to relieve anxiety. And in addition to relief from tension, they sought the pleasures of the senses that a moderate amount of alcohol could provide. Enveloping the pleasant package were companionship and religious meanings. Many ancient civilized peoples doubtless had some reasons for drinking that were similar to those of the primitives. A remark made by novelist Sholem Asch might be considered to have a universal application to drinking: "Not the power to remember, but its very opposite, the power to forget, is a necessary condition of our existence."[13] A Guatemalan Indian expressed this even more briefly: "A man must sometimes take a rest from his memory."

WHAT IS AN ALCOHOLIC? Definitions vary. The Rutgers University Center for Alcohol Studies suggests one like this: Alcoholics are people who are unable to consistently choose whether they will drink or not, and who, if they do drink, are consistently unable to choose to stop or not.

The accompanying box contains a questionnaire designed to determine if an individual has an alcohol problem. Such questionnaires may help an individual know whether he or she needs help. Help, obtained early, can prevent endless problems with alcoholism. The average alcoholic has been drinking too much for about ten years before he or she seeks and obtains help.

Two out of three adults in this country drink some kind of alcoholic beverage. There is some early evidence that U.S. drinking habits are changing. People now seem to be drinking more wine and vodka than other alcoholic beverages. However, this change will not decrease our alcohol problem. Wine is the national drink of France, and alcoholism is one of that nation's major problems. And in Russia, where the national drink is vodka, drunkenness among the population is a known fact. In this country, about ten million people abuse alcohol creating a cost to society of over $44 billion per year. Alcoholism is thought by some to be the world's third greatest problem, following only war and hunger. There is increasing evidence that many teenagers regularly drink to intoxication and, indeed, become dependent on alcohol. For many high-school students alcohol is no longer merely a taste of adulthood; it is an ongoing way of life.

For about one person of every eleven who use alcohol, the drug is a poison. That one person is an alcoholic. Without treatment the person may become human backwash, gutted and guttered.

Could You Be in Danger?

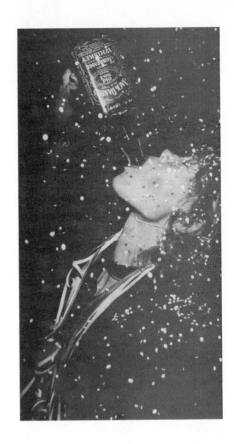

EARLY SYMPTOMS: (the first stage of alcoholism)

YES NO

☐ ☐ Are you beginning to lie or feel guilty about your drinking?

☐ ☐ Do you gulp your drinks?

☐ ☐ Do you try to have a few extra drinks before joining others in drinking?

☐ ☐ Must you drink at certain times—for example, before lunch or a special event; after a disappointment or quarrel?

☐ ☐ Do you drink because you feel tired, depressed, or worried?

☐ ☐ Are you annoyed when family or friends talk about your drinking?

☐ ☐ Are you beginning to have memory blackouts and occasional passouts?

MIDDLE SYMPTOMS: (an extension of early symptoms)

☐ ☐ Are you making more promises and telling more lies about your drinking?

☐ ☐ Are there more times when you need a drink?

☐ ☐ When sober, do you regret what you have said or done while drinking?

☐ ☐ Are you drinking more often alone, avoiding family or close friends?

☐ ☐ Do you have weekend drinking bouts and Monday hangovers?

☐ ☐ Have you been going "on the wagon" to control your drinking?

☐ ☐ Are memory blackouts and passouts becoming more frequent?

LATE SYMPTOMS: (the advanced stage of alcoholism)

☐ ☐ Do you drink to live and live to drink?

☐ ☐ Are you obviously drunk on important occasions—for example, a special dinner or meeting?

☐ ☐ Do your drinking bouts last for several days at a time?

☐ ☐ Do you sometimes get the "shakes" in the morning and think it helps to take a "quick one"?

☐ ☐ Do blackouts and passouts now happen very often?

☐ ☐ Have you lost concern for your family and others around you?

SOURCE: *Harvard Medical School Health Letter*, Vol. 3 (August 1978). Reprinted by permission of Ayerst Laboratories.

Why can one person drink alcohol sociably, while another becomes an alcoholic? There are no simple answers. In some cases the reasons reach back into childhood. People with problems—especially if their work or social environment condones drinking—may turn to alcohol either to boost their courage or to avoid dealing with their inadequacies. Many people drink too much because they are bored, or because they are unhappy, or because they are under too much pressure, or because it is expected of them. A young person's friends may have a profound influence on drinking patterns.

Some researchers suggest that alcoholism tends to run in families, or to have a genetic basis. Some recent studies do suggest that different susceptibilities to alcohol may be due to differences in rates of metabolism among various racial groups.[14] And family-history studies have shown high rates of familial incidence of alcoholism.

An alcoholic ceases to have control over how much he or she drinks. And without adequate treatment, loss of control marks the beginning of a downhill journey. The problem, however, is that the individual often does not recognize, or admit, that control is gone. "I can stop anytime I want to. I don't really need this stuff—just a few drinks to relax and be sociable." But the alcoholic does not—cannot—stop. Bottles are stashed away in hiding places. Drinking is done secretly so that family and friends will not know how much is being consumed.

The body, long resentful, is now in angry protest. Hoarseness develops from a swollen throat; eyes are bloodshot, the skin pasty, the nose red. Vitamin-deficiency diseases develop. Without alcohol, *delirium tremens* may develop (the abstinence syndrome). Five percent of alcoholics develop delirium tremens. Without attention, perhaps 25 percent of those with this syndrome die. With care, less than 5 percent die.

Other signs of vitamin deficiency may occur. Prickly burning of the hands and feet signify the pain and paralysis of nerve disease. Prompt treatment with vitamin B can prevent permanent disability. One form of psychosis (also seen with diseases other than alcoholism) is characterized by periods of amnesia, which are filled in by the alcoholic with all sorts of preposterous tales. Alcoholism may also bring on another collection of signs and symptoms that result from abnormal brain tissue metabolism. Again, vitamin B therapy can likely improve this condition.

In addition, recent research suggests that the long-term ingestion of alcohol plays a part in heart disease. It is now believed that alcohol is directly toxic to the heart.

There is no evidence that moderate consumption of alcohol causes brain damage, but this does occur with long-term, excessive intake of alcohol. Studies support the conclusion that, with prolonged use, it is alcohol and not only malnutrition (as was previously thought) that inflicts liver damage. Recent work also suggests that problems of blood circulation caused by alcoholism also contribute to brain disease.

THE FATE OF ALCOHOL IN THE BODY Once swallowed, alcohol stops first at the stomach. The walls of this frequently mistreated organ promptly help its owner by allowing only about 20 percent of the alcohol to be absorbed into the circulatory system. Absorption is delayed by foods rich in protein and fats (milk, eggs, meat) and by dilution (water, juices). It has been said that for this reason Russian diplomats drink large quantities of milk before trying to impress their foreign guests with their ability to "hold their vodka" at state banquets. Alcohol not absorbed through the stomach lining must await entrance into the small intestine. There, complete absorption is quick regardless of the presence of food. But this entrance is slowed or even temporarily halted (depending on the amount of alcohol taken) by the rapid closure of the sphincter at the juncture of the stomach leading to the small intestine. The delay prevents a sudden absorption (and a walloping dose) of the total amount of ingested alcohol into the blood circulation. Whether absorbed into the circulatory system from the stomach or the small intestine, alcohol in the blood means rapid access to the next stop, the liver. It is in the liver that most (90 percent) of the ingested alcohol is processed. Relatively little passes out through the lungs as expired air or via the kidney as urine.

Alcohol is a toxin, or poison. *Detoxification*, the destruction of alcohol's poisonous properties, is accomplished by *oxidation*, a chemical process involving the body's oxygen. During the body detoxification of alcohol, three oxidation processes occur.

1. The first oxidation process occurs in the liver. Because the liver receives much more alcohol than it can handle at one time, it oxidizes a tiny amount of its received alcohol into a chemical called *acetaldehyde*. (The fate of this irritating substance is detailed in 2. below.) The rest of the alcohol leaves the liver utterly unchanged. It is then carried by the blood to the right side of the

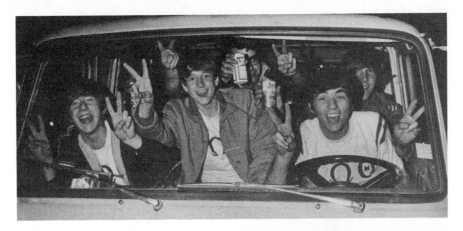

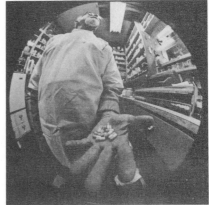

PHOTO ESSAY
Why do people turn to drugs?
The reasons are as varied as the
individuals who use them; among
them are peer influence, availability,
stress or anxiety, idleness, poverty,
and loneliness.

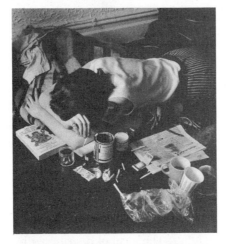

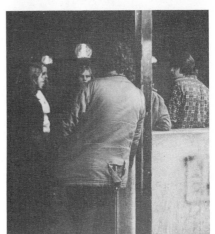

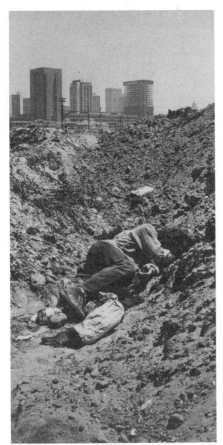

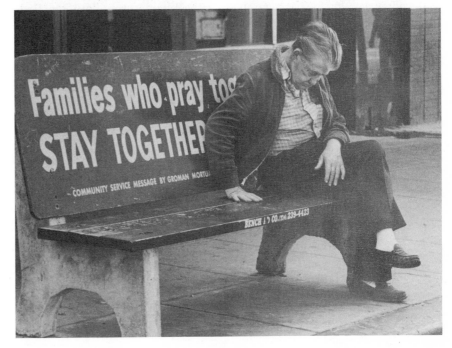

Families who pray to
STAY TOGETHER
— COMMUNITY SERVICE MESSAGE BY GROMAN MORTU

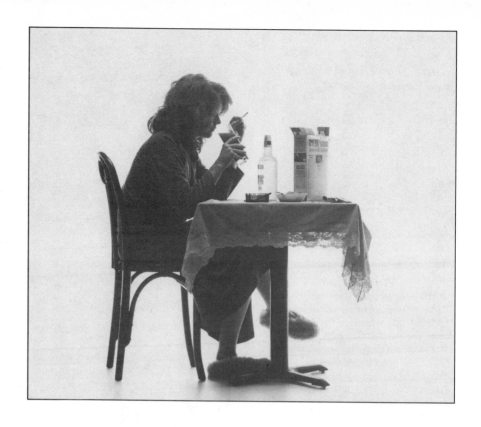

heart, and from there it continues on to the lungs. As the blood in the lungs goes through its usual process of exchanging carbon dioxide waste for fresh oxygen, it also rids itself of a very little of its freeloader, alcohol. Thus, a tiny amount of alcohol is evaporated with breathing. This is not the alcohol that can be smelled, though it can be accurately measured. The alcohol that can be smelled is that which has rinsed the mouth.

From the lungs, the alcohol that has not evaporated on the breath (and this is, by far, the greatest part of it) returns, with the newly oxygenated blood, to the left side of the heart. Then, not yet detoxified, still not oxidized, the alcohol is pumped throughout the body.

So, the hitch is in the liver. It cannot oxidize all the alcohol it gets in one fell swoop. The liver

works slowly, oxidizing alcohol a little at a time. The rest gets into the circulation via the heart and lungs. The alcohol distributed by the blood throughout the body must wait its turn for bit-by-bit detoxification by the liver. It is during that waiting period that the famed reactions to alcohol occur. Thus, alcohol acts with relative rapidity, but it leaves the body slowly.

2. While alcohol travels unchanged over the circulatory route, the liver busily, but slowly, oxidizes a few drops at a time to acetaldehyde. The acetaldehyde is very toxic. Fortunately, it quickly undergoes a second oxidation, so that acetic acid is formed. This occurs not only in the liver but throughout the body.

3. The third, and final, oxidation is to water, carbon dioxide, and caloric energy.

How do hangovers happen? Alcohol causes the body cells to lose fluid. There is thirst. Circulatory changes cause headaches. Decreased inhibitions promote overactivity, resulting in fatigue. The alcohol irritates the stomach, promoting nausea. And the assault of alcohol on the nervous system is responsible for dizziness.

THE EFFECTS OF ALCOHOL Although alcohol is a depressant, most people who drink spirits moderately do not seem depressed. On the contrary, they are relaxed, even happy. And those who drink quite a bit seem highly stimulated. Benjamin Rush, a Quaker doctor and one of the signers of the Declaration of Independence, described people who had drunk too much as "singing, hallooing, roaring . . . tearing off clothes . . . dancing naked."[15]

Depression only comes later. Why

the delay? Alcohol does indeed depress and anesthetize the nervous system. But it also releases inhibitions. Carried by the blood through the brain, alcohol courses through the cerebral cortex, where the numberless nerve connections of learning are laid. Alcohol numbs them. If one has learned to hold one's tongue, for example, alcohol loosens it. If it is loosened enough, one may even halloo.

Alcohol also releases sexual inhibitions. Unless a couple desires a child, alcohol in moderate amounts before sexual intercourse is not contraindicated. However, routine use of alcohol to diminish anxiety about sexual intercourse may signal a need for professional help. Confirmed alcoholics eventually lose interest in sexual intercourse. Male alcoholics often become impotent. The porter in Shakespeare's play *Macbeth* correctly says of alcohol, "It provokes and unprovokes. It provokes the desire, but it takes away the performance." Marriages complicated by excessive drinking are seven times as likely as other marriages to end in separation or divorce.

The harmful effects of excessive alcohol intake on the unborn child have long been known. However, only in recent years has it become clear that even *moderate amounts* of alcohol (two or three cocktails a day) taken early in pregnancy may harm the embryo, resulting in an abnormal fetus.[16] A one-time drinking binge may also have this result. More alcohol seems to cause more abnormalities. It is advised that women do not partake of alcohol (whether whiskey or wine) when they plan to become pregnant or as soon as they suspect or know they are pregnant.

The *fetal alcohol syndrome* is a collection of a considerable number of signs and symptoms. Among

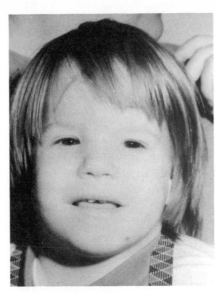

Fetal alcohol syndrome.

these are smallness at birth, underdeveloped head, abnormal spacing between eyelids, abnormal nose formation, small nails, limited joint movements, heart murmurs, ear abnormalities, and possible mental retardation.

As a depressant of the brain and central nervous system, alcohol impairs muscle control and coordination and also the ability to make sound judgments. Thus driving, even with low to moderate amounts of alcohol in the bloodstream, is a particularly dangerous activity. This statement is supported by statistics that show that more than half the fatal traffic accidents in this country involve a driver who has been drinking. In Wisconsin, it was found that among young people aged sixteen to twenty the death rate from this cause was more than twice that of the general population.

Several chemical tests are available for measuring the alcohol content in the system. The spinal fluid, saliva, blood, urine, and breath all have been accurately tested. Such evidence can, of course, be used in court.

Before driving, a drunken person may be walked around the block a couple of times to "sober him up." This is a useless exercise. Muscle tissue cannot use alcohol. Exercise will not materially reduce the level of alcohol in the blood.

Two final grim statistics attest to the effects of alcohol: One-half of all murders and one-fourth of all suicides may be associated with alcohol abuse.

ALCOHOL, CALORIES, AND MALNUTRITION Because the calories contained in alcohol are not directly stored as fat, alcohol, in itself, does not cause obesity. The body does, however, use alcohol's calories for energy instead of food calories, so that the latter are stored as fat. So unless the drinker cuts down on food calories to the same extent that he or she intakes alcohol calories, the person will become overweight.

The calories contained in alcohol supply no vitamins and minerals. There is less appetite for needed foods, and malnutrition is a common and serious problem among alcoholics. The malnutrition of acute alcoholism contributes to increased fat deposition in the liver. The cells of a fatty liver are only mildly injured. However, with the more serious liver inflammation of *hepatitis*, numerous liver cells are killed. Sometimes the hepatitis itself is fatal. When it is not, the healing process causes normal liver tissue to be replaced with scar tissue. *Cirrhosis of the liver* may result. And since the fibrous scar tissue cannot function as normal tissue, the liver's functions are severely impaired. Cirrhosis of the liver is in part the result of malnutrition, in which alcohol plays an important role. It is not surprising that an alcoholic's life span is, on the average, shortened by ten to twelve years.

TREATMENT OF ALCOHOLISM

The treatment of alcoholism must begin with evaluation of the physical, emotional, social, and cultural factors influencing both the alcoholic *and his or her family.* According to the patient's needs, either inpatient or outpatient services may be used. All methods must be carefully supervised. Treatments for alcoholism include *aversion therapy, Antabuse,* and *adjustment* help, as well as *Alcoholics Anonymous* and *Al-Anon/Alateen.*

In **aversion therapy** the patient is first given injections of a nauseant drug, and then drinks of various kinds of liquor are fed to the patient. The goal of this type of treatment is to establish in the alcoholic an association between alcohol and nausea so that an *aversion* (intense dislike) to alcohol is created. For many, this treatment has been successful. **Antabuse** is a drug that when combined with alcohol produces a toxic reaction. With Antabuse, even a small amount of ingested alcohol can be a dangerous experience—the patient may become seriously ill. Some clinicians feel that another drug, called pyribenzamine, reduces the dangers. Various tranquilizers may also be used.

The patient may achieve psychological **adjustment** with the aid of group therapy. **Alcoholics Anonymous (AA)** is an organization designed to offer psychological and spiritual support for alcoholics. AA has had much success in keeping its members sober. There are AA organizations in almost every city in the United States. **Al-Anon** and **Alateen** are groups designed to help the families of alcoholics. The need for such groups was emphasized by a 1977 Gallup Poll that revealed that the number of families troubled by excessive drinking had risen 50 percent since 1974. This increase had been accompanied by a sharp rise in women drinkers. In Al-Anon/Alateen, it is the family members' reaction to the alcoholic that is explored and shared. There is emphasis on the fact that one cannot help the alcoholic until one helps oneself deal with the problem. Futility, resentment, pity, and control of family members are explored. Al-Anon also has a spiritual aspect. Some may find this difficult to accept, but many learn that it helps to submit one's own will to a higher power. Alateen is an offshoot organization of Al-Anon especially for teen-agers. Its purpose is to help young people cope with the problem of an alcoholic mother or father. There are many branches of Al-Anon/Alateen in both the United States and Canada.

The best approach to the treatment of alcoholism seems to be one that combines the various methods. Many health departments have embarked on combination alcoholism prevention and treatment programs.

Stimulants

Stimulants, like depressants, work on the central nervous system, but they excite psychic and motor activity rather than reduce it. For this reason, **hallucinogens** (drugs that produce hallucinations), such as LSD, are discussed with the stimulant group, along with the amphetamines. Nevertheless, although the amphetamine-type abusers ("speed freaks") and the LSD abusers ("acid heads") both take a type of stimulant, their choice of drug is quite different—and largely the result of different needs and personalities. Each of these stimulants, however, has potentially dangerous effects.

The Amphetamine Type of Drug Dependence

Amphetamine abusers seek one result; LSD abusers another. The amphetamine-type drug abuser takes the drug primarily to experience a "flash" or "rush," which is sometimes experienced as a "full body orgasm." The acute anxiety, hallucinations, and paranoia associated with heavy abuse of amphetamines are secondary symptoms. This psychic storm may combine with a temporary increase in physical strength to produce potentially violent and dangerous behavior. The LSD abuser, on the other hand, typically seeks a quieter, more introspective experience.

Rather than seeking a *flash* or a thrill as do the speed freaks, the chronic LSD user develops a complex set of motivations for his drug use, involving self-psychoanalytic, pseudoreligions and creative aspirations. [The speed freak is often violent; this the acid head rejects. Thus] speed always drives out acid.[17]

Although amphetamines have been available for close to forty years, their legitimate medical uses are still not completely defined. For many years they were widely prescribed to help control obesity and depression, but as we will see below, their disturbing side effects left their value open to question. They are, however, useful in treating some **hyperkinetic** (abnormally overactive) children with learning disorders (see below), and also in the treatment of **narcolepsy** (uncontrollable sleepiness). But since these two disorders are rather uncommon, there is no justification for the production of mass quantities of the drugs.

In 1967, the governments of Britain and Sweden set strict limits on the types of disorders for which amphetamines could be prescribed. And in 1970, the United States Food and Drug Administration prohibited physicians from prescribing amphetamines for anything except narcolepsy, hyperkinetic behavior disorders in children, and short-term treatment of obesity. Now ten years later, even stricter government control of amphetamines is being considered.

A NOTE ABOUT THE HYPERKINETIC CHILD

The child behaves "as if there were an inner tornado."[18] Hyperactivity, hyperexcitability, a short attention span, frequent impulsiveness, temper tantrums, learning and reading disabilities, and low tolerance to frustration are all symptoms of hyperkinesis. A hyperkinetic disorder (or "minimal brain dysfunction," as it is sometimes called) may have many causes, but it is believed by some to result from a disorder of the mechanisms in the central nervous system that inhibit behavior. In other words, stimuli that are not essential to the task at hand, and that would ordinarily be filtered out, are permitted to enter

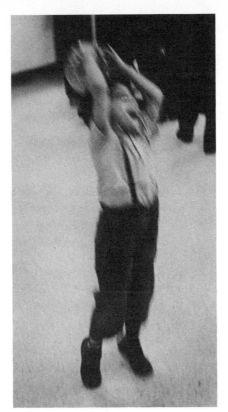

A hyperkinetic child.

the consciousness, leaving the child at the mercy of all environmental stimuli. Because hyperkinetic children are disruptive at home and in the classroom—often displaying the same behavior patterns as children with emotional problems—it is important to distinguish them from those who are responding to stresses at home, poor teaching, overcrowded classrooms, or frustrated, rigid, punishing adults who respond with disfavor to active, questioning children of high intelligence. In fact, of the estimated 3 percent of all U.S. children who have been classified as hyperkinetic, most are believed to have normal or superior intelligence.

Amphetamines, or amphetamine-type drugs, have the paradoxical effect of acting as tranquilizers for many hyperkinetic children. For them, stimulant drugs seem to activate or strengthen the inhibitory

mechanisms in the central nervous system. In this country, more than 150,000 children are now being treated with these drugs. Large-scale screening and testing programs for hyperkinesis are now being proposed because some experts believe that the stimulant drugs are too often used without real justification or adequate supervision. Others point to limited studies that indicate that children treated between the ages of eight and eleven continue to have severe behavioral problems in their teens. And still others suggest that "the basic flaw of drug treatment is that it cannot teach a child anything, and it is not yet established that drug treatment makes the child more accessible to other intervention techniques."[19] Although most of those who work with hyperkinetic children would not discontinue drug treatments of properly selected and supervised cases, all are agreed on the need for more caution and research in this area. Amphetamine-like dependence from the careful use of this treatment has not been proved.

AMPHETAMINE: THE BITTER PILL

Some of the common trade names for methamphetamine central nervous system stimulators are Methedrine and Desoxyn. For dextroamphetamine, they are Dexedrine and Benzedrine. In street terminology, amphetamines are often referred to as "speed," "crystal," "meth," "bennies," "dexies," or "whites."

Unlike the opiates or barbiturates, amphetamines do not create physical dependence; withdrawal is, therefore, neither dangerous nor painful. However, the potential for psychological dependence and

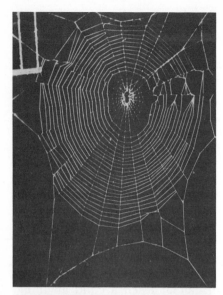

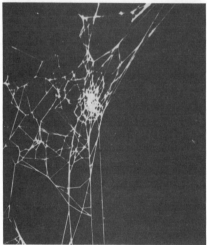

The spider, perhaps the greatest architect among living creatures, loses its cunning when given "speed." Top: A normal web. Bottom: A web spun twelve hours after the spider was given a dose of dextro-amphetamine.

tolerance is marked. A long-time abuser may gobble as many as 150 "pep pills" or "uppers" a day to attain the effect first experienced with just one.

When swallowed, amphetamines are tasteless, but they can become a bitter pill. Long-term abuse causes prolonged sleeplessness, extreme restlessness and anxiety, bizarre mood changes, paranoia, and hallucinations. Even relatively moderate doses may cause such profound behavioral and emotional changes as to make the individual unable to carry out normal routines. Chronic amphetamine abuse has led to brain damage.

Most amphetamine abusers take the drug in pill or capsule form, but some individuals go on to "shoot" the drug into their veins. After many injections, "shooters" develop scars along their veins called "tracks." Tolerance develops quickly, and before long the drug is injected about every two to four hours around the clock. During this period, which may last from three to six days, the abuser remains continuously awake. This is called a "run" or "speed binge." The abuser then "falls out." Tremulous, disorganized, hallucinating, and paranoid, the exhausted individual finally falls into a deep sleep from which he or she cannot be awakened. Following a three- or four-day run, a drug abuser may sleep twelve to eighteen hours. Upon awakening, hunger is intense, and the paranoia is largely gone. But there is now deep depression. Barbiturates or opiates often are taken to relieve the unpleasantness of the "coming down," or "crashing," period. Sometimes they are combined with amphetamines during a run to control anxiety, hallucinations, and paranoia.

Paranoia may appear with the first injection, though usually it is delayed several days. Everyone is suspect. Friends "bug" the phone; every car is a police cruiser; behind every tree is a detective. The abuser is likely to become violent toward those whom he considers his enemies.

During a run, the amphetamine abuser may display purposeless compulsions. One abuser may shine shoes, again and again, all day long. Another will take a radio or an automobile motor apart. Completely absorbed, the abuser seems untroubled by the lack of coordination and the failure to "repair" it. For extended periods a male abuser may engage in nonejaculatory intercourse. Eventually this will lead to the inability to get or maintain an erection at all. With discontinuance of the drug, the impotence disappears, but the psychotic symptoms often persist. In the female, the functional parallel to the male erection is vaginal lubrication. But amphetamines have a drying effect on the vaginal lining. If the woman engages in prolonged intercourse under such conditions, the result may be an eroded and extremely painful lower vagina. Even the labia may feel sore.

During a period of chronic abuse, twenty to thirty pounds may be lost. Commonly seen, and in part because of malnutrition, are abscesses, nonhealing ulcerations, and brittle fingernails. Among those who inject amphetamine, serum hepatitis is common, caused by a virus spread by dirty needles and syringes. The death rate from this liver disease is much higher than that from infectious hepatitis.

It is estimated that in the major cities of this nation, thousands of young people take amphetamines intravenously. And those who want to stop often find it difficult to do so. Why? "Speed freaks" generally share living quarters with one another, and friendships are formed often as the result of their common need for the drug. Yet in this human need for companionship, there is an ironic complication. Amphetamine toxicity seems to be increased in a crowded ecosystem. For example, experiments done with animals have shown that crowding increases the toxicity of amphetamine fourfold. Among humans, too, it has been observed that taking the drug in a high-density population setting increases its toxic effect.

The Hallucinogen (LSD) Type of Drug Dependence

The drugs causing dependence of the hallucinogen (psychedelic or "mind revealing") type include *LSD* (lysergic acid diethylamide), *PCP* (phencyclidine), *psilocybin* (a drug found in a particular Mexican mushroom), and *mescaline* (found in the buttons of a small cactus—mescal or peyote—and in the seeds of certain varieties of the morning-glory plant). In this country, some Indian tribes are legally permitted to use the mushrooms, cactus buttons, and morning-glory seeds as part of their religious rites, as has been their custom for centuries. They may also be used for treatment purposes by their medicine men. Like amphetamines, hallucinogens have the capacity to induce tolerance. This, however, is not characteristic of cannabis, or marijuana. Thus, there is cross-tolerance between LSD, mescal, and peyote but not between these three and marijuana (see page 213).

LSD

The effective dose of LSD is tiny. One ounce would provide 300,000 adult doses. Two pounds, distributed equally, would be enough to cause mental and emotional disturbances in millions of people.

LSD begins to have noticeable effects about twenty to forty-five minutes after it is swallowed. These effects reach a peak in about four hours, and they are usually gone anywhere from six to twelve hours after the drug is ingested. Tolerance to LSD is rapidly developed. Unlike tolerance to opiates, LSD tolerance may be developed in a few days; however, it is usually lost in two or three days. Thus, if LSD is taken regularly over a period of days, some users may build up a tolerance from 100 to 1,000 or 2,000 micrograms (sometimes even more). Then, if the drug is not taken again for a week or so, the average dose (150 to 250 micrograms) regains its effectiveness. There is no evidence of physical dependence on LSD.

PSYCHIC EFFECTS The first effects of LSD, or "acid," as it is commonly called, may be slight dizziness or nausea. This is generally followed—or accompanied by—a sense of well-being or euphoria and marked perceptual alterations. The individual may feel that he or she is becoming an actual part of a chair or a fireplace or of another person. There is often an orgy of vividly colored shapes and patterns, some beautiful, others bizarre. These are called "pseudohallucinations," meaning that the individual knows the altered perceptions have no basis in external reality but sees them anyway. The environment is not exactly different; rather its shapes, colors, and meaning have changed. A flower, for example, may seem to breathe visibly, or a painting may seem to come alive. These are not strictly hallucinations, since the stimuli for the perceptions do exist in reality.

Many individuals remark that they have "really seen the world for the first time" during an "acid trip." *Synesthesia*, the translation of one type of sensory experience into another, may occur. For example, music may be felt as body vibrations, or colors may beat in rhythm with music. The sense of time is also distorted. Rapid thought sequences and mood changes seem to make time slow down. Others claim feelings of *transcendence*—of being above and beyond earthly things or even beyond the universe. And personal insights, or glimpses of the self without the usual defense mechanisms, are another commonly reported experience.

There is no explanation for the *"flashback" phenomenon* of an LSD experience. Weeks or months after the last ingestion of the drug, an individual may have spontaneous recurrences of LSD-like hallucinations. One woman told of "terrifying involuntary illusions of people decomposing in the street in front of her and . . . nightmares in vivid color. She continued to have these experiences five months after her last drug experience."[20]

Research on the psychic effects of LSD indicates that, in a controlled situation, it may enhance, though not replace, skilled psychotherapy. And it has been used successfully with terminally ill patients as a way of getting them to come to terms with their approaching death. With one woman, four LSD treatments combined with psychotherapy had a beneficial effect on her attitude toward her knowledge that she was dying of cancer. Previously, she had been markedly depressed. After the treatments she

left the hospital in good spirits and was able to participate actively in her daughter's wedding.

She fulfilled her desire to walk down the aisle without the aid of even a cane, and during the reception she amazed all the guests by dancing with her husband. Her sister said she had been the life of the party.[21]

The patient died soon afterward, but her last days had been made immeasurably happier.

PHYSICAL EFFECTS In determining whether LSD has lasting physical effects, scientists have sought the answers to four questions:

1. Does LSD damage the chemical structure of the hereditary material of genes that are part of the chromosomes?
2. Does LSD cause cancer (is it carcinogenic)?
3. Does LSD cause genetic changes or mutations? Does it cause modifications or new combinations of genes or chromosomes that are transmissible from one generation to another?
4. Does LSD have a *teratogenic* effect? That is, does it produce physical defects in offspring while in the uterus?

Much of the scientific literature related to these questions has been reviewed by a group of researchers in the field. Some years ago they examined sixty-eight studies and case reports that had been published over a period of four years. They concluded: "From our work, and from a review of the literature, we believe that pure LSD ingested in moderate doses does not damage chromosomes in vivo [within the living body], does not cause detectable genetic damage, and is not a teratogen or a carcinogen in man."[22] It was noted that "in a study of human pregnancies, those exposed to illi-cit [probably impure] LSD had an elevated rate of spontaneous abortions."[23] These investigators, therefore, suggested that, other than during pregnancy, there was no present reason to stop the controlled experimental use of pure LSD. They noted in addition that a further review of fifteen studies resulted in conclusions similar to their own.

PCP

"Devil dust" would be a better name for PCP than "angel dust." Phencyclidine (PCP for short) has been around for almost a quarter of a century. On the basis of experiments conducted with animals, the government once approved it as an anaesthetic for humans. But among members of the medical community, PCP soon lost its popularity. Too many of their patients were waking up with weird reactions. So the Detroit pharmaceutical house that manufactured PCP asked the government to limit its use to an animal tranquilizer only. The government complied. But PCP can easily be made in makeshift kitchen or garage laboratories, and it is cheap. In San Francisco PCP gained popularity on the street and became known as the "peace pill." In New York it was called "hog." By 1978, "angel dust" was being widely used, even by younger teen-agers. Because of its dramatically potent effects, taking the drug became a sign of bravery: If you used angel dust you could do just about anything— including losing your mind.

PCP is a powerful hallucinogen. Nobody knows why some people react to the first dose of it while others do not. It is most commonly laced with marijuana or sprinkled on parsley or mint leaves. It can also be dissolved in liquid or taken as a tablet. It can have a combination of effects that can kill an abuser or an innocent bystander. First, there is a loss of any feeling of pain. Add to this a sense of superhuman strength. Mix these two with an unpredictable violence, and add a deep feeling that everyone is out to hurt you (paranoia). To these add a loss of caring about the self, other people, and external events. The result is that use of this chemical can cause explosive personality disorders and extreme behavior changes.

The chemicals needed to make a pound of PCP cost $150. On the street, this pound can bring more than $8,000. For illegal manufacturers and dealers that means a profit; for the user it may mean homicide, suicide, paranoia, schizophrenia, or permanent brain damage. It all depends on how much of the drug is taken and how the user happens to react to it.

OTHER HALLUCINOGENS

One disturbed twenty-four-year-old man "first learned of the hallucinogenic effects of morning-glory seed ingestion through a newspaper article cautioning against the use of the seeds."[24] Before going into shock, he experienced a variety of hallucinations. Four months later, hallucinations were still occurring—both at will and against his will.

Recent years have seen a revival of interest in the use by North American Indians of **peyote**, the hallucinogenic plant containing mescaline (see page 209). Considered Mexico's original "peyote tribe," about ten thousand Huichols have lived for centuries (separated from European culture) in the remote regions of the high Sierra Madre mountains. Their *nearikas*

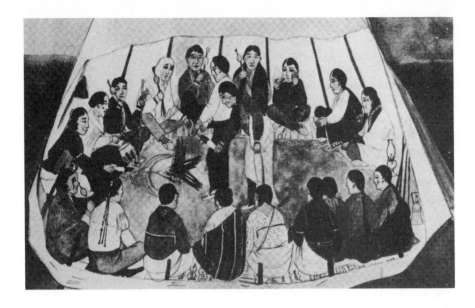

A peyote ceremony being celebrated by the Plains Indians. Once the peyote is ingested, the participants stay awake all night, singing, shaking rattles, and waiting for visions.

—wool paintings based on visions resulting from ingesting peyote—are collectors' items. Unlike some other North American Indian tribes who use peyote rituals to relieve frustration and despair, and who have often abused the drug, the Huichols are temperate and disciplined in their ritual use of peyote.

The use of peyote and whiskey by the Indians of the Plains, however, has a different history, and one in which the white man played an evil role. There is an old Indian legend that when Henry Hudson landed at the southern tip of Manhattan Island, he opened a keg of whiskey and fed it to the Indians. The Indian name *Manhattannick* means "the place where we all got drunk." Until the coming of the white man, the Plains tribes did not use hallucinogenic plants, such as mushrooms and Jimson weed. Even tobacco was used only in a few ritual puffs. However, the Indians of the Plains tribes greatly respected visions, and to achieve them they would inflict dreadful self-tortures, imploring the spirits to pity their suffering. Peyote was native to northern Mexico. It spread from one

tribe to another as far north as the Canadian plains. At first, it provided a new way for the Indians to seek visions. Later, it provided escape from the humiliations inflicted by the white man.

Today, the Native American Church of North America comprises religious Indian groups from almost all tribes. Members of the Native American Church believe that the cactus plant peyote is a God-given sacrament. During their religious ceremonies they eat considerable amounts of it. One population of Navajo Indians was studied for rates of emotional illness that might be traced to their ceremonial ingestion of peyote. The rate was found to be very low, "probably because the feelings evoked by the drug experience are channeled by church belief and practice into ego-strengthening directions and there are built-in safeguards against bad reactions."[25]

OVER-THE-COUNTER HALLUCINOGENS

Not all hallucinogens are illegal. In recent years, a number of reports have been made of cases of psy-

chedelic-like experiences following ingestion of a considerable diversity of over-the-counter products. Many, such as some cold tablets, cough suppressants, and sleep inducers, are intensely advertised. These products should be kept "under the counter" and sold only by prescription.

Cocaine

The street name for **cocaine** is "snow" or "coke" or "girl." It is derived from the leaves of certain coca plants growing high on the eastern slopes of the Andes Mountains in Peru and Bolivia. Indians native to these regions have chewed coca leaves for centuries, both to increase their stamina in the high altitudes and for the pleasurable effects the drug provides. Coca leaves also play a significant role in the Indians' religious ceremonies.

In the early part of this century, cocaine was legal in this country, and small quantities were contained in some soft drinks and patent medicines. In some factories it was provided to workers to increase their rate of production and their endurance for working long hours under extremely unpleasant conditions. In recent years cocaine has largely been replaced by synthetic derivatives. It is, however, gaining increasing popularity as an illegal "street" drug, particularly among the upper-middle-class population, who are more likely to be able to afford its extremely high price. (One gram of cocaine currently sells for about $100 on the street.)

Cocaine is a central nervous system stimulant, and its effects are similar to those of the amphetamines. Cocaine intoxication is marked by lack of fatigue, talkativeness, a sense of well-being, and an increased feeling of physical and mental power. With very large doses, it may produce a headache, a sudden rise in temperature preceded by a chill, or nausea. Cocaine can be highly toxic. Why? It is absorbed from all sites of application, including the mucous membrane. The rate at which the body absorbs the drug may exceed the rate at which it leaves, thus building up to dangerously high levels. This does not occur when cocaine is swallowed, however, because in the gastrointestinal tract the drug undergoes chemical changes. The majority of users sniff the powdery drug into their nostrils through a straw or small spoon, because it is rapidly absorbed through the mucous membrane of the nose. Chronic abusers may inject dissolved cocaine directly into their veins to obtain a more intense reaction.

As with the amphetamines, chronic cocaine abuse can lead to extreme weight loss, general physical and mental deterioration, anxiety, and unfocused hyperactivity. Cocaine sniffers report that the drug is a sexual stimulant, but the fatigue and numbness that follow its abuse may be accompanied by the temporary inability to have an orgasm. Also reported among chronic cocaine sniffers is an inflammation of the mucous membrane of the septum (dividing wall between the two sides of the nose). Furthermore, there may be a reduced resistance to infection (caused, perhaps, by chronic fatigue and poor eating habits).

Overdoses of cocaine can cause hallucinations, delirium, paranoia, and dangerously high increases in blood pressure and heart rate.

Marijuana

The annual *Cannabis sativa* plant, the source of **marijuana** and **hashish,** grows wild in most temperate and tropical areas, and almost everywhere in the United States. It is in the young, small leaves surrounding the seeds of the plant, and in its flowering tops, that most of the mind-affecting ingredients are found. Figures as to the extent of marijuana use in the United States vary considerably; however, experts in the field estimate that several million people use the drug regularly (daily to weekly). Apparently, millions of others try it and discontinue its use. Reasons for stopping vary from boredom with the drug to concern about its illegality.

The leaf is most often cut and crushed and rolled into a thin cigarette, usually called a "joint." It is also smoked in a pipe, baked in brownies or other food, and boiled in water to make a tea. Hashish usually appears as a hard brown cake. It is five to ten times more potent than marijuana and is most often smoked in a pipe. However, it, too, may be eaten or drunk. Hashish is also sold as an oil. In this form, its potency is greatly increased, and it is often sprinkled on marijuana and smoked. Today, the great majority of cannabis users in this country use marijuana rather than hashish, and smoke it rather than swallow it.

Experienced marijuana and hashish smokers are able to control the dose and, therefore, the effect of the drug. They obtain some effect within a few minutes. The "high" usually begins in about fifteen minutes and lasts about three hours.

When ingested, there is no control over the dose. The effects of oral intake of cannabis begin after one-half hour to two hours, reach a peak in about three to four hours, and continue in a diminishing fashion for about eight hours.

The Fate of Marijuana in the Body

The effect of delta-9-tetrahydrocannabinol (THC), one active ingredient of the cannabis plant, on the human being is not easy to determine. In part, this is because of the difficulty in determining the dose taken. When marijuana is smoked as a cigarette or in a pipe, 20 to 50 percent (perhaps even less) of the THC in a marijuana cigarette is absorbed via the lungs. Thus the dose of THC that is actually delivered to the smoker varies greatly.

Marijuana: A Drug in a Class by Itself

Marijuana is hard to classify (see footnote 3 to Table 7–1). Many experts consider it to be, like alcohol, an ultimate depressant. Others disagree; they think of marijuana as a basic stimulant, classified with no other drugs. Still others classify it as a hallucinogen, but different from LSD. In the laboratory, its effects are puzzling. When a mouse is given a barbiturate depressant, it sleeps. When both a barbiturate and marijuana are administered, the two drugs together produce a greater depressant effect than the barbiturate alone. The marijuana has increased the depressant effect of the barbiturate. When a mouse is given a stimulant amphetamine, it becomes excited. When both an amphetamine and marijuana are administered, the two drugs have a greater stimulant effect than the amphetamine alone. The marijuana has increased the stimulant effect of the amphetamine. When the combined effect of two drugs is greater than the effect of either drug used alone, a phenomenon called *potentiation* has occurred. Thus, paradoxically and remarkably, "marijuana potentiates both barbiturate sleeping time and amphetamine excitement in mice."[26]

Marijuana is also unique in the matter of tolerance.

TOLERANCE

Unlike many lower animals, people develop only a slight tolerance to marijuana. By no means is it as great as tolerance to opiates, bar-biturates, and alcohol. Numerous long-time marijuana smokers report that they need less—not more—of the drug to achieve the same effect. This phenomenon is called *reverse tolerance.*

WHY REVERSE TOLERANCE? SOME POSSIBLE REASONS

In the body THC is thought to break down into simpler chemical compounds. These are called *metabolites.* The metabolites of THC continue to be excreted in the urine and feces of a chronic marijuana smoker for several days. This suggests that repeated intake of marijuana results in an accumulation of the drug's active chemicals in the body tissues. Therefore, residues of the drug remain in the body of the chronic user for considerable periods. For this reason it is possible that reverse tolerance would develop—that the drug would have increasing effects with repeated smaller doses. Still another reason for reverse tolerance is the fact that people must "learn" how to smoke marijuana efficiently and what effects to expect from it. *Suggestibility,* or the user's anticipation of the effect of the drug, plays a major role in this learning process. Long-time users frequently report a marijuana high after they have smoked *placebos*—"marijuana" cigarettes from which, unbeknown to them, all the active ingredients have been removed. They are thus deceived into anticipating an effect. It may be that this "learned sensitization" to marijuana, based on prolonged past experience, minimizes the mild tolerance to it that actually may occur.

CROSS-TOLERANCE

In large doses, marijuana can cause hallucinations in some peo-ple. So can the stimulant hallucinogens LSD, PCP, mescaline, and peyote. But LSD, mescaline, and peyote show a cross-tolerance for one another, while marijuana shows no cross-tolerance with any of these three hallucinogens.*

Psychic Effects

This old Persian tale is still told today in southwestern Asia:

Three men arrived at Ispahan at night. The gates of the town were closed. One of the men was an alcoholic, another an opium-addict, and the third took hashish. The alcoholic said, "Let us break down the gate"; the opium smoker suggested, "Let us lie down and sleep until tomorrow"; but the hashish-addict said, "Let us pass through the keyhole."

At doses ordinarily used, smokers report that within seconds to minutes they feel jittery "rushes." Then comes *euphoria*—a pleasant relaxed tranquility. Time seems to pass slowly. As has been noted, space may seem lessened. So are inhibitions. Attention is dulled. Thought processes fragment. The user may be either hilarious and friendly or silent and distant. There is an awareness of being intoxicated not unlike that produced by alcohol. The user becomes acutely conscious of certain stimuli to the extent that the whole attention is focused, immersed, and at times lost with the sensory experience. Less commonly, dizziness and a sense of lightness are reported. Increased hunger has also been experienced. The increased hunger, like some other

---

*It is worth noting, however, that delta-9-THC shows a cross-tolerance for delta-8-THC, even though delta-8-THC has few psychoactive effects.

symptoms, may be due in part to the increased suggestibility to the actions of others.

What symptoms occur with *higher than ordinary doses*? Depersonalization—loss of the sense of personal ownership of one's body—has been reported. Visual distortions and imagery are also common. For example, colors may appear to shimmer. The higher the dose of marijuana, the more likely it is that such symptoms as depersonalization and hallucinations will occur. (A very few marijuana smokers experience these effects with small doses.)

Panic, depression, and toxic (poison-induced) psychoses, although extremely rare, may occur, especially among inexperienced users. Panic is the most common of these reactions. The floating feeling of unreality, the eerie sense that the body has lost its place in space, frightens some people. The best treatment is quiet, nonjudgmental, nonthreatening reassurance. As a rule, panic, depression, and psychoses disappear. They occur more frequently among those who are new to the drug or who attach much emotional meaning to the use of it. Possibly the drug precipitates these reactions in individuals already predisposed to emotional disorders.

Physical Effects

The immediate physical signs of marijuana smoking are few. The *conjunctiva* (see page 248) may become red. The pulse rate may increase. These signs may last as long as the psychic effects of the drug. (It is not the smoke that causes the red conjunctiva; taking cannabis by mouth has the same effect.) Some impairment of muscle strength and mild unsteadiness have also been reported. Both smoked marijuana and orally taken delta-9-THC cause dilation of airways lasting as long as sixty minutes and six hours, respectively.

With people who are new to the drug, moderate doses of marijuana significantly impair reading comprehension and impede performance on learning tests. Even with experienced abusers, the drug interferes with logical thinking processes. Thus cannabis impairs the understanding and reasoning function. The impairment increases as the dose increases or the task becomes more complex.

Marijuana: Delusion of Early Adolescence

As a child approaches adolescence, he must begin to

> relinquish his dependence on his parents for emotional support and learn to base his self-esteem on his own achievements. These achievements not only involve success in the path towards his profession, but also social and sexual success. . . . The adolescent . . . has to deal with many disappointments, frustrations, feelings of helplessness and wishes to escape. . . . The question now is how are these inevitable conflicts of adolescence going to be settled? . . . Is he going to be able to base his self-esteem on his own achievements? Or is he going to fall back on external "magic" [such as marijuana] that can elevate his self-esteem at command just as the traditional objects [such as a teddy bear or a blanket] that he used when he was a toddler . . . .?[27]

It may be argued that many adults also use alcohol, tobacco, and marijuana for some emotional support. True. The difference lies in this: Usually the adult has already established the realistic patterns of his or her life, whereas the adolescent has yet to do so. Yet the temptation of the adolescent to rely on the "magic" of marijuana is much greater than that of the adult. Although the use of alcohol and tobacco has caused much human harm, it is doubtful "that Margaret Mead and some others are justified when they criticize parents and ask, 'What do parents expect if they tell their teen-age children not to smoke marijuana when they themselves have a martini in one hand and a cigarette in the other?'"[28]

The Amotivational Syndrome

Some chronic marijuana smokers develop a disinterest in the self and in their social improvement. These characteristics are known as the *amotivational syndrome*.[29] There is much disagreement over the causes of the syndrome. Numerous individuals regularly smoke mild preparations of marijuana without such personality changes. Others state that the drug has not been used long enough in this culture to permit such an evaluation. Many chronic users of marijuana exhibit the amotivational syndrome.

In one study of Jamaican farmers, the work records of thirty chronic marijuana smokers did not differ significantly from those of thirty nonsmokers. But there is disagreement as to whether the study is basically scientific. For example, the question is asked whether Jamaican workers would do repetitive and boring tasks without the drug. After all, work demands on Jamaican farmers are different from those on U.S. truck drivers or students, for example. More carefully controlled studies in this country are indicated. But they must never lose sight of individual responses. No matter what the results turn out to be, if they are not clearly applicable to a considerable number of people, they will be the kind of "proof" upon which to concentrate doubts.

Marijuana and Increased Awareness

Many marijuana abusers report increased sensitivity to and appreciation of music. Some tests (such as for pitch discrimination) of nonmusicians do not support this claim. Nor do some available tests support the commonly described marijuana-increased awareness of touch, taste, and smell. However, it may be that the tests are inadequate to measure such responses. It may also be that increased suggestibility and the environment (set and setting) account for some of the reports by many users. Moreover, a person normally ignores a stimulus that is not needed for a particular activity. In some way, marijuana causes a loss of the ability to ignore extraneous stimuli. This loss, plus the user's frequently changing sense of time and space, may well account for some of the sensory novelty caused by marijuana.

Marijuana: Stepping Stone to Other Drugs?

Does marijuana abuse lead to the abuse of other drugs, including heroin? Those who answer negatively base their reply on two points:

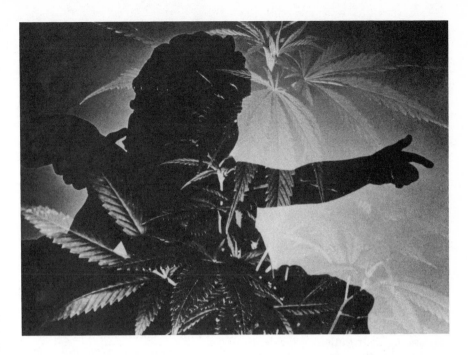

1. There is nothing in the pharmacological action of cannabis per se that causes an abuser to turn to other drugs.
2. Millions of people in this and other countries use marijuana and other cannabis products regularly without regularly using other drugs.

The first of these statements is probably correct. The degree of its truth depends largely on the chemical formulas of the various drugs in the plant. The accuracy of the second statement depends not on the nature of the drug, but on the nature of people. And unlike drugs, there are no formulas for people. Numerous studies[30] support the following two statements:

1. "No one has failed to find a statistical relation between marijuana and the use of other drugs—legal and illegal."[31]
2. "Use of other drugs is clearly related to frequency of marijuana use.[32]

So, there is no evidence that the pharmacological properties of cannabis per se lead to the abuse of other drugs. Such secondary drug abuse appears to be due to the personality and environment of the individual. Many people who use marijuana do not abuse other drugs. Many do.

Can Cannabis Be a Medicine?

Because marijuana decreases pressure within the eye, it may be helpful in treating glaucoma (see page 249).[33] It is also being used experimentally in the treatment of selected cancer patients who respond adversely to drug or massive radiation treatment that is necessary with some kinds of leukemia and other cancers.

Marijuana and the Law

Today, cannabis is governed in this country by narcotics laws. But it is not a narcotic. In recent years, several states have decriminalized the use of marijuana, and there is considerable public opinion favoring its legalization. What are some of the arguments on which this view is based? How do they stand up under scrutiny?

1 Enforcement of marijuana laws is costly.

True. Arresting and imprisoning thousands of marijuana offenders costs the government millions of dollars a year. Yet outright legalization of marijuana would hardly be cost-free. Licensing, production, processing, distribution, and sale of marijuana all would need to be government-controlled so as to prevent overpricing, adulteration, and other abuses. Bureaucracies, similar to those needed for alcohol, would be required. "Then tax marijuana to pay for government control," say the proponents of legalization. But, as with alcohol, the cost does not stop there. Should chronic marijuana abuse, like alcoholism, be responsible for an amotivational syndrome, it (combined with the proved association with other drug abuse) would inevitably increase welfare costs. In addition, all taxpayers would have to pay the costs of treatment and rehabilitation of those whose dependence on various other drugs would be associated with freer availability of marijuana. Of course, millions of people who use no drug but marijuana today would never need treatment, rehabilitation, or welfare after legalization—but many people might. This much seems clear: Those who do not want marijuana legalized would have to pay at least as much for its use as those who do.

2 Use of marijuana is nobody else's business.

There is no such thing as a purely private drug problem. A person who overindulges in drugs affects the lives of others because he or she is less available for civic obligations.

3 Marijuana is no more harmful than alcohol.

Mounting evidence, though incomplete, tends to support this statement. However, alcohol is rooted in Western culture. Indeed, for many it is part of a religious sacrament. Nevertheless, the cost of alcohol to society includes about ten million emotional and physical cripples. What is the cost in money? Every year alcoholism drains the U.S. economy of billions of dollars. Marijuana is not yet completely ingrained in this culture. Why risk adding to the already massive problems of society?

4 Tobacco is more harmful than marijuana.

No responsible observer can ignore the tobacco disaster. But the evils of one drug do not necessarily prove the virtues of another.

Does marijuana smoking cause cancer? When applied to the skin of mice, it does cause cancerlike cellular changes. That marijuana smoke must be retained in the lungs for effect would seem to increase its cancer-producing capabilities. On the other hand, marijuana now seems less likely than tobacco to cause cancer because the number of marijuana cigarettes consumed by the average user is small compared with the number of tobacco cigarettes consumed by the average tobacco smoker.

5 Since marijuana can be made more cheaply and acts more quickly than alcohol, legalization would drive the alcohol industry out of business.

This is not likely. When cannabis was legal in India, that country still had serious alcohol problems. In addition, people who use alcohol do so for reasons different from those who use marijuana. Moderate alcohol users do not take the drug for the express purpose of getting "stoned." Marijuana users do. In this culture, moderate use of alcohol is involved with its palatability and the social activities of which it is a part. One needs to justify marijuana use in its own right, separate from the social conventions that include a moderate use of alcohol.

6 People of other countries use marijuana without problems.

This is not true. The use of marijuana is now legally restricted in almost every country in the world. After twenty-five centuries of use, during which cannabis became part of its religious life, India has undertaken a program aimed at the elimination of its "pot skid rows." (It is worth noting that the United States is a cosigner of the United Nations treaty controlling marijuana. To legalize the drug, this nation would have to abrogate the treaty.)

7 In the doses ordinarily taken in this country, marijuana is usually harmless.

The psychological harm that prolonged marijuana use does to some people has yet to be accurately evaluated. As with alcohol, many people may begin moderate marijuana use only to find themselves trapped in chronic abuse. The use of cannabis in this country may not long be limited primarily to marijuana, any more than alcohol consumption is limited to 3.2 percent beer. As yet, relatively little is known about chronic abuse of stronger cannabis preparations, such as hashish.

8 Present marijuana laws are unenforceable and unfair.

Government regulation of drugs is necessary. Legal restrictions apply to both alcohol and tobacco. Protection of the public demands no less. The controversy surrounding laws against marijuana is rooted in criminal sanctions presently directed against abusers. It is argued that if anyone should be prosecuted, it is the grower and seller. Another objection to present marijuana laws is that, in their enforcement, constitutional guarantees of privacy are violated. Many who are not generally deviant have suffered the stigma of arrest. Penalty structures are also said to be unfair because they are unduly harsh and because they vary from state to state. Moreover, the ease with which marijuana can be grown makes uniform enforcement impossible. Bootlegging of beer and wine is possible, but not easy. Anyone with a window box can grow marijuana.

"Laws and institutions are constantly tending to gravitate. Like clocks, they must be occasionally cleansed and wound up, and set to true time."[34] Marijuana exploded on the national scene so suddenly that there was no time to adjust existing laws. Nevertheless, much responsible opinion has urged that marijuana laws be revised to avoid making felons out of people. Today in several states the possession of up to one ounce of marijuana is a minor violation.

Purposeful Pollution of Drug Crops

In the mountainous areas of Mexico, farmers grow opium poppies and marijuana plants. By early 1978, thousands of tons of marijuana and heroin were being smuggled into the United States. The Mexican farmers who grew opium and marijuana increased their income twenty-five times. Mexican soldiers and narcotics agents fought a losing battle against growers. Fertile grounds were hundreds of miles from highways. And high-altitude drug-fields were impossible to conquer.

In 1973, U.S. money, training, and technology were put to Mexican use. Herb killers (used in Vietnam), helicopters, and other specialized aircraft were put at the disposal of Mexican officials. The herbicide *paraquat* was sprayed on the marijuana crops. Another herbicide— 2,4-D—was thought to be most destructive to the opium poppy. In 1977, thousands of acres of Mexican poppy and marijuana plants were destroyed.

But to destroy the marijuana plant, paraquat needed at least twenty-four hours in the sun. Mexican farmers began to harvest their marijuana crop on the same day it was sprayed. It was then packed into "bricks" and smuggled across the border. The result was that a percentage of the estimated fifteen million U.S. marijuana smokers were being exposed to a dangerous herb killer.

It seems agreed that the U.S. State Department has violated federal law since the program began. It is now said that the Mexican government alone is carrying out the paraquat program. What effect has the program had on the supply of marijuana in the United States? Probably very little, since now Colombian marijuana is being smuggled almost uncontrolled into this country via the vast coastline of Florida.

Tobacco

Before we can properly study the effects of tobacco on the human body, we must first know something about the part of the anatomy that is most directly affected by tobacco —that is, the **respiratory system.**

The Normal Respiratory Tree

Inhaled air passes through the nasal and (if the mouth is open) oral cavities, on past the *pharynx* and the *larynx*, to reach the hollow, stiff *respiratory tree* (see Figure 7–2 and Body Charts 11 and 12). This is indeed a tree, albeit an upside down one, with its branches spreading out on each side of the chest cavity.

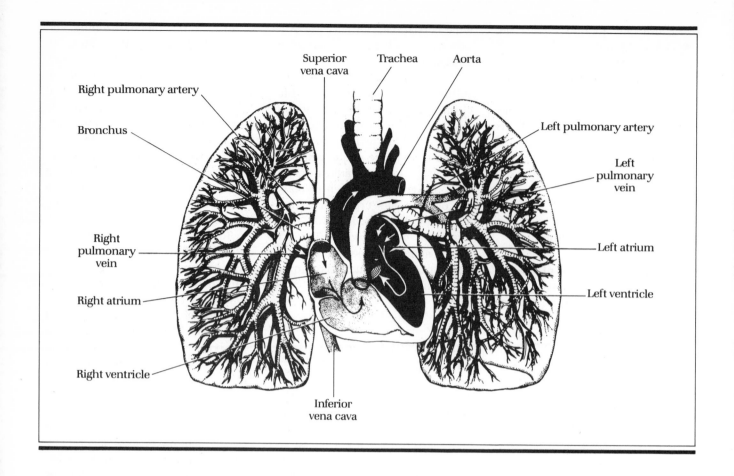

FIGURE 7–2
The respiratory tree.

The main trunk, the four-inch-long *trachea* (windpipe), divides into two main branches, called the *bronchi* (singular, *bronchus*). Division and subdivision continue until tiny twigs, called the *bronchioles*, are reached. These end in thin-walled air sacs, the *alveoli* (see Figure 7–3). There, through the capillary network embedded in the alveolar walls, life-giving oxygen is absorbed into the blood, and poisonous carbon dioxide is eliminated.

The trachea and bronchi are kept rigid and open by regularly spaced, C-shaped rings of hard fibrous tissue called *cartilage*. The bronchioles, however, are not held open by cartilage but by *elastic fibers*. Thus, they get larger with inhalation and smaller with exhalation.

Covering the whole respiratory tract, from nose to bronchioles, is a thin, moving film of *mucus*. Every day about three ounces of mucus are produced by glands in the lining of the air passages. The mucus is kept moving toward the throat by countless sweeping, hairlike *cilia*. Like millions of tiny brooms, the cilia project from the lining of the bronchial tubes (see Figure 7–4). The moving mucus blanket keeps the air passages moist and protected from inhaled dust, germs, and other foreign particles, which stick to the mucus blanket and are swept away by the ciliary "brooms." Anything that interferes with this ciliary action interferes with the normal housekeeping and, hence, functioning of the respiratory system. This is where tobacco enters the story.

Cigarette Smoking: Harbinger of Sickness and Death

On January 11, 1964, the report of the Advisory Committee to the Surgeon General of the Public Health Service, *Smoking and Health*, was released. In 1967, a second report, *The Health Consequences of Smoking*, was made available by the Surgeon General, and supplements to it were issued in 1968, 1969, 1971, and 1973. In 1978, statements made by the Commissioner of Health, Edu-

FIGURE 7–3
Alveoli: air sacs that are terminals of the lung's bronchioles. Oxygen is supplied to the blood through the capillary network embedded in the walls of the alveoli.

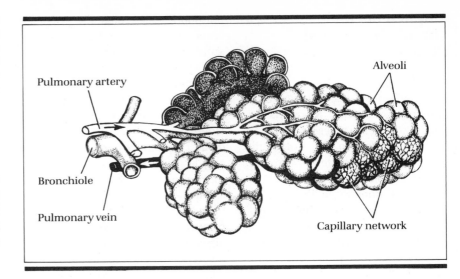

cation and Welfare reinforced the earlier reports. And in 1979 the U.S. surgeon-general released yet another comprehensive report on smoking and health.[35] What are some of the accumulated findings?

1. Because of illness, cigarette smokers spend over a third again as much time away from their jobs as persons who never smoke. Women who smoke are sick in bed 17 percent more often than women who never smoke.

2. The death rate for all age groups is nearly 70 percent higher for cigarette smokers than for nonsmokers. And the more one smokes, the higher the death rate. For example, for those who smoke forty or more cigarettes daily, the death rate is 120 percent higher than that of nonsmokers. The ratio of smoker to nonsmoker death rates is greatest between the highly productive ages of forty and fifty. Furthermore, life expectancy among young men is reduced by an average of eight years for heavy cigarette smokers (those who smoke over two packs a day) and an average of four years for those who smoke less than one-half pack per day.

3. The death rate from cancers of the lung, larynx (voice box), oral cavity, esophagus, kidney, urinary bladder, and pancreas are all markedly higher for cigarette smokers than for nonsmokers.

FIGURE 7–4
Respiratory epithelial cells resting on connective tissue. When the surface layer of epithelial cells is damaged, the damaged cells are cast off and replaced by upgrowing deeper cells, which grow cilia when they reach the surface. Although the epithelial cells lie at different levels, they all reach the underlying connective tissue and are in contact with the nerves in connective tissue, which control the beat of the cilia. The columnar cells reach the connective tissue by narrowing. The cells of this type of respiratory epithelium are found throughout the entire respiratory tract except in the alveoli and in the smallest air passages leading directly to the alveoli. The extremely thin epithelium in the alveoli is unlike the rest of the respiratory epithelium to permit an efficient exchange of oxygen and carbon dioxide gases. In addition, cilia are absent in the passage of the vocal cords. Were they present there, voice production would be hampered. Therefore, this passage is cleared by clearing the throat or by a slight cough.

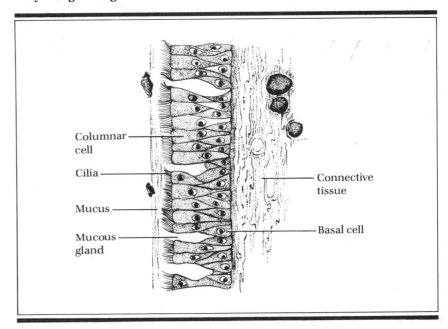

Emphysema and Chronic Bronchitis: Chronic Obstructive Lung Disease

The smoke from cigarette combustion produces gases. More than a dozen of these gases contribute further poison to the polluting smoke. Even cigarettes low in tar and nicotine may still contain dangerous amounts of these gases. The three most poisonous are hydrogen cyanide, nitrogen oxides, and carbon monoxide. Leading filter cigarettes may produce more of the killing trio of gases than do leading nonfilter brands. It is these poisonous gases plus the particles (especially tar) in the cigarette smoke that interefere with the proper action of the cilia. When the cilia cannot move as they should, neither can the mucus. In the bronchioles, a traffic jam is created. How? Remember that the bronchioles expand with inhalation. This enables air to squeeze in past the unmoving mucus. But as air is exhaled, the bronchioles diminish in size. They clamp down on the trapped, accumulated mucus, and air cannot get out. The trapped air stretches the air sacs (alveoli), which balloon and form large air blisters. Some of these blisters rupture, causing the destruction of lung tissue. Breathing efficiency is diminished. To accommodate the damaged, overstretched lung, the entire bony chest cage enlarges. Then the *diaphragm*, the breathing muscle separating the chest and abdomen, also loses efficiency. This sequence of events characterizes the serious lung disease **emphysema**.

The accumulation of mucus and the loss of efficiency of the cilia combine to prevent the elimination of germs. These, in turn, infect the bronchial tubes, causing bronchitis. **Chronic bronchitis**, which may lead to emphysema, is caused primarily by cigarette smoking.

Six Psychological Reasons for Smoking (Horn's Test)

Each person's habit is unique. Thus, there is no truly "typical" smoker. However, according to the American Cancer Society, smokers do fit roughly into one or more of six smoking types, depending on how their habit has developed. Horn's test shows how smokers use their cigarettes to manage their emotions. Smoking may be characterized by one, or a combination, of these factors. After reading the descriptions below, take the test on page 221 to determine what smoking type you are.

- Stimulation (10 percent). This type of smoker is stimulated by the cigarette. It helps him to wake up in the morning, to organize his energies, and to keep him going. Many smokers report that while smoking they experience a sharpening of intellectual capacity and an increase in impulse control.
- Handling: Sensorimotor Manipulation (10 percent). This type enjoys manipulating the cigarette with his hands, watching the smoke curl as he exhales, and making a production of lighting the cigarette, holding it, and flicking the ashes.
- Pleasurable Relaxation (15 percent). This smoker gets real, honest pleasure from smoking, especially after a dinner or with a cocktail. He tends to smoke to accentuate or enhance pleasurable feelings accompanying a state of well-being.

  Comment: The above stimulation-handling-relaxation positive-effect smokers characteristically smoke under pleasant circumstances that are relaxing. They usually require an adequate substitute for quitting and often find that it is not too difficult to stop.
- Crutch: Tension Reduction (30 percent). This negative-effect type of smoker uses cigarettes for the sedative or tranquilizer effect in moments of stress, fear, shame, disgust, discomfort, or pressure. He uses cigarettes to help him cope with problems. Substitutions will generally not help this smoker, and success is gained from learning how to properly manage the situations that produce the bad feelings in the first place.
- Craving: Psychological Addiction (25 percent). This type of smoker feels totally dependent upon his cigarettes, and alternates between an increase of positive feelings and a decrease of negative feelings. He is constantly aware when he is not smoking and begins the craving for the next cigarette when he puts out the present one. Tapering off doesn't seem to work; the only solution is to quit "cold turkey."
- Habit (10 percent). The habitual smoker gets very little satisfaction from his habit and performs it somewhat automatically. He may smoke a cigarette without realizing it or even wanting it. There is very little emotional component to his smoking activity and a minimal amount of awareness. It is important for him to develop this awareness and to understand the pattern of his smoking.

NOTE: The Smoker's Self Test is available from local units of the American Cancer Society and from the National Office on Smoking and Health, Department of Health, Education and Welfare.

SOURCE: Arden G. Christen and Kenneth H. Cooper, "Strategic Withdrawal from Cigarette Smoking," *CA—A Cancer Journal for Clinicians*, Vol. 29 (March–April 1979), pp. 97–99.

Why Do You Smoke?

Here are some statements made by people to describe what they get out of smoking cigarettes. How *often* do you feel this way when smoking them? Circle one number for each statement. *Important:* Answer every question.

	Always	Frequently	Occasionally	Seldom	Never
A. I smoke cigarettes in order to keep myself from slowing down.	5	4	3	2	1
B. Handling a cigarette is part of the enjoyment of smoking it.	5	4	3	2	1
C. Smoking cigarettes is pleasant and relaxing.	5	4	3	2	1
D. I light up a cigarette when I feel angry about something.	5	4	3	2	1
E. When I have run out of cigarettes I find it almost unbearable until I can get them.	5	4	3	2	1
F. I smoke cigarettes automatically without even being aware of it.	5	4	3	2	1
G. I smoke cigarettes to stimulate me, to perk myself up.	5	4	3	2	1
H. Part of the enjoyment of smoking a cigarette comes from the steps I take to light up.	5	4	3	2	1
I. I find cigarettes pleasurable.	5	4	3	2	1
J. When I feel uncomfortable or upset about something, I light up a cigarette.	5	4	3	2	1
K. I am very much aware of the fact when I am not smoking a cigarette.	5	4	3	2	1
L. I light up a cigarette without realizing I still have one burning in the ashtray.	5	4	3	2	1
M. I smoke cigarettes to give me a "lift."	5	4	3	2	1
N. When I smoke a cigarette, part of the enjoyment is watching the smoke as I exhale it.	5	4	3	2	1
O. I want a cigarette most when I am comfortable and relaxed.	5	4	3	2	1
P. When I feel "blue" or want to take my mind off cares and worries, I smoke cigarettes.	5	4	3	2	1
Q. I get a real gnawing hunger for a cigarette when I haven't smoked for a while.	5	4	3	2	1
R. I've found a cigarette in my mouth and didn't remember putting it there.	5	4	3	2	1

How to Score:

1. Enter the numbers you have circled to the Test 3 questions in the spaces below, putting the number you have circled to Question A over line A, to Question B over line B, etc.
2. Total the 3 scores on each line to get your totals. For example, the sum of your scores over lines A, G, and M gives you your score on *Stimulation* — lines B, H, and N give the score on *Handling*, etc.

Totals

$$\overline{}_{A} + \overline{}_{G} + \overline{}_{M} = \overline{}$$ Stimulation

$$\overline{}_{B} + \overline{}_{H} + \overline{}_{N} = \overline{}$$ Handling

$$\overline{}_{C} + \overline{}_{I} + \overline{}_{O} = \overline{}$$ Pleasurable Relaxation

$$\overline{}_{D} + \overline{}_{J} + \overline{}_{P} = \overline{}$$ Crutch: Tension Reduction

$$\overline{}_{E} + \overline{}_{K} + \overline{}_{Q} = \overline{}$$ Craving: Psychological Addiction

$$\overline{}_{F} + \overline{}_{L} + \overline{}_{R} = \overline{}$$ Habit

Scores of 11 or above indicate that this factor is an important source of satisfaction for the smoker. Scores of 7 or less are low and probably indicate that this factor does not apply to you. Scores in between are marginal.

How? There is some evidence that the nitrogen oxide contained in cigarette smoke lowers the efficiency of the cellular *macrophages* in the lung-cleansing system. It will be remembered that macrophages are major fighters of infection (see pages 57–58). The persistent infections of the bronchi result in a chronic condition.

For those people who have chronic bronchitis and emphysema, and who continue to smoke cigarettes, the death rate is much higher than it is for nonsmokers. This deadly duo constitutes the major elements of *chronic obstructive disease* of the bronchi and lungs. And in the past twenty years, the number of deaths from these conditions has increased more than sixfold. Moreover, smoking is a much more significant cause of these diseases than is air pollution or occupational exposure to pollutants.

The role of cigarette smoking as an actual cause of asthma is not entirely clear. But it is beyond dispute that smokers are more likely to die from asthma. The fact that asthma is a result of allergy and bronchial swelling (see page 63)—permitting air to enter the breathing system but interfering with air getting out—is doubtless part of the grim picture not only for those with asthma who smoke but also for those with asthma who do not smoke but are exposed to it.

Smoking and Cancer

The following statement was issued by the Public Health Service as long ago as July 1969:

Additional evidence substantiates the previous findings that cigarette smoking is the main cause of lung cancer in men.

Smoking is a significant factor in the causation of cancer of the larynx and in the development of cancer of the oral cavity. Further data strengthen the association of cigarette smoking with cancer of the bladder and cancer of the pancreas.[36]

Recently, the relationship between cigarette smoking and lung cancer has been studied more intensively. These are some of the findings: (1) The cigarette tars and other particulate matter are the likely irritating causes of lung cancer. (2) The average male cigarette smoker has nine to ten times the chance of the nonsmoker of developing lung cancer. For heavy smokers this risk doubles. (3) If smoking is discontinued, the risk of dying from lung cancer sharply decreases. (4) Since 1930, the lung cancer death rate in women has increased more than 400 percent. This increase continues. At present rates lung cancer exceeds breast cancer as the major cancer cause of death among U.S. women. (5) Only one of twenty diagnosed lung cancers is now cured. Of all the common malignancies, lung cancer offers by far the least hope of cure. (6) About 100,000 specimens of microscopic lung tissue (taken from people who had either died or who were undergoing lung surgery) were compared with the smoking history of their donors. The results are as follows:

1. Those who had never smoked had normal lung tissue.
2. "Precancerous lesions" were found in proportion to the amount of cigarettes smoked.
3. The tissue of those who had smoked and stopped showed less lung disease changes, indicating that reversibility is possible when smoking is stopped.

The relationship between smoking and lung cancer is no longer open to serious question. In one definitive study, cancer of the lung was produced in dogs made to smoke (via an incision in the trachea) seven cigarettes a day for a two-year period. The dogs had learned to enjoy the tobacco, "begging and wagging their tails for a cigarette."[37]

Smoking and the Heart and Blood Vessels

Increasing evidence indicates that cigarette smoking contributes to the development of cardiovascular disease and particularly to premature death from coronary heart disease. Here, too, the risk increases with the number of cigarettes smoked.

How does cigarette smoking affect the heart? Nicotine causes the release of chemicals influencing the body's nerve centers, which in turn release chemicals controlling blood pressure and heart rate. The results are an increase of tension in the heart wall, a more rapid heart rate, a rise in blood pressure, some heartbeat irregularity, and other evidences of increased demands on the heart. The heart muscle must work harder because it needs more blood, for only by an increased blood supply can more oxygen and other nutrients be brought to the more active heart. Ironically, having created the need for more blood, cigarette smoking decreases the body's ability to supply it in several ways.

The fact that nicotine increases the work of the heart is but part of a series of heart-threatening events. The blood hemoglobin carries oxygen to all the tissues. But cigarette smoking means the inhaling of carbon monoxide gas (cigarette smoke is 3 to 4 percent carbon monoxide). Smokers generally have 3 percent to 7 percent of their blood hemoglobin saturated with carbon monoxide. Carbon monoxide then interferes with the ability of the heart to take oxygen from the blood. The combination of *increased oxygen requirement* and *decreased oxygen availability* leads to a diminished amount of oxygen to the heart muscle. This situation is particularly dangerous for patients with coronary artery disease. In addition, owing to the impaired functioning of the lungs that cigarette smoking causes, not enough oxygen is delivered to the tissues, and the heart is further short-changed.

If the coronary arteries are partially blocked by atherosclerosis, the danger is multiplied. Atherosclerotic arteries have lost some elasticity and cannot dilate enough to bring more blood and other nutrients to the heart. It is believed that the absorbed nicotine and carbon monoxide gas from cigarette smoking contribute to the progression of atherosclerosis. Nor are the harmful effects of cigarette smoking limited to the heart, lung, hemoglobin, and blood vessels. It is now thought that cigarette smoking makes *platelets*, a type of blood cell involved in clotting (pages 90–91), more adhesive. As a result, clots may be formed more readily within the coronary arteries that bring blood to the heart. And with the blood flow obstructed by clots, the possibility of a heart attack is greatly increased.

Cigarette smoking delivers blow after blow to the heart. It is not surprising that those more likely to have coronary disease who smoke have heart attacks more often—and recover less often. A pending fatal heart attack may be precipitated by a single cigarette. In such a situation, "the patient can be told not

merely that he is killing himself slowly but that the next cigarette could be his last."[38]

More Facts about Smoking

Peptic ulcers (see page 285) afflict the mucous membrane of the esophagus, stomach, or duodenum. Such ulcers are more prevalent among cigarette smokers than nonsmokers. And stomach ulcers have a stronger association with cigarette smoking than do duodenal ulcers. Furthermore, cigarette smoking reduces the effectiveness of medical and surgical treatment of both types of ulcers. For instance, complications following surgery for peptic ulcers are more frequent among cigarette smokers, and smokers also are more likely to have a recurrence of the peptic disease.

Periodontal disease (particularly gum inflammation, bony-tissue destruction, and loss of teeth) is much more common among smokers than nonsmokers. As an example, women smokers between the ages of twenty and thirty-nine have twice the chance of losing their teeth as do nonsmoking women in that age group. Among men who smoke, the chance of becoming toothless between the ages of thirty and fifty-nine is double that of nonsmokers.

Smokers complicate the physician's task. For example, a test for *colon cancer* may result in dangerously misleading results. Why? Because the amount of a certain chemical in smokers without colon cancer may reach the same high levels as in people with colon cancer. Also, the *concentration of circulating white blood cells* is higher in the blood of smokers than in nonsmokers. The physician must be on guard to this result because many infections also result in a rise in white blood cell concentration.

Nutrition, particularly of pregnant patients, is also altered by smoking; there may be changes in the body's use of carbohydrates and proteins with smokers, and smoking may impair protein metabolism. Smokers may also have increased needs for vitamins C, B_{12}, and B_6, and for bone minerals.

For those who take *oral contraceptives*, the risk of heart damage is increased. Cigarette smoking increases that risk even more. A recent study showed that women taking oral contraceptives who smoke thirty-five or more cigarettes a day have a rate of heart damage twenty times higher than women who have never smoked.

The action of some drugs is changed by smoking. Thus for some smokers certain drugs must be given in different doses and frequency than for patients who do not smoke. And if the patient reduces or stops smoking, the dose and frequency of a drug may need to be altered. It is nicotine that is believed to cause a person's dependency on tobacco, and it is nicotine that is the root of increasing difficulties in administering necessary drug treatments to smokers.[39]

SMOKING AND WOMEN

Once it became socially acceptable for women to smoke in public, it did not take the tobacco companies long to capitalize on this lucrative new market. Over the years, many advertising campaigns have been directed specifically to the female audience. But as of January 1, 1971, radio and television advertising for cigarettes was outlawed in the United States. One reason for this action was the influence of such ads on children.

Meanwhile, women smokers have indeed increased in numbers, and they are beginning to smoke at an earlier age. And younger smokers become heavier smokers. Moreover, compared with nonsmoking women, they are spending more time sick in bed, have a greater incidence of chronic diseases, are losing more time from work, and have increased their risk of dying (from lung cancer, for example) by at least 20 percent.

SMOKING AND PREGNANCY

Smoking during pregnancy apparently increases the risk of complications of pregnancy, delivery of a child before term, spontaneous abortion, and stillbirth. Children born of women who smoke during pregnancy are more likely than babies born to nonsmoking women to die during the early weeks of life. (Women who give up smoking by the fourth month of pregnancy sharply reduce the risk to their babies.) The chances of a newborn being underweight and having congenital heart disease may be greater if the mother smokes during pregnancy.

Why is the unborn child so affected? The evidence suggests that smoking causes the flow of blood through the placenta to decrease; increases the poisonous carbon monoxide gas content of the placental blood; and decreases the supply of oxygen and other nutrients to the baby. In addition, the nicotine in cigarette smoke is believed to have a directly poisonous effect on the fetus. It has, moreover, been noted that cigarette smoking results in a lesser weight gain of the pregnant woman because the fetus gains less weight during the pregnancy.

ARE PIPES AND CIGARS SAFER THAN CIGARETTES?

Cigar and pipe smokers run the risk of developing cancers of the mouth, pharynx, and larynx. Their chances of developing such cancers are higher than those of nonsmokers and about the same as or slightly lower than those of cigarette smokers. As with cigarettes these cancers are due to particles in the smoke that contain nicotine, tars, and other chemical cancer initiators. The gaseous phases of the smoke also contain nicotine and other cancer causers.

It is in both the gaseous and particulate phases of the smoke that chemicals are present that interfere with the function of the cilia. "Little cigars" are dangerous. They also contain hydrocyanide and carbon monoxide gases, as well as other harmful chemical compounds such as tar. Pipe smokers are particularly prone to oral cancer, especially cancer of the lip. There is an unduly high incidence of cancers of the bladder and kidney among pipe and cigar smokers. Some smokers are trying to escape smoking by the use of snuff and chewing tobacco; however, both are distinct causes of cancer of the oral cavity.

THE BEST TIP

Do filters strain out some of the harmful contents of cigarettes? Recent studies indicate that they do. The risk of developing cancer of the lung and larynx are reduced by about 25 percent in long-term smokers of filter cigarettes (ten years) as compared with smokers of nonfilter cigarettes. The risk of heart attack and blood-vessel disease of the extremities is also diminished. There is a suggestion that charcoal-filtered cigarettes help to lessen coughing.[41] However, it should not be inferred that filter cigarettes will lessen the risk of disease as much as will complete abstinence from smoking.

The best tip, then, is to quit smoking.

For Most Nonsmokers There Is No Escape — As Yet

In this country, state and local legislators are making some progress in their efforts to pass laws limiting cigarette smoking in public places. Adverse reactions to tobacco smoke are the bane of many allergic people. And the carbon monoxide in cigarette smoke may be hazardous to nearby nonsmokers. The carbon monoxide content of polluted city air rarely contains more than thirty parts of carbon monoxide per million parts of air, while the cigarette smoker exposes those nearby to about four hundred parts per million (p.p.m.) of carbon monoxide. Among relatively healthy people, a ninety-minute exposure to only fifty p.p.m. of carbon monoxide can result in diminished hearing discrimination. Visual acuity, particularly at low levels of light intensity, is also lessened. These hazards must be added to those already suffered by individuals with diseases of the heart, bronchi, and lungs.

An increased concentration of carbon monoxide may present a genuine threat, further aggravating the problems that are already part of their disease. It is believed that adult nonsmokers who spend several hours in smoke-filled rooms are inhaling the equivalent of one or two cigarettes a day. This may be enough to double their chances of dying from lung cancer. There is, moreover, mounting evidence that exposing children to cigarette smoke is harmful.

It is little wonder that antismoking activity is increasing in countries all over the world. Japanese experts have questioned the value of warnings on cigarette packages. They feel that cigarettes should instead be prohibited from sale. Governments are hesitant to do this because of the revenue from taxes on cigarettes that would be lost. Thus the experts have said that governments are "putting the national treasury before the national health."

Helping the Smoker to Quit

People may learn to stop smoking. One method is as follows: Smokers are instructed to double their normal amount of cigarettes for four days and then to treble it for two days. For the next few days, at least, not smoking is more a relief than a trial. Another similar technique requires smokers to smoke almost continuously—at least four packs a day—for several days. Eventually, smoking even one more cigarette becomes almost overwhelmingly distasteful.

Other techniques to teach dislike of smoking have been used with some success. In one method, smokers take a puff on a cigarette every six seconds. At the same time a smoke machine blows hot puffs of smoke into their faces. Their noses and throats burn; eyes water; coughing is almost constant; the smokers want to vomit. After a brief rest, the process is repeated. For this course of treatment the smokers pay a deposit. If the course is quit instead of the smoking, the deposit is lost.

Electric shock has also been tried. In a laboratory setting, smokers occasionally and unpredictably receive electric shocks as the cigarette is brought to the mouth and inhaled. Pain and anxiety, rather than comfort and peace, become associated with smoking. What if smokers persist with cigarettes away from the laboratory? The use of a special cigarette case is recommended. It is electrically wired so that reaching for a cigarette results in painful shock.[42]

The English writer Charles Lamb once rhymed: "For thy sake, tobacco, I/ Would do anything but die."[43] Every year thousands of smokers go him one better.

Summary

Drugs have been used throughout history for a variety of reasons. *Drug dependence* can be either physical or psychological, or both, and means that the person develops a need for the drug after periodic or continued use. *Drug abuse* is excessive drug use inconsistent with or unrelated to medical practice. *Withdrawal symptoms* become evident when the effects of a drug on which one is physically dependent are interrupted. *Tolerance* occurs when one needs increasingly larger doses of the drug to achieve the effect obtained with beginning doses. If tolerance to one drug results in tolerance to another, *cross-tolerance* is said to have occurred.

Depressants are drugs that act on the central nervous system to reduce psychic and motor functioning. The *morphinelike drugs,* derived from the opium poppy, include *opium, morphine, codeine, and heroin.* Both physical dependence and tolerance result with use of these drugs. Various types of treatment are used, including withdrawal, or *detoxification* —either with or without ("cold turkey") medical involvement—group therapy, and treatment centers. Another form of treatment, methadone maintenance, is, unfortunately, losing support. The discovery that the brain produces its own morphinelike drugs may eventually lead to a new understanding of morphine-type dependence. The *barbiturates* and *tranquilizers*—both classified as sedatives—are widely abused. Barbiturates account for many suicides and deaths from overdose every year. They are especially dangerous when taken with alcohol. This is also true of methaqualone (Quaalude), a nonbarbiturate that is being increasingly abused in this country.

Alcohol has been with us from earliest recorded history, and so has its problems. Alcohol is a toxin, or poison, and detoxification, or destruction of alcohol's poisonous properties, is accomplished very slowly by the liver. Dependence upon alcohol is known as *alcoholism*. Alcoholics are often unable to choose whether they will drink or not, and if they do drink, are consistently unable to choose to stop. It is not certain why people become alcoholics; childhood experiences, unhappiness, and familial causes are among the reasons. Some problems associated with alcoholism are delirium tremens, vitamin deficiency, malnutrition, brain damage, and depression. Drinking alcohol during pregnancy can cause a child to be born with a collection of abnormalities that make up the *fetal alcohol syndrome.* The best treatment for alcoholism is a combination of methods, including *aversion therapy, Antabuse, adjustment help,* and the support of such groups as *Alcoholics Anonymous* and *Al-Anon/Alateen.*

Stimulants act on the central nervous system to excite psychic and motor activities. Amphetamines, which are no longer used in medical treatment of obesity and depression, are now used primarily for treatment of *hyperkinesis* and *narcolepsy.* Amphetamines produce no physical dependence, but psychological dependence and tolerance are probable. Prolonged sleeplessness, anxiety, bizarre mood changes, and hallucinations are among the effects of these drugs.

Another group of stimulants are the *hallucinogens*—drugs that cause hallucinations. These include LSD, PCP, psilocybin, and mescaline, as well as many over-the-counter products. LSD usage might be accompanied by the "flashback" phenomenon, a spontaneous recurrence of LSD-like hallucinations. Some research indicates that LSD may enhance psychotherapy. There has been much concern about the physical effects of LSD, but recent studies indicate that pure LSD does not cause damage. Phencyclidine, called PCP or "angel dust," is a powerful and dangerous hallucinogen that can cause unpredictable violence, extreme behavior changes, and brain damage. *Peyote* has long been used by North American Indians as part of their religious ceremonies. Rates of emotional disturbance from such use are low.

The effects of *cocaine*, another stimulant, are very similar to those of the amphetamines. Cocaine can be extremely toxic because it leaves the body much more slowly than it is absorbed.

One active ingredient of *marijuana* is delta-9-tetrahydrocannabinol, or THC. There is much confusion as to how marijuana should be classified, since it potentiates the effects of both barbiturates and amphetamines and also has hallucinogenic effects. Long-time users often report reverse tolerance; that is, they need less of the drug to achieve the effects of beginning doses. The psychic effects of marijuana range from euphoria and increased suggestibility to depersonalization and toxic psychosis. Physically it can increase the pulse rate, impair muscle function, and interfere with logical thinking processes. The amotivational syndrome— a disinterest in oneself and one's social improvement—has been reported in chronic users of marijuana. Studies show that those who smoke marijuana tend to abuse other drugs as well. The relationship probably lies in the personality and environment of the individual rather than in the pharmacological properties of the drug. There are many agruments both for and against decriminalization of marijuana, but the trend toward reducing marijuana possession to a minor violation will most likely continue. One potential danger to marijuana smokers is the recent spraying of these plants with the herb killer paraquat.

Tobacco smoking has been determined to be dangerous to health because of its harmful effects on normal body functions. The poisonous gases in its smoke—such as hydrogen cyanide, nitrogen oxide, and carbon monoxide—and other polluting substances—such as tar and nicotine—can cause such diseases as *emphysema, chronic bronchitis,* and *lung cancer.* Nicotine can contribute to the development of cardiovascular disease by raising heart pressure, causing heartbeat irregularity, and increasing demands on the heart. Moreover, the carbon monoxide in cigarette smoke can replace the oxygen in hemoglobin, thus decreasing the oxygen available to the heart. Other health problems associated with cigarette smoking are peptic ulcers and periodontal disease. Smoking can complicate a physician's task by giving misleading results on tests, such as for colon cancer and for white blood cell levels. Taking oral contraceptives and smoking increases the risks of heart disease. Smoking during pregnancy can cause such problems as premature delivery, spontaneous abortion, and stillbirth, and it also increases the baby's chances of being underweight or having congenital heart disease. Pipes and cigars have not been found safer than cigarettes. Smoking them increases the risks of developing cancers of the mouth, pharynx, larynx, bladder, and kidney. Nonsmokers who are exposed to cigarette smoke can suffer from allergic reactions and an increased chance of developing lung cancer; many health problems may be aggravated by the smoke. The methods developed to help the smoker quit this habit include forms of aversion therapy and electric shock.

References

1. Cecil E. Johnson, "Mystical Force of Nightshade," *International Journal of Neuropsychiatry*, Vol. 3 (May–June 1967), p. 274.
2. H. V. Morton, *Ghosts of London* (New York, 1940), pp. 33–34.
3. Lucia Masson, *La Belle France* (New York, 1964), p. 23.
4. Ann Parker and Aaron Neal, "What a Way To Go!" *Ciba Journal*, No. 39 (1966), pp. 20–29.
5. Nathan B. Eddy et al., "Drug Dependence: Its Significance and Characteristics," *Bulletin of the World Health Organization*, Vol. 32 (May 1965), p. 722.
6. *WHO Expert Committee on Drug Dependence, Sixteenth Report*, World Health Organization Technical Report Series, No. 407 (Geneva, 1969), p. 6.
7. Ibid., pp. 721–733.
8. John C. Kramer, "Methadone Maintenance for Opiate Dependence," *California Medicine*, Vol. 113 (December 1970), pp. 7 and 10.
9. "Probing Schizophrenia with Naloxone," *Science News*, Vol. 114 (July 15, 1978), p. 38.
10. Ibid.
11. R. Jeffry Smith, "Study Finds Sleeping Pills Overprescribed," *Science*, Vol. 204 (April 20, 1979), pp. 287–288.
12. Sir E. A. Wallis Budge, "The Dwellers on the Nile," cited in "Alcoholism as a Disease," *World Health* (January 1966), p. 21.
13. Sholem Asch, *The Nazarene*, tr. by Maurice Samuels (New York, 1939), p. 3.
14. D. Fenner, L. Mix, O. Schefer, and J. L. Gilbert, "Ethanol Metabolism in Various Racial Groups," *Canadian Medical Association Journal*, Vol. 104 (1971).
15. Benjamin Rush, "Inquiry into the Effects of Ardent Spirits upon the Human Body and Mind," reprinted in *Quarterly Journal of Studies in Alcohol*, Vol. 4 (September 1943), p. 325.
16. Sterling K. Clarren and David W. Smith, "The Fetal Alcohol Syndrome," *The New England Journal of Medicine*, Vol. 298 (May 11, 1978), pp. 1063–1067; and Sterling K. Clarren and David W. Smith, "Even Moderate Drinking May Be Hazardous to Maturing Fetus," *Journal of the American Medical Association*, Vol. 237 (June 13, 1977), pp. 2585–2587.
17. David E. Smith, "Speed Freaks vs. Acid Heads," *Clinical Pediatrics*, Vol. 8 (April 1969), pp. 187–188.
18. "Amphetamine-Type Drugs for Hyperactive Children," *The Medical Letter*, Vol. 14 (March 31, 1972), p. 21.
19. Arthur R. DeLong, "What Have We Learned from Psychoactive Drug Research on Hyperactives?" *American Journal of Diseases of Children*, Vol. 123 (February 1972), pp. 177–180.
20. Saul H. Rosenthal, "Persistent Hallucinosis Following Repeated Administration of Hallucinogenic Drugs," *American Journal of Psychiatry*, Vol. 121 (September 1964), pp. 24–41.

21. Walter N. Pahnke, Albert A. Kurland, Stanford Unger, Charles Savage, and Stanislav Grof, "The Experimental Use of Psychedelic (LSD) Psychotherapy," *Journal of the American Medical Association*, Vol. 212 (June 15, 1970), p. 1860.

22. Normal J. Dishotsky, William D. Loughman, Robert E. Mogar, and Wendell R. Lipscomb, "LSD and Genetic Damage," *Science*, Vol. 172 (April 30, 1971), p. 439.

23. Ibid.

24. P. J. Fink, M. J. Goldman, and I. Lyons, "Morning-Glory Seed Psychoses," *Archives of General Psychiatry*, Vol. 15 (August 1966), p. 210. Many experts hold that the wide publicity concerning dangerous drugs has piqued the curiosity of the vulnerable and promoted drug use.

25. Robert L. Bergman, "Navajo Peyote Use: Its Apparent Safety," *American Journal of Psychiatry*, Vol. 128 (December 1971), pp. 51–55.

26. Richard Colestock Pillard, "Marihuana," *New England Journal of Medicine*, Vol. 283 (August 6, 1970), p. 295.

27. Klaus Angel, "No Marijuana for Adolescents," *The New York Times Magazine* (November 30, 1969), pp. 170–178.

28. Ibid.

29. W. H. McGlothlin and L. J. West, "The Marijuana Problem: An Overview," *American Journal of Psychiatry*, Vol. 125 (September 1968), pp. 370–378.

30. *The Use of Cannabis*, report of a World Health Organization Scientific Group, p. 12, citing the following: R. H. Blum and associates, *Drugs, II, Students and Drugs* (San Francisco, 1969); E. Goode, "Multiple Drug Use Among Marihuana Smokers," *Social Problems*, Vol. 17 (1969), pp. 48–64; M. I. Soueif, unpublished data.

31. Pillard, "Marihuana," p. 30.

32. "The Marijuana Problem," an edited transcription of the Clinical Case Conference arranged by the Department of Psychiatry at the UCLA School of Medicine, moderator: Norman Q. Brill. This excerpt is from the discussion by Evelyn Crumpton. Reprinted in *Annals of Internal Medicine*, Vol. 73 (September 1970), p. 43.

33. R. S. Hepler and I. R. Frank, "Marijuana Smoking and Intraocular Pressure," *Journal of the American Medical Association*, Vol. 217 (September 6, 1971), p. 1392; "Marijuana Works in a Legal Study, Too," *Medical World News*, Vol. 14 (September 14, 1973), pp. 20–21.

34. Henry Ward Beecher (1813–1887), *Life Thoughts.*

35. United States Department of Health, Education, and Welfare, Public Health Service, *Smoking and Health*, report of the Surgeon General (January 1979). Summarized in *Population Reports*, Series L, No. 1 (March 1979), pp. L1–L34.

36. "Summary of the Report," *The Health Consequences of Smoking*, 1969 supplement, p. 4.

37. *Newsweek* (February 16, 1970), p. 86.

38. "Sudden Death by Cigarette," *New Scientist*, Vol. 53 (March 2, 1972), p. 462.

39. Department of Health, Education, and Welfare, Public Health Service, Food and Drug Administration, "Clinical Implications of Surgeon General's Report on Smoking and Health," *FDA Drug Bulletin*, Vol. 9 (February–March 1979), pp. 4–6.

40. George E. Moore, "Hazards of Snuff," *Journal of the American Medical Association*, Vol. 223 (January 15, 1973), p. 336.

41. E. L. Wynder and D. Hoffmann, "Tobacco and Health," *The New England Journal of Medicine*, Vol. 30 (April 19, 1979), pp. 898–899.

42. Edward Lichtenstein, "How to Quit Smoking," *Psychology Today*, Vol. 4 (January 1971), pp. 42ff.

43. Charles Lamb, "A Farewell to Tobacco," in *Bookman's Pleasure*, comp. by Holbrook Jackson (New York, 1947), p. 164.

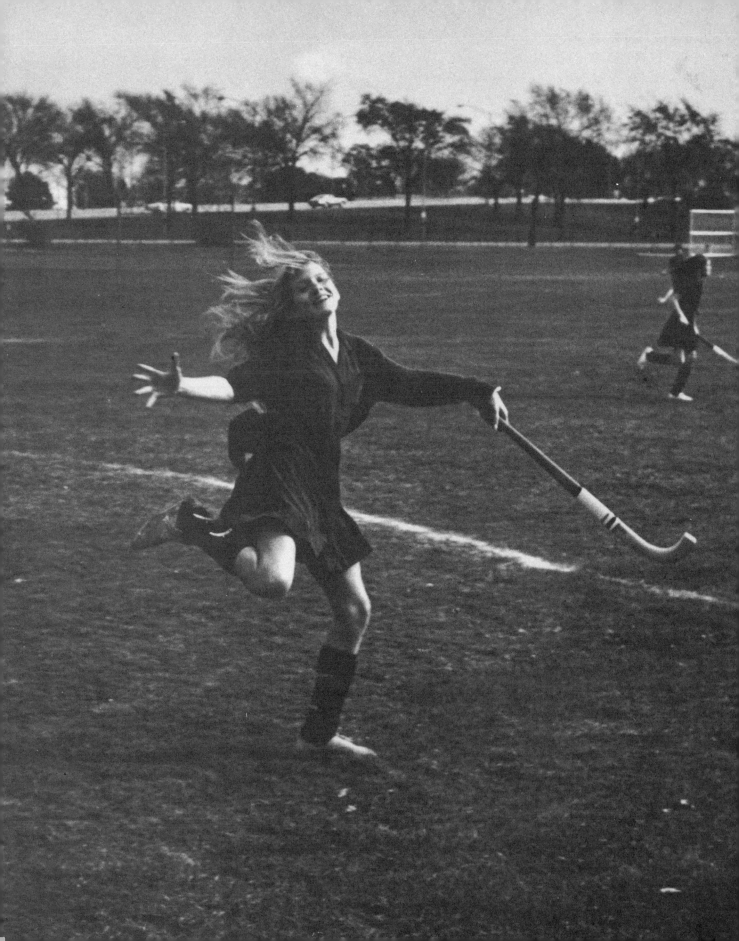

8

Physical Fitness and Some Special Body Structures

More than 250 years ago a German reporter on assignment in the United States wrote an article for the readers back home about someone who had invented a horseless carriage that would drive a distance of fourteen miles in two hours. If true, nothing came of this speedy machine for over a century and a half. When it finally did become part of the U.S. scene, nobody imagined how much it would interfere with the population's physical condition. Over the years, human legs have been used less and less. Muscles have softened. Nor is physical fitness and health improved by ending an inactive day munching calories in front of a television set. Movement is one of the basic features of life itself. Physical fitness by means of exercise must again become a part of people's lives. How this may be accomplished and what results may be expected are the subjects of the first part of this chapter.

Fitness: The Meaning of the Term

Generally, fitness may be defined as the state of being healthy enough to actively adjust to the many demands made by the physical, emotional, and social environments of which one is a part. But, as we saw in Chapter 1, different people have different desires, needs, tasks, rhythms, requirements for relaxation, and levels of fatigue; they also vary in age, gender, occupation, emotional and physical make-up, mood, and in numerous other ways. To some extent, then, fitness must be an individual matter. And as much as possible, the efforts to achieve it must be tailored to meet the abilities and needs of the individual person. These efforts can be either specific or general.

Specific Fitness

Specific fitness is the degree to which one is able to perform some particular task. Even slight differences in body structure can make one person more fit for a particular task than another. Differences in bone length or in the ways tendons are attached to bones, for example, will help to make one person a superior sprinter and another a better jumper or weight lifter. But body structure alone is not the only criterion for fitness. An understanding of the mechanics of movement—that is, which movements are most efficient—combined with practice to improve movement efficiency can bring satisfying results. "The most beautiful motion," wrote Plato, "is that which accomplishes the greatest result with the least amount of effort."

Consider, for example, the movements of a ballet dancer and a baseball pitcher. The specific fitness required for the tasks they perform is not so different as you might think. The dancer, leaping in the air, completing two 360° turns, and landing gracefully on the toes of one foot, has trained many years to make that single action possible. The baseball pitcher—a less elegant character, perhaps, with a ball of gum pouching his cheek and sweat running down his back—has also spent much of his life in training. It is only after long years of practice that the muscles of the arm

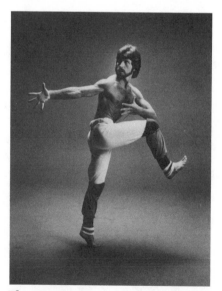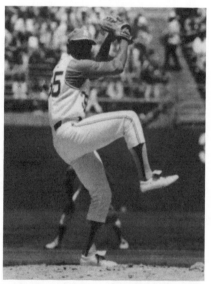

The movements—and the physical training—of dancers and athletes are very similar.

are able to achieve their greatest strength, their peak control, just before the ball leaves the hand; that is, *before* the automatic follow-through motion that sends the arm forward.

Most people will not be great athletes or dancers, perhaps not even good ones. But everyone can seek the greatest efficiency of movement within his or her limitations and often be happily surprised by the heightened ease of movement and the lessened fatigue that result from careful and committed training.

General Fitness

General fitness implies the ability to meet with all the tasks of life, including its emergencies. Moreover, a person who is generally fit has enough remaining energy at the end of a workday to enjoy active forms of relaxation. And with those pleasures passed, such a person is not too tired or too tense to spend the night in refreshing sleep. It is doubtful that a perfect level of general fitness is ever reached by the average person. But a practical level of general fitness is within the reach of nearly everyone.

Striated Muscles

Almost all the individual muscle fibers a person will ever have are formed before birth. General muscle growth, then, is due to an increase not in the number but in the size of individual muscle fibers or cells. All these muscle fibers or cells are able to contract and thereby cause movement. There are two types of muscles: *smooth* and *striated*. For a brief description of **smooth muscles,** see text appearing with Body Charts 4 and 13. At this

point, however, we will focus our attention on the **striated muscles,** for it is these muscles that are directly involved in physical activity.

There are more than four hundred skeletal, or striated, muscles in the human body, accounting for as much as 42 percent of the body's weight. They are called skeletal because they are attached to bone (see Body Chart 6), and they are also called striated because (unlike smooth muscles) under a microscope they are seen to have alternating light and dark stripes (see Figure 8–1). When skeletal muscles contract, they force two regions of the skeleton closer together. In this way they are able to move a joint (see Body Charts 3 and 5). Each muscle is a unit; that is, it has its own supply of nerves, arteries, veins, and lymphatic channels. Nevertheless, muscles usually contract in groups, and they do so in response to stimuli from the central nervous system. Striated muscles are made for *voluntary contraction.* That is why with prolonged inaction they wither.

But where do muscles obtain their capacity to contract, to do their work? For activity, they need a source of energy, or fuel. This is accomplished by a complicated set of chemical reactions within each muscle cell. And although oxygen does not start the chemical reactions within the muscles, it is basic to their completion. Oxygen is necessary for burning food into the energy needed for the exercise that leads to physical fitness. (Table 8–1 lists several common everyday activities and the amount of energy in calories each activity expends.) Now, the body can store extra food, but oxygen cannot be stored. Why not? After all, is there not more than sufficient oxygen available in ordinary air? Normal lungs can surely

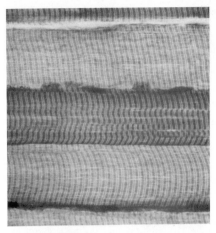

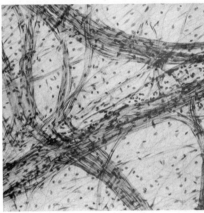

FIGURE 8–1
Striated (top) and smooth muscle fibers (bottom).

TABLE 8-1
Energy Expenditures for Various Everyday Activities

ACTIVITY	CALORIES PER POUND PER HOUR
Asleep	.4
Bicycling, moderate speed	1.7
Cello playing	1.1
Dancing, mildly active	2.2
Dishwashing	1.0
Dressing and undressing	.9
Driving a car	1.0
Eating a meal	.7
Horseback riding, trot	2.6
Ironing	1.0
Laundry, light	1.1
Lying still, awake	.5
Painting furniture	1.3
Piano playing, moderate	1.2
Playing ping-pong	2.7
Reading aloud	.7
Running	4.0
Sewing, on a machine or by hand	.7
Sitting quietly, watching TV	.6
Skating	2.2
Standing	.8
Sweeping, vacuum cleaner	1.9
Swimming, 2 m.p.h.	4.5
Tailoring	1.0
Typing rapidly	1.0
Walking, 3 m.p.h.	1.5
Walking, 4 m.p.h.	2.2
Writing	.7

NOTE: Energy is the ability to do work. It is thus required to accomplish the activities of the body. People get all their energy from the plant and animal foods they eat. The possible energy value of foods (proteins, carbohydrates, and fats) as well as the energy exchanges that go on in the body are expressed as *calories*. A calorie is a unit of heat; it is the amount of heat necessary to raise the temperature of one gram of water one degree Centigrade (for instance, from 15° to 16°). (For an expanded discussion of calories, see page 270 in Chapter 9.)

SOURCE: Adapted from C. M. Taylor, Grace Mac-Leod, and M. D. S. Rose, *Foundations of Nutrition*, 5th ed. © 1956, Macmillan Publishing Co., Inc. Reprinted by permission.

hold enough oxygen for the body's needs. A normal heart muscle indeed has sufficient strength to pump enough oxygen-carrying blood through decreasingly smaller arteries to the capillaries to feed oxygen to the muscles and to other cells. But it is at the capillary-cell level that the hitch occurs. For oxygenated blood to reach the capillaries, energy must be used. But for the oxygen to leave the red blood cells, pass through the capillaries, and enter the cells through their watery medium, no energy is used. This process does not need to be hurried by energy. Also, when a muscle contracts, the pressure within it increases. Blood vessels are compressed. Bloodflow to the muscle is hindered. When the muscle relaxes, bloodflow to it is increased. In these ways, a steady state—an inner ecological balance—is reached: Oxygen is brought to the muscles and to other cells only as rapidly as it is needed.

So to become truly physically fit, the breathing apparatus must be in excellent working order. Routine exercises that use the cardiovascular and respiratory systems will enable the body to operate at peak efficiency. (Aerobic exercises, discussed a bit later in this chapter, will accomplish just this.)

Strength, Flexibility, and Endurance

The basic elements of physical fitness are *strength, flexibility*, and *endurance*. Each one influences the other two. And they, in turn, are each influenced by a variety of other factors. Among these are body build, reaction time, the ability to use one's senses, and mood or emotional state. Reaction time, for example, is hardly as important for weight lifting as it is for tennis. And endurance is surely necessary for long-distance running, but when running to avoid a car, good perception and quick reaction time are the crucial factors. And who could deny that a player's emotional state influences one's game, whether it be basketball, tennis, football, or any other activity? On the other hand, one's emotional state can certainly be influenced by exercise and other physical activities. Skiers, for example, often speak of the "sense of freedom" they experience flying "on the wind" across the snow.

Strength: Through Isometrics and Isotonics

Isometrics is a method of exercise in which one group of muscles pushes or pulls against another set of muscles or against an object that cannot be moved. When done routinely and repeatedly (several times a week with a maximum of exertion), isometrics will increase the size of the used muscles, their strength, and their endurance.

Wisely emphasizing the importance of a complete physical examination before any exercise program is begun, Columbia Medical Center bone and joint specialist (*orthopedist*) Professor Keith L. McElroy recommends three simple and safe isometric exercises to increase muscle strength.[1] No special equipment is required. These exercises, McElroy suggests, should be done briefly and often rather than in one long, strenuous period.

1. Lying face down over an ordinary armless chair, the exerciser places the waist at the center of the seat. For stability the hands may touch the floor or hold onto the chair legs. Keeping the knees straight, both legs are raised until they are parallel to the floor. The legs are kept in a horizontal line with the body. This position is held as long as the exerciser is able. Then the toes are permitted to drop to the floor. When first attempted, the position may be held for about ten seconds. After a few months of effort, however, a maximum of three minutes in the position may be reached.

2. The second exercise is the same as the first; the only difference is that the exerciser lies in a face-up position.

3. Standing upright, the exerciser flattens his or her spine against a door or wall. Slowly, the body is permitted to slip down until the thighs, from the hip to the knee, are in a horizontal line that is parallel to the floor. The lower legs, from the knee down, are kept vertical and parallel to the wall. Not all people will be able to achieve this position with ease. It should, however, be held as close as possible to the described position. McElroy recommends a gradual increase in the length of

time during which the position may be held. Beginning with fifteen seconds, the exerciser may repeat the exercise until a maximum of four minutes pass. After the exercise is completed the exerciser returns to a standing position.

These activities may be supplemented by others. Muscle warm-up exercises should be alternated with resting periods. The exerciser should stop any exercise if pain occurs. A passing ache lasting a minute or so is no reason for concern. However, aches and pains that last an hour or more mean that the exerciser is overdoing.

Isometric exercises do not increase the efficiency of the heart and blood vessels nor of the breathing apparatus. Also, when overdone, some isometric exercises might possibly result in hypertension. Although not necessarily lasting, this can be of some danger to people whose blood pressure already borders on upper levels or to those who have severe atherosclerosis. Certain isometric exercises may also constrict arteries. This lessens the blood supply to organs, especially the heart and lungs. Vigorous isometric exercise can also be dangerous to people with possible heart disease.

Isotonics is a form of exercise in which a group of muscles work (contract) against a *moving* resistance. For the average person, isotonics is preferable to isometrics. If the objects moved are of gradually increasing resistance, such as a set of weights, muscle strength will also increase gradually. Calisthenics, which involve body movements (see Figure 8–2), are a lighter form of isotonic exercise. Calisthenics increase muscle strength, flexibility, and coordination. Although they,

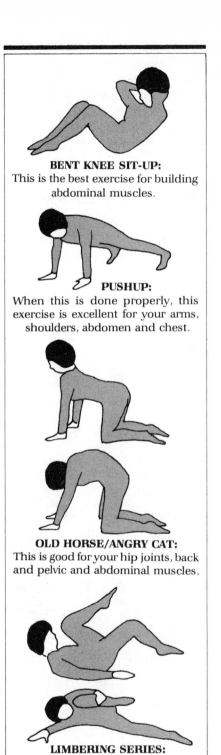

BENT KNEE SIT-UP:
This is the best exercise for building abdominal muscles.

PUSHUP:
When this is done properly, this exercise is excellent for your arms, shoulders, abdomen and chest.

OLD HORSE/ANGRY CAT:
This is good for your hip joints, back and pelvic and abdominal muscles.

LIMBERING SERIES:
These are for the relief of backache caused by tension.

FIGURE 8–2
Calisthenics.

like isometrics, do little for the cardiovascular and respiratory systems, calisthenics are valuable as "warm-up" exercises. Thus they may be used as part of an oxygen-dependent exercise program, which will be discussed on pages 238–241.

Isometric and isotonic exercises together are good training for the weight lifter. They are, for example, the important elements in the training of those whose ambitions are similar to those of Teenage Mr. America, Jim Yasenchok (see the accompanying boxed insert).

In 1978, Jim Yasenchok held the title of Teenage Mr. America. Yasenchok's extraordinary physique is the result of isometric and isotonic exercises, plus a little prodding from his trainer.

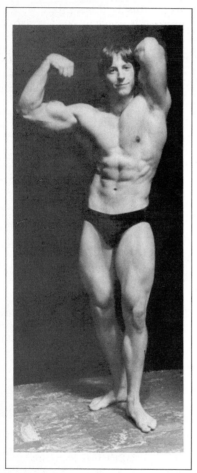

D o you want muscles that bulge and ripple? In a *Coast Dispatch* article, Melanie Kaestner reveals the training secret confided to her by Jim Yasenchok, Teenage Mr. America: First, his coach ties the youngster's arms and legs to the heavy weights that he trains with. Then, when Yasenchok "reaches the point where he thinks he can't go on [lifting], the trainer sticks him with a [20,000-volt] electric cattle prod, sending shocks through his body that ... make one hundred additional lifts seem like nothing in comparison."

Just before each contest, Teenage Mr. America also "takes anabolic steroids under a doctor's supervision" and meditates so as to visualize "prepictures" of how he'll perform during the contest. "When I won [my title]," Yasenchok says, "all the crying and yelling and trying to kick the trainer was worth it."

Now Yasenchok's goal of goals is to become Mr. America within the next five years—a piece of news that should make the local electric power companies happy.

SOURCE: "Shocking Secrets," *Saturday Review*," Vol. 5 (March 4, 1978), p. 8.

Flexibility: Bending Without Breaking

In his *Just So Stories*, the English writer Rudyard Kipling (1865–1936) rhymed:

*The Camel's hump is an ugly lump
Which well you may see at the Zoo;
But uglier yet is the hump we get
From having too little to do.*[2]

Kipling's little poem may be applied to people whom the ancient Roman orator Cicero described as being "in perpetual repose."

One of the longest natural periods of repose occurs before we are born—within the narrow space of the mother's uterus. Therein curls the fetus, backbone flexed, head bent onto the chest, and extremities flexed at the shoulder and hip joints. The fetus can accommodate so easily to the limited living quarters because of the elasticity and flexibility of the developing supporting tissues. But upon birth from the watery ecosystem of the uterus, the newborn is in a sharply changed environment. For one thing, there is no longer fluid on which to remain afloat. And gravity is a factor to be reckoned with.

With increasing growth and control of the striated muscles, the infant soon can bring the head, then the back, upward, by pulling and straining. Next the baby sits, temporarily supporting the shift of weight on the arms. Growing stronger, the child crawls, and at last, never idle, stands and walks. The life of the toddler is not one of "perpetual repose," but of seemingly perpetual motion. Unfortunately, as the child grows older, such constant activity often is replaced by long, hypnotizing hours in front of a television set. By the time the child

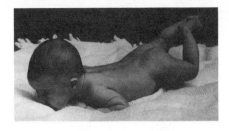

PHOTO ESSAY
Stages of muscle development from infancy to childhood. These pictures are all of the same little girl.

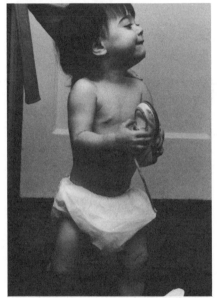

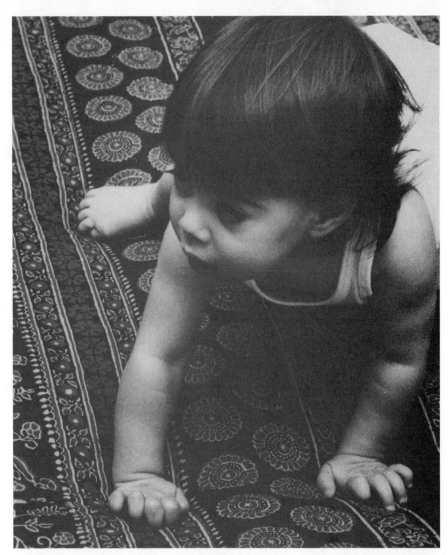

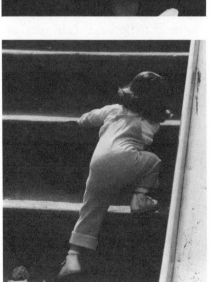

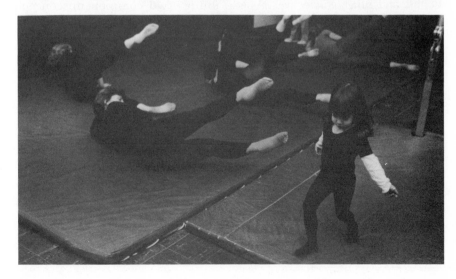

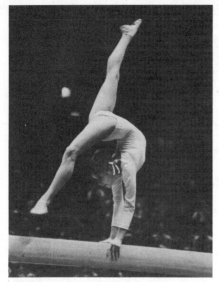

Olga Korbut, the Soviet gymnast who won three gold medals at the 1972 Olympic Games, affords a visual definition of the word flexibility.

FIGURE 8–3
Flexibility exercises.

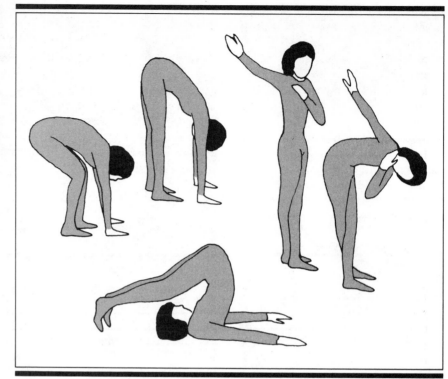

reaches high school, thousands of inactive, fattening hours have been spent watching television, and the once-flexible muscles of early childhood have lost a degree of flexibility.

Flexor muscles (those that cause joints to bend), **ligaments** (which connect the ends of muscles to bone), and other connective tissue must all be capable of being extended. And muscles that oppose the bending must lengthen. Because of differences in body structure, not all people have equal ranges of motion. Moreover, flexibility varies enormously among the various joints of a normal body.

Flexibility can be improved by specialized exercises (see Figure 8–3). Slow, controlled, stretching exercises require less energy, possibly result in less muscle soreness, and provide more relief from muscle pain than do fast, jerky, and violent exercises. Recommended exercises to increase flexibility involve stretching slowly to the point of mild discomfort—then stretching a little more. Moreover, the opposing muscles should be actively stretched. No form of exercise demands more help from a specialist than those designed to increase flexibility. Two common misconceptions should be laid to rest at this point. The idea of the "muscle-bound" person who loses flexibility as strength is gained is false. So is the Victorian notion that exercise will transform a "feminine" woman into a muscular, manlike creature.

Endurance:
Aerobic Exercises

Aerobic means requiring oxygen to live. Thus, **aerobic exercises** are any activities, especially certain sports, that are designed to gradually in- crease the functioning abilities of the pulmonary and cardiovascular systems. Swimming, long-distance running, jogging, rowing, tennis, bicycling, and rapid walking are among the best aerobic exercises. The ability of these exercises to promote the transfer of oxygen from the lungs to the sites of chemical activity in the working tissues is indeed essential to physical fitness and health. (Recall from our earlier discussion the vital role that oxygen plays in muscle activity.)

A person runs a long-distance race. The effort is as great as possible, but it is measured and rhythmic. However, as the end of the distance nears, the energy required to finish becomes enormous so does the need for oxygen. This greatest oxygen intake—the amount of oxygen a person can take from the air under the most extreme circumstances—is known as the *maximum aerobic capacity.* The greater a person's aerobic capacity, the greater will be his or her endurance. *And the regular exercises that contribute the most to endurance fitness are the ones that most benefit the heart and lungs (the cardiovascular-respiratory systems)—aerobic exercises.*

To be of value, aerobic exercises must make regular demands on the cardiovascular and respiratory systems. These exercises should be preceded by an isotonic calisthenic warm-up. Then, according to age and physical condition, as determined by a physician, aerobic exercises can begin. Even for a person in acceptable physical condition the vigor of aerobic exercise should increase gradually. However, for continuing good health, increasingly more strenuous exercises are important. A leisurely stroll down a long-forgotten wooded path may produce a nostalgic sigh, but it will not exercise the lungs or the belly, and though it may warm the heart, it will do little to strengthen it. For a normal person, the motion of isotonic exercise should increase the heart rate to about 130 or 135 beats a minute.

Some Measurements of Physical Fitness

There are many measurements of physical fitness, but some lack scientific proof. The story is told, for example, of a world-famous symphony conductor who insisted that his heart rate was normal. This despite a life full of stress, constant cigar smoking and traveling, and, except for conducting, nearly complete inactivity. How could his heart be abnormal? he asked his physicians. His heart rate kept time with the tempo of one of his favorite passages in Beethoven's Second Symphony. The conductor died at a relatively young age after suffering his fourth heart attack. A check of the tempo of the musical passage showed it to be about 116 beats per minute—considerably above the normal heart rate.

Another example of an inaccurate measurement of physical fitness fortunately has a happier ending. An enthusiastic horsewoman wanted to know of Dr. Kenneth H. Cooper, originator of the Aerobic Exercise Method (see the following section), how much aerobic credit she earned by riding for one hour. "You don't get any credit," he told her. "It all goes to the horse."

Sometimes even scientific efforts at measuring physical fitness can be misleading at first. Some years ago, members of the Philadelphia 76ers, a professional basketball team, became disheartened and despondent when they learned that their star player, 7-feet-2-inch Wilt Chamberlain, showed signs and symptoms of a heart attack. He complained of severe chest pain; his electrocardiogram (electrical tracings of the heart's action) and blood studies suggested heart damage due to a lack of blood supply to the heart. However, repeated and reexamined electrocardiograms showed that Chamberlain's heart action was normal *for him*. (His abnormal blood chemistries were apparently due not to heart damage, but to an inflammation of the pancreas.) Like others among his teammates, Chamberlain has a heart rate of only fifty beats per minute—considerably below the average. A lower-than-average pulse rate is normal in a person who is in superb physical condition. Such a person's heart does not have to beat so fast to get its work done. Indeed, the heart is saved many extra beats (and thus some extra work) in a given period of time.

Cooper's Aerobic Measurements: Testing Toward Fitness

Accurate measurement of endurance fitness—maximum oxygen consumption—is normally a laboratory procedure. But Kenneth H. Cooper has developed a method whereby people can measure their own maximum oxygen consumption merely by determining how far they can run and walk in twelve minutes.

The person first warms up by means of isotonic exercises, such as calisthenics (see the box on page 240); then he or she begins the test by running. When the individual gets short of breath, the run is reduced to a walk, but running should begin again as soon as possible. Cooper has established standards, shown in Table 8–2 on page 241, to determine fitness as it relates to various age groups among adult males. (Table 8–3, shows the corresponding figures for women.) Once the person determines his or her fitness category, a series of gradually increasing exercises may

The Warm-up

Here is a 7- to 10-minute warm-up routine we recommend:

Arm circles. Arms extended straight out to the sides, rotate them counterclockwise 10 times, then clockwise 10 times. The circle described by your hands should have a diameter of at least 2 feet.

Twisters. Same position, arms extended, legs apart about 30 inches. Twist trunk all the way to the right, then all the way to the left, 10 times.

Trunk circles. Legs apart about 30 inches, hands together above head. With both hands together, touch the outside of your left foot, then the ground between the legs, then the outside of the right foot, then return to erect position, hands above your head. Repeat 10 times.

Toe touches. Sit with legs apart and flat on floor or ground. Reach for your toes with both hands, bringing your forehead as close to your knees as possible. Don't "bounce," even if you're not reaching your feet; just stretch, slowly, a total of 10 times.

Knee-chest. Lie flat on the floor on your back with the legs extended. First pull one knee up to the chest, hold for a count of 5, and then repeat with the other knee. Relax, then pull both knees together up to the chest. Hold for a count of 5. Repeat the cycle 5 times. This is not only a good stretching exercise, but also good for the back.

Sprinter. Assume a squatting position and then extend one leg straight back as far as possible, hands touching the floor. Hold momentarily and then repeat with the other leg. Repeat the cycle 5 times.

Achilles tendon stretcher. Lean forward, body straight, palms against a wall at about eye level. Step backwards, supporting your weight with your hands, staying flat-footed until you can feel your calf muscles stretching. Hold for 15 seconds. Repeat 5–10 times. Again, don't "bounce," just stretch out those calf and ankle tendons, *slowly.*

SOURCE: From THE AEROBICS WAY by Kenneth H. Cooper, M.D., M.P.H. Copyright ©1977 by Kenneth H. Cooper. Reprinted by permission of the publisher, M. Evans and Company, Inc., New York, New York, 10017.

begin. As fitness increases and the individual progresses to categories higher on the scale, his or her oxygen consumption increases. However, the exercises must be vigorous enough to produce a "training effect." In this respect Cooper's research has led him to establish two principles:

1. If the exercise is vigorous enough to produce a sustained heart rate of 150 beats per minute or more, the training-effect benefits begin about five minutes after the exercise starts and continue as long as the exercise is performed.

2. If the exercise is not vigorous enough to produce or sustain a heart rate of 150 beats per minute, but still demands oxygen, the exercise must be continued considerably longer than five minutes, the total amount of time depending on the oxygen consumed.

Thus, activities that are sustained for longer than five minutes demand more of the body's oxygen-transporting system (the cardiovascular system) than do short bursts of energy. This is why the hundred-yard dash, for example, cannot offer the same endurance-training effect that can be gained from long-distance running. One of the advantages of the Cooper Aerobic System of exercise is that it presents a goal toward which the out-of-condition person can strive. In order to earn thirty points a week (five points for each of six days a week), a man must be able to run a mile in less than eight minutes six days a week. This is equivalent to Category IV on Cooper's scale.

Because the average woman's size and aerobic capacity are smaller than the average man's, Cooper's aerobic test for women is not the same as that for men. The average woman has a lesser amount of circulating blood and, thus, fewer red blood cells and less hemoglobin. Cooper does not believe that the twelve-minute test is essential for the average woman; all she need do to achieve physical fitness is earn twenty-four points a week.

Walking

Undoubtedly, the most enjoyable, least costly, and yet least practiced of all aerobic isometric exercises is walking. There is abundant evidence to indicate that a daily brisk walk can be more than healthful: It can actually be lifesaving. Those who say they cannot find the time for walking might at least consider this question: "What do you usually do with the time you save?" Time set aside for walking cannot be better spent.

Feet and Shoes

The foot of the average U.S. citizen typically is in bad shape. It has endured much mistreatment. Excessive weight, poor posture, lack of exercise, high heels, and pointed toes all have taken their toll. Some foot problems need the attention of a medical specialist. A long walk will tire normal feet, but it will not hurt them. A tepid (lukewarm) footbath will relieve aching muscles. Moreover, dancers and other athletes advise that, after long periods of inactivity, foot use should at first be moderate. Conditioning is important.

The twenty-six bones of each foot are held together by **ligaments** and work by muscles attached to them by **tendons,** as illustrated in Figure 8–4. In some places, where parts of the foot might otherwise move upon each other, there are little fluid-filled sacs called **bursae** (*bursa* is the singular form). Bursae act as protective cushions, and there is a particularly prominent bursa at the heel. One arch (the **longitudinal arch**) runs lengthwise from the heel to the toes; the other (**transverse arch**) runs across the foot behind the toes. When weight is placed on the foot, the arches yield, and when the weight is lifted, they spring back. In the adult, defective arches may result in flat feet, which are not necessarily painful or disabling. In infants, flat feet are normal.

Hurting feet are not localized pains. When you damage or strain your feet, you will hurt elsewhere too. Pain in your legs and back may also be added to your discomfort. In standing, walking, and running, your feet are a basic weight-bearing link in your body mechanism. That is why wearing proper shoes is so essential to your well-being. Unfortunately, what are often considered stylish shoes are often not healthy shoes.

When buying shoes for daily wear, try both of them on. Your two feet are not exactly alike. Also, stand up and walk about in them. Your feet will then spread and will give you a better idea as to how the shoes fit.

The ball of your foot should rest over the shoe's widest part. A ¾-inch heel is about as high as anyone should use. Higher heels throw your body forward; your normal center of gravity is changed. This causes pressure on the transverse arch, with resulting pain. In addi-

FIGURE 8–4
The anatomy of the foot.

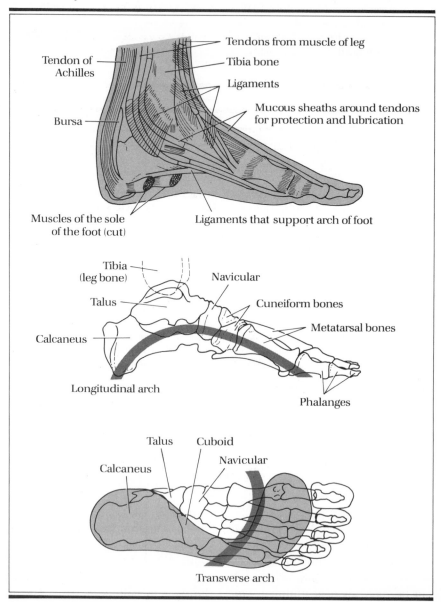

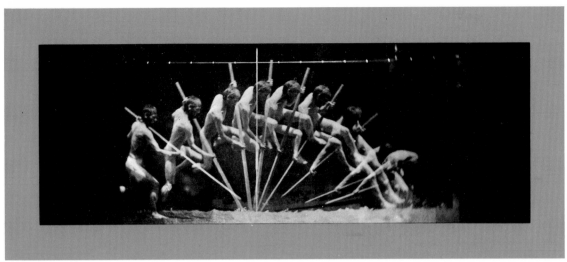

Multiple-exposure photograph by Thomas Eakins (1844–1916).

the human body

GUIDE TO CONTENTS

The numbers are the numbers of the body charts.

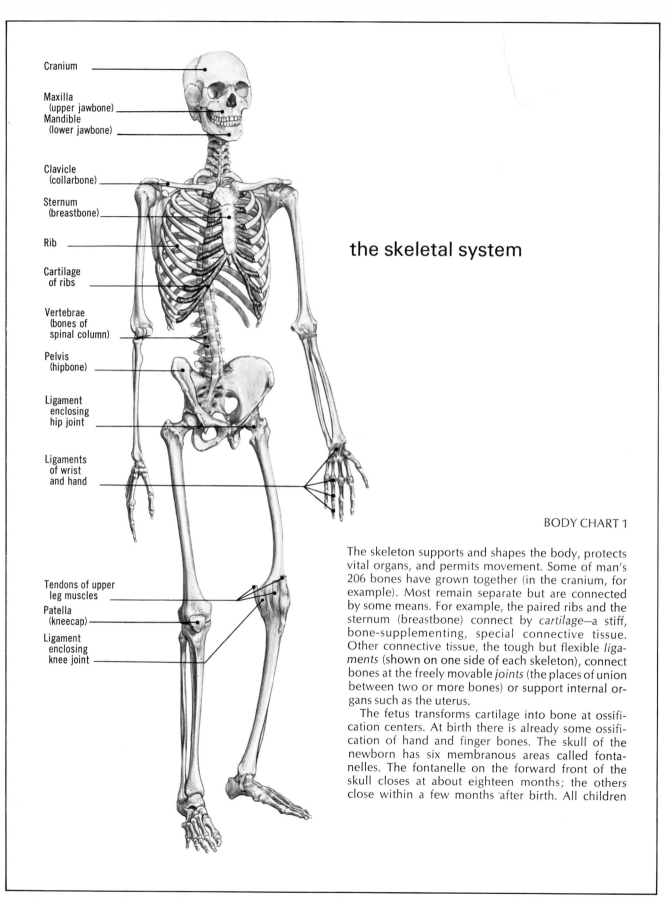

Cranium

Maxilla
(upper jawbone)
Mandible
(lower jawbone)

Clavicle
(collarbone)

Sternum
(breastbone)

Rib

Cartilage
of ribs

Vertebrae
(bones of
spinal column)

Pelvis
(hipbone)

Ligament
enclosing
hip joint

Ligaments
of wrist
and hand

Tendons of upper
leg muscles

Patella
(kneecap)

Ligament
enclosing
knee joint

the skeletal system

BODY CHART 1

The skeleton supports and shapes the body, protects vital organs, and permits movement. Some of man's 206 bones have grown together (in the cranium, for example). Most remain separate but are connected by some means. For example, the paired ribs and the sternum (breastbone) connect by *cartilage*—a stiff, bone-supplementing, special connective tissue. Other connective tissue, the tough but flexible *ligaments* (shown on one side of each skeleton), connect bones at the freely movable *joints* (the places of union between two or more bones) or support internal organs such as the uterus.

The fetus transforms cartilage into bone at ossification centers. At birth there is already some ossification of hand and finger bones. The skull of the newborn has six membranous areas called fontanelles. The fontanelle on the forward front of the skull closes at about eighteen months; the others close within a few months after birth. All children

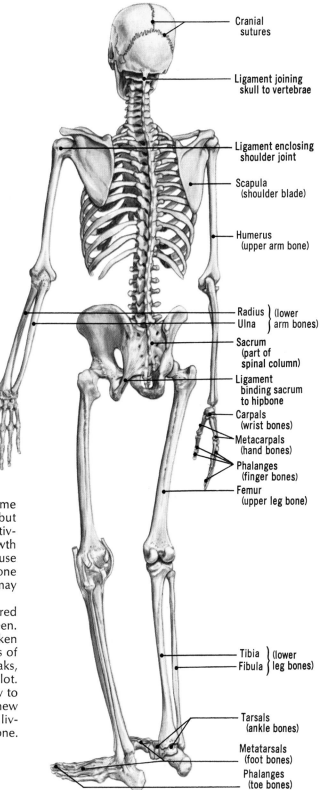

Cranial
sutures

Ligament joining
skull to vertebrae

Ligament enclosing
shoulder joint

Scapula
(shoulder blade)

Humerus
(upper arm bone)

Radius } (lower
Ulna } arm bones)

Sacrum
(part of
spinal column)

Ligament
binding sacrum
to hipbone

Carpals
(wrist bones)

Metacarpals
(hand bones)

Phalanges
(finger bones)

Femur
(upper leg bone)

Tibia } (lower
Fibula } leg bones)

Tarsals
(ankle bones)

Metatarsals
(foot bones)

Phalanges
(toe bones)

BODY CHART 2

ossify bones in the same order but not at the same rate. Order and rate are genetically established, but rate is influenced by nutrition, endocrine gland activity, and disease. Adverse effects on cartilage growth from pituitary or thyroid gland disease can cause dwarfism. Insufficient vitamin D may retard bone formation and development in children and may promote rickets.

Before bone structure appears in the fetus, red blood cells are formed mostly in the liver and spleen. As bone develops, red blood cell formation is taken over by marrow, the soft tissue filling the cavities of the bones (see body chart 6). When a bone breaks, the gap between the fragments fills with a blood clot. From unimpaired blood vessels, new vessels grow to bring the clot food. From surrounding tissue, new cells invade the clot. The nonliving clot becomes living tissue and the groundwork for repair of the bone.

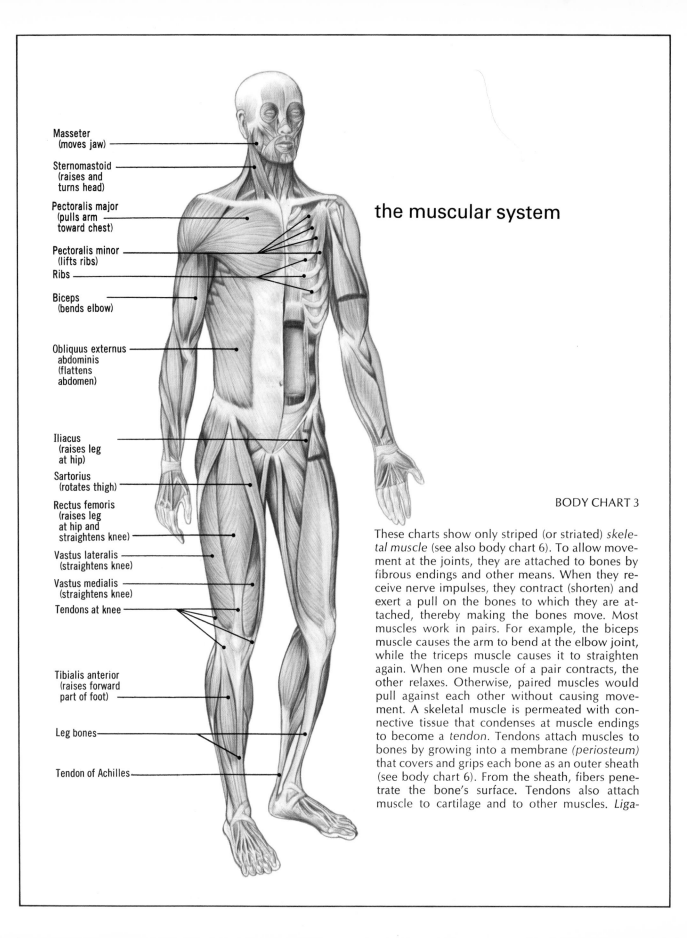

Masseter
(moves jaw)

Sternomastoid
(raises and
turns head)

Pectoralis major
(pulls arm
toward chest)

Pectoralis minor
(lifts ribs)

Ribs

Biceps
(bends elbow)

Obliquus externus
abdominis
(flattens
abdomen)

Iliacus
(raises leg
at hip)

Sartorius
(rotates thigh)

Rectus femoris
(raises leg
at hip and
straightens knee)

Vastus lateralis
(straightens knee)

Vastus medialis
(straightens knee)

Tendons at knee

Tibialis anterior
(raises forward
part of foot)

Leg bones

Tendon of Achilles

the muscular system

BODY CHART 3

These charts show only striped (or striated) *skeletal muscle* (see also body chart 6). To allow movement at the joints, they are attached to bones by fibrous endings and other means. When they receive nerve impulses, they contract (shorten) and exert a pull on the bones to which they are attached, thereby making the bones move. Most muscles work in pairs. For example, the biceps muscle causes the arm to bend at the elbow joint, while the triceps muscle causes it to straighten again. When one muscle of a pair contracts, the other relaxes. Otherwise, paired muscles would pull against each other without causing movement. A skeletal muscle is permeated with connective tissue that condenses at muscle endings to become a *tendon*. Tendons attach muscles to bones by growing into a membrane *(periosteum)* that covers and grips each bone as an outer sheath (see body chart 6). From the sheath, fibers penetrate the bone's surface. Tendons also attach muscle to cartilage and to other muscles. *Liga-*

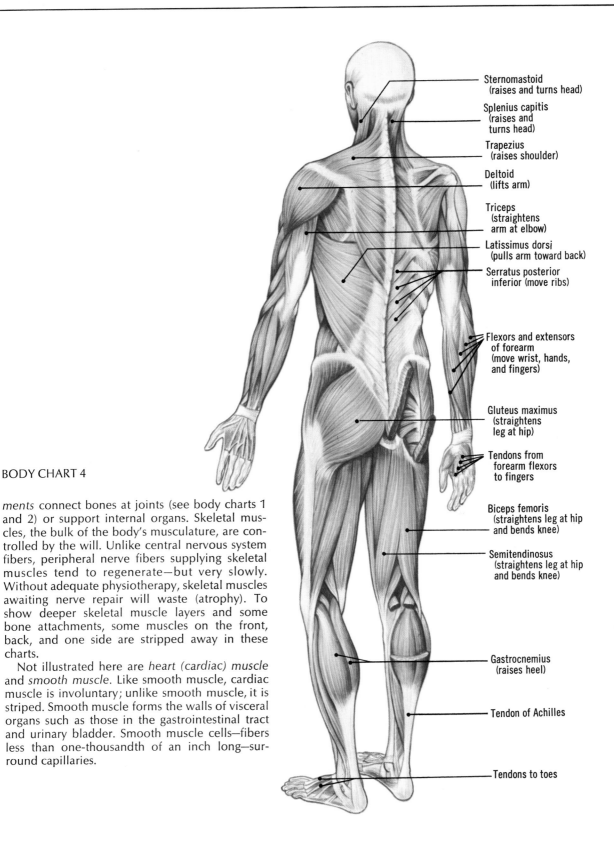

Sternomastoid
(raises and turns head)

Splenius capitis
(raises and
turns head)

Trapezius
(raises shoulder)

Deltoid
(lifts arm)

Triceps
(straightens
arm at elbow)

Latissimus dorsi
(pulls arm toward back)

Serratus posterior
inferior (move ribs)

Flexors and extensors
of forearm
(move wrist, hands,
and fingers)

Gluteus maximus
(straightens
leg at hip)

Tendons from
forearm flexors
to fingers

Biceps femoris
(straightens leg at hip
and bends knee)

Semitendinosus
(straightens leg at hip
and bends knee)

Gastrocnemius
(raises heel)

Tendon of Achilles

Tendons to toes

BODY CHART 4

ments connect bones at joints (see body charts 1 and 2) or support internal organs. Skeletal muscles, the bulk of the body's musculature, are controlled by the will. Unlike central nervous system fibers, peripheral nerve fibers supplying skeletal muscles tend to regenerate—but very slowly. Without adequate physiotherapy, skeletal muscles awaiting nerve repair will waste (atrophy). To show deeper skeletal muscle layers and some bone attachments, some muscles on the front, back, and one side are stripped away in these charts.

Not illustrated here are *heart (cardiac) muscle* and *smooth muscle*. Like smooth muscle, cardiac muscle is involuntary; unlike smooth muscle, it is striped. Smooth muscle forms the walls of visceral organs such as those in the gastrointestinal tract and urinary bladder. Smooth muscle cells—fibers less than one-thousandth of an inch long—surround capillaries.

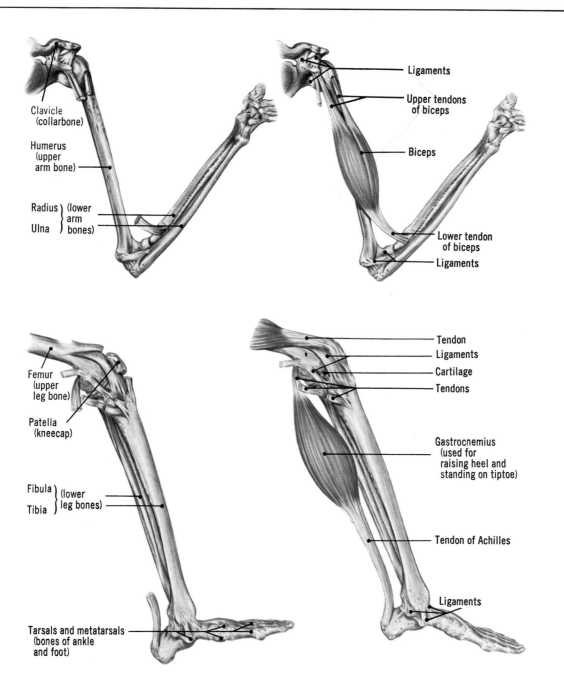

Clavicle
(collarbone)

Humerus
(upper
arm bone)

Radius } (lower
arm
Ulna } bones)

Ligaments

Upper tendons
of biceps

Biceps

Lower tendon
of biceps

Ligaments

Femur
(upper
leg bone)

Patella
(kneecap)

Fibula } (lower
leg bones)
Tibia }

Tarsals and metatarsals
(bones of ankle
and foot)

Tendon
Ligaments
Cartilage
Tendons

Gastrocnemius
(used for
raising heel and
standing on tiptoe)

Tendon of Achilles

Ligaments

the bone-muscle relationship

The structure of an arm and leg clarifies the bone-muscle relationship. Muscles bending a limb at a joint (elbow, knee) are called *flexor* muscles; those that straighten the limb are *extensor* muscles. For movement to occur, bones must be joined at joints, and muscles must pull upon bones by contracting (shortening). Furthermore, the tendons at the opposite ends of each muscle must be attached to different bones. For example, the lower tendon of the biceps is attached to a bone of the forearm. Since the elbow is a freely movable joint, contraction of the biceps will cause the arm to bend. (Muscle fibers of the biceps are six to seven inches long and are among the body's longest cells.)

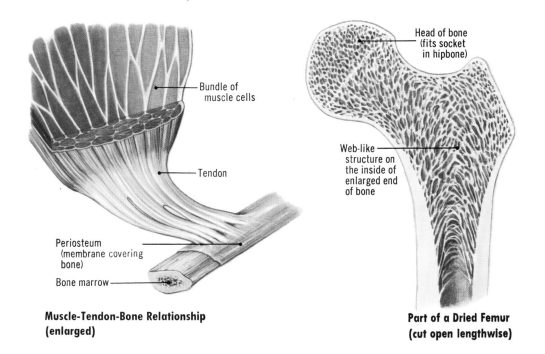

Muscle-Tendon-Bone Relationship
(enlarged)

Part of a Dried Femur
(cut open lengthwise)

Head of bone
(fits socket
in hipbone)

Web-like
structure on
the inside of
enlarged end
of bone

Bundle of
muscle cells

Tendon

Periosteum
(membrane covering
bone)

Bone marrow

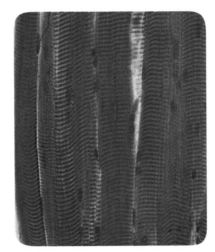

Small Parts of Several Stained Skeletal
Muscle Cells (as seen under the microscope)

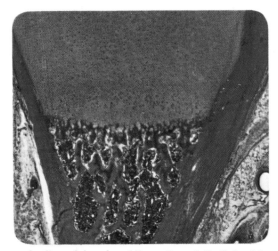

Cartilage (above) and Young Bone Cells (below) in
Stained Fresh Bone (as seen under the microscope)

BODY CHART 6

The most versatile joint is that of the shoulder; it has the greatest range of movement. The knee is both the largest and weakest joint of the body. When a tendon rides over a bony surface, a small sac (a bursa) containing fluid protects it. These bursae are found at such places as about the elbow and knee joints and at the back of the heel. Between the kneecap (patella) and the skin is a bursa. Like other bursae, it may become inflamed (bursitis).

The muscles of adult men are stronger than those of women both because the muscles are larger and because men have a higher rate of oxygen consumption per pound of body weight than do women.

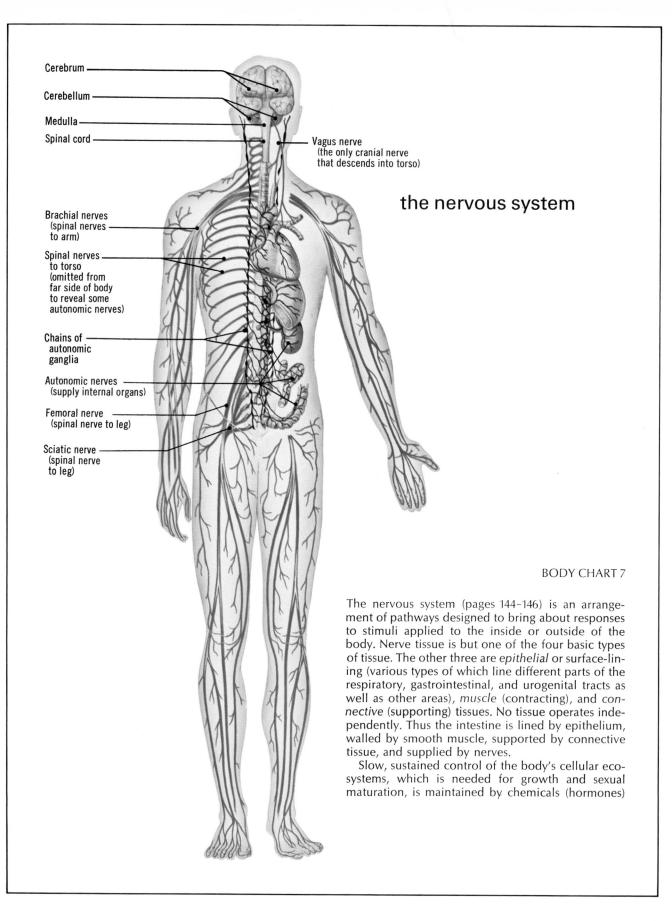

Cerebrum

Cerebellum

Medulla

Spinal cord

Vagus nerve
(the only cranial nerve
that descends into torso)

the nervous system

Brachial nerves
(spinal nerves
to arm)

Spinal nerves
to torso
(omitted from
far side of body
to reveal some
autonomic nerves)

Chains of
autonomic
ganglia

Autonomic nerves
(supply internal organs)

Femoral nerve
(spinal nerve to leg)

Sciatic nerve
(spinal nerve
to leg)

BODY CHART 7

The nervous system (pages 144–146) is an arrangement of pathways designed to bring about responses
to stimuli applied to the inside or outside of the
body. Nerve tissue is but one of the four basic types
of tissue. The other three are *epithelial* or surface-lin-
ing (various types of which line different parts of the
respiratory, gastrointestinal, and urogenital tracts as
well as other areas), *muscle* (contracting), and *connective* (supporting) tissues. No tissue operates independently. Thus the intestine is lined by epithelium,
walled by smooth muscle, supported by connective
tissue, and supplied by nerves.

Slow, sustained control of the body's cellular ecosystems, which is needed for growth and sexual
maturation, is maintained by chemicals (hormones)

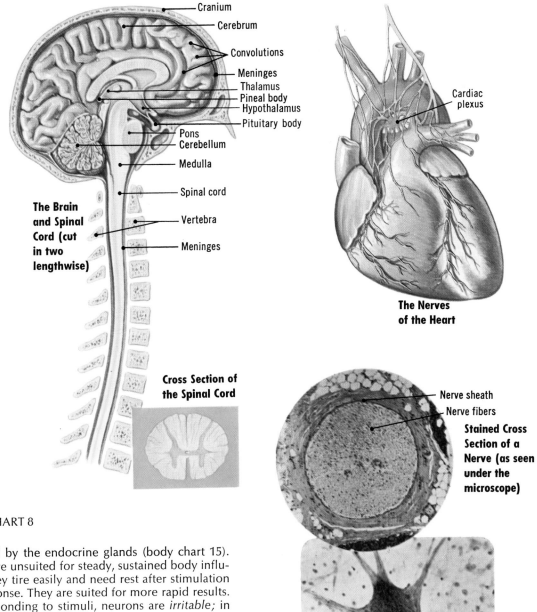

Cranium
Cerebrum
Convolutions
Meninges
Thalamus
Pineal body
Hypothalamus
Pituitary body
Pons
Cerebellum
Medulla
Spinal cord
Vertebra
Meninges

The Brain and Spinal Cord (cut in two lengthwise)

Cardiac plexus

The Nerves of the Heart

Cross Section of the Spinal Cord

Nerve sheath
Nerve fibers

Stained Cross Section of a Nerve (as seen under the microscope)

Nucleus
Cytoplasm

Stained Cell Body of an Efferent (Motor) Neuron (as seen under the microscope)

BODY CHART 8

produced by the endocrine glands (body chart 15). Nerves are unsuited for steady, sustained body influence. They tire easily and need rest after stimulation and response. They are suited for more rapid results.

In responding to stimuli, neurons are *irritable;* in transmitting impulses, they are *conductive.* These two properties combine with their ability to *correlate* and *evaluate* on the basis of memory to make nerve tissue the most specialized of the four basic tissue types. It has been written that the hand without a thumb is but a hook, for it can no longer grasp. But a hand that loses its nerve function loses more than its ability to participate in creation; it loses the more primitive ability to warn its owner of surrounding dangers.

the circulatory system

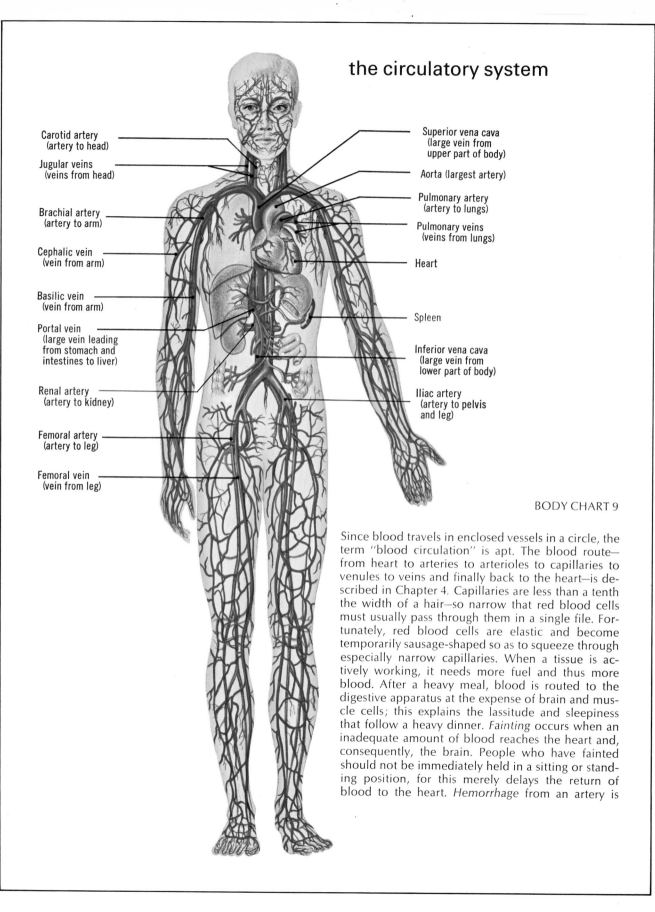

Carotid artery
(artery to head)

Jugular veins
(veins from head)

Brachial artery
(artery to arm)

Cephalic vein
(vein from arm)

Basilic vein
(vein from arm)

Portal vein
(large vein leading
from stomach and
intestines to liver)

Renal artery
(artery to kidney)

Femoral artery
(artery to leg)

Femoral vein
(vein from leg)

Superior vena cava
(large vein from
upper part of body)

Aorta (largest artery)

Pulmonary artery
(artery to lungs)

Pulmonary veins
(veins from lungs)

Heart

Spleen

Inferior vena cava
(large vein from
lower part of body)

Iliac artery
(artery to pelvis
and leg)

BODY CHART 9

Since blood travels in enclosed vessels in a circle, the term "blood circulation" is apt. The blood route—from heart to arteries to arterioles to capillaries to venules to veins and finally back to the heart—is described in Chapter 4. Capillaries are less than a tenth the width of a hair—so narrow that red blood cells must usually pass through them in a single file. Fortunately, red blood cells are elastic and become temporarily sausage-shaped so as to squeeze through especially narrow capillaries. When a tissue is actively working, it needs more fuel and thus more blood. After a heavy meal, blood is routed to the digestive apparatus at the expense of brain and muscle cells; this explains the lassitude and sleepiness that follow a heavy dinner. *Fainting* occurs when an inadequate amount of blood reaches the heart and, consequently, the brain. People who have fainted should not be immediately held in a sitting or standing position, for this merely delays the return of blood to the heart. *Hemorrhage* from an artery is

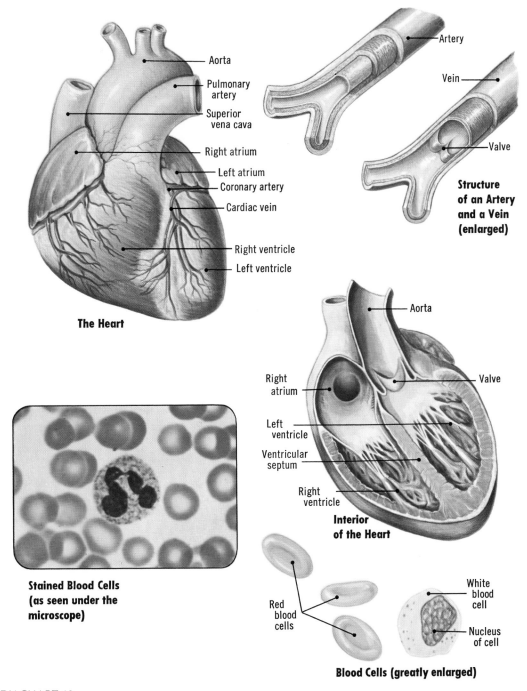

Aorta

Pulmonary artery

Superior vena cava

Right atrium

Left atrium

Coronary artery

Cardiac vein

Right ventricle

Left ventricle

The Heart

Artery

Vein

Valve

Structure of an Artery and a Vein (enlarged)

Aorta

Right atrium

Valve

Left ventricle

Ventricular septum

Right ventricle

Interior of the Heart

Stained Blood Cells (as seen under the microscope)

Red blood cells

White blood cell

Nucleus of cell

Blood Cells (greatly enlarged)

BODY CHART 10

bright red because the blood has been oxygenated. Arterial blood spurts because it escapes under pressure. The spurt may be stopped by the application of pressure between the point of bleeding and the heart. Most venous blood is bluish-red. With hemorrhage, it seeps or wells up into a wound. This bleeding can be stopped only by applying pressure beyond the bleeding point. Escaping capillary blood merely oozes and clots quickly. When serious hemorrhage occurs, rest is important. Alcohol should not be given. By increasing the force of the heartbeat and raising the blood pressure, both activity and alcohol increase bleeding. Moreover, by dilating the blood vessels, alcohol is certain to facilitate the escape of blood.

the respiratory system

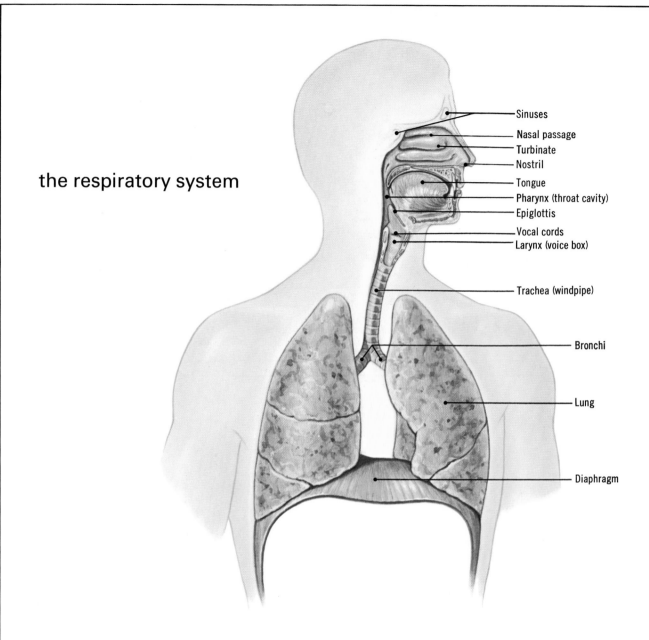

- Sinuses
- Nasal passage
- Turbinate
- Nostril
- Tongue
- Pharynx (throat cavity)
- Epiglottis
- Vocal cords
- Larynx (voice box)
- Trachea (windpipe)
- Bronchi
- Lung
- Diaphragm

BODY CHART 11

The nasal cavity extends deep into the skull and is separated into right and left by a septum. Rarely, the septum deviates so much that only surgery permits proper breathing. Each side wall of the nasal cavity supports three shell-like projections called *turbinates,* and the furrowlike *nasal passages* run between these small mounds. The duct carrying tears empties into the lowest of these furrows. Also emptying into the nose are various sinus spaces.

The nose is an efficent filtering and air-conditioning system. Larger particles are trapped by coarse hairs in the nostril. The entire nasal cavity, including the sinuses, is covered with mucous membrane, which is kept moist by mucus. Mucus also picks up foreign particles and, aided by the sweeping motion of hairlike cilia, moves the particles toward the pharynx to be swallowed. In the upper part of the nasal cavity, the ciliated cells are replaced by specialized receptor nerve cells. This is the olfactory "organ"; bundles of axons run from neurons in this area through the bony roof of the nose and on to the brain. The mucous membrane covering the septum and that of the middle and lower turbinates is thick and full of blood vessels. When inflamed, this mu-

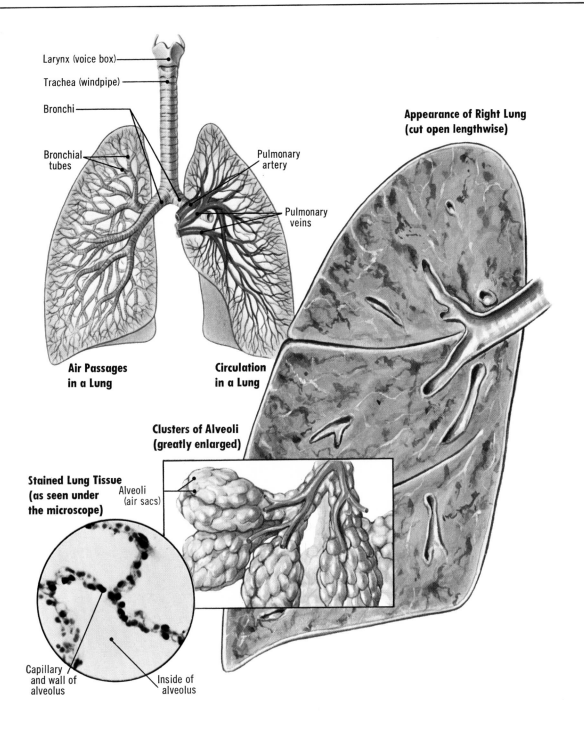

Larynx (voice box)

Trachea (windpipe)

Bronchi

Bronchial tubes

Appearance of Right Lung (cut open lengthwise)

Pulmonary artery

Pulmonary veins

Air Passages in a Lung

Circulation in a Lung

Clusters of Alveoli (greatly enlarged)

Stained Lung Tissue (as seen under the microscope)

Alveoli (air sacs)

Capillary and wall of alveolus

Inside of alveolus

BODY CHART 12

cous membrane swells and blocks the nasal passages. Swollen mucous membrane in the sinuses may also block drainage. The veins in the mucous membrane of the middle and lower turbinates dilate to become venous spaces. With sexual excitement these venous spaces become engorged with blood in much the same way as does erectile tissue of the genital organs. Because of its great vascularity, this area bleeds easily. This very vascularity also makes the nose an excellent ventilating system, for cold air about the capillaries is warmed before entering the lungs. The respiratory tract is further discussed on pages 217–218.

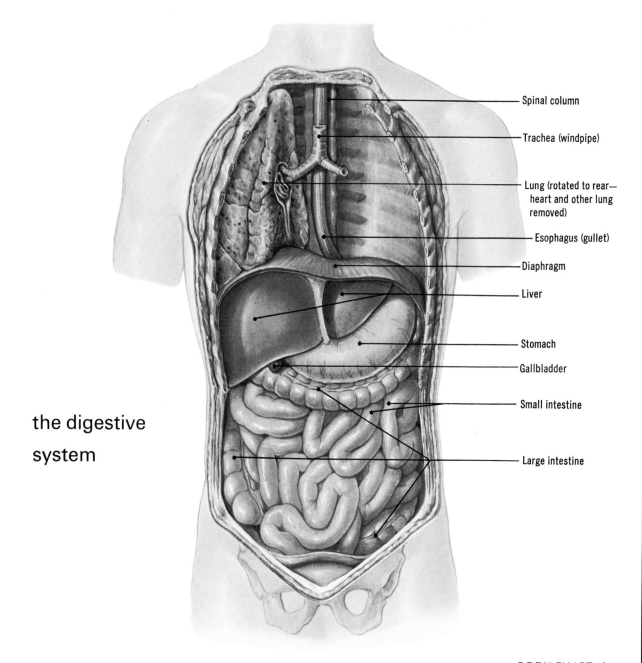

the digestive system

Spinal column

Trachea (windpipe)

Lung (rotated to rear—heart and other lung removed)

Esophagus (gullet)

Diaphragm

Liver

Stomach

Gallbladder

Small intestine

Large intestine

BODY CHART 13

The seventeenth-century English satirist Samuel Butler sardonically described the human body as "a pair of pincers set over a bellows and a stewpan and the whole fixed upon stilts"; he doubtless saw the teeth as pincers and the remaining digestive system as a stewpan. This system is somewhat more comprehensively described in Chapter 9.

From the lips to the anus the adult digestive tract is about 30 to 32 feet long. Two basic kinds of tissue contribute to the wall of the digestive tract from the lower part of the esophagus to the lower end of the small intestine—involuntary *smooth muscle* and the *mucous membrane* lining the muscle. This muscle contracts more slowly than skeletal muscle, and it is able to sustain rhythmic contraction without tiring. The mucosal lining of the digestive tract protects and lubricates. In the small intestine, its absorptive inner surface is unique.

The digestive tract provides the excretory apparatus for food residue; it also excretes other body

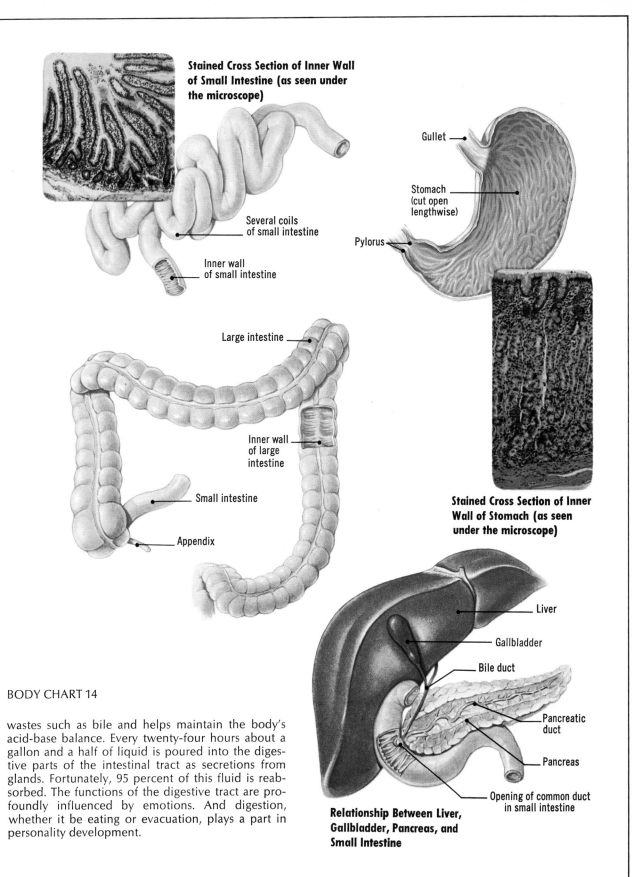

Stained Cross Section of Inner Wall of Small Intestine (as seen under the microscope)

Several coils of small intestine

Inner wall of small intestine

Gullet

Stomach (cut open lengthwise)

Pylorus

Large intestine

Inner wall of large intestine

Small intestine

Appendix

Stained Cross Section of Inner Wall of Stomach (as seen under the microscope)

Liver

Gallbladder

Bile duct

Pancreatic duct

Pancreas

Opening of common duct in small intestine

Relationship Between Liver, Gallbladder, Pancreas, and Small Intestine

BODY CHART 14

wastes such as bile and helps maintain the body's acid-base balance. Every twenty-four hours about a gallon and a half of liquid is poured into the digestive parts of the intestinal tract as secretions from glands. Fortunately, 95 percent of this fluid is reabsorbed. The functions of the digestive tract are profoundly influenced by emotions. And digestion, whether it be eating or evacuation, plays a part in personality development.

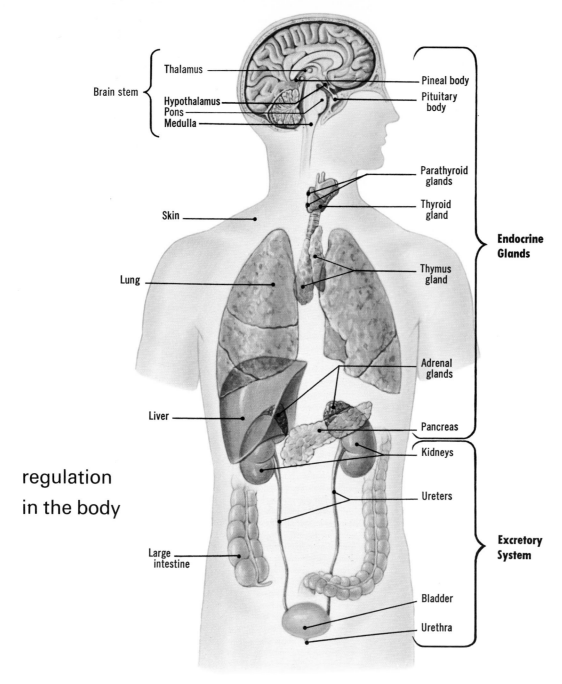

Thalamus

Pineal body

Brain stem

Hypothalamus
Pons
Medulla

Pituitary
body

Parathyroid
glands

Thyroid
gland

Skin

**Endocrine
Glands**

Lung

Thymus
gland

Adrenal
glands

Liver

Pancreas

Kidneys

Ureters

**Excretory
System**

Large
intestine

Bladder

Urethra

regulation
in the body

BODY CHART 15

"The stability of the interior environment," wrote the nineteenth-century French physiologist Claude Bernard, "is the essential condition of free and independent life…all vital mechanisms, however varied they may be, have only one object: that of preserving constant the conditions of life in the interior environment." This chart illustrates some of the most important body regulators involved in maintaining a harmonious balance among the internal human ecosystems. But one can consider these inner ecosystems of man only as they relate to his outer ecosystems. An unhealthy external environment interferes with the ecological health of the internal environment. Man cannot long safely subject the sensitive organs regulating his "interior environment" to the gross pollutions with which he surrounds himself.

tion, high heels shorten the stride length. This tends to disrupt the normal range of motion at the knee and ankle. The hind portion of the shoe should fit firmly, but neither too loosely nor too tightly. Otherwise there will be damage to the heel bone. If the hind portion of the shoe is too loose, blisters may result. Avoid clog shoes. You are unstable in them, and this often leads to injury. The sole of the shoe should not be too stiff because this will interfere with the functioning of the transverse arch. Both sole and heel of hard rubber are more flexible than those of leather. Should a shoe for daily wear have laces? Yes, but two eyelets are not enough. Three to four eyelets will provide better support. Are tennis shoes suitable for general wear? For adults they are *if* they have an adequate arch support (as must all shoes). This can be determined by looking and feeling for the arch. The bottom of the shoe should not be flat. Some sneakers taper in the front, crowding the toes, and should, of course, not be worn. There is a make of shoe in which the heel is lower than the rest of the shoe. You can compare this to walking in the sand, and, essentially, it is not a natural foot position. Such shoes often have other desirable features, such as a cushioned arch-support system and a wide front providing plenty of toe room, but because of the unnatural foot position, conservative experts are reluctant to recommend them.

Shoes for regular two- to five-mile walking and jogging have much in common. They should be structurally firm, pliable, but not rigid. Examine the shoe for an arch support. Notice the shape of the shoe. Since it will provide the "floor" for your foot, it should be the shape of your foot. If the shape is straight,

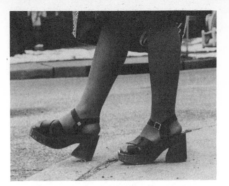

The wearer of platform shoes always risks injury, even when she—or he—is merely stepping off a curb.

you do not have the proper shoe for you. Next, how do your toes fit in the shoes as you stand and walk in them? Pay particular attention to the big toe. If possible, trace an outline of your foot on some paper. Then trace an outline of a shoe you might buy. If they match, the chances are good that you have found a well-fitting shoe.

Much of your rapid walking and jogging will land on the heel of your shoe. Sponge rubber for both heels and shoes are not adequately shock-proof. Nylon and hard rubber are too hard for most people. Buy the shoe that combines sponge for shock absorption and hard rubber for stability. Crepe rubber will do very well for the heel, as will gum rubber. What of rippled soles? They are fine, but giant ripples hamper good control. Some soles are rubber studded. These improve traction.

For regular long-distance (two- to five-mile) walking or running, the shoes that are lower in the heel than your ordinary shoes are best avoided. Such a shoe adds strain on the Achilles tendon (see Figure 8–4) at the back of the foot. However, be sure that the heel is not too high, for, as has been pointed out, it will upset your body balance, throwing your weight forward. The heel should also have a cup that

firmly embraces the heel; the cup (called a *counter*) must be strong and supportive. When trying on the shoes check them for the following points while standing:

How does your big toe fit? It should be about three-quarters of an inch from the front of the shoe. Your feet should fit snugly but not too tightly in the shoe, and only you can judge that. However, it will help to have the shoe clerk measure the width of your foot. Finally, buy a pair of shoes that breathe; they will do this if there are well-placed holes in the body of the shoe.

So, buying shoes for your particular purpose takes care, patience, and knowledge. But when you consider that an estimated 70 percent of this nation's adult population have foot problems due to improperly fitting shoes, it is well worth the trouble.

Preparing for a Walk

Climate, of course, varies from one part of the country to another and from season to season. But except in extreme conditions, there are few times and places unsuitable for walking. In warm weather, light-colored clothes are cooler because they reflect both heat and light waves. A brimmed hat will do as well as sunglasses — and will also shade the back of the neck. (Unusually prolonged skin exposure to the sun promotes wrinkling of the skin; in the case of blonds, such long-term overexposure may hasten the development of skin cancer.) Normal eyes are equipped to adjust to both light and shade, and the eye muscle needs exercise too. Exposure to glare from snow or sand, however, does require good sunglasses. For winter weather, sports shops sell

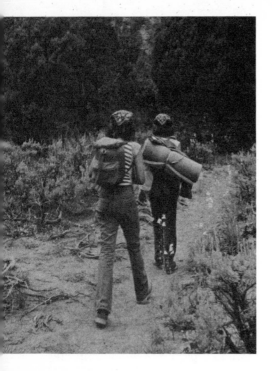

hooded waterproof and water-repellent parkas that weigh less than a pound, and rainsuits are also available. Modern thermal underwear is well-designed and comfortable. What are the essential parts of the body to keep warm? The extremities and the head and neck. A hat, scarf, warm sleeves, and thermal underwear under warm slacks or trousers are good insurance against the cold. Two pairs of socks have been recommended for serious walkers—a thin inner pair of cotton (or even silk) and a thicker outer pair of wool or textured cotton. Nylon is nonabsorbent and is not as flexible as silk or cotton. The outer wool or thick cotton hose are both sweat-absorbers and cushioning agents. They are also a warm comfort against inhospitable cold. And it should not be forgotten that rapid walking in itself helps keep the body warm.

Setting the Pace

A mile is exactly 5,280 feet. An average man's walking stride is two feet per step. Thus, 2,640 steps will carry him a mile. Moreover, the average healthy man can walk three miles an hour. Small women of perhaps 5 feet, 2 or 3 inches will find that speed hard going because their legs are shorter. But most women can walk as fast as most men, unless the man is unusually tall.

From a psychological point of view, a mile-long walk can be either long and dull or short and interesting. Everybody develops his or her own technique for making walking time pass quickly. One infantry soldier clipped a few pages out of his Bible every day and stuffed them into his helmet. When the walks seemed long, he would ponder, even memorize, a passage or two. "And

he found that the rolling King James rhythms made remarkably fine marching music."[3]

How can you increase your walking pace without increasing your fatigue? Lengthen your stride and increase your speed. But do these gradually. Soon, tense muscles and stiff joints will loosen, the body's flexibility will improve, and so will your ability to negotiate the down-pulling force of gravity. All this will help to prevent the fatigue and the aches and pains so common with the inexperienced walker. There is a rhythm, a beat to walking. That beat is part of the joy of walking, and it comes with experience.

Also to be considered is the placement of the feet. This can be determined by walking in sand or on a thick carpet, or by stopping while walking to observe which way the toes point. Interestingly, if the toes point out, so do the hands. The toes should be pointed in the direction of the body's movement—neither in nor out. This does not mean a tightrope walk. The good walker swings a trifle to one side as the corresponding foot takes a forward step, and the opposite arm swings forward to keep the body from moving too far from the center line. Good walkers do not waddle. They do not walk a tightrope. And the toes are pointed straight ahead.

"I have two doctors," an English writer wrote long ago, "my left leg and my right."[4] For him, as for all regular walkers, there were the advantages of making your own appointments and an inexpensive way of promoting good health. Although the first is not possible for today's doctors, the second is recommended by all of them. For the beginning walker, all that is needed are clothes to suit the climate and a comfortable pair of shoes. When should you walk? If you make a point of planning time you will be surprised at how regular walking can easily be fitted into your schedule. Perhaps you have an hour between classes. Take about twenty minutes of that time for a basic walk, and you cover a mile or so. Don't walk so fast that you become breathless, but don't saunter either. After a few weeks increase your distance. How? If you drive to college, park ten blocks away. True, that means rising half-an-hour earlier, but ten blocks a day each way will add a couple of miles to your distance. And you might avoid a stressful parking problem, too. If you like movies, walk to them. Walk after dinner, before you watch television, to the house of a friend, and anytime you can avoid driving. What routes should you follow? There again you are the chooser. Why, for example, fight traffic on a heavily traveled street when a few blocks away there may be a friendly neighborhood of lawns, trees, an occasional garden, or some interesting houses? Within a few months, with some planning, taking advantage of all your opportunities to walk, and a little knowledge of distance, you should be able to fit three to four miles of walking into your day. Before long you will notice this: If you miss a day or two of walking, you won't feel quite so well. Your body has become accustomed to a healthier life style of regular exercise.

Jogging

With attention to these details, a good walk can be enough fun to make one break into a jog. As with walking, there is some individuality to jogging. But there are some general suggestions that are worth following: (1) you should stand erect with the back kept as straight as is naturally comfortable; (2) the head should be kept erect and the eyes not focused on the feet; (3) the arms should be held a bit away from the body; and (4) the elbows should be bent so that they and the hands are about the same distance from the ground. Occasionally the arms and shoulders should be shaken and relaxed while running. This helps reduce any tightness that may develop. The foot should hit the ground heel first, then the body should rock forward so that the weight is on the ball of the foot when beginning the next step. If this is too uncomfortable, you might land with most of your weight on the ball of the foot instead of the heel. But landing with *all* your weight on the ball of the foot will cause soreness of both your feet and legs. Hard surfaces are not for beginning joggers. Ungiving cement or asphalt may cause muscle strain.

Some Practical Results of Exercise

Relief of Stress

Exercise makes people feel better. One reason may simply be that it is fun to take part in such competitive games as tennis, handball, and basketball. But another reason is that exercise often relieves harmful stress.

To be sure, not all stress is harmful. In its broadest definition, stress is just the body's reaction to any demand made of it. A tennis game or a passionate embrace, for example, may be stressful but usually not harmful. So it is not stress, as such, that is injurious. It is the *kind* of stress and a person's *way of cop-ing* with it that can be harmful to health.

An increasing number of physicians believe that the constant striving for success, now so much a part of modern life, may be a contributing cause of heart attacks. People who are slaves to the clock, who are overly competitive, who are constantly under social and economic pressures are not living a life; they are suffering a life. And it is this kind of suffering, it is theorized, that can lead to a heart attack. Recent animal experiments seem to support this theory. They suggest that emotional factors can make the electrical mechanism of the heart unstable, which could account for sudden death.

The famed expert on stress, Hans Selye, writes:

*Fight for the highest attainable aim
But do not put up resistance in vain.*[5]

His meaning is not unlike that in these Oriental lines:

*For three things I pray:
The serenity to accept that which
    cannot be changed;
The courage to change that which
    can be changed;
And the wisdom to tell the one from
    the other.*

Improved Body Posture

People do not often think of posture as a form of movement, yet rarely does anyone stand completely still. One researcher concluded that standing is movement upon a stationary base."[6] People, she discovered, sway constantly, if slightly. Such swaying (not done consciously) helps both in returning venous blood to the heart and in bringing sufficient blood to the brain.

Exercise is part of the growth process that results in the ability to stand erect. Earlier in this chapter we saw that growth and control of striated muscles are a precondition for infant development. But the reverse is also true: Developmental movements (exercise) enable the muscles to develop properly. As the child grows taller, the muscles will increase in length. If exercise is inadequate, the muscles will grow anyway, but they will be thin and underdeveloped. The child will not have the muscle strength to hold his or her body erect in its most efficient posture. Moreover, the bones, which are still pliable, may be improperly shaped and molded.

Poor posture results not only from inadequate exercise during childhood, but also because children have a natural tendency to mimic grown-ups. Observations of students' postures on high school and college campuses suggest that, sadly, the imitation has been only too accurate. Poor posture is unattractive. Whether casual or not, clothes fit better on a body whose segments are well aligned. When the body segments sag—head and shoulders drooping, hips forward, upper back rounded and trunk listing backward—it is as if the person would fall were he not held together

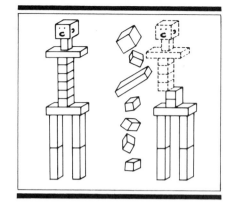

FIGURE 8–5
Like this figure of blocks, the human body is made up of segments. The blocks will stand as long as they are centered on top of one another (left). Move one block, however, and its center is no longer over the blocks below. The figure of blocks collapses (right). When a person's posture is good, then each body segment is centered over the base that supports it. When a person's posture is poor, the body does not collapse, because muscles and ligaments hold the segments together; rather, the body sags, which promotes fatigue.

by bone and ligaments. Indeed, one expert refers to this posture of fatigue as "hanging on the ligaments."[7] So stretched are both muscles and ligaments that much body adjustment has to be made before efficient movement can be achieved. Moreover, prolonged poor posture can eventually cause chronic pain due either to pressure on a firm structure, such as bone or a taut muscle on part of a nerve, or to severe tension on a structure, such as a tendon or ligament.

Other writers have emphasized this by pointing out that the force of gravity has a tendency to cause the skeletal framework of the body to collapse, to buckle at the ankle, knee, and hip. To counteract these buckling tendencies, certain muscle groups work together to hold the

body erect (see Figure 8–5). Exercise of these muscle groups is of importance in any body-conditioning program.

How Much Can Exercise Accomplish?

For normal people, the answer to this question depends on two basic factors: *heredity* and *the effort of exercise.* From the strictly hereditary point of view, nothing can be done to improve the tissues' supply of oxygen. It is, therefore, necessary for a person to concentrate on the effort of exercise for this purpose. Most people do not maximize their potential to use oxygen because of lack of enough regular aerobic exercise. Are the lungs able to get as much oxygen as possible from the air to deliver to the heart? Is the cardiovascular system able to carry the maximum amount of oxygenated blood to the tissue cells? Does the oxygen efficiently leave the red blood cells and pass through the capillaries to the needy tissue cells? Are the cellular chemicals able to make the best use of the oxygen that does reach them? For each of these questions the answer is this: In normal young people, yes—but each function can be improved with regular aerobic exercise. Now, if an exercise program will improve the use of oxygen, there is a decreased need for the heart to work so hard to get oxygen to the tissues. Such was the case with Wilt Chamberlain. The pulse rate, heart rate, and heart effort of a well-conditioned person will be less than that of a poorly conditioned person for the same amount of work. However, the ability to use oxygen at its fullest is not developed during a single hour of exercise. If a person spends most of his or her time inactively, it will take months of regular aerobic exercise before the greatest and most efficient use of oxygen is possible. Years of inactive neglect are not overcome in an hour. Indeed, a sudden strain on the heart may be dangerous. It is always best to have a physician check your physical condition before *any* exercise program is begun. For many people, the attainment of physical fitness involves changing a whole life style from one of regular inactivity to one of regular activity.

It has been often claimed that a regular program of exercise will increase the number of capillaries (and thus the amount of blood flow) in the normal heart muscle. Moreover, this has been touted as one of the benefits of aerobic exercise. There is no evidence to show that this happens. *If* the arterial blood supply to the heart is constantly lessened because of atherosclerosis or actual coronary blockage, the heart muscle is damaged and stressed by a decreased lack of blood and oxygen. It is believed that only to meet a seriously reduced blood supply to the heart with actual heart damage will an added number of capillaries develop (a *collateral* circulation). So regular aerobic exercise, begun in childhood, cannot be expected to supply a collateral circulation to prevent heart disease later in life. However, this does not decrease the other real benefits of habitual aerobic exercise begun early in life. They are, as has been pointed out, very considerable.

Another common error is the belief that deep breathing exercise will improve lung functioning. Not so. However, habitual aerobic exercises, such as swimming, bicycle riding, tennis, and jogging, will increase the spread of available oxygen into lung tissue (*diffusion*). This is probably due to the increased flow of blood

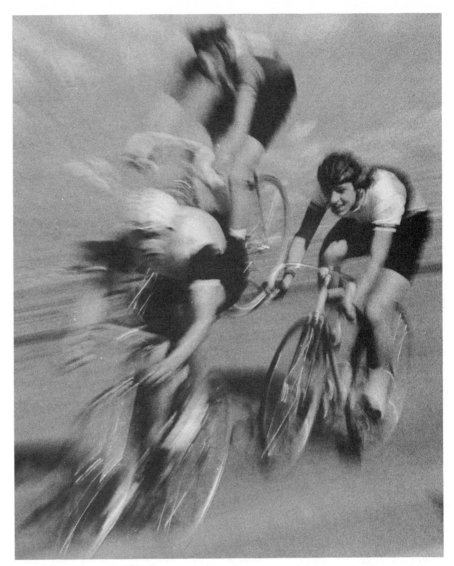

Bicycling is an excellent way to increase one's aerobic capacity, even when one is not a top-speed racer.

through the capillaries that is promoted by exercise.

To this point we have discussed ways of achieving fitness as it applies to the body as a whole. We have described widespread body structures, such as muscles, tendons, and ligaments, and, moreover, we have discussed ways of exercising them that would lead to whole-body well-being. In addition, we have stressed the beneficial effect of aerobic exercises on the body's heart and its connected system of blood vessels. Now let us turn our attention to fitness of some of the special body parts — in particular the eyes, ears, and teeth. We will continue in the same general way. First the physical make-up and functions of the structures will be described, and then we will discuss ways to keep them healthy and to correct any malfunctions that may occur.

Sight: A Special Sense

The light of the body is the eye.
MATTHEW 6:22

The Eye's Structure

Each eyeball is protected from shock by its surrounding fat-padded socket. Its movements are controlled by muscles. Its fluid is contained by a three-layered wall. These three layers, or coats, are the **sclera**, **choroid**, and **retina** (see Figure 8–6). The tough, outer layer, the sclera, is the white of the eye. The transparent **cornea** is the front continuation of the sclera. As the window of the eye, the cornea covers the *pupil* and *iris* like a crystal covers the face of a watch. Overlying the sclera and cornea in front is a loose membrane, the **conjunctiva.**

The **iris** is the front continuation of the middle layer of the eyeball, the choroid. The choroid contains the capillaries that bring nourishing blood to the eye's living tissue. The opening in the iris of the eye is the **pupil.** The iris gives the eye its color, and the pupil is the round dark spot in its center. In the iris are delicate muscles that automatically open and close the iris. In this way, light that gets through the covering cornea and passes through the opening in the iris—the pupil—is controlled.

Inside the eye are two chambers. The smaller *front chamber* contains a salty, clear, watery fluid called the **aqueous humor.** This fluid is constantly provided to and drained from the eye by capillaries. It leaves through a *filtration area.* Behind the front chamber, just behind the pupil and iris, is the **lens.** The lens focuses an image on the eye's light-sensitive surface in the same way as does a lens in a camera. In the eye, that light-sensitive surface is one of the layers of nerve tissue in the *rear chamber* that make up the retina. The shape of the eye's lens is also controlled by muscles. This makes it possible to focus and to clearly see objects at various distances. The retina in the rear chamber of the eye ends in a large nerve (the **optic nerve**) leading to the brain.

Some Eye Problems

EYESTRAIN

When the muscles controlling the eyeballs or the iris are overworked, they get tired. Pain around the eyes, headache, twitching eyelids, oversensitivity to light, blurred vision, even dizziness and a sick feeling in the stomach are all symptoms of muscle fatigue, or *eyestrain.* Often this is caused by reading without enough light. Resting the eyes by looking at a distant object or a blank wall can help relieve eyestrain. Of course, continuous symptoms of

FIGURE 8–6
The eye.

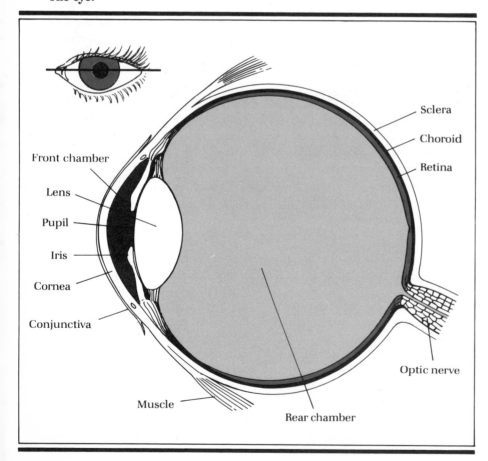

Front chamber

Lens

Pupil

Iris

Cornea

Conjunctiva

Muscle

Rear chamber

Sclera

Choroid

Retina

Optic nerve

eyestrain should mean an early visit to an *ophthalmologist* (or *oculist*)— a physician who specializes in the care and treatment of the eyes.

INJURY AND INFECTION

Injury and infection commonly occur to the exposed parts of the eye. Looking *directly* at the bright sun is always a serious mistake, for it can cause severe eye damage. To avoid eye injury from the sun, one should wear nondistorting sunglasses. Foreign bodies that lodge in the eye can also have damaging consequences. Often the objects can be removed by pulling the upper lid over the lower one or by rotating the eyeball. If not, the help of a doctor may be necessary. While working in an area in which there are many dust particles, wearing a pair of protective goggles is wise.

Conjunctivitis is an inflammation of the conjunctiva (refer back to Figure 8–6). A common form, a condition called *pink eye*, can be treated by the family doctor. One virus disease that attacks the cornea is also treatable. In fact, it is one of the few viruses for which there is now an effective drug. Nevertheless, some injuries to and illnesses of the cornea do result in blindness. In these cases it is sometimes possible to perform transplant surgery using a cornea willed to a corneal bank.

GLAUCOMA

Glaucoma results when the fluid (aqueous humor) in the front chamber of the eye cannot escape through the filtration area. There are many causes for the obstruction of the filtration area, all of which result in increased pressure in the eye, which in turn damages the delicate nerve cells and fibers. Headaches, loss of side vision (see

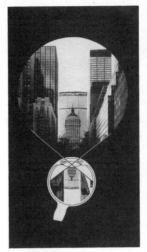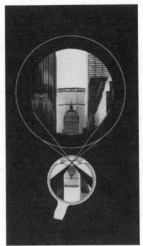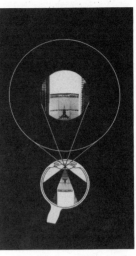

FIGURE 8–7
Glaucoma narrows vision: normal vision (left), early glaucoma (center), and advanced glaucoma (right). Without adequate treatment, the person may eventually lose all sight.

Figure 8–7), and halos around lights may all be among the signs and symptoms of glaucoma. When the disorder progresses rapidly, severe pain and blindness can occur quickly. Emergency drug treatment can relieve the pressure, but for some kinds of glaucoma surgery is necessary.

There is a hereditary tendency to some forms of glaucoma. Blood relatives of such individuals should be regularly examined. Most often glaucoma develops very slowly with only a mild increase of pressure inside the eye. There is no warning pain, and loss of vision is very gradual. A simple test for measuring pressure in the eye is an important preventive part of any eye examination.

PROBLEMS OF THE LENS

Cataracts can occur as part of the aging process. They are a cloudiness of the lens that results when the lens hardens and is no longer able to respond well to muscle control. The

cloudy areas prohibit light from passing through the lens, and where light cannot get through, there is no vision. Blindness may result without corrective surgery. Fortunately, surgery for this condition has a high rate of success. The procedure is to remove the cloudy lens and replace it with a contact lens that substitutes for the natural lens. Until recently, vision after surgery could only be corrected with eyeglasses. However, the spectacle lens does not work as well because of its excess magnification and the difficulty the other eye has in adjusting to the larger images. In selected cases, the surgical insertion of a plastic lens may replace the contact lens. But by no means does the insertion always turn out well. The decision to do the operation is never made lightly. It may be accompanied by corneal swelling, inflammation, and hemorrhage. Also, vision with plastic lenses may be reduced.

Far less serious but much more common eye conditions are **near-**

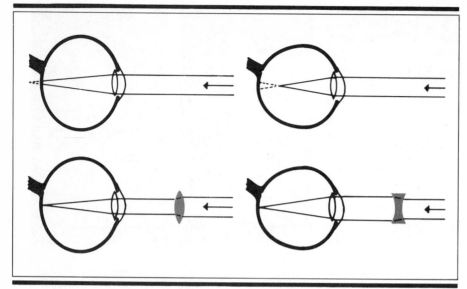

FIGURE 8–8
Farsightedness (top left) and its correction with a convex lens (bottom left), and nearsightedness (top right) and its correction with a concave lens (bottom right). In both cases, the corrective lens makes images fall on the retina.

sightedness (*myopia*), **farsightedness** (*hyperopia*), and a third called **astigmatism**, which can accompany either of the first two. Now, the word *refract* refers to the ability to bend light. The most important refracting part of the eye is the *cornea*. It is also, therefore, the principal focusing part of the eye. The crystalline *lens* is also a powerful part of the eye. To increase the focusing power of the eye, the lens must have the ability to change its shape. Focusing for object distance is called *accommodation*. So the lens is a way of accommodating the eye to see at various distances. How does the lens accomplish its purpose? Its shape is indirectly changed by the ciliary muscle attached to an elastic capsule that surrounds it. When the eye is nearsighted, parallel rays of light from a distant object will focus in front of the retina. When it is farsighted, they will focus behind the retina. With astigmatism, some light rays focus in front of the retina,

while others focus behind it, so that part of the image is out of focus. How do these three conditions occur?

There are several theories for nearsightedness. One states that it is a natural result of the eye's growth and development. When the eyeball grows too long, nearsightedness is the result. (See Figure 8–8, right.) Tied in to this theory, then, is heredity. The refractive ability of the eye is inherited just as is height, hair color, and other genetic features of people. A second theory for nearsightedness is that it occurs with extra use of the eyes during the school years. Because of excessive strain, the accommodation mechanism of the eye does not relax properly, so nearsightedness results. Certainly there is a relationship between schoolwork and an increase of nearsightedness.[8] This condition tends to get worse, particularly when it goes uncorrected. Also, with aging and progressive drying, the lens loses

some of its ability to bend light (accommodate), and the nearsightedness worsens.

At birth most eyes are farsighted, but this improves quickly during the first few years of life. By the time puberty is reached little farsightedness remains. Farsightedness becomes a problem when the elements of the eye are inadequate to the task of focusing *nearby* objects on the retina. This will be the case if the eye does not grow long enough. (See Figure 8–8, left.)

Astigmatism occurs most commonly when the curvature of the cornea is unequal and light passing through it cannot focus on a single point image on the retina, as shown in Figure 8–9. A slight degree of astigmatism can also occur when there is a faulty curvature of the lens. Severely astigmatic eyes can seriously distort vision. (See Figure 8–10.)

These conditions can be adjusted for by corrective eyeglass lenses or with contact lenses. Some people achieve better vision with spectacle lenses, others with contact lenses.[9] Modern contact lenses are usually made of plastic and are not notice-

FIGURE 8–9
Astigmatism. Because two adjacent portions of the cornea have different curvatures, light rays focus improperly.

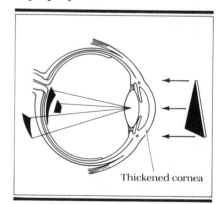

Thickened cornea

able. This, however, is but one of their advantages. There are no frames or lenses to break, and some people find fitting frames uncomfortable. Also, the progression of the eye condition of some people is halted by contact lenses. Contact lenses have the disadvantages of expense and they are often lost (requiring insurance). Eye irritation occurs with some who wear contact lenses and focusing problems when doing close work can be another complication. Blurring can occur because of the stagnation of tear fluid and the formation of tiny bubbles behind the lens. Moreover, a thin contact lens can warp, become distorted, or flattened and thus interfere with vision. Careful attention to the proper fit and performance of the contact lens, therefore, is essential to good vision.

In the future it may be possible to cure nearsightedness by surgery. A promising surgical procedure has been developed by a Russian physician and is now being tried on patients in the United States, particularly in Detroit.[10]

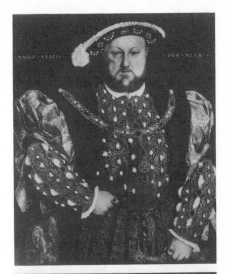

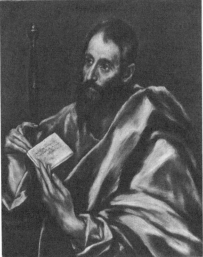

FIGURE 8–10
The severe astigmatism of two great Renaissance artists, Hans Holbein (1497?–1543) and El Greco (1541?–1614?), is believed by some to account for the distortion of their painted figures. For centuries these distortions, in themselves so beautiful and so characteristic of the artists' respective styles, have been widely and rightly admired. Top: Holbein's "Henry VIII." Bottom: El Greco's "St. Paul."

Hearing: Another Special Sense

The ear is the road to the heart.
VOLTAIRE (1694–1778)

For a sound to reach the brain where it is interpreted into something meaningful, each of three main parts of the ear must fulfill its purpose. These parts are the *outer*, *middle*, and *inner* ear (see Figure 8–11).

The Outer Ear

The *outer ear* is made up of the fleshy external ear (or **auricle**). It collects sound waves and directs them into the 1¼-inch-long funnel-shaped ear (or **auditory canal**). This canal ends blindly. It is closed off by the outer wall of the middle ear, the membranous **eardrum** (or *tympanic membrane*).

The Middle Ear

Except for the membranous eardrum, the walls of the middle ear chamber are bone. Across the middle ear is strung a connected chain of the three smallest bones in the body. These bones are named for their shape. The first is the **hammer** (or *malleus*). The handle of the hammer is attached to the inside of the eardrum. The second bone is the **anvil** (or *incus*). The third little bone is the **stirrup** (or *stapes*).

Connecting the middle ear to the back of the nose is the **Eustachian** (or **auditory**) **tube**. Ordinarily this tube is closed. With swallowing it opens. Were it not for this tube, a great increase in pressure in the auditory canal would push the eardrum into the middle ear. A decrease in pressure in the auditory canal would push the eardrum out. Normally, air pressure changes little within the auditory canal, but a loud noise, such as a pistol shot near the ear, can cause enough pressure within the auditory canal to rupture the eardrum. When the mouth is kept open, the pressure against the eardrum comes from both sides (auditory canal and Eustachian tube), which may prevent eardrum damage.

The Inner Ear

The *inner ear* is a tiny chamber totally encased in protective bone. In the bony wall closest to the middle ear are two small openings—the **oval window** above and the **round window** below. The foot plate of the stirrup in the middle ear fits into the top oval window. As explained below, the function of the tiny middle ear bones is to carry along the motion of the eardrum to the oval window.

Chiseled in bone, the inner ear is made up of tiny, tunneled bony canals. Contained within these bony canals are membranous canals. And within both the bony and membranous canals is a thin fluid. So the membranous canals are surrounded by this fluid and also contain it.

One part of the bony canals is molded into a pea-sized snail-shaped passage making a two-and-three-quarters turn; this is the bony **cochlea**. (A second part of the bony canals has nothing to do with hearing. It is concerned with balance.) Within the membranous structure inside the bony cochlea is the basic organ of hearing, the spiral-shaped **organ of Corti**. The organ of Corti contains cells with little hairs on their tops. These little hair cells are supplied with delicate nerve fibers. These countless nerve fibers collect to become the brain's nerve of hearing (the **acoustic nerve**). So it is the organ of Corti that receives the stimuli of sound to send to the brain.

How Hearing Happens

Sound waves are gathered by the external ear and then directed into the auditory canal. The sound waves strike the eardrum, which sets the eardrum to vibrating in time with the sound waves. The vibrations of the eardrum then tremble on along the three tiny bones in the middle ear. The stirrup pushes into the oval window, producing pressure waves in the fluid within the bony cochlea. These gently rippling waves stimulate the hair cells within the membranous structure of the cochlea. Finally, the stimulated hair cells of the organ of Corti cause impulses to be received by the surrounding nerve fibers that join to become the acoustic nerve. These impulses are then carried to the brain by the acoustic nerve. Thus is sound energy carried through air, membrane, bone, and fluid to become, in the inner ear, nervous impulses to be sent to the brain for interpretation.

The round window is not directly involved in the transmission of sound energy. Located below the oval window, it is a membrane-covered window of adjustment. As the bones of the middle ear are stimulated by sound waves, the vibrating foot plate of the stirrup pushes the oval window slightly inward. As was just described, this disturbs and displaces the fluid within the cochlea. But fluid cannot be compressed. The displaced cochlear fluid must go somewhere.

FIGURE 8–11
The ear. Not visible in the illustration is the membranous cochlear duct, which is housed in the bony cochlea. It is the cochlear duct that, in turn, contains the organ of hearing — the spiral organ of Corti. And it is the organ of Corti whose stimulated hair cells will induce the impulses on the surrounding acoustic nerve fibers. These impulses will reach the brain as sound.

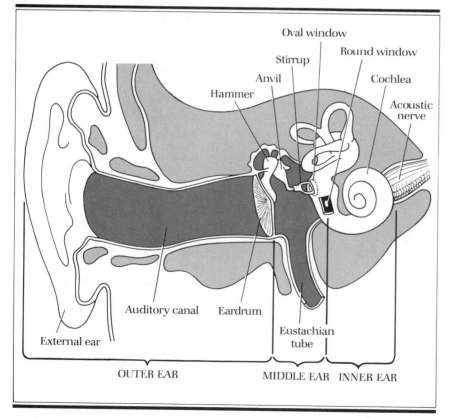

External ear
Auditory canal   Eardrum
Hammer
Anvil   Stirrup
Oval window
Round window
Cochlea
Acoustic nerve
Eustachian tube
OUTER EAR   MIDDLE EAR   INNER EAR

It is accommodated by the membrane of the round window, which allows the fluid to push outward. When the foot plate moves outward, the fluid can move inward. So, the tiny adjusting membrane of the round window, by permitting the stirrup to move, permits hearing.

Sound Measured As a Physical Force

Sound waves traveling through air cause pressure changes within it. Sound is measured in **decibels** (dB). What are decibels? They are the units by which sound **intensity** or **loudness** is measured. The "bel" in the word is from the name of the inventor of the telephone, Alexander Graham Bell. "Deci" originates from the Latin word *decem*, meaning "ten." As the decibels go up, it means that the intensity or loudness of sound increases by multiples of ten. Zero decibels is known as the *threshold of hearing*. It is the smallest intensity of sound that can be heard by the healthy ear. Ten decibels are ten times more intense, or louder, than one decibel. Twenty decibels are ten times more intense than ten decibels. Thirty decibels (a whisper) are ten times more intense than twenty, and so on. At one hundred feet a jet plane taking off is ten times louder than a pneumatic riveter, and the noise will hurt (see Figure 8–12). As decibels increase, sound energy multiplies fantastically. The greater the energy is, the more discomfort a person will experience. Of course, this will also depend on how far a person is from the source of the sound. Thus, at a rock concert, the music has a decibel level of 120 at its source on the stage. This sound level will be more harmful to the ears of the playing musicians than it will be to a lone listener standing one hundred feet away. Above 85 decibels, excessive noise can cause damage to the hair cells and membrane within the inner ear.

Notice that dB is the usual abbreviation for decibels. The abbreviation dBA is now gaining some use. It refers to the decibel measurement on the A-scale of a special noise-level measuring meter. This special measuring meter records annoying higher **frequencies** of sound. Frequency refers to the **pitch**. An example of a high-pitched sound is the harsh screech of an animal or of chalk going the wrong way on a blackboard. When the pitch is great, the frequency of sound vibrations is higher too.

The third characteristic of sound waves (besides intensity and pitch) is **quality,** or **timbre**. The timbre of a sound refers to the form of its sound waves. Pleasant musical notes have equal-appearing waves. Harsh sounds result in helter-skelter sound waves (see Figure 8–13).

Some Ear Problems

Hearing, like sight, is a precious gift. Along with the hundreds of joys it affords, it also protects us. For instance, before we see danger, we usually hear it. Like blindness, deafness is a harsh handicap. Yet, millions in this nation are chronically deaf to some degree. Among older age groups, hearing defects occur in astronomical numbers. These defects may take the form of partial or complete hearing loss or they may be the inability to understand speech and other sounds clearly.

Conductive deafness means there is an interference with sound transmission through the outer or middle ear. As simple a matter as

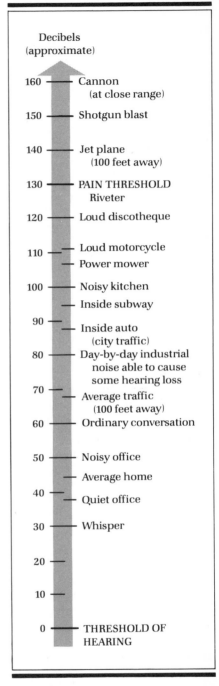

**FIGURE 8–12
The decibel scale of loudness.**

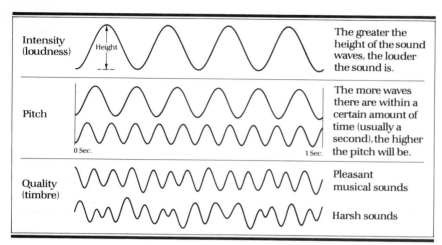

Intensity (loudness)	[waveform] Height	The greater the height of the sound waves, the louder the sound is.
Pitch	[waveforms] 0 Sec. — 1 Sec.	The more waves there are within a certain amount of time (usually a second), the higher the pitch will be.
Quality (timbre)	[waveforms]	Pleasant musical sounds
	[waveforms]	Harsh sounds

FIGURE 8–13
The characteristics of sound waves: intensity, quality, and pitch.

excessive earwax may cause conductive deafness. Its removal by a physician will restore hearing. Its removal by an amateur with a hairpin, or some other sharply pointed instrument, may pierce the eardrum. "He has not so much brain as earwax," wrote Shakespeare. This pronouncement might be made of one who, in the above manner, senselessly risks deafness. Largely because of the use of antibiotics, infection of the middle ear, which sometimes accompanies or follows a childhood communicable disease, used to be a more frequent cause of conductive deafness than it is today.

Hearing loss by way of the Eustachian tube is not uncommon. As was mentioned on page 251, the Eustachian tube is open only during swallowing. In this way an equal pressure on both sides of the eardrum is maintained. During descent in an unpressurized airplane, the passenger should repeatedly swallow. Otherwise, the high-altitude air pressure, trapped in the middle ear, will fail to correspond to the increasing atmospheric pressure on

the outside of the eardrum. The eardrum may then rupture. An upper respiratory infection may, moreover, cause swelling around the opening and within the Eustachian tube. Sometimes this causes temporary deafness. An attempt to open the tube by vigorously blowing the nose may force infectious material into the middle ear. Indiscriminate use of nose drops or nasal sprays may promote such infection. The consequences may be serious and chronic.

Sometimes infection will cause stiffening of the joints between the three little bones in the middle ear. The bones become rigid, limiting their normal ability to vibrate. Without the vibration, sound waves cannot be transmitted through them to the fluid of the inner ear. Hearing is diminished, even lost. But sound waves *can* be transmitted through *the skull to the fluid in the inner ear*, and it is on this principle that the hearing aid works. The power-packed transistor hearing aid has been greatly improved since its invention and has helped many people with hearing problems.

Children born deaf will not learn to speak unless they are taught through some pathway other than the ear. But a deaf child need not be a dumb child. Schools and individual therapists that specialize in teaching deaf or hard-of-hearing individuals to communicate have allowed those who are handicapped to lead normal, productive lives.

The Teeth and Their Supports

Who hath aching teeth hath ill tenants.

JOHN RAY (1628–1705)

At twenty-four, George Washington had his first tooth extracted; at fifty-seven, he lost his last tooth. A sad comment on earlier times? Hardly. In the United States today about half of all persons over fifty have lost their natural teeth. For all ages, the figure is one person of eight.

Yet despite these sobering statistics, the fact is that teeth are far less destructible than their owners. (We will examine some of the reasons for their decay, and what can be done about it, later in this section.) Their durability, combined with the fact that teeth are arranged in a highly individual way from person to person, have made dental charts an indispensable means for establishing positive identification of burn victims.

Growth and Structure

At six weeks, the human embryo begins to form tooth buds for the twenty temporary **deciduous** ("baby") **teeth**. Shortly thereafter, the buds of the thirty-two perma-nent teeth (see Figure 8–14) begin to form. At birth, the unerupted de-ciduous teeth are almost complete, and beneath the deciduous teeth some permanent teeth now begin to gain calcium.

About six months after birth, babies show their first tooth. Before their third birthday, they have a mouthful of deciduous teeth. These will be shed at various times over the next several years. Nevertheless, neglect of temporary teeth may re-sult in permanent problems. The

FIGURE 8–14
Teeth: a longitudinal section of a molar (left), the dentition of a six-year-old child (top right), and the dentition of an adult (bottom right).

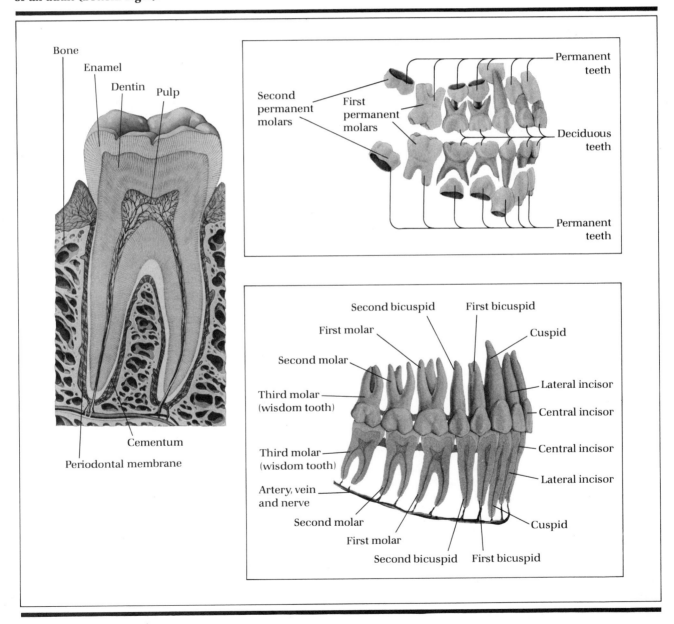

temporary teeth guide the permanent teeth beneath them. Loss or decay of temporary teeth may result in crooked permanent teeth, chewing and speech problems, and psychological problems. Between the ages of 2½ and 3 years, a child should see the dentist for the first time.

Usually the first, or "six-year," molars are the first permanent teeth to erupt. At about this time, the child is losing the front deciduous teeth. The position of the first molars helps determine the position of the other teeth and profoundly influences the shape of the whole lower face. As soon as the first molar erupts, this tooth, the "keystone of the dental arch," should be examined by the dentist.

Some Dental Problems

Dental cavities (or **caries**) share with the common cold the doubtful distinction of being the most common human health problems. How does a cavity form in a tooth? Three things are necessary: a susceptible tooth, sugar, and certain bacteria.

Most teeth are usually covered by a filmy **dental plaque**. This slimy coating gathers and holds together an untidy collection of mucus, food bits, and bacteria. The plaque is about the same color as the teeth. Some, but not all, of the dental plaque may be temporarily removed by brushing. But plaque is not easily removed, and it provides the medium for tooth decay. It is within and around the plaque that the bacteria live and are protected. It is against the plaque that the basic attack on dental caries must be made. This is how plaque harms teeth.

From simple sugars formed by the breakdown of food in the mouth, some of the mouth's bacteria make more complex sugars.

Between feedings, the bacteria get energy by changing the stored complex sugars to destructive acids. How much time do the bacteria need to transform sugar to erosive acid? Within fifteen or twenty minutes most of the damage is done. That is why rinsing or brushing the teeth immediately after eating is so helpful. The bacteria are a common part of dental plaque. The acid in the saliva, formed by bacterial action on sugar, first destroys the tooth **enamel**, the outside surface of the tooth. At this stage there is usually no warning pain. Only later, when destruction has reached the **dentin** (the inside layer of the tooth), is there toothache. An unchecked cavity may get to the **pulp** (the soft, innermost tissue of the tooth, which is surrounded by the dentin). Infection sometimes travels from the pulp toward the tissues surrounding the **root**, contained inside the bone beneath the gum. At this stage, abscess formation may occur. Pus may then spread through the blood vessels, causing a swelling of the adjacent soft tissues.

What Can Be Done?

Following are some commonly accepted practices for regular care of the teeth.

1. If at all possible, teeth should be brushed after each meal. Even rinsing with a warm drink helps remove food particles. Mouthwashes are not substitutes for brushing. Many dentists recommend water-under-pressure equipment to be used after (but not instead of) brushing. Electric toothbrushes are not more effective than the manual kind. *The use of dental floss after each meal is extremely important and*

should not be neglected (see Figure 8–15).

2. To find cavities and arrest their progress, regularly scheduled visits to a dentist are essential.

3. During the period within the uterus, the mother's nutrition is of particular importance to herself and her unborn child. Her diet provides minerals for the developing teeth of the child within her. Should her diet be lacking, the child obtains some minerals not from the mother's teeth, but from her bones. It is after birth that permanent teeth are calcified. So the child's diet (especially during the first eight years) should include foods rich in calcium and phosphorus as well as vitamins A, C, and D (see pages 264–268). Moreover, all living tissue needs and contains protein. An adequate diet, so essential for general health, is also an absolute necessity for development of normal tooth structure.

Do adult teeth, permanent and calcified, need calcium? No, but the bone that holds the teeth in place cannot remain healthy without calcium. Does adult dental health require an adequate diet? Indeed it does. Without enough protein for tissue replacement, for example, mouth structures would quickly suffer. And the destructive effect on adult oral health of shortages of vitamins B and C has long been recognized.

4. For centuries sugar in the Western world was a luxury, available only to the rich and sold to them by pharmacists by the ounce. It has been a significant part of diets in this country only for less than a century. Yet today, the average person in this country consumes about two pounds of sugar (sucrose) every week, usually in the

**FIGURE 8-15
Dental flossing.**

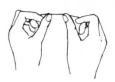

Wind most of 18 inches of floss around one middle finger.

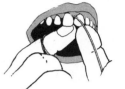

Wind the rest around the middle finger of the other hand.

Use thumbs and forefingers to guide floss.

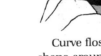

Insert floss between teeth with *gentle* sawing motion.

Curve floss into C shape around tooth at the gum line.

Scrape the floss up and down. Repeat for all five surfaces of every tooth.

form of jams and jellies, cakes and cookies, frozen and canned fruits and desserts, and bottled beverages. And as pointed out earlier, sucrose, as a sugar, is used by oral bacteria to promote caries. So to prevent caries, avoidance of these sweet foods is essential. Of particular importance is the frequency and duration of exposure to sucrose. Thus sucrose-containing foods that stick to the teeth are particularly harmful: A piece of chocolate cake is not quite as apt to cause cavities as is a piece of caramel, but it is best to avoid them both. Modification of diet, so that carbohydrates are obtained from starchy foods instead of from sweets, would surely help to reduce the incidence of caries. Unfortunately, people do have cravings for sweets, and it has been suggested that many artificial sweeteners may cause other problems. What is needed is a sweetener that has been proved totally harmless.

For over forty years the effect of **fluoride** on human health in general, and on dental health in particular, has been carefully investigated through massive studies carried out in communities across the entire North American continent. It is a proven fact that properly fluoridated drinking water will result in at least a two-thirds reduction in tooth decay and will not harm human health.

Today, in this country, more than four thousand communities, totaling about ninety million people, have fluoride fed directly into their drinking water supplies. Two-thirds of the major cities in the United States, including New York, Chicago, Philadelphia, and Detroit, have adopted controlled fluoridation. In some cities a vocal minority has succeeded in confusing enough people to delay fluoridation of the water supply. By their misguided action, they condemn millions to needless pain, expense, and disability due to dental problems.

Over one-fifth of the U.S. population (about forty-four million people) have no access to a public water supply. For them, it would be advisable to add fluoride to such widely consumed foods as salt, flour, and milk. Fluoride solutions applied to the teeth of children have resulted in a 75 to 80 percent reduction of cavities. But these treatments are more expensive and time-consuming than water fluoridation. Fluoride *tablets* and *drops* taken during the early years of life can be ingested only if prescribed. Although the beneficial results of tablets and drops are comparable to those obtained from water fluoridation, they cannot provide a reliable method of cavity prevention because many people simply do not cooperate on a long-term basis. Fluoride-containing toothpastes may help.

Periodontal Diseases

Disorders of the tissues surrounding and holding the teeth in their sockets are called **periodontal diseases.** For people under thirty-five, most tooth loss is caused by cavities. But after thirty-five, periodontal disease is the major cause. It can vary from a mild gum inflammation to actual bone destruction.

Periodontal disease can develop in various ways. The initial signs of inflammation of the gums (**gingivitis**), such as redness, swelling, and bleeding, are usually painless. Poor oral hygiene, the accumulation of hard deposits such as **tartar** (or **calculus**), and **malocclusions** (the inefficient and improper meeting of the upper and the lower teeth) are common causes. Less ordinary evidences of periodontal disease are conditions such as diabetes, leukemia, and deficiencies of vitamins B and C. **Vincent's angina** ("trench mouth"), caused by two different bacteria, can be treated with penicillin and good dental hygiene.

Periodontitis (or **pyorrhea**), the inflammation of the tissues supporting the teeth, can be related to the presence of tartar or calculus. Calculus appears when *bacteria-laden plaque* calcifies and hardens. The resulting irritation and infection causes the pyorrhea. Malocclusion can be corrected by a dental specialist—an *orthodontist*. Periodontitis may also be started by damage caused by toothpicks.

Summary

Fitness, or being healthy enough to adjust to environmental demands, varies from person to person because of individual differences. The basic elements of physical fitness are strength, flexibility, and endurance. Strength can be gained through *isometric* and *isotonic* exercises. Flexibility is increased by doing slow, controlled stretching exercises. Finally, endurance, which involves improvement of the cardiovascular and respiratory systems, is gained through *aerobic exercises*, such as jogging, bicycling, and swimming.

One of the best methods for measuring endurance fitness, or maximum oxygen consumption, is Cooper's aerobic measurements. By evaluating oneself according to certain established standards, one can determine one's fitness and then undertake an exercise program to accomplish a desired goal of fitness.

Besides accomplishing fitness, exercise can provide two other important effects: relief of stress and improved body posture. It is important to remember that though one's potential for fitness is limited by heredity, exercise can help maximize this potential. But the benefits of exercise can only be attained by a consistent program that slowly, but constantly, increases the demands upon the body.

Just as the entire body must be kept in shape, so must particular body parts be subjected to a program of regular fitness.

The eye is composed of three layers: The *sclera* continues at the front of the eyeball as the *cornea*; the *choroid* continues as the *iris*; and the *retina* is the light-sensitive surface on the inside back of the eye that allows us to see. The cornea overlays the iris, which is the colored portion of our eye. The iris contracts or expands to allow varying amounts of light through the *pupil*. The front chamber is filled with fluid, which leaves the chamber via a filtration area. We are able to see because muscles change the shape of the *lens* to focus an image upon the retina.

The eyes are subject to many problems; eyestrain, glaucoma, and cataracts are but a few. But the most common eye problems are *nearsightedness*, *farsightedness*, and *astigmatism*, which are caused by the inability of the lens to bend in a way that properly focuses an image upon the retina. Common-sense measures such as using a proper reading light and wearing protective goggles will help maintain the fitness of one's eyes. And though many conditions are not preventable, a program of regular eye examinations, use of corrective lenses, and, when necessary, surgery can help to provide one with proper vision for a lifetime.

The ear is considered to have three parts—outer, middle, and inner. The external ear, or *auricle*, collects sound waves, which travel through the *auditory canal* to the *eardrum*. The sound waves vibrate the eardrum, and these vibrations pass through the three small bones of the middle ear—the *hammer*, the *anvil*, and the *stirrup*—to the *oval window* of the inner ear. Here the vibrations cause pressure waves in the fluid of the *cochlea*, which in turn stimulate the hair cells of the *organ of Corti*. Nerve fibers of these hair cells collect and travel as the *acoustic nerve* to the brain, where their impulses of sound are interpreted.

The *loudness*, or *intensity*, of sound is measured in *decibels*. Sound of sufficient loudness can damage one's hearing. Other characteristics of sound are *pitch*, measured in terms of *frequency*, and *quality*, or *timbre*.

Deafness or other hearing problems can result if something interferes with the transmission of sound within the ear (*conductive deafness*) or if a structure of the ear has been damaged, as by infection or by uneven pressure on the eardrum. Proper medical care and use of ear protectors around loud noises can prevent hearing problems. Hearing aids have greatly benefited those with impaired hearing.

Human beings have two sets of teeth during their life—their *deciduous* ("baby") *teeth* and their *permanent teeth*. Unless the deciduous teeth are well cared for, a person can have problems with the permanent teeth. *Dental cavities*, or *caries*, are the most common dental problem. These form when bacteria, found in *plaque* in the mouth, break sugars down into an erosive acid that can destroy the *enamel*, *dentin*, and *pulp* of the tooth. Proper brushing and regular flossing remove the plaque, preventing tooth decay and many other dental problems. A diet rich in minerals and vitamins, especially during the early years, will develop strong teeth. Limiting sugar intake and drinking *fluoridated* water will help to reduce the incidence of tooth decay.

References

1. The remainder of this section is based on an article by Nancy Beach, "Health and Beauty: A Medical View," *The New York Times Magazine* (March 5, 1978), pp. 93–94, 96.
2. Rudyard Kipling, *Just So Stories* (New York, 1912.)
3. Aaron Sussman and Ruth Goode, *The Magic of Walking* (New York, 1967), p. 83.
4. G. M. Trevelyan, quoted in Aaron Sussman and Ruth Goode, *The Magic of Walking*, p. 15.
5. Reprinted from Hans Selye, "The Evolution of the Stress Concept," *American Scientist*, Vol. 61 (November–December 1973), p. 699.
6. Quoted in Marion Broer, *Efficiency of Human Movement* (Philadelphia, 1973), p. 129.
7. Marion Broer, *Efficiency of Human Movement*, p. 129, citing Katherine F. Wells, *Kinesiology* (Philadelphia, 1971), p. 382.
8. James R. Gregg and Gordon G. Heath, *The Eye and Sight* (Boston, 1966), p. 41.
9. Irvin M. Borish, *Clinical Refraction* (Chicago, 1970), p. 992.
10. "'Myopia Cure' Is Several Cuts Above Eyeglasses," *Medical World News*, Vol. 20 (June 11, 1979), pp. 18 and 20.

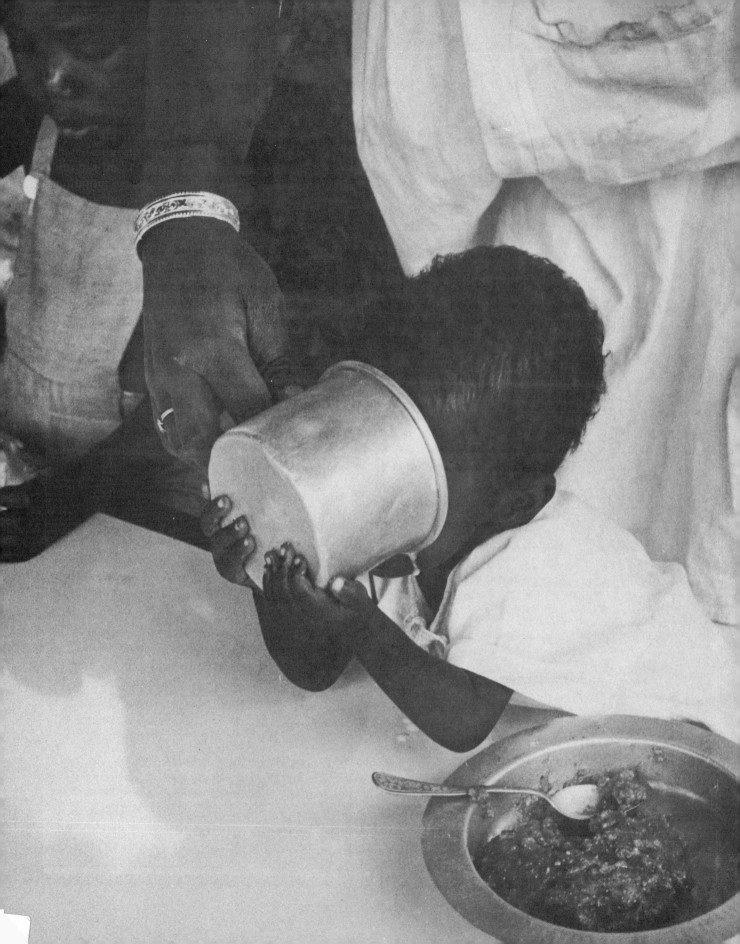

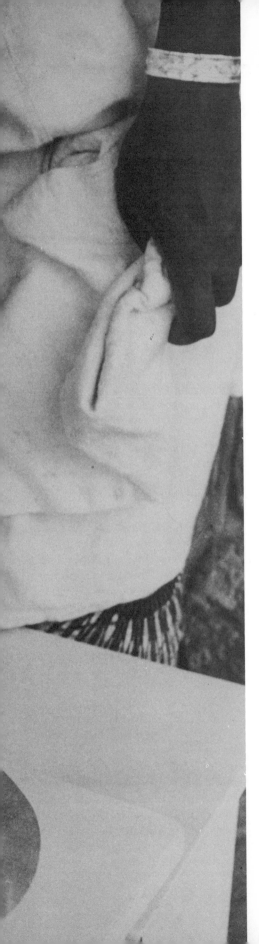

9

Nourishment

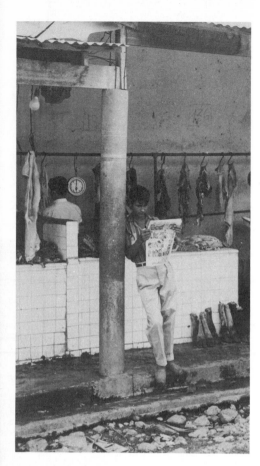

An open-air meat market in the cattle town of Villavicencio, Colombia. The white meat is tripe; the cow feet are used to make soup and gelatin.

Taste:
For Which There Is Some Accounting

Although it happened years ago, many citizens of Peoria, Illinois, still remember the deed with horror. To make matters worse, it had been perpetrated by an officer of the U.S. Army. What had Lieutenant Andrew O'Meara done to so arouse his community?

To demonstrate one means of military survival to some friends, he had killed and skinned a stray dog, and then put it on a spit to cook. The lieutenant was prosecuted, and a judge—under considerable public pressure—fined him the maximum $200 for cruelty to animals. The animal had been killed not cruelly, but by a sudden blow. The lieutenant could have pleaded innocent, but the furor resulting from his demonstration that dog meat could prevent starvation was too intense. He did not contest the case.[1]

Food taboos have a long history. Hebrew biblical instruction forbidding swine, for example, is specific. "Of their flesh shall ye not eat and their carcase shall ye not touch: they are unclean to you." It was doubtless people's affectionate domestication of the dog that led to strong feelings against consuming the meat of the family pet. The people of the Western world have had over twenty centuries to learn to abominate dog meat. And they are not alone. An ancient religious group of Iran considered dogs holy and the eating of them a sin. Moslems also reject dog meat. But in some cultures puppy hams are a delicacy. Those who consider eating "man's best friend" a savage act should know that, until recently, dog flesh was relished among the Chinese, and their great culture has extended over fifty centuries.

Poorly prepared foods are long remembered. Spoiled food provoked the Harvard Butter Rebellion of 1766, which was accompanied by the following announcement:

And it came to pass in the ninth month of the 23rd day of the Month, that the Sons of Harvard murmured and said:

Behold! Bad and unwholesome butter is served out unto us daily; now therefore let us depute Asa the Scribe, to go out unto our Rulers and seek redress.

Then arose Asa, the Scribe, and went unto Belcher, the Ruler, and said behold our butter stinketh and we cannot eat thereof; now give us, we pray thee, butter that stinketh not.[2]

But no matter how fresh the dish, members of many cultures today still reject certain food because of dietary taboos. The Hindus will not eat beef, since the cow is sacred to them. To the Moslems, the pig is unclean; they refuse pork. Milk is the favorite food of soldiers in the U.S. Army, but to the Dravidians of Southern India it is comparable to urine.

Mingled with the vast array of cultural and individual emotional factors that determine food tastes are the endlessly subtle sensory perceptions of food. Some people smack their lips over coffee with "body." It provides a pleasurable resistance in the mouth. Most people relish color; hence, the sprig of green parsley on the plate. In the Bible, food without salt is deplored by

Job. "Can that which is unsavory be eaten without salt?" Creamy substances mixed with air are smoothly delicious. A "rough" chocolate insults exquisitely sensitive mucous membranes. Crisp biscuits are tastier than tough meat. Good bread pleases the palate. Clearly there is more to food than eating.

The digestive process is often described in terms of combustion machines and hydraulic pressures. As book illustrations, these are useful. But digestion is deeply influenced by the mind. Hunger is not the same as appetite. And food can cause effects totally unrelated to either hunger or appetite. "Mine eyes smell onions," old Lafew remarks in Shakespeare's *All's Well That Ends Well.* Centuries before Pavlov's drooling dogs, Shakespeare, in four short words, had already begun to define the conditioned response.*

Shakespeare also understood well the effect of the mind on digestion. "Unquiet meals make ill digestions," says the Abbess in Shakespeare's play *The Comedy of Errors.*

All hungry animals enjoy food, but only humans savor sharing meals. Appetite is a human quality. "The infant cannot be fed by food alone," writes Dorothy V. Whipple, "he needs to dine. . . . He cannot eat until the conditions of dining have been met . . . the infant relaxes and is eager to eat when picked up by gentle, warm, comfortable arms."[3] These are the observations of a pediatrician, but the emotional needs of dining have also been re-

*A conditioned response is a learned, or acquired, response to a stimulus that did not originally evoke the response. The Nobel Prize-winning Russian scientist Ivan Pavlov conditioned dogs to salivate at the sound of a bell or the sight of a light by repeated pairings of these stimuli with the presentation of food. Eventually the light or bell alone came to evoke the salivation response.

corded by geriatricians—those who treat the aged. Elderly people often forget to eat because they are alone and food has lost its meaning. From the first infant intimacy of mother's warmth to the last suppers of the aged, humans learn this: People may eat alone, but they dine with others.

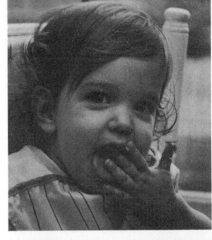

To eat is not necessarily to dine.

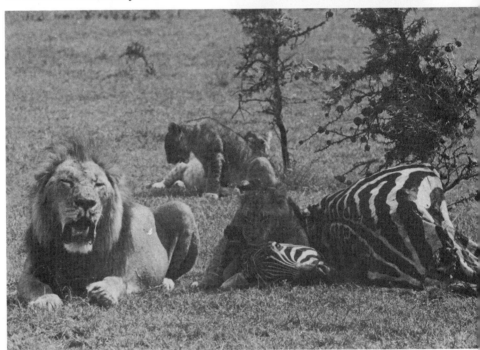

The Basic Constituents of Foods

There are six basic constituents of foods: *carbohydrates, fats, proteins, vitamins, minerals,* and *water.* In health, all work together. A healthy body is made up of delicately balanced ecosystems, which are helped maintained by a balanced diet. Ten of the major nutrients, including their important nutritional sources, are listed in Table 9–1.

"All Flesh Is Grass": Carbohydrates, Fats, and Proteins

All human food ultimately comes from green plants. From the air, plants take carbon dioxide, which is carbon and oxygen. From the soil, plants take water, which is hydrogen and oxygen. From the sun, they

TABLE 9–1
Ten Leading Nutrients

NUTRIENT	IMPORTANT SOURCES OF NUTRIENT	SOME MAJOR PHYSIOLOGICAL FUNCTIONS	
		Build and maintain body cells	Regulate body processes
Protein	Meat, poultry, fish Dried beans and peas Eggs Cheese Milk	Constitutes part of the structure of every cell, such as muscle, blood, and bone. Supports growth and maintains healthy body cells.	Constitutes part of enzymes, some hormones and body fluids, and antibodies that increase resistance to infection.
Carbohydrate	Cereal Potatoes Dried beans Corn Bread Sugar	Supplies energy so protein can be used for growth and maintenance of body cells.	Unrefined products supply fiber—complex carbohydrates in fruits, vegetables, and whole grains—for regular elimination. Assists in fat utilization.
Fat	Shortening, oil Butter, margarine Salad dressing Sausages	Constitutes part of the structure of every cell. Supplies essential fatty acids.	Provides and carries fat-soluble vitamins (A, D, E, and K).
Vitamin A (Retinol)	Liver Carrots Sweet potatoes Greens Butter, margarine	Assists formation and maintenance of skin and mucous membranes that line body cavities and tracts, such as nasal passages and intestinal tract, thus increasing resistance to infection.	Functions in visual processes and forms visual purple, thus promoting healthy eye tissues and eye adaptation in dim light.
Vitamin C (Ascorbic Acid)	Broccoli Orange Grapefruit Papaya Mango Strawberries	Forms cementing substances, such as collagen, that hold body cells together, thus strengthening blood vessels, hastening healing of wounds and bones, and increasing resistance to infection.	Aids utilization of iron.
Thiamin (B_1)	Lean pork Nuts Fortified cereal products		Functions as part of a coenzyme to promote the utilization of carbohydrate. Promotes normal appetite. Contributes to normal functioning of nervous system.
Riboflavin (B_2)	Liver Milk Yogurt Cottage cheese		Functions as part of a coenzyme in the production of energy within body cells. Promotes healthy skin, eyes, and clear vision.
Niacin	Liver Meat, poultry, fish Peanuts Fortified cereal products		Functions as part of a coenzyme in fat synthesis, tissue respiration, and utilization of carbohydrate. Promotes healthy skin, nerves, and digestive tract. Aids digestion and fosters normal appetite.
Calcium	Milk, yogurt Cheese Sardines and salmon with bones Collard, kale, mustard, and turnip greens	Combines with other minerals within a protein framework to give structure and strength to bones and teeth.	Assists in blood clotting. Functions in normal muscle contraction and relaxation, and normal nerve transmission.
Iron	Enriched farina Prune juice Liver Dried beans and peas Red meat	Combines with protein to form hemoglobin, the red substance in blood that carries oxygen to and carbon dioxide from the cells. Prevents nutritional anemia and its accompanying fatigue. Increases resistance to infection.	Functions as part of enzymes involved in tissue respiration.

SOURCE: Ruth M. Leverton, *A Girl and Her Figure* (Rosemont, Ill., 1976), pp. 10–11. Courtesy of National Dairy Council.

get energy. Chlorophyll in the leaves of green plants uses carbon dioxide, water, and the energy from the sun to form the chemical formaldehyde and its related acids. (These acids account for the sour taste of unripe fruit.) With continued chemical change—that is, with ripening—acids become sweet sugars. These, in turn, combine into starches. Then starches combine to form cellulose. These three—sugars, starches, and cellulose—are the most important forms of food **carbohydrates.** Cellulose and maple sugar are found in the leaves, wood, and bark of trees; grains contain starch, cellulose, and some sugars; fruits and vegetables contain all three carbohydrates.

But not all carbon dioxide and water in plants become carbohydrates. Some combine to form complex acids, the *fatty acids*. These are the chief constituents of **fats.*** Unlike carbohydrates and fats, **proteins** contain nitrogen. The nitrogen originally comes from air, which is essentially a mixture of oxygen, nitrogen, a small amount of carbon dioxide, and some rare gases. Twenty-three nitrogen-bearing acids, the **amino acids**, make up the body proteins. According to DNA instructions (Chapter 14), these twenty-three known amino acids are arranged in hundreds to thousands of ways to become the thousands of body proteins. Of these twenty-three, ten cannot be synthesized in the human body. Since they must be provided in the diet so that the body can make the proteins essential to life, these ten are called the *essential amino acids*. From these ten the body is able to build the remaining thirteen. Since a variety of animal proteins are sources of

the ten essential amino acids, they are generally superior to the vegetable proteins.

Thus, carbohydrates, fats, proteins—the three basic food constituents—are all manufactured, either directly or indirectly, by green plants. Normally, when consumed, carbohydrates and fats combine with body oxygen (a process called oxidation) to produce the energy the body needs to support life. With a diet deficient in carbohydrates and fats, the body must resort to using proteins for energy instead of using them for body growth and maintenance. Growth—indeed, basic health—is then impossible. Present in adequate amounts, carbohydrates and fats free the proteins from energy-producing duty and save them for body building.

Before an animal can begin to use the carbohydrates, fats, or proteins obtained from another plant or animal, it must break them down or *digest* them. Why? For two reasons. First, ingested food must be reduced to a size small enough to enter body cells. Second, within the far-flung billions of cell factories, the raw material must be reconstructed to resemble more closely the tissues to be rebuilt.

And so the processes of nutrition can become quite complex. However, in part, it remains simple: As stated in the Bible, "All flesh is grass."

The Vital Amines

VITAMIN C

With *scurvy*, a disease of dietary deficiency, there is bleeding of the gums as well as under the skin surfaces and into the exquisitely tender joints. Prevention and treatment of scurvy are accomplished by the use of vitamin C (ascorbic acid).

---

*Cholesterol, which is involved in fat digestion, is thought to be related to diseases of certain arteries, as was noted in Chapter 4.

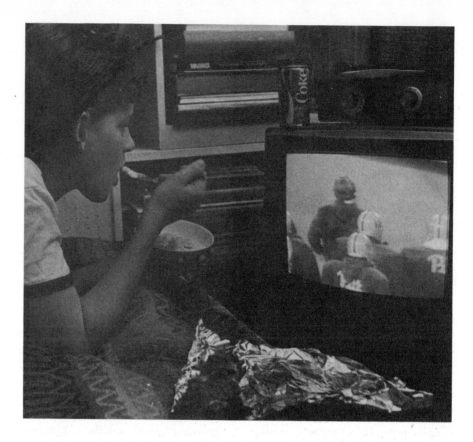

Inadequate nutrition is by no means a problem limited only to those with low incomes. Eating quick snacks that appease hunger but that are low in nourishment can be a dangerous practice.

The human body cannot manufacture an adequate supply of vitamin C, so we must depend on our diets to obtain it. Many commonly used fruits and vegetables (listed in Table 9–1) are rich in this vitamin. Unfortunately, vitamin C is unstable, easily destroyed. To prevent its being destroyed in the cooking process, vegetables should be dropped (undamaged) into a minimal amount of already boiling water and then immediately covered with a lid so that air will be kept out (and oxidation reduced). Since even slight alkalinity destroys vitamin C, soda should not be added to food that is being cooked. Modern food canning and freezing procedures retain most of the vitamin C contained in foods.

There are many who believe that large doses of vitamin C help to lessen the duration and complications of the common cold. Proof of this contention, however, today remains inadequate. Furthermore, it must be emphasized that large doses of vitamin C may be hazardous for some people. For example, long-term ingestion of large doses of vitamin C may have a bad effect on the way the body handles calcium and phosphorous.[4]

VITAMIN B

At the turn of the century, two Dutch doctors stationed in Java noted a curious coincidence in a prison yard. Prisoners and some hens in the prison yard shared both a diet of milled rice and a disease called beriberi. After a series of classic experiments, the doctors proved that the "rice polishings"—the germ and outer layer of rice, which are removed by milling—prevented the disease. It is now known that the outer husky portion of the rice grain contains B vitamins, particularly thiamine (vitamin B_1). In infants, beriberi is so rapidly fatal that an afflicted child may die only a few hours after being seemingly well. Even today beriberi is common among breast-fed children in Thailand, Malaysia, and Vietnam. When the mothers are given thiamine, recovery is dramatic.

NIACIN

In 1914, an American, Joseph Goldberger, turned his attention to *pellagra* (from Italian—*pelle*, "skin," + *agra*, "rough"). He proved that this disease, then common among many people in the southern United States, was due to the deficiency in the diet of a factor later named *niacin*, a member of the vitamin B complex. Opponents of Goldberger's dietary concept of pellagra insisted that the disease was infectious. In a series of human experiments begun on April 25, 1916, twenty men and two women—including Dr. and Mrs. Goldberger—swallowed capsules of concoctions of blood, feces, and urine of pellagra patients, which would surely have contained a variety of infectious agents. None of the human volunteers developed pellagra.

VITAMIN D

As dietary deficiency diseases, scurvy and beriberi are hardly alone. During the first few decades of this century, science shed light on more old dietary mysteries. The softening of children's bones from *rickets* had long been noted. The relationship of the illness to inadequate sunlight and its cure by cod-liver oil therapy was established many years before 1918, when an antirickets vitamin was first described. It required more years to prove that this vitamin—vitamin D—is manufactured in skin that is exposed to sunlight. Now it is known that vitamin D also is essential to maintaining the correct balance of calcium in the body. Calcium is important not only in the manufacture of bone, but in normal nerve functioning and in many important body reactions. When vitamin D is ingested, both the liver and kidneys take part in the complex process of maintaining the body's calcium balance. This helps explain why people with diseased kidneys lose bone calcium and fail to absorb calcium from the intestine.

VITAMIN E

Discovered more than half a century ago, vitamin E was noted to be necessary in the diet of female rats if

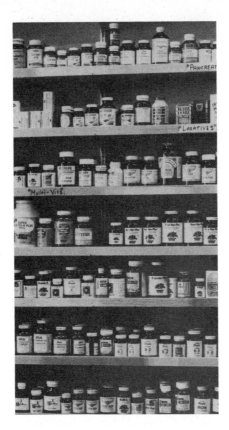

they were to reproduce normally. The vitamin was identified as an alcohol and given the name *tocopherol*. It is an essential nutrient, but in normal people whose diet is average, disease from vitamin E deficiency does not occur. Despite this fact, and despite the presently incomplete knowledge about the action of vitamin E in the human body, sales of it as a veritable cure-all are enormous. It is claimed that vitamin E improves the complexion and sexual potency, protects against miscarriage, pollution, and heart disease, and performs a host of other miracles. As yet, there is no scientific evidence to support such claims.

VITAMIN K

Vitamin K is essential for the manufacture of substances neces-

sary for normal blood clotting. Much of it is made by bacteria in the large intestine, and it is then absorbed into the circulatory system. When certain antibiotics are ingested orally, the intestinal ecosystem of these vitamin K-producing bacteria changes, so they may not survive. The interruption of the beneficial action of these bacteria in the human intestine can result in vitamin K deficiency—a good argument against self-medication.

MORE ABOUT VITAMINS

In 1912 the Polish biochemist Casimir Funk summed up what was known about vitamins at that time. Certain substances containing nitrogen are known as *amines*. There are four amines that are vital to life, Funk stated. These vital amines he called *vitamines*, and he held that each specifically prevents beriberi, scurvy, rickets, or pellagra. Funk was right, as far as he went. Now it is known that there are more than four such vital substances. Since new factors have been discovered, the "e" has been dropped in "vitamines."

Each vitamin is either water- or fat-soluble. The water-soluble vitamins are A, D, E, and K.

Vitamin pills never make up for an inadequate diet. Furthermore, their unwise use can be harmful. Folic acid (one of the B vitamins) and vitamin B_{12} are both needed by the bone marrow to make red blood cells. Used in high doses, folic acid relieves some of the symptoms of pernicious anemia. But folic acid does not halt the progressive destruction of the nervous system caused by pernicious anemia. For a while, a self-medicating individual with the disease may feel better. But that person has been lulled into a false sense of security. By the time medical care is sought, it may be too late to correct the error. The toxicity of excessive doses of vitamin D provides another example of the hazards of self-medication. Nausea, vomiting, and diarrhea may occur. Intake of too much vitamin A may cause serious signs and symptoms, including loss of appetite, irritability, abnormal skin pigmentation, dry skin, loss of hair, and bone and joint pains. Individuals should seek the advice of a physician about the use of vitamin pills.

Necessary Elements

The relative amounts of essential minerals in the human body vary greatly. An average-sized man has about two-and-three-fourths pounds of calcium in his body but a mere trace of iron. Although human requirements of most of the **trace elements** (elements that are essential to the organism although present only in minute quantities) have not yet been established, tiny amounts are known to exert an enormous influence. Zinc deficiencies, for example, have resulted in retarded adolescent growth and sexual maturation.[5] Some trace elements, though essential to life, may be harmful in larger amounts.

It is in calcium and iron that the diet of this nation's people is often poor. Foods with enough protein and calcium usually contain adequate phosphates too. Some foods (milk, for example) contain more calcium than others (such as eggs); some (milk, again) contain calcium that is more readily absorbed than the calcium in other foods (such as spinach).

Women need more iron than men. Periodic blood loss during menstruation and the increased needs during pregnancy account for the greater iron requirements of women. Iron deficiency among women is common. Also, during the growth years from infancy to adolescence, the need for iron is particularly great.

Water

People can live for weeks without food but only for days without water. Water accounts for more than half the adult body weight. It is the medium in which all chemical reactions of the body take place. Cells waiting to receive food are bathed in water. Two-thirds of the body's water is inside the cells, and one-third is outside. Nutrients are brought to the cells by the blood, which is about 80 percent water. After food has been used by the cells, there are waste products. These are transferred through watery solutions to the blood and excreted via the kidney in the urine, which is about 97 percent water. In the discussion of water pollution (in Chapter 2) it was pointed out that many industries now recycle their waste water, purify it, and use it again. The normal kidney has always done this efficiently. Large volumes of water carry waste to the kidney, but in passing through the kidney most of the water is reabsorbed and reused. The urine that is excreted is a concentrated watery solution of the body's waste products (see page 106).

Water has even more functions. In its involvement with the movements of the internal organs of the abdomen, and in the lubrication of the joints, water is essential to body mechanics. Too, water helps regulate body temperature.

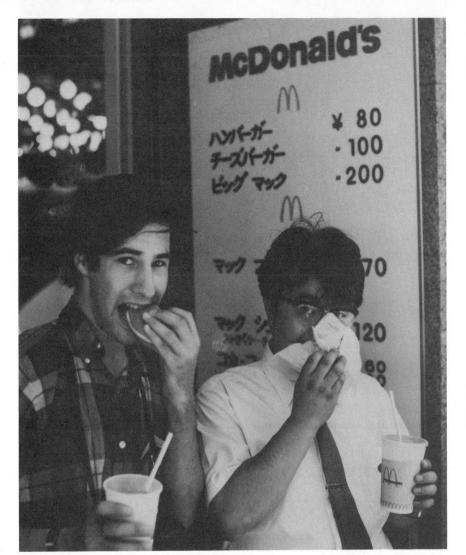

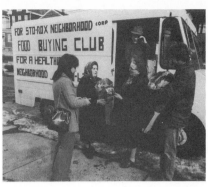

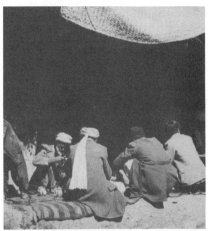

PHOTO ESSAY
Fast-food establishments are of many varieties and may be found in some very unlikely places.

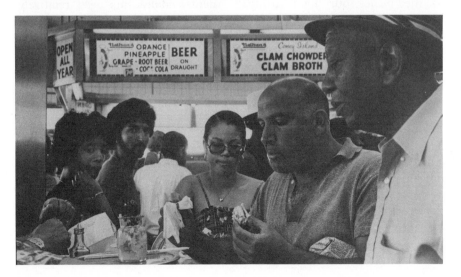

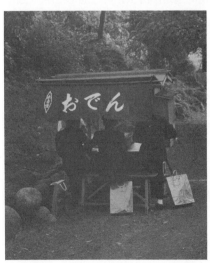

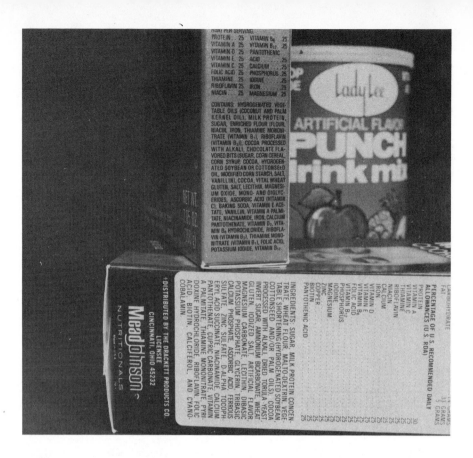

Undoubtedly, the federal law that requires content labeling on all food packages is a boon to consumers. But although we now know what is in our food, often the problem is understanding exactly what it does. Who, for instance, would know the effects to the body of D-alpha tocopheryl acid succinate or cyanocobalamin?

Some Measures of Nutrition

Calories

A **calorie** is the amount of heat required to raise the temperature of one gram of water one degree Centigrade. Because this is such a tiny unit of heat, nutritionists use instead the large **kilocalorie**, which is a thousand times greater than the calorie. The term "calorie" is now so commonly used, however, that the "kilo" is dropped in ordinary usage.

Caloric contents of food vary enormously. A given weight of fat contains over twice as many calories as an equal weight of carbohydrates or proteins. Proteins and carbohydrates each have four calories per gram. In a gram of fat there are nine calories.

What is adequate nutrition for the normal, nondieting person? One may rely on the food groups. Table 9–2 provides caloric values in single servings of representative samples of the basic four food groups —milk, meat, vegetable-fruit, and bread-cereal. It also includes representative fats and sweets. Table 9–3 gives the caloric values of some snacks. (Tables 9–4 provides another measure of adequate nutrition—the U.S. Food and Drug Administration's recommended daily allowances of certain nutrients.) A major advance in human nutrition is the statement of the nutritional content of foods in containers. In this way the customer can tell what nourishment is being bought.

With physical activity, calorie requirements increase. But age, sex, body size, and climate also influence the number of calories a person uses. Because of growth requirements, adolescents need relatively more calories than adults. The aged need fewer calories than the young. Women usually need fewer calories than men. Pregnancy and lactation increase caloric demands. A hot day, mostly because it decreases activity, decreases caloric needs.

Weights and Measures

It has been found that the people who are of average or slightly less than average weight at twenty-five are healthier and live longer if they maintain that weight for the rest of

TABLE 9—2
Caloric Values for Representative Foods, Classified by Food Groups

FOOD[1]	WEIGHT OR APPROX. MEASURE	CALORIES	FOOD	WEIGHT OR APPROX. MEASURE	CALORIES
MILK GROUP			**FRUIT GROUP**		
Cheese, Cheddar	1⅛ in. cube	115	Apple, raw	1 medium	70
Cheese, cottage, creamed	¼ cup	60	Apricots, dried, cooked	½ cup	135
Cream	1 tbsp.	35	Banana, raw	1 small	85
Milk, fluid, skim (buttermilk)	1 cup	90	Cantaloupe	½ melon	40
Milk, fluid, whole	1 cup	165	Grapefruit	½ medium	50
			Orange	1 medium	70
MEAT GROUP			Orange juice, fresh	½ cup (small glass)	60
Beans, dry, canned	¾ cup	250	Peaches, canned	2 halves with juice	90
Beef, pot roast	3 oz.	245	Pineapple juice, canned	½ cup (small glass)	60
Chicken	¼ small broiler	185	Prunes, dried, cooked	5 with juice	160
Egg	1 medium	80	Strawberries, raw	½ cup	30
Frankfurter	1 medium	155			
Haddock	1 fillet	135	**BREAD-CEREAL GROUP**		
Ham, luncheon meat	2 oz.	170	Bread, white, enriched	1 slice	60
Liver, beef	2 oz.	120	Cornflakes, fortified	1⅓ cup	110
Peanut butter	1 tbsp.	90	Macaroni, enriched, cooked	¾ cup	115
Pork chop	1 chop	260	Oatmeal, cooked	⅔ cup	100
Salmon, canned	½ cup	120	Rice, cooked	¾ cup	150
Sausage, salami	1 slice	135			
			FATS GROUP		
VEGETABLE GROUP			Bacon, crisp	2 strips	95
Beans, snap, green	½ cup	15	Butter or fortified margarine	1 tbsp.	100
Broccoli	½ cup	20	Oils, salad or cooking	1 tbsp.	125
Cabbage, shredded, raw	½ cup	10			
Carrots, diced	½ cup	20			
Corn, canned	½ cup	85	**SWEETS GROUP**		
Lettuce leaves	2 large or 4 small	5	Beverages, cola type	6 oz.	80
Peas, green	½ cup	55	Sugar, granulated	1 tbsp.	50
Potato, white	1 medium	90			
Spinach	½ cup	20			
Squash, winter	½ cup	50			
Sweet potato	1 medium	155			
Tomato juice, canned	½ cup (small glass)	25			

1. Foods on this list are in forms ready to eat. All meats and vegetables are cooked unless otherwise indicated.

SOURCE: From NUTRITION IN ACTION, Second Edition, by Ethel Austin Martin. Copyright © 1965, 1963 by Holt, Rinehart and Winston, Inc. Reprinted by permission of Holt, Rinehart and Winston.

TABLE 9–3
Caloric Values for Common Snacks

FOOD	AMOUNT OR AVERAGE SERVING	CALORIES	FOOD	AMOUNT OR AVERAGE SERVING	CALORIES
SANDWICHES	With bread:		CANDIES		
Hamburger	3-in. patty	330	Chocolate bars:		
Peanut butter	1 tbsp.	330	Plain, sweet milk	1 bar (1 oz.)	155
Cheese	1 oz.	280	With almonds	1 bar (1 oz.)	140
Ham	1 oz.	320	Chocolate-covered bar	1 bar	270
Pizza, cheese	⅛ pie	180	Chocolate fudge	1 piece 1-in. sq.	90–120
BEVERAGES			Caramels, plain	2 medium	85
Carbonated drinks,			Lifesavers	1 roll	95
soda, root beer, etc.	6-oz. glass	80	Peanut brittle	1 piece 2½ ×	
Pepsi-Cola	12-oz. glass	150		2½ × ⅜ in.	110
Club soda	8-oz. glass	5	DESSERTS		
Chocolate malted milk	10-oz. glass	500	Pie:		
Ginger ale	6-oz. glass	60	Fruit	⅙ pie	375
Tea or coffee, black	1 cup	0	Custard	⅙ pie	265
Tea or coffee, with			Mince	⅙ pie	400
2 tbsp. cream and			Pumpkin with		
2 tsp. sugar	1 cup	90	whipped cream	⅙ pie	460
ALCOHOLIC DRINKS			Cake:		
Ale	8-oz. glass	155	Chocolate layer	3-in. section	350
Beer	8-oz. glass	110	Doughnut, sugared	1 average	150
Highball (with ginger ale)	8-oz. glass	185	SWEETS		
Manhattan	average	165	Ice cream:		
Martini	average	140	Plain vanilla	⅙ qt.	200
Wine (muscatel, port)	2-oz. glass	95	Other flavors	⅙ qt.	260
Sherry	2-oz. glass	75	Orange sherbet	½ cup	120
Scotch, bourbon, rye	1½-oz. jigger	130	Sundaes, small chocolate		
			nut with whipped cream	average	400
FRUITS			Ice-cream sodas,		
Apple	1 medium	70	chocolate	10-oz. glass	270
Banana	1 small	85	MIDNIGHT SNACKS		
Grapes	30 medium	75	Cold potato	½ medium	65
Orange	1 medium	70	Chicken leg	1 average	88
Pear	1	65	Milk	7-oz. glass	140
SALTED NUTS AND			Roast beef	½ in. × 2 in. ×	
POTATO CHIPS				3 in. piece	130
Almonds, filberts,			Cheese	¼ in. × 2 in. ×	
hazelnuts	12–15	95		3 in. piece	120
Cashews	6–8	90	Leftover beans	½ cup	105
Peanuts	15–17	85	Brownie	¾ in. × 1¾ in.	
Pecans, walnuts	10–15 halves	100		× 2¼ in.	140
Potato chips	1 serving	108	Cream puff	4 in. diam.	450

SOURCE: Adapted from Helen S. Mitchell *et al.*, *Cooper's Nutrition in Health and Disease*, 15th ed. (Philadelphia: J. B. Lippincott Company, 1968), pp. 282–283. Data provided by Smith, Kline, and French Laboratories.

TABLE 9–4
U.S. Food and Drug Administration Recommended Daily Allowances
for Certain Vitamins and Minerals

VITAMIN OR MINERAL	UNIT	INFANTS (0–12 MONTHS)	CHILDREN UNDER 4 YEARS	ADULTS AND CHILDREN 4 OR MORE YEARS	PREGNANT OR LACTATING WOMEN
Vitamin A	IU	1500	2500	5000	8000
Vitamin D	IU	400	400	400	400
Vitamin E	IU	5	10	30	30
Vitamin C	mg	35	40	60	60
Folic acid	mg	0.1	0.2	0.4	0.8
Thiamine (B_1)	mg	0.5	0.7	1.5	1.7
Riboflavin (B_2)	mg	0.6	0.8	1.7	2.0
Niacin	mg	8	9	20	20
Vitamin B_6	mg	0.4	0.7	2	2.5
Vitamin B_{12}	mcg	2	3	6	8
Biotin	mg	0.05	0.15	0.3	0.3
Pantothenic acid	mg	3	5	10	10
Calcium	g	0.6	0.8	1.0	1.3
Phosphorus	g	0.5	0.8	1.0	1.3
Iodine	mcg	45	70	150	150
Iron	mg	15	10	18	18
Magnesium	mg	70	200	400	450
Copper	mg	0.6	1.0	2.0	2.0
Zinc	mg	5	8	15	15

SOURCE: *FDA Drug Bulletin*, December 1973.

their lives. (Table 9–5 lists desirable weights, by height and bone structure, for men and women aged twenty-five and older.) In addition, after one's maximum height is achieved, there is no need to gain more weight. Moreover, fat, muscles, organs, bones, and fluid all contribute to weight. Thus, a muscular athlete may weigh more than is recommended because of the weight of larger muscles. Such a person is heavy, but the problem is not excessive fat. Although modern charts attempt to correct this by adding body build to weight charts, the best way to determine actual body fatness is by measuring skinfold thickness with *calipers*. Norms for this measurement have yet to be completely agreed upon.

What is meant by overweight? The term does not mean excessive fat. A better term might be overheaviness. However, many nutritionists would agree that someone who weighs 10 to 20 percent over the desirable body weight is overweight. *Obesity* is a general term, commonly denoting 20 percent or more above the desirable weight. It results from an increase in the amount of fatty tissue. A person who is obese has three to five times more fat cells than one who is not. In addition, the fat cells of an obese person are greater in size. Fat cells of obese children six years old have been observed to have attained adult size.[6] By proper dieting and exercise, an obese person can lose weight. This is accomplished not by

reducing the number of fat cells, but by decreasing the fat content within these cells.

It is believed by some nutritionists that most fat cells are laid down during three different stages of life: first, during the late fetal stage; second, in the first year of life; and third, during early adolescence. Pinpointing, through research, the time of greatest multiplication of fat cells may well make the prevention or early treatment of obesity more likely. However, dietary limitations during these periods of fat-cell multiplication should be approached with great caution. It must be remembered that these are periods of significant growth, and unwise dietary practices during these times can cause much harm.

TABLE 9–5
Desirable Weights in Pounds for People Twenty-five or Over[1]

MEN HEIGHT[2] Ft.	In.	SMALL FRAME	MEDIUM FRAME	LARGE FRAME	WOMEN HEIGHT[2] Ft.	In.	SMALL FRAME	MEDIUM FRAME	LARGE FRAME
5	2	112–120	118–129	126–141	4	10	92–98	96–107	104–119
5	3	115–123	121–133	129–144	4	11	94–101	98–110	106–122
5	4	118–126	124–136	132–148	5	0	96–104	101–113	109–125
5	5	121–129	127–139	135–152	5	1	99–107	104–116	112–128
5	6	124–133	130–143	138–156	5	2	102–110	107–119	115–131
5	7	128–137	134–147	142–161	5	3	105–113	110–122	118–134
5	8	132–141	138–152	147–166	5	4	108–116	113–126	121–138
5	9	136–145	142–156	151–170	5	5	111–119	116–130	125–142
5	10	140–150	146–160	155–174	5	6	114–123	120–135	129–146
5	11	144–154	150–165	159–179	5	7	118–127	124–139	133–150
6	0	148–158	154–170	164–184	5	8	122–131	128–143	137–154
6	1	152–162	158–175	168–189	5	9	126–135	132–147	141–158
6	2	156–167	162–180	173–194	5	10	130–140	136–151	145–163
6	3	160–171	167–185	178–199	5	11	134–144	140–155	149–168
6	4	164–175	172–190	182–204	6	0	138–148	144–159	153–173

1. These figures are based on the person's wearing indoor clothing. For nude weight, women should subtract two to four pounds; men, five to seven pounds. Girls between the ages of eighteen and twenty-five should subtract one pound for each year under twenty-five.

2. Height is measured with shoes on: one-inch heels for men, two-inch heels for women.

SOURCE: Courtesy of Metropolitan Life Insurance Company. Derived primarily from data of the Build and Blood Pressure Study, Society of Actuaries, 1959.

Weighing Too Much

Why Do People Weigh Too Much?

A relatively small number of people are obese because of an endocrine gland disturbance. Specific tests help make such a diagnosis. There are others who, although spared an actual endocrine dysfunction, nevertheless have a hereditary tendency to being fat. This cause of obesity is said to be widespread. However, there is much about the problem of obesity that remains a mystery. It is surely true that some people can eat gluttonously without putting on weight; others, exercising just as little (or as much), gain weight on a relatively modest diet. The glutton's body metabolism is such that he or she handles food differently.

However, for a good many people, the problem is simpler. Their overweight is due to excessive eating and lack of exercise. Thus, their caloric intake exceeds their energy needs. The excess is stored as fat, and excess fat is detrimental to health. Labor-saving devices have eased life, but the food intake of the average U.S. citizen has not decreased along with energy needs. The customary snack between meals has added to the problem of weight control for the people of this nation. Small children and teen-agers may need between-meal fuel to help meet their growth needs. But it should be remembered that snacks represent calories, and calories do add up rather quickly.

Today, obesity caused by overeating is usually the result of intemperance. A vegetarian, the dramatist George Bernard Shaw was tall and thin. Greeting him on a London street one day, the short, stout writer G. K. Chesterton said, "From the looks of you, George, one would think there was a famine in England."

"And from the looks of you," replied Shaw, "one would think you had caused it."

Obesity: A Heavy Load for Mind and Body

To the emotional stress of the obese, one must add physical hazards. Fat people are more susceptible than the thin to sickness and death from heart disease, stroke, kidney disease, diabetes, and various diseases of the digestive system, such as gallstones and a variety of liver conditions. And the fat do not live as long as the lean. The only agent known to be capable of doubling rodent lifespan is caloric restriction.[7]

How to Reduce Weight Problems

EXERCISE

The child's training in weight control begins at home and may continue at school. People settling into the routines of their late twenties and early thirties often find them-

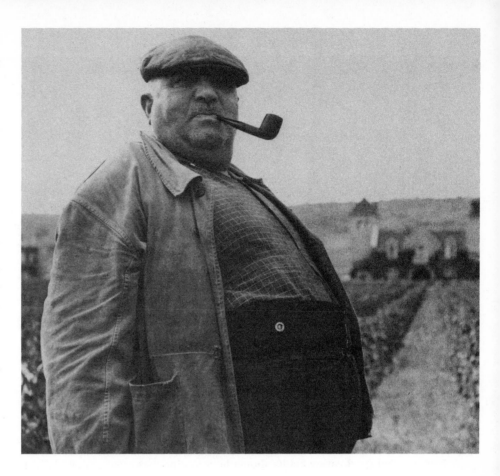

selves fitting tightly into their clothes. It is then that fewer calories are needed to maintain usual weight. A proper diet and exercise (see Chapter 8) should have been woven into the lifetime pattern long before this.

Moderate exercise over a *prolonged period* is an excellent reducer. Half an hour a day of vigorous handball or racquetball burns up, in a year, the equivalent of sixteen pounds of fat. (Table 8–1 on page 234 gave the caloric loss per hour resulting from various activities.) That moderate exercise increases appetite is a mistaken notion. Moreover, exercise improves muscle tone, creates a feeling of well-being, and relieves frustrations and tensions that tend to cause overeating. Not all exercise is equally effective, however. Far superior to weight lifting and sit-ups, for example, are swimming, bicycling, jogging, and walking.

DIETING

The would-be dieter is often exposed to a barrage of poor advice. Reliance on quacks, diet fads, and self-medication may all end disastrously. However, for many people, calorie counting ought to become a way of life. Nothing is more discouraging than repeated weight losses followed by repeated gains. Also, for many growing children, weight loss may be undesirable. During the growing period, good weight control may mean either maintaining the same weight for several months or decreasing the weight gain. The success of dieting, at that time, should not be measured by actual weight loss.[8] Dramatic weight losses during this stage of life are dangerous and should not be expected. But what is learned about being overweight during the growing years can later be put to good use.

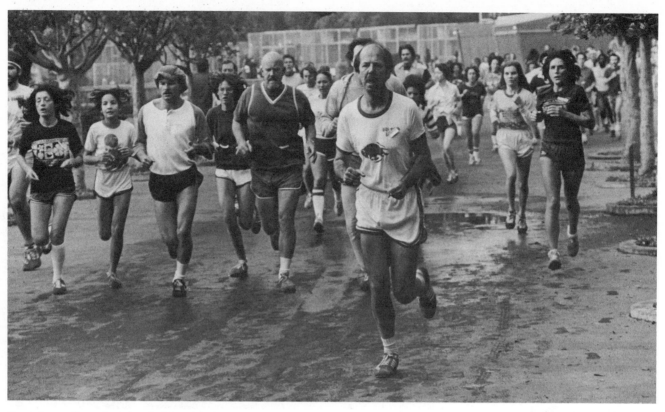

Exercise and good eating habits should be a routine part of everyone's daily life.

A varied, tastefully prepared diet is essential to morale. A snack one hour before a meal may be helpful to the dieter in reducing the appetite for the large meal. A lot of energy is required to use up relatively few calories (refer again to Table 8–1). For the dieter, exercise is essential, and vitamin supplements also are necessary for adults on weight-reduction diets.

To maintain their present weight, most normally active people need 15 calories per pound of weight per day. Assume that a man weighs, and wishes to stay at, 150 pounds. To *maintain* this desired weight, he may eat

150 × 15 = 2,250 calories per day

However, consider the individual who wishes to *reduce* his weight to 150 pounds. He wants to lose one pound a week. In each stored pound of fat there are 3,500 calories. Every day he must do with 500 calories less to lose one pound a week. The formula:

150 pounds (the desired weight)
× 15 calories
2,250 calories per day needed
      to maintain 150 pounds
− 500 calories per day to lose
      3,500 calories (1 pound)
      per week
1,750 total calories permitted
      per day to lose one
      pound per week

To lose *two* pounds a week, the same dieter would have to reduce his caloric intake by twice as much, or by 1,000 calories per day, which means he would be permitted to consume only 1,250 calories per day.[9]

It should be reemphasized that adolescent and adult overweight are not based on the same problem. All adolescents gain weight while growing. Increased fatty tissue (see page 273) is the problem.[10] The average growing teen-ager should not expect large amounts of fat to be lost. It is more realistic in early and middle adolescence to prevent further gain of body fat by eating what the rest of the family eats, whether it be pizza or potatoes, but in *smaller portions*. Nobody should go on a strict diet without first consulting a physician. Without close supervision, losing two pounds a week may be hazardous. Patients on diets of less than 1,000 calories per day are often admitted into a hospital for supervision of their diet.

Weighing Too Little

Justified concern with obesity has made the social life of the underweight individual much more pleasant than it was in former days. Even in comparison to persons of average weight, the thin person has better resistance to cardiovascular and renal diseases, to diabetes, and to accidents.

There is a hereditary aspect to being underweight; being lean often is a familial characteristic. However, when adults are more than 10 percent underweight, particularly if they are in their twenties, a physician's advice is indicated. By increasing their attention to some details, moderately underweight people usually gain weight. Among these details are elimination of infections, particularly of the appendix, teeth, and tonsils. Overactivity of the thyroid gland may need correction. Increased amounts of rest or a change to a job involving less tension may be indicated. Moreover, some people eat less because of anxiety or depression. These emotional problems will need to be treated before weight gain can be expected. Appetite-dulling tobacco is contraindicated.

High-protein drinks are especially helpful. There are several commercial preparations that provide an "instant breakfast." These are generally nutritious, and a glass or two of such a drink at each meal will substantially increase one's daily caloric intake.

The Hurt of Hunger

Retardation—whether physical, mental, or both—has multiple causes, varying from hazards within the uterus to those within the slums. The brain of a three-year-old weighs 80 percent of what it will weigh in adulthood, but the body weight at that age is only 20 percent of its adult weight. It is believed that during the early years of life malnourishment can do its greatest permanent damage. Childhood malnutrition is often the result of poverty, and since malnutrition can be one of the causes of retardation, the tragedy is doubled by the fact that the retarded child is unequipped to someday better his or her circumstances. Adult malnutrition results in inefficiency but is not thought to cause mental retardation.

Brain growth of protein-starved infants is markedly impaired. Chronic protein deficiency results in an apathy that translates into diminished learning potential. It is estimated that over 350 million children are affected. This equals about seven out of every ten children under the age of six throughout the entire world.

Are children in this country affected? An alarming prevalence of characteristics associated with undernourishment has been found. Indeed, 10 to 15 percent of all the children examined showed retarded growth levels and were therefore considered a high risk in terms of retardation of mental and physical performance.

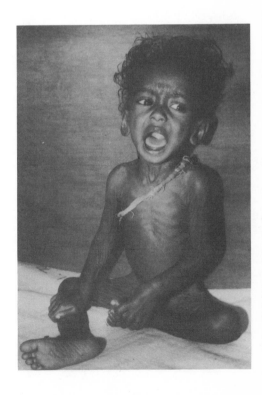

A hungry person is not free. This richest nation, which finds the means to war and explore, cannot afford to permit millions of its children to be permanently crippled by malnutrition and hunger; yet government programs to solve this problem are grievously inadequate.

Food Fads and Fancies

Organic Foods

Organic, natural, and *health foods* are not identical. **Organic foods** are those grown in soil that has been treated with organic matter, such as manure, vegetable compost, or natural and mineral fertilizers. Pesticides, antibiotics, and hormones are not used. Such foods are not processed; that is, they are prepared without the use of artificial food additives. Sometimes, however, processed foods are sold as organic because they were grown with the use of organic fertilizers and without pesticides.

Natural foods are not necessarily organically grown. They are merely neither refined nor processed, and thus they contain no additives. Examples of natural foods are honey, molasses, brown (unpolished) rice, and grains, whole or ground into flour.

The meaning of the term **health foods** is both unclear and misleading. This doubtless helps make them so profitable. Many buyers believe that products sold as health foods are both organic and natural and are therefore more healthful than other foods. This is not necessarily true.

Much of the current interest in organic foods is based on fears that conventionally grown foods are nutritionally inferior and dangerously contaminated by pesticides. What claims are made for organic foods? And what are the facts?

1 **The nutritional value of organic foods is higher than that of similar foods produced under ordinary conditions.**

The nutrient content of a plant is controlled not by soil conditions or type of fertilizer but by its genetic structure. Soil that is deficient in essential nutrients simply will not support plant growth. Fertilizers increase crop size, not nutrient value.

2 **The use of pesticides makes consumption of inorganially grown foods dangerous.**

Pesticides are sprayed on foods, not in them. They are easily washed or peeled off.

3 **Organic foods are always freer of contaminants such as bacteria, pesticides, natural toxins, and heavy metals (lead and mercury).**

Not so. Organic foods may have pesticides on them that were blown over from neighboring orchards and farms. Foods grown without pesticides are quite likely to have insect markings; therefore, damaged produce grown under ordinary conditions can easily be sold as organic. It is worth noting that long-estab-

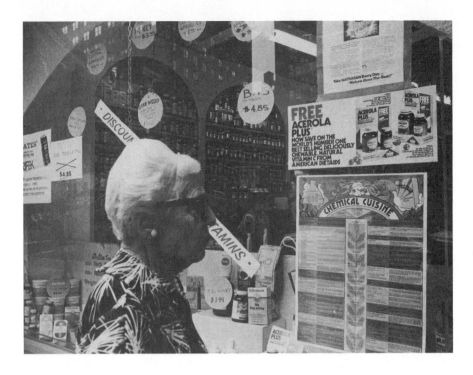

lished labeling and inspection standards regulate the quality of conventionally grown foods, but no such standards yet apply to the multimillion dollar organic food industry that supplies thousands of stores in the nation.

4 Organic foods can supply most of the food needed by the nation's population.

This impractical notion fails to consider that most people live in cities and that they desire foods grown in different climates. Such foods must be harvested before ripening, protected by pesticides, processed, and shipped great distances in order to make a variety of foods available year-round.

5 "Natural" or "organic" vitamins are superior to those manufactured by a reliable pharmaceutical company.

This claim is a fraud. Whether ex-tracted from a natural product, as is ascorbic acid (vitamin C) from rose hips, or made in the laboratory, the vitamin acts exactly the same in the body. Any specific vitamin has only one chemical structure.

Vegetarianism

The English dandy Beau Brummel was once asked if he ever ate vegetables. He replied, "I once ate a pea." Nevertheless, vegetarians abound in this and other cultures. Their reasons vary. For Bible Christians and Seventh Day Adventists, the reasons are religious. For Mahatma Gandhi, vegetarianism was a means of "calming the spirit and allaying animal passion." Others believe that a vegetable diet promotes intellectual capacity.

Vegetarians must endure considerable spoofing. Glancing at one of George Bernard Shaw's meals of vegetables drowned in oil, an observer once inquired of the dram-atist whether he was going to eat it or had already eaten it. A more serious problem for vegetarians is that of finding alternative sources of protein. Meats ordinarily contain ten essential amino acids; a single vegetable is rarely adequate in this respect. To meet daily protein needs, vegetarians must add other foodstuffs to their diets, such as milk, cheese, enriched corn and wheat, Brazil nuts, and soybean products. Soybeans are known to be a particularly valuable source of protein; they are also rich in phosphorus, iron, and calcium, and contain substantial amounts of vitamins A, B_1, and B_2. Calcium and iron are abundant in milk, cheese, fruits, and vegetables. Kidney beans, lima beans, whole wheat, peanut butter, and leafy vegetables are good sources of iron. There is no shortage of vitamin sources for the vegetarian: Spinach, turnips, dandelion greens, and broccoli are rich in vitamin A; soybeans, lima beans, peas, wheat germ, and salad greens provide B_1; B_2 can be obtained from milk, soybeans, spinach, and asparagus; a medium-sized orange or grapefruit supplies more than the presently accepted daily requirement of vitamin C. Complete vegetarians do not eat meat, fish, eggs, or milk products. Such individuals should be encouraged to eat a mixture of cereals, legumes, and nuts, and to take vitamin B_{12} supplements. Diets including milk products are usually adequate.[11]

Thus, there is considerable reason to believe that a well-balanced vegetarian diet can be adequate for health. Millions of the earth's inhabitants, however, are vegetarians not by choice, but by economic necessity. They suffer chronic protein shortages. Modern nutrition research leading to protein-enriched food products and high-protein strains of wheat, corn, and rice promises to make their diets adequate.

The Process of Nourishment

Nourishment depends on an intricate interplay of many organs and body chemicals. A special area in the brain's hypothalamus tells people whether they are hungry or full (see Body Chart 15 in the color section). Destroy the satiety center in an animal (that part of the brain that tells it that it has eaten more than enough), and it will gorge itself to obesity; damage the brain area signaling hunger, and the animal will die of starvation. However, the functions of nutrition begin even before food is ingested. It is now known, for example, that hunger is rarely the stimulus causing an ordinarily obese person to eat. It is the "hungry eye or nose."

Once food is ingested it enters the *digestive system** (illustrated in Figure 9–1), so the mouth and its associated structures contribute to the digestive process. For the moment, skip the first part of the digestive system and consider food in the small intestine. Nerves stimulate the contraction of the outer layers of muscle of the small intestine. This *mechanical* process propels the food within it and breaks it down into finer particles. Stimulated by nerves and hormones, intestinal glands in the lining of the inside of the small intestine produce *enzymes.*** The enzymes attack the food, breaking it down into even finer particles. This is a *chemical* reaction. So *digestion* is both a mechanical and a chemical process by which nutrients are broken down into smaller units. The digestive process makes possible the transfer of nutrients primarily from the small intestine into the blood and lymph channels. This transfer is called *absorption* and, like digestion, it is part of the nourishment process. After absorption, nutrients must be *transported* by the blood to the tissue

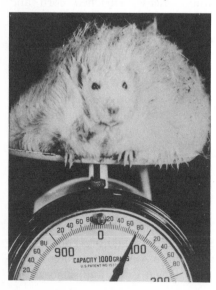

The fat rat in this photo weighs three to four times its normal weight. A small part of its hypothalamus was destroyed, and with it the ability to determine hunger and satiety.

*The *digestive system* includes the mouth and its associated structures, the pharynx, the components of the digestive tube, and the organs and glands associated with digestion. The *alimentary tract* or *canal* is that part of the digestive tract formed by the esophagus, stomach, and small and large intestines. The *gastrointestinal tract* includes the stomach and intestines. *Gastric* pertains only to the stomach.

**All plants and animals produce thousands of *enzymes.* These are proteins that increase the rate of a reaction without becoming a part of the products of the reaction. Since they are used up in the body's chemical processes, enzymes are continuously produced by the living cells.

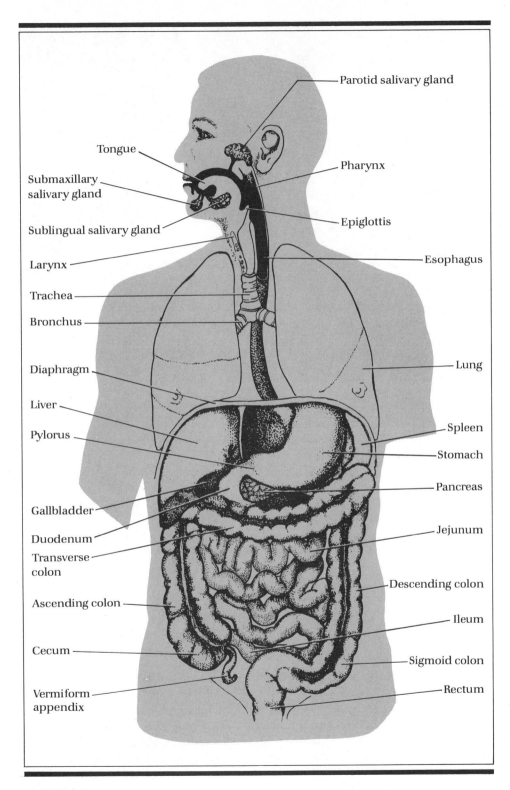

FIGURE 9–1
The digestive system. Parts of the respiratory system are also labeled here.
See also Body Chart 13.

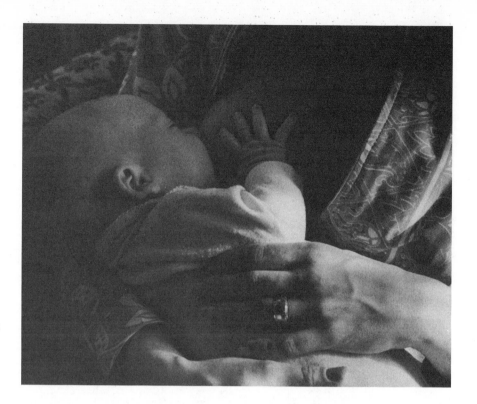

Infants often "practice" for this first meal while still in the womb. The sucking reflex begins to appear as early as the twelfth week of fetal development.

cells. By means of a *metabolism*, a complex chemical activity within the tissue cells, nutrients are converted into energy and are used to create new molecules for tissue. But not all nutrients are immediately used. Some, such as fat and vitamin A, are *stored* within specific cells. Other nutrients (proteins) are held in *reserve.*

Digestive Activity in the Mouth

Even on the first day of life, newborns drink sugar water or their mothers' early milk, making good use of their lips. Composed of muscle fibers, the lips are surrounded by a circular band of still more muscle, the *orbicularis oris.* The "little circle around the mouth" (translated from the Latin) curls the lips snugly about the nipple, sealing off air, making

sucking possible. The *orbicularis oris* is a sphincter muscle. "Sphincter" is Greek for "that which binds tight." Body sphincters do just that. By constricting a passage, the sphincter keeps it closed. It relaxes temporarily to permit some material to continue through the passage. For example, a constricted sphincter prevents food from prematurely leaving the stomach for the small intestine. When the sphincter relaxes, it helps to govern the amount of food that goes from one part of the passage to the next.

One cannot help admiring the constant labor of the heart. Consider, however, the *mouth.* It is used in talking, breathing, chewing, singing, whistling, coughing, vomiting, laughing, kissing, yawning, spitting, and other activities. But, through it all, one function is constant. The adult human mouth is not diverted from being the receptacle for a daily total of about two pints of saliva.

Food is taken into the mouth, passing under the nostrils. Then taste begins. Eliminate vision and smell and one cannot differentiate between wine and lemonade or between apples and potatoes.

The muscular *tongue* is covered with a great many fine, wartlike *papillae*. Within the walls of the papillae are the *taste buds*. The buds at the back of the tongue are sensitive to bitter; at the tip, sweet; at the sides, sour. In the tongue's center, the "zone of silence," there is no taste. People may make much of their cultivated taste, but compared with the cow's thirty-five thousand taste buds, our three thousand buds are few. Nevertheless, the tastes of human beings (including intermingled smell) are refined enough to recognize the finest size of grains, the subtlest body of liquids, the most piquant wines.

Skillfully guided by the muscular, shoveling, kneading tongue, the incisor teeth cut, the canines tear, and the molars masticate (chew) the solid food (refer back to Figure 8–14). In this maceration and fragmentation, the *salivary glands* have already begun to help. The mere thought of tasty food sets the brain to instruct the salivary glands to increase secretory activity. There are many salivary glands about the lips, cheeks, and tongue. Three pairs of them have been named: the largest of these are the *parotid glands* (in front of and below the ears); the others are the *sublingual glands* (in the floor of the mouth, beneath the tongue) and the *submaxillary glands* (under the jaw). (See Figure 9–1.) All their ducts empty into the mouth.

Since fish eat moist food, they neither have nor need salivary glands. But in one day, a drooling cow, confronted with a dry feed, can muster two hundred quarts of soft-ening saliva. For dry toast people need, and so produce, more saliva than for milk. In the human, to replace swallowed saliva and thus to keep the mouth moist, salivary secretion is continuous. In one ordinary lifetime, the specialized microscopic salivary cells secrete over fifty thousand pints of saliva—more than enough to fill two large swimming pools. This secretory activity, like all other body activities, requires energy available only through food.

Glands throughout the entire lining of the gastrointestinal tract secrete a slimy substance called *mucus*. Its chief chemical constituent is called *mucin*. Mucus lubricates the lining of the gastrointestinal tract in order to help the passage of its contents. In so doing it protects the inner lining of the tract from damage. Moreover, it can neutralize both acids and bases. Its value, for example, in protecting the stomach from the erosive action of the hydrochloric acid liberated there, is obvious. About half the saliva is mucus, and its mucin makes it sticky. The lubricative action of salivary mucus makes possible the swallowing of food. The other half of the saliva is a solution of a protein enzyme, *ptyalin*. This enzyme breaks down starch into simple sugars (maltose and dextrins). Thus does digestion begin in the mouth. It is in the mouth that food is rendered into a liquid or a semiliquid.

The mouth is an anatomic exception. All other body structures or cavities are lined with an unbroken layer of skin or mucous membrane. But in the mouth, that protective mucosal layer is penetrated by the erupted teeth. Also, nowhere else but in the mouth are there such anatomic connections as there are between tooth and soft tissue or between tooth and bone. Nor does the oral ecosystem promote tooth health. Swarming with microorganisms, often containing a bewildering variety of food chemicals, tolerating wildly fluctuating temperatures ranging from hot soup to frozen ice cream, containing gold, silver, cements, and plastics, enduring endless pollution and even small electric currents between dissimilar metals in the electricity-conducting saliva, the oral ecosystem is a challenge to dental survival. The teeth profoundly affect nourishment and health. (A discussion of these special body structures appeared in Chapter 8.)

Swallowing

Having been cut and ground to a pulp by the teeth, moistened by the saliva, and partly digested by salivary enzymes, the soft food mass is ready to be swallowed. *Swallowing* is the last voluntary digestive act. When the food is slid by the tongue into the *pharynx*, digestion becomes involuntary, automatic. The pharynx is in the neck, as is a small portion of its continuation, the muscular *esophagus*. The pharynx is a muscular passageway for both food and air. Above, it opens into the nasal passages; below, into the larynx. During swallowing, both of these openings, above and below, must be shut off. The *soft palate* and *uvula* (Latin, "little grape") shut off the upper nasal part of the pharynx. The *epiglottis* covers the larynx. Thus, without being forced back into the nose or into the larynx and bronchi,* swallowed food safely

---

*The *bronchi* are the larger air passages in the lungs and are continuations of the windpipe (page 218).

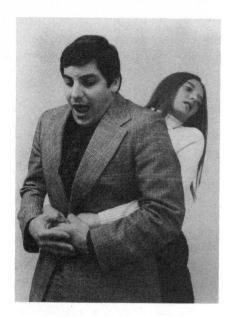

The Heimlich maneuver. This technique is used to prevent death by choking, which can happen when an individual's airways become obstructed by a piece of inadequately chewed food.

reaches the esophagus. This organ also secretes and is protected by mucus.

Food, even when liquid, does not swiftly drop down the ten-inch esophagus. The food dilates the esophagus, causing muscular contractions, or *peristalses.* Unless food is too hot or too large, it is not felt in the esophagus. The esophagus travels down the chest behind the heart, between the lungs, and through the *diaphragm* into the abdomen, where it empties into the stomach. Normally it takes about seven seconds for food to pass from the mouth through the esophagus and into the stomach.

The Stomach and Duodenum

The often-abused *stomach* is a muscular, distensible, bottle-shaped tube in the left abdomen. It is separated from the major chest contents (heart and lungs) by the *diaphragm.* Its usually empty upper portion, the *cardia*, may fill with gas, which can be expelled by belching. The stomach is closed off from the esophagus by the *cardiac sphincter* and from the small intestine by the *pyloric sphincter.*

Before leaving the stomach for the small intestine, some food may remain in the stomach for three to four hours. Other foods are fed into the small intestine within a few minutes. What determines this? The nature of the food. In their early digestive stages, meats tarry in the stomach. Soft drinks bubble on into the small intestine. For this reason, meats provide a greater sense of satiety, or fullness, than do soft drinks.

The inner mucous lining of the stomach contains millions of microscopic *gastric glands.* Their juice

contains three enzymes—*rennin, pepsin,* and *lipase.** (Rennin, a milk-coagulating enzyme, is found in the human infant, but not in the adult.) *Hydrochloric acid*** is also a part of gastric juice, as is a substance named the *intrinsic factor.* Without this factor, vitamin B_{12} would not be absorbed. This vitamin is necessary for red blood cell formation.

The entrance of liquid and semi-liquid food from the esophagus (through the open cardiac sphincter) into the stomach is the signal for the gastric glands to produce their juice. This secretion, in turn, stimulates the muscular stomach walls to begin peristaltic waves. (Peristalsis may also occur when the stomach is empty.) Food is then slowly and thoroughly churned with the acidic gastric juice. During this process, trapped gas in the stomach may move about, causing the stomach to rumble. Gas pressure against the stomach wall causes "hunger pangs."

It is in the stomach that an important problem is solved by nature. The problem is this: How can the stomach secretions carry out their basic function of beginning the digestion of proteins without also digesting the protein stomach lining itself? Part of the answer lies in the great amount of protective mucus secreted by the stomach. When its production is inadequate to deal with an increase of acid, an ulcer soon develops (see the following section). Another reason for the resistance of the stomach lining to digestion by its own secretions has to

*Refer back to the definition of enzymes in the footnote on page 281.
**The normal stomach is insensitive to the acid in the gastric juice. However, the "heart burn" that occurs with regurgitation of hydrochloric acid proves the esophagus to be quite sensitive.

do with the structural arrangement of its cells.

So the food is prepared in the stomach for its intermittent entrance into the approximately foot-long *duodenum*, the upper part of the small intestine. This happens at intervals, or from time to time, and not all at once. The opening of the stomach leading to the duodenum is called the *pylorus*. Only a small amount of food at a time is passed into the duodenal section of the small intestine. Food that is adequately mixed with acidic gastric juice causes the pyloric sphincter to open. As soon as food touches the alkaline intestine, the pyloric sphincter closes. Thus the acid stomach and the alkaline intestine are regulated to provide for intermittent opening and closing of the pyloric sphincter. And the extra mucin, made at the top part of the duodenum, protects the duodenum lining from the acid contents of the stomach.

PEPTIC ULCERS

A **gastric ulcer** is a break in the tissue of the stomach lining. Much more common, but similar, is the **duodenal ulcer.** Both are referred to as **peptic ulcers,** and they are treated similarly. Either ulcer may break into or erode a blood vessel, causing hemorrhage. Either may penetrate the wall of the involved organ, necessitating emergency surgery. Because some types of gastric ulcers are more likely to become cancers than are duodenal ulcers, the former can be particularly dangerous.

Peptic ulcers may occur at any age, even among children. Usually a peptic ulcer is first noted in the early thirties. Males suffer them four times more frequently than females. However, the increasing number of women exposed to the stresses of the competitive business world is causing this ratio to change. Although these ulcers do occur in relatively relaxed people, they are far more common in conflict-ridden, striving individuals. For this reason a duodenal ulcer is called the "executive's" disease.

Significantly, ulcers occur only in those areas of the digestive tract that come in contact with high concentrations of hydrochloric acid—the stomach, the duodenum, and the lower esophagus. The burning or gnawing abdominal pain of peptic ulcer usually begins two or three hours after meals. Occasionally pain will awaken an individual during the night. Milk, alkali, or food relieves the pain. Several hours after eating there is no food in the stomach to neutralize the excess acid secreted by the mucous membrane of the stomach. And it is the free excess acid that acts upon the ulcer, causing the pain. An X-ray usually reveals the ulcer, and laboratory analysis of the gastric juice shows abnormally high levels of acid. A reduction of stress-provoking stimuli; frequent intake of bland foods, such as milk and milk products; and complete abstinence from tobacco, alcohol, and coffee help recovery.

The Pancreas: A Double Gland

The head of the **pancreas** nestles in the duodenal loop, and its long body lies beneath the stomach (see Figure 9–1). Although it is the second largest body gland, the pancreas weighs only one-twentieth as much as the body's largest gland, the liver. Along with the duct from the liver, the *pancreatic duct* opens into the duodenal part of the small intestine.

Through the pancreatic duct pour the alkaline enzymes produced by the pancreas—*trypsin, amylase,* and *lipase.* Specialized cells of the pancreas also produce a carbohydrate-regulating protein called *insulin.* These cells are scattered throughout the tail of the pancreas as islands, and they are called the *islets of Langerhans.* They do not secrete into the pancreatic duct. Insulin is secreted directly into the blood. Thus, the pancreas is both an exocrine (ductal) and an endocrine (ductless) gland (see page 348). Failure of the islets of Langerhans to secrete enough insulin results in *diabetes mellitus*—a condition that will be discussed in detail in the Epilogue (page 476–479).

The Four-Lobed Liver

The multipurpose human **liver** fits under the diaphragm and occupies most of the upper abdomen, particularly on the right. It is truly a chemical factory. Not only does it produce bile, but it also chemically treats carbohydrates, proteins, and fats, preparing them for human cellular use. It detoxifies poisons, such as alcohol (see pages 202 and 204) and caffeine. It destroys bacilli. Like the muscles, it stores glycogen, a sugar. It manufactures carbohydrates from fats. It is also influenced by the emotions. Anger may temporarily stop the flow of bile, robbing one of an important body juice. Infections, such as viral hepatitis (see pages 76–77), may seriously threaten liver function.

The Sometimes Troublesome Gallbladder

Another name for the yellow, bitter bile secreted by the liver is *gall.* Before reaching the duodenum, bile stops to be stored and concentrated in a two- or three-inch pouch located under the right side of the liver. This is the **gallbladder** (see Figure 9–1). Concentration of bile in the gallbladder is accomplished when part of its water is absorbed by the mucous membrane of the gallbladder and returned to the bloodstream.

With entrance of food into the duodenum, the fat in the food stimulates the duodenal wall to liberate a hormone (cholecystokinin) into the bloodstream. This hormone, in turn, causes the muscular gallbladder to contract. Bile is thus forced from the gallbladder into its duct (*cystic duct*) and by way of the continuation of the cystic duct into the *common bile duct.* From the common bile duct bile enters the duodenum. Just before the common bile duct enters the duodenum, it is joined by the *pancreatic duct.* Thus, one duct carries both bile and pancreatic juice into the duodenum.

Bile contains three major constituents: *bile salts, cholesterol,* and *lecithin.* Bile salts hasten fat digestion by helping the moving intestine to break up (*emulsify*) large fat globules in the duodenum. The smaller, broken-up fat globules have more surface. This increased surface makes the fat more susceptible to the digestive action of the pancreatic enzyme, lipase. Cholesterol is a fatlike substance found in all animal fats; it is, therefore, a part of the normal diet. Moreover, certain body tissues synthesize cholesterol. Thus, there is a normal level of cholesterol in the human body. It is when the dietary intake of cholesterol is high that concern about it as a cause of atherosclerosis occurs (see pages 97–99). Lecithin is found not only in bile but also in nerve tissue, semen, and blood. A pigment called *bilirubin* gives bile

its golden-yellow color. Bilirubin is produced as the result of the ordinary destruction of worn-out red blood cells. The normal amount of bile pigment in the blood gives urine its characteristic straw color.

GALLSTONES

Some animals, such as the elephant, whale, horse, camel, and rat, do not have a gallbladder. Women, men, and mice have cause to envy them. Normal human gallbladder bile is 85 percent aqueous (prepared in watery solution). This aqueous solution of bile can ordinarily carry the solid 15 percent of bile salts, lecithin, and cholesterol in solution. However, the bile's ability to dissolve cholesterol (and thus keep it in solution) depends on the relative concentrations of bile salts and lecithin. Perhaps for genetic reasons, in many people this delicate balance functions inadequately. The excess cholesterol precipitates into tiny crystals, which adhere to one another, forming gallstones (see Figure 9–2).

Most gallstones do not cause symptoms. They may pass harmlessly from the gallbladder into its duct and, via the continuation of the cystic duct into the common bile duct, into the duodenum. They will then proceed down the intestine without incident. Often, however, they cannot pass through the ducts. The ensuing pain is agonizing.

Until recently, the only cure for symptomatic gallstones was surgical removal of both gallbladder and stones. The gallbladder is not an essential organ. Persons who have been surgically parted from their gallbladders are still able to adequately digest a fatty meal. It is estimated that over twenty million people in the United States have

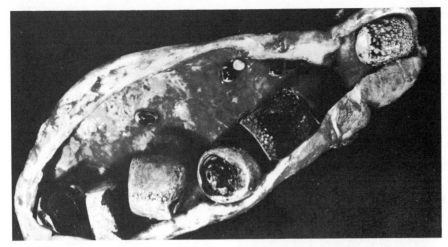

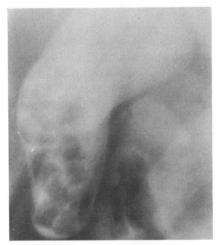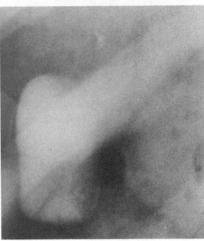

FIGURE 9–2
Top: Gallstones within a surgically removed gallbladder. Bottom left: X-ray of a gallbladder showing numerous gallstones. Bottom right: X-ray of the same gallbladder after a year of drug therapy that "dissolved" the gallstones.

The Tortuously Coiled Intestine

The *intestine* (see Figure 9–1) is divided into the long, narrow *small intestine* and the shorter but wider *large intestine*. Below the point of entrance of the small intestine into the large intestine is the dilated intestinal pouch, the *cecum*. From the cecum projects a narrow tube, the *vermiform appendix*.* The entire intestine of a dead human is about twenty-eight feet long. During life, however, the ability of the muscle layer of the intestine to contract (*tonus*) shortens the intestine to about ten feet. The large intestine, or *colon*, terminates in the four or five inches of *rectum*.

THE SMALL INTESTINE

The **small intestine** is the major digestive organ. Within it, digestion is completed. In its lower portion, absorption of the products of digestion into the bloodstream takes place. Encouraged by intestinal peristalsis, food morsels from the duodenum are mixed with pancreatic juice and bile. They are then pushed into the *jejunum* and then to the *ileum*, the final three-fifths of the small intestine.

Covering the inner lining of the small intestine are millions of *villi*

gallstones. These are about four times as common in women as in men, and they occur most frequently in middle age. Almost half a million operations for the removal of gallbladder and gallstones are performed yearly in the United States; of these, about six thousand people die postoperatively. For selected patients, chemical treatment may replace surgery. In an attempt to increase the bile's ability to dissolve stone, the use of a chemical

compound is being tried. Results at Minnesota's Mayo Clinic and in London are encouraging. Given before symptoms occur, the drug has been known to dissolve gallstones within one or two years. After symptoms appear, however, surgery is necessary because the drug requires so much time to be effective. Sometimes stones cannot be easily removed with surgery. A new chemical has been tried to finish the job successfully.[12]

*The opening of the cecum to the appendix is usually small. Cecal contents are ejected into the intestine with difficulty. The appendix may become plugged. Then its wall ulcerates. Inflammation (*appendicitis*) progresses. Eventually, the appendix may rupture. If this occurs, its spilled, bacteria-laden contents cause *peritonitis*—inflammation of the peritoneum. (The peritoneum is the membrane lining the walls of the abdomen and pelvis. Peritonitis also occurs with a perforated peptic ulcer.) To prevent all this, it is essential that a diseased appendix be surgically removed (*appendectomy*) as soon as possible. Appendicitis occurs more often in children than in adults, but the disease is more serious in adults.

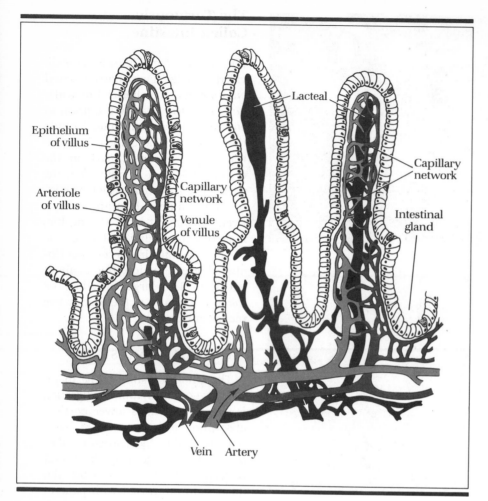

FIGURE 9–3
Villi in the small intestine. The villus at the left shows only the blood vessels; the villus in the center, only the lymph vessel (the lacteal); the one at the right is complete, showing both the blood and lymph vessels.

Labels in figure: Epithelium of villus; Arteriole of villus; Capillary network; Venule of villus; Lacteal; Capillary network; Intestinal gland; Vein; Artery

lymph vessels. The ingested food has been broken down. It can now be transported by the blood and lymph to the liver and from there, via the blood, to the body cells to be built up again into the carbohydrates, fats, and proteins of the human type. The products of carbohydrate and protein digestion first go directly to the liver and then to the other body cells. Not all the products of fat digestion follow this route. About 60 percent of the fat is first absorbed into the lymphatic system and then travels on to tissue. The rest goes directly to the liver. As droplets, fat may be stored in connective tissue cells. These storage cells make up *adipose* tissue.

About twenty million glands in the small intestine secrete an average of a gallon and a half of intestinal juice daily. Every day about 10 percent of the body's total water and salt enters the small intestine. Ninety percent of the total secretion is reabsorbed by the body tissues. What is lost is easily replaced. Thus not only digestion and absorption of food take place in the small intestine but also reabsorption of fluid. Usually it takes between three to four hours for food to pass through the small intestine into the large intestine.

(from the Latin *villus*, meaning "tuft of hair"). Villi are tiny finger-like projections extending into the intestinal canal (see Figure 9–3). It has been estimated that the total surface of the villi is about three thousand square feet. Combined with the intestinal folds and coiling, the villi enormously increase the digestive and absorptive surface of the small intestine. But that is not all. The surface of each villus is further increased by *microvilli*, which are visible under the electron microscope. These further increase the effective absorptive surface of the intestine thirty-fold. At the base of each villus, the *intestinal glands* secrete the intestinal juices. Carbohydrate-digesting enzymes, as well as enzymes for fat and protein digestion, are secreted in the small intestine. And along the entire inner surface of the small intestine is secreted a protective film of mucus.

It is from this remarkable inner surface of the small intestine that food is absorbed into the blood and

THE LARGE INTESTINE

Entering the **large intestine,** or the **colon** (see Figure 9–1), from the small intestine, through the ileo-colic sphincter, is a semifluid material.* Bereft of nutrient, it is waste—largely water. However, salt, bile, and undissolved (even un-

*A chronic ulceration of the colon (*ulcerative colitis*) occurs in both children and adults. Its cause remains unclear. Many physicians consider it of psychosomatic origin.

digested) food are contained in it. As in the esophagus, digestion does not occur in the large intestine. Water absorption in the large intestine causes the contents to solidify and to form *feces* (from the Latin *faeces*, meaning "refuse").

Fecal material should be soft and formed like a column. Consistently fluid adult feces (*diarrhea*) or small pieces expelled with difficulty (*constipation*) merit investigation by the physician. If severe diarrhea occurs, digestive enzymes enter the large intestine. Since they do not normally belong there, they are irritating.

Here again the protective mucus secreted by the large intestine is helpful. Feces are expelled from the rectum through the rectal opening, the *anus*. Regulating this passage of waste material from the body is the anal sphincter. With this, the process of digestion is completed.

Summary

Taste is determined by a number of factors, including cultural and individual emotional preferences and the color and texture of food. While any animal may have hunger, only humans can have appetite. This is because only humans impart emotion to the sharing of a meal.

The six basic constituents of food are carbohydrates, fats, proteins, vitamins, minerals, and water. All human food ultimately comes from green plants. The chlorophyll of these plants uses water, carbon dioxide, and the sun's energy to produce, either directly or indirectly, carbohydrates (sugars, starches, and cellulose), fats, and proteins. These are ingested by animals and reconstructed to fulfill their body needs.

Vitamins are nitrogen-containing substances that are vital to life. They may be either water-soluble (as are vitamins A, D, E, and K) or fat-soluble. Vitamin C, or ascorbic acid, is found in fruits and vegetables and is necessary to prevent scurvy. The B vitamins, found in unmilled grains, prevent beriberi. Niacin, a member of the vitamin B complex, also prevents a skin disease called pellagra. Without vitamin D, the body is unable to maintain the correct balance of calcium, which is necessary to bone manufacture, nerve function, and many body reactions. One disease of vitamin D deficiency is rickets. Sunlight and cod-liver oil help prevent this disease. Disease from vitamin E deficiency is uncommon with an adequate diet. Vitamin K, manufactured by bacteria in the large intestine, is essential to the process of blood clotting. Vitamin pills cannot make up for an inadequate diet, and self-medication can be quite hazardous.

Trace elements are minerals that are essential to the organism although present in minute amounts. Some of the minerals needed by the human body are calcium, zinc, and phosphorus. Women need more iron than men. Water must be ingested much more frequently than food. All chemical reactions of the body take place in water. Water is also essential to body mechanics and the regulation of body temperature.

A calorie is the amount of heat required to raise the temperature of one gram of water one degree Centigrade. Nutritionists actually use the kilocalorie, which is one thousand times greater. All foods have their own caloric value. The number of calories required by a person is a very individual matter, depending on age, sex, body size, climate, and physical activity.

Although endocrine gland dysfunction and heredity can cause a person to be overweight, the problem usually arises when calorie intake exceeds the body's energy needs. Being above one's optimum weight results in emotional and physical stresses, and it can shorten one's life expectancy. Weight is best reduced by moderate exercise over a long period of time and by a sensible, balanced diet that cuts caloric intake enough to lose one to two pounds a week. Dramatic weight losses through fasting or fad diets will not be maintained and can also be dangerous.

Being underweight may have a hereditary aspect. However, this condition may also be caused by infection, an overactive thyroid gland, anxiety, depression, tension, or even smoking.

Malnourishment is common in children throughout the world, even in the United States. These children run a great risk of being both mentally and physically retarded. Malnourished adults suffer from inefficiency but not retardation.

Organic foods are those grown without the use of pesticides, antibiotics, or hormones; they are not processed. Natural foods are not necessarily organically grown, but they also are not processed. Health foods are generally assumed by the buyer to be organic and natural, but this may not be true. Organic foods and vitamins are not necessarily freer of contaminants than, or nutritionally superior to, ordinarily grown food.

The reasons for a vegetarian diet vary widely, though they are often religious in nature. A well-balanced vegetarian diet can be adequate for health, but such a diet requires more care, especially in finding alternative sources of protein.

Digestion is both a mechanical and a chemical process that breaks nutrients down into units small enough to be transported from the intestine by blood circulatory channels to the tissue cells. Here the nutrients are either stored or converted into energy and used to create new molecules for tissue.

Digestion begins in the mouth, where food is ground up by the teeth and mixed with saliva. Saliva both softens the food, allowing it to be swallowed, and breaks starch down into simple sugars. Swallowed food is moved through the pharynx and the esophagus by muscular contractions, or peristalses. (The epiglottis prevents food from going into the larynx.) Then the food passes through the cardiac sphincter into the stomach, where it is acted upon by hydrochloric acid and three enzymes—rennin, pepsin, and lipase. (In some people, especially those under much stress, the acidic stomach juices may eat through the mucous membrane of the stomach, lower esophagus, or the duodenum, causing an ulcer.) Food that is adequately mixed with the gastric juices passes through the pyloric sphincter into the duodenum, the upper part of the small intestine. The pancreas releases into the duodenum alkaline enzymes—trypsin, amylase, and lipase—which neutralize the acidic gastric juices. Bile, produced in the liver and stored in the gallbladder, also enters the duodenum. Bile hastens the digestion of fat. Intestinal peristalsis moves the contents of the duodenum into the remaining sections of the small intestine—the jejunum and the ileum. Millions of fingerlike projections called villi cover the inner lining of the small intestine. These and the microvilli on them greatly increase the digestive and absorptive surface of the small intestine, which is already long and greatly coiled. Intestinal glands at the base of the villi release enzymes that further digest carbohydrates, fats, and proteins. The fully digested food is now absorbed by the small intestine's surface and transported by lymph and blood to the liver, and then by blood to the body cells. Fats may not follow this route but may instead go directly by lymph to the fat cells. The remaining waste material passes into the large intestine, or the colon, where its water is absorbed so that feces are formed.

References

1. *Wisconsin State Journal* (August 11, 1959), cited in Frederick J. Simoons, *Eat Not This Flesh* (Madison, Wis., 1961), p. 91.
2. Quoted in C.A. Wagner, *Harvard—Four Centuries and Freedoms*, cited in Adelia M. Beeuwkes, E. Neige Todhunter, and Emma Seifert Weigley, eds., *Essays on History of Nutrition and Dietetics* (Chicago, 1967), p. 154. Asa the Scribe, whose real name was Asa Dunbar, was the grandfather of Henry Thoreau.
3. Dorothy V. Whipple, *Dynamics of Development: Euthenic Pediatrics* (New York, 1966), pp. 368–369.
4. R.G. Brown, "Possible Problems of Large Intakes of Ascorbic Acid," *Journal of the American Medical Association*, Vol. 224 (June 11, 1973), p. 1530.
5. Michael Hambidge and Donough O'Brien, "On Developmental Nutrition: Trace Metals," *Ross Laboratories*, No. 7 (March 1973), citing J.A. Halsted et al., "Zinc Deficiency in Man," *American Journal of Medicine*, Vol. 53 (1972), pp. 277–284.
6. "Control of Hypercellularity Held 'Best Hope' in Obesity," *Pediatric Currents* (Ross Timesaver), Vol. 22 (May 1973), p. 1, citing J.L. Knittle, *Journal of Pediatrics*, Vol. 81 (1972), p. 1048.
7. Alex Comfort, "Eat Less, Live Longer," *New Scientist*, Vol. 53 (March 30, 1972), p. 689.
8. Johanna T. Dwyer, Caroline V. Blonde, and Jean Mayer, "Treating Obesity in Growing Children," *Postgraduate Medicine*, Vol. 51 (May 1972), p. 93.
9. Council on Foods and Nutrition, American Medical Association, *The Healthy Way to Weigh Less*, cited in Mort Weisinger, "How to Stick to Your Diet," *Today's Health*, Vol. 51 (July 1973), p. 35.
10. Felix P. Heald, "Treatment of Obesity in Adolescence," *Postgraduate Medicine*, Vol. 51 (May 1972), p. 112.
11. "Vegetarian Diets," *The Medical Letter*, Vol. 21 (July 27, 1979), p. 63.
12. "Cholesterol Stones Dissolved Harmlessly," *Medical World News*, Vol. 19 (November 13, 1978), p. 28.

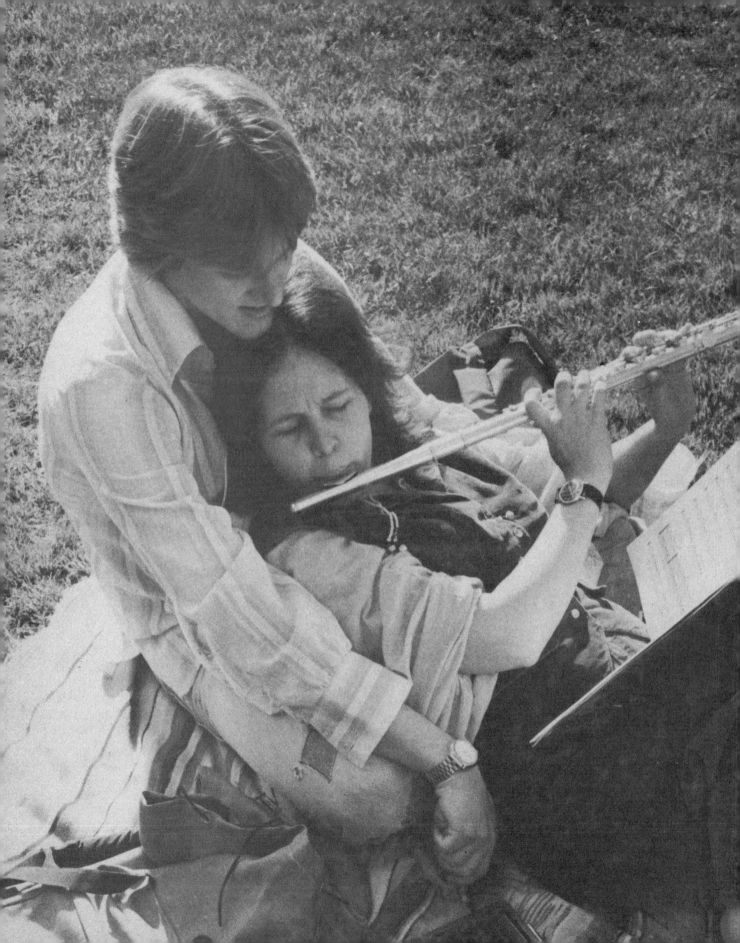

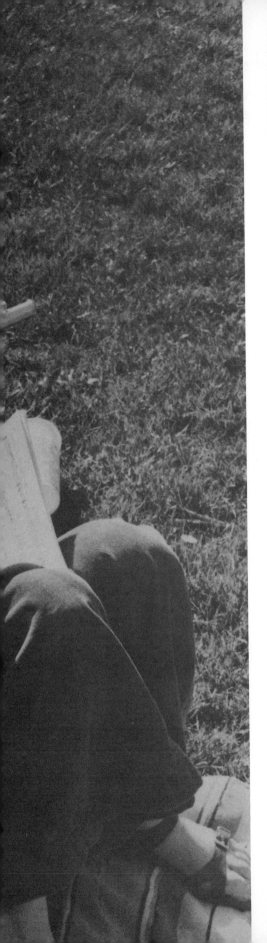

10
Courtship and Marriage

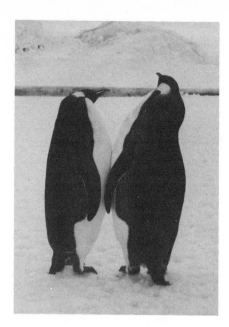

Penguins courting.

Courtship and Conquest:
Animal Instinct, Human Learning

*They dream in courtship, but in wed-
   lock wake.*

ALEXANDER POPE

"The snail is a hermaphrodite: male
and female are incorporated into
one; there is no he and no she.
Perhaps that is why snails are so
sluggish; they have nothing to stir
them, nothing to fight for, nothing
to pursue, nothing to win."[1] Almost
all other creatures, however, actively differentiate between the sexes,
and engage in elaborate mating rituals too. For elegance and variety,
nonhuman courtship is both instructive and humbling. The fighting fish of Siam do an underwater
courtship ballet, the color, grace,
and timing of which would delight
the most exacting dancing master.
And the female cricket knows true
devotion. Responding to a phono-
graph record playing the ardent
chirp of a long-dead male cricket,
she will desert locally available
swains. Hurrying a considerable distance, she will lovingly seek an approach into the record player.[2] Gift
giving, too, is not unknown to creatures that go courting. Indeed, with
some species of spider, an empty-
handed male may become a snack.
So, instinctively, he often arrives
with a fly, carefully gift-wrapped in
silk. Dancing a specific pattern and
displaying his markings, he can only
trust to luck. As for higher animals,
the complex courtship that goes on
among penguins, for example, or
among monkeys and apes has long
fascinated zoologists.

And so, all in season, the nonhuman world is a rhythmic maneuvering of courtship, a pervasive,
instinctive planning for new life. Instinctive, not learned. But people
need to be taught the art of courtship and love. Among earth's creatures, people are almost alone in
becoming confused by such matters.
Our confusion is created by our
culture.

Social Codes and Health:
A Review

This culture is based on Judeo-
Christian traditions. These can be
traced to the age of the biblical Hebrews. The family was established
as an institution to provide stability
and protection for the group. In the
home of the ancient Hebrews, the
father was the head and the mother
the heart of the family.

From the Hebrews, the early
Christians got a model for building
a stable family structure. From the
Romans, they learned the price of
excessive societal laxity and disrup-
tion of normal family life. Three
Punic Wars against Carthage (in the
second and third centuries B.C.) occupied Rome for over a century.
These had made many Roman
families enormously rich. Roman
sons were constantly off at war.
Fathers consequently placed their
daughters in positions of wealth and
indirect power. Roman women of
leading families began to vie with
one another and with men for
power. The Roman statesman Cato
the Elder, reflecting on the sexism of
that age, complained bitterly: "All
men rule over women, we Romans
rule over all men, and our wives rule
over us." Contemptuously, Roman
men rejected marriage. "Why do I

not marry a rich wife?" asked a Roman writer. "Because I do not wish to be my wife's maid."[3] Laws penalizing celibacy were to no avail. The upper classes, remaining childless, customarily adopted children for purposes of inheritance. Divorce, previously rare, became widespread. Marriage became a cynicism. Slaves cared for children, and the children were spoiled. "Expressions which would not be tolerated even from the effeminate youths of Alexandria," wrote the Roman teacher Quintilian, "we hear from them with a smile and a kiss."[4] The family structure crumbled. Luxury and laziness replaced the formerly strict family life. The public amorality of the highborn also became a way of life for the middle classes. Other factors, such as widespread malaria and an overextended economy, certainly helped to enfeeble the once mighty empire. But a basic flaw marred Rome. The vitality of the family had been wasted. Rome collapsed, and upon its ruin, Christianity began to build.

The year 312 saw Christianity legally recognized by the decaying Roman Empire. Observing the social disarray about them, the early Christians were determined not to repeat the errors of their predeces-

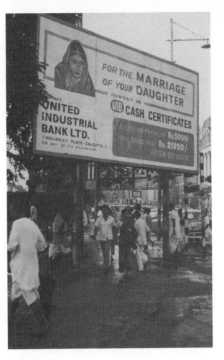

Marriage customs differ the world over. In the United States— apparently unlike in India—we usually subscribe to Shakespeare's notion (from his play *King Lear*) that "she is herself a dowry."

sors. Polygamy, practiced by the Hebrews, was rejected. Roman sexual looseness was condemned, as were the abortion and infanticide and the divorce and adultery of the Greeks and Romans. In this atmosphere, sexual permissiveness was out of the question. In fact, sexuality was sinful. Centuries passed before

even marital sexual intercourse became more than a need to be tolerated only because it provided children.

This is not to say that rigid sexual regulations immediately took hold in the Christian world. Controls developed gradually. It was not until 786 that the Anglo-Saxon Synod passed a decree ensuring permanence to marriage. Indeed, up to the Reformation, one year's trial marriage was practiced in Scotland. The Church, however, held fast. Gradually its precepts took hold. Yet, restrictive rules were retained. Those who took short cuts found society harsh indeed. Why? Because their actions threatened the family as the basic unit of society and, therefore, threatened society itself. If the way of life was to survive, it was essential that sexuality and mating be controlled.

The Judeo-Christian culture, then, established basic marriage codes that have endured for the Western world. Often, these codes have been supported by threat and guilt, two powerful tools of Western society. But guilt promotes anxiety. Prolonged, unresolved guilt may become disease. That is why the origins of marital codes merit some exploration in a health book.

The Lover, Whom All the World Does Not Love

Primitive Courtships

The tribulations of love and courtship vary from culture to culture. Among the Macusis of British Guiana, a young swain may not choose a wife until he has proved his courage. One way to demonstrate it is by allowing himself "to be sewn up in a hammock full of fire ants."[5]

The hopeful Arab bridegroom of Upper Egypt displays his valor by undergoing a severe whipping by the bride's relatives.[6] The romantic maneuvering among the young of one Bolivian Indian tribe is no less hazardous:

Ordinarily young people of nubile age are supposed to be shy

of one another, and while tending herds pass one another by many times without apparently seeing each other. Around Camata, if a boy . . . wishes to take notice of a girl, he picks up a handful of fine earth or dust and throws it at her. This is a first step of courtship. . . . The next time they meet, the boy picks up some fine gravel, and the girl may do likewise. If they continue to be interested this goes on until finally they throw rocks at each other. Informants told me that there were two cases of deaths in Camata during the last four years from such a cause; one woman received a fractured skull and the other a broken back.[7]

Yesterday's Courtships

In 1700 the British Parliament enacted the following:

> That all women of whatever age, rank, profession or degree, whether virgin maid or widow, that shall from and after such Act impose upon, seduce and betray into matrimony any of His Majesty's subjects by means of scent, paints, cosmetic washes, artificial teeth, false hair, Spanish wool, iron stays, hoops, high-heeled shoes or bolstered hips, shall incur the penalty of the law now in force against witchcraft and like misdemeanors, and that the marriage upon conviction shall stand null and void.[8]

It was perhaps such legislation that prompted the degree of cautious honesty, if not outright optimism, so often proclaimed as proper in eighteenth-century English books on model letter-writing. One such volume, the *New London Letter Writer*, includes a model letter entitled, "From a Young Lady After Having Smallpox to Her Lover." Apparently, the young man had led her to believe that "the beauties of my person were only exceeded by the perfection of my mind." She was, therefore, not regretting too much the loss of her good looks, for "it gives you a happy opportunity to prove yourself to be a man of truth and veracity."[9]

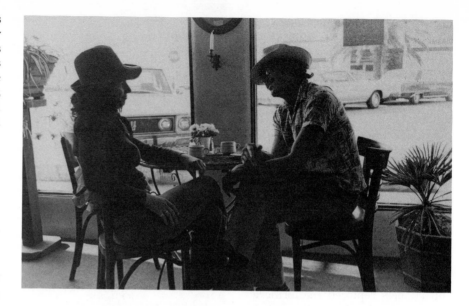

Many years later, in the nineteenth century, English lovers, for reasons of their own, were wont to go skating. Since chaperones rarely skated, they were benched on the sidelines. But they kept a keen eye on the action. A Mrs. Burton Kingsland, composing for the *Ladies Home Journal* (circa 1900), prepared this brief, but presumably effective, speech to be made by a young lady whose debauched swain had slipped his arm about her waist: "Don't you think it rather cowardly for a man to act toward a girl as you are doing when she has trusted him and is in a measure powerless to resist such familiarity?"[10]

Things have changed.

Modern Courtship

Perhaps it is during a shopping tour with their parents that modern children gain the first unconscious tips for random dating. Random dating is just shopping around. One does not have to buy. There is time for window-shopping. If one chooses, one may come in and browse. Sometimes, a small investment is made. By telephone, one learns a lot and overcomes much. Everybody gets stung a little, some more than others. But one gets to know the game. And, in the end (with luck), one sees enough and adds up enough experience to get some idea of what one needs, what to look for, and what commitment may be safely made. People of some other countries view random dating with astonishment. For them, the sheer number of dates per teen-ager is fickleness amounting to immorality. And the absence of a chaperon is regarded as an open invitation to family dishonor.

It is in the turbulent, searching years of adolescence that a person must begin learning the mating game. It is in this anxious time of searching for a self-acceptable self, of trying to settle on a life's work, of attempting to cope with overwhelming bodily changes, and of beginning a separation from one's parents that the dating dilemma occurs. The dilemma is this: Without being clearly told what is expected of them, teen-agers are nevertheless given to understand that much is expected of them. "Grow up," they are told, yet they are forbidden to do what they see grownups do. Driven by urges they have not yet learned to understand or control, they attempt to answer them as grown-ups do. With the paraphernalia of sexual activity, such as cars and condoms, readily available, what is missing? A chaperone? In this society, she is all but extinct.

Strict rituals of courtship are still routinely followed in some countries; indeed in some places, parents and families play a large role in them. In this country, however, there has been a tendency for the ways of courtship to be largely decided by the two people involved. Courtship—the time spent in preparation for marriage—has become a somewhat more casual understanding between couples. In many, though not all, cases, formal engagements are no longer considered necessary. There is some data that is almost ten years old suggesting that formal engagements are less inclined to be terminated than informal understandings. Whether this is still true today needs continued study. In any event, some form of courtship lasting at least a year is a valuable way of learning something about the potential partner. Something. Not all. Too often couples do not take advantage of the courtship period to gather useful information about each other. Instead, they drift from a dreamy romance into an all too realistic marriage. The awakening can be quite rude. It is essential to a good marriage for each partner to know what the other expects of marriage, and for both to realize that it cannot be one long romantic song. As we shall see, this does not mean that marriage need be a crashing bore, but it does mean that one should have some idea of what one is getting into.

Why Marry?

Over 90 percent of the people in this nation marry at least once in their lives, and about four out of five of those who divorce marry again. What makes marriage so popular?

There is no single reason why people marry. Some unmarried men seek wives, and single women husbands, so that they will not be alone. Other reasons include social pressure, a wish to share ideas and experiences, sexual desire and satisfaction, and financial security. But the majority of people marry because they seek a meaningful, sharing relationship with another.

To want and be wanted by someone, to share confidences, and to give and receive affection are universal human needs. A successful marriage cannot be an escape from a lonely, self-centered, downbeat emotion. It is a positive and creative opportunity for the maximum self-realization of two people. Successfully married people can take and give affection. They can confide in each other without fear of harsh judgment. They can cry together and not be ashamed. They can disagree, even quarrel violently, and know it is not the end. They are busy, not only with each other, but with a variety of life's challenges in and out of the home. They respect and enjoy each other's minds and bodies. In no other human relationship can this kind of mutuality be developed. But the skills involved in building and sustaining such a relationship are not easily acquired. Successful marriages require work. And, to be effective, that work needs love. It is love that stirs the human heart. What can be said about love?

Love: The Substance of Life

There is a land of the living and a land of the dead and the bridge is love, the only survival, the only meaning.[11]

Life begins and ends with separation. Both are inevitable. Each has its own poignancy.

There is separation at birth. Filling the gulf is love. Without mothering, without embracing love, the infant suffers. Yet, mothering is not smothering. True mother love teaches further separation. The constancy of the mother's love, even after her child's departure, is mirrored by the child's ability to learn to love others in later life.

During the course of normal learning, children explore their bodies and come to love themselves. This self-love is not necessarily selfish.

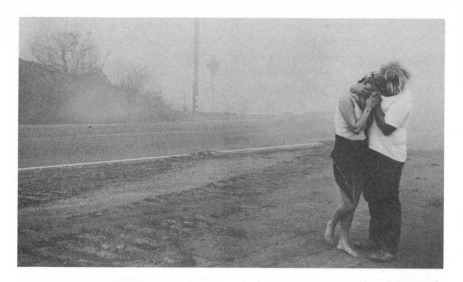

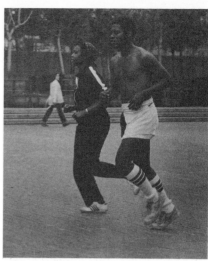

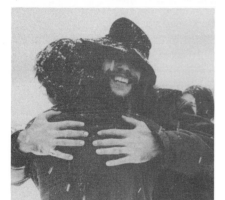

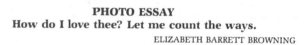

PHOTO ESSAY
How do I love thee? Let me count the ways.

ELIZABETH BARRETT BROWNING

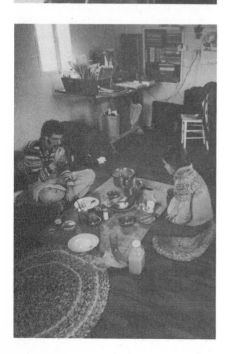

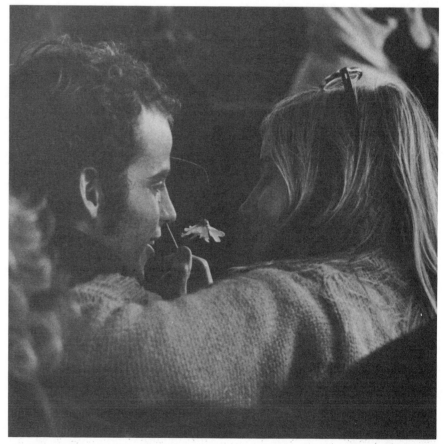

Children are born selfish, but that selfishness will remain only if they learn to hate themselves. But if children learn self-worth, love of a worthy self is possible. And, through giving of their worthy selves, children will be able wholeheartedly to enter into the long learning process of loving others. People must, for example, learn to love their neighbors. Were people born with this ability, they would not have had to be commanded.

But how do children learn to hate themselves?

Self-hate comes through being taught that they are evil. If they are told a thousand times that they are naughty, that they are bad, that they should be ashamed of themselves, children believe this to be true. They become devalued. And devaluated children devaluate themselves still further. Such children are cruelly robbed of life's paramount need—the need to give a worthy love. Of course, when it is necessary, children

should be corrected, even punished, but this should occur briefly and to the point—never heartlessly. Children must never be made to feel unloved.

Love is not lust. Love gives. Lust takes. It is true that both love and lust find expression through coitus; yet coitus satiates lust and furthers love. And although love is not a prerequisite for coitus, most people consider it desirable. Sexual desire may result from loneliness, vanity, social status, a desire to conquer or be conquered, or to hurt or be hurt. Any strong emotion (of which love is but one) can stimulate sexual desire.[12] Once desire is satiated, the individual may experience physiological relief. But if such desire has not been an expression of love, he or she often will not be emotionally satisfied. That person has given the least of the self. Tenderness has not been shared; greed has not been given up. Such an individual remains separate and alone.

The techniques of sexual intercourse are important; however, they do not replace the art of loving. Both may be learned. But just as food without love leaves the infant emotionally starved, so does sexual intercourse without love leave the adult still hungering. Only love can solve the anxiety of separation.

Entering adolescence with self-esteem unshaken, convinced of a wholesome personal value, the young person can further develop the vital enrichments that are possible because one is human. Since there is self-respect, there is respect for others. In these years, slowly, now clearly, then beclouded, but ever recurring, there comes to the youth a new perception: that love is the art of giving. And part of the art of giving love lies in taking it without exploitation. Having learned to give and to take love, the young person is ready for adulthood. Prepared to exchange separation for union, a mate is sought.

Searching for Someone to Marry

At twenty, one can hardly contemplate fifty years of living, let alone fifty years of marriage. And since a majority of marriage choices are made at about this age, the wonder is not that one of three marriages in this country ends in divorce but that there are not even more failures. There are those, like the English writer H.G. Wells, who consider it foolhardy to leave so vital a decision "to flushed and blundering youth . . . with nothing to guide it but shocked looks and sentimental twaddle and base whisperings and cant-smeared examples."[13] Yet this time Wells, who wrote so much

about the future, was, to some extent, writing about the past. It is surely more possible for modern young people to make intelligent decisions about marriage than it was for their earlier counterparts. True, today's youth live among more rapid changes, and what they see and hear can cause anxiety, but the very fact that they have access to so much information enables them to choose with more wisdom.

In considering marriage, people today consider a multitude of factors. Among the most important of these are the rising divorce rates, to be discussed later in this chapter.

Indeed, by the time children in the United States reach the age of 16, more than one-third will have spent part of their childhood living in a single-parent home as the result of a disrupted marriage.[14]

Other factors that must be considered include increased family mobility; alternatives to marriage, such as couples living together unmarried, or people choosing to live alone; the long overdue, yet still far-from-adequate, liberation of women; the greater proportion of women in the working force; the changing roles of men and women in family and society; the declining birth rate;* and the high cost of supporting children, which is higher now (and still increasing) than the figures shown in Table 10–1.

Courtship: Reflexive, Reflective, or Both?

The right person can mean contentment. The wrong one can indeed entwine two lives in grief. "Though thou canst not forbear to love," wrote Sir Walter Raleigh to his son, "yet forbear to link."[15] The brilliant Elizabethan knight was not advising against marriage, he was advising caution. Of three elemental events in human life—birth, death, and marriage—marriage is the most open to intelligent personal decision. Love has been too simply defined as a conflict between reflex and reflection.[16] But reflection can enrich the expressions of love that mold a good marriage. Following are some thoughts and questions that should occur to the person who is considering someone as a potential mate.

1. How confident are both members of the couple that their marriage will be successful? Studies show that lack of confidence in this respect is a good indicator of future failure.[17]
2. Does the relationship survive loss of glamor? In the moonlight most girls look lovely. In a similar light most young men get by pretty well. However, how do

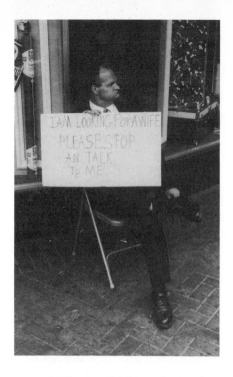

matters seem when one of the parties is miserable with a bad cold?
3. How is conflict handled? Do the inevitable problems that erupt during a disagreement always get buried only by mutual physical attraction? Or do conflicts teach insight and better understanding of each other? It is as important to learn from a quarrel as it is to make up. But the courting couple whose quarrel-

ing is constant and unresolved will find little happiness in marriage.
4. Is conversation easy? Perhaps the pair have never really talked to each other. Can one endure the occasional long silence of the other when necessary?
5. What happens when the pair is with a group? Does either of them embarrass or persistently criticize the other? Is one ashamed of the other? Do they avoid groups altogether? Why? Courting is a private affair, but most married people have get-togethers with friends.
6. How are decisions made? Does one member of the pair expect the other to "like it or lump it"? Some couples say that "we have been married for forty years and have never had a word of disagreement." When two people agree on everything, only one is thinking. Has there been a frank and open discussion about some of the possible misunderstandings that may arise during a marriage? How will the division of labor in the home be handled—who will be responsible for what and when? Will there be children? How many? Will the

*A Stanford University researcher suggests that divorce is directly related to the declining birth rate since 1961, which is due largely to use of the pill and the IUD. He reasons that during the first five years of marriage childless couples are twice as likely to divorce as those with young children. (See "Dealing in Divorce: Is Birth Control to Blame?" *Human Behavior*, Vol. 7 [November 1978], p. 37.)

TABLE 10–1 Total Direct Costs of a Child in the U.S., about 1977				
COST LEVEL	CHILDBIRTH	COSTS TO AGE 18[1]	4 YEARS OF COLLEGE	TOTAL
Low-cost	$1,443[2]	$35,261	$7,452	$44,156
Moderate-cost	2,194	53,605	8,416	64,215

1. Based on U.S. average for urban areas.
2. Assumed to be in the same proportion to the moderate-cost childbirth figure as the respective costs to age 18.

SOURCE: Thomas J. Espenshade, "The Value and Cost of Children," *Population Bulletin*, a publication of the Population Reference Bureau, Inc., Vol. 32 (April 1977). Compiled from various sources.

responsibility for them be shared, and how? If the woman wants a career, will it be as important as her husband's? Should one's career require a transfer to a job in a different state, the other's career could be endangered. How would that be handled? Should there be a signed agreement about important matters?

7. Is that knitting or stamp collecting or watching pro football or endless chattering on the telephone going to be bearable for fifty years?

8. What is the home life of the possible life partner like? How does the potential partner treat his or her parents? How do the in-laws-to-be react to the potential son- or daughter-in-law? Studies have repeatedly shown that people from relatively happy homes are the best marriage risks. (There is the exception, of course, of the child of divorced parents who works all the harder to make a marriage succeed. Too, there is the occasional case of the marital partner who sacrifices an entire life to the wounding memory of a parental divorce. Fearful of marriage failure, he or she may scrupulously avoid all disagreement and never express individual feelings.)

9. What are his or her best friends like? Off-beat? If so, it is well for the marriage partner to be a trifle off-beat too. Of course, there may be limits. Some time ago, a Boston woman "sued for final separation because her husband insisted on coming to bed with his pet monkey wrapped around his neck," and a Seattle woman complained that her husband "maintained a spring-fed trout pool in their marital bedroom, together with pipelines providing wine and beer on tap."[18]

10. What is the physical health of the potential marital partner? A slight anemia may add a bewitching pallor to the complexion, but perpetual illness may become wearing after a few years of marriage.

11. How self-sufficient is the proposed mate? How dependent? There is a difference between depending and being dependent on someone. How much dependency does one potential marriage partner need of the other? Overdependency can become an illness. Manifesting itself in marriage, overdependency may, for example, cause one partner to unconsciously expect the other to be a substitute parent. The second partner may reject this role. Frustrated, the dependent partner may seek attention by becoming a hypochondriac or an alcoholic. When this happens, the marriage is endangered.

12. What role does each potential marital partner expect the other to play? One man may want to marry a pretty girl who is a good housekeeper. He understands and insists on the responsibility of making the money to support his family. Other men emphasize companionship and continued education and want their wives to participate in the business and professional world. Some men want some of both. Those who contemplate marriage then, need to examine the role they want to play and the role they want their intended partner to perform in the marriage situation.

13. Has the relationship been frequently broken off and renewed? Such a relationship does not promise a happy marriage.

14. Is the potential partner a compassionate person? Passion needs compassion. There are bound to be hurts during a marriage. Is the partner capable of extending needed extra care and consideration? Importantly, can he or she say "I'm sorry"?

15. How does each member of the couple feel about the self? A lack of self-esteem hinders one's ability to solve marital problems. Almost five hundred years ago the Dutch religious thinker Erasmus wrote:

I ask you: will he who hates himself love anyone? Will he who does not get along with himself agree with another? Or will he who is disagreeable and irksome to himself bring pleasure to any? No one would say so, unless he were himself more foolish than Folly.[19]

Some Special Premarital Considerations

The wonderful conglomeration of people in this country marry and reproduce in a society dominated by a belief in the sanctity of the individual. A clash of interests is inevitable, for the satisfaction of individual needs may be thwarted by the demands imposed by one's cultural background. Marriages often cannot survive in the face of such conflict.

INTERFAITH MARRIAGES

People of different religious faiths often fall in love and marry. Rebellion or status seeking by no means accounts for all interfaith marriages. But even among couples who are in love, interfaith marriages seem somewhat less likely to suc-

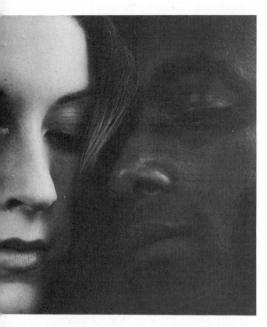

Whether the chances for success of a black-white marriage are any less than those for a racially nonmixed marriage is hard to know. But we do know that in the United States, the number of black-white marriages has increased from about 50,000 in 1960 to about 112,000 in 1977.

ceed than marriages in which the couple is of the same religious belief.

There are signs of growing permissiveness among some members of the major religious bodies. However, the general reaction of the religious leadership in the United States to interfaith marriage remains negative.

What are some major sources of disharmony in interfaith marriages? Despite ardent premarital agreements, conflicts often occur over the religious training of children. (This may account, for example, for the high divorce rate of couples of which the wife is Protestant and the husband Catholic.) For many people religion is a way of life. Even those whose relationship to their own faith is casual may find the rituals of another faith an imposition.

Although many interfaith marriages succeed, it is wise to remember that love alone does not necessarily conquer all.

INTERRACIAL MARRIAGES

Those contemplating an interracial marriage would do well to carefully consider all the issues, varying from personal motivations to the possibilities of differing values, whether they be social, ethical, educational, or religious. Of course, these considerations, among others, are important in all marriages. As to the potential for marital success of interracial marriages, adequate appraisal awaits more intensive study.

Neither has enough research been given to the children born of interracial marriages. There is some reason to suggest that the quest for identity of the child of a black-white marriage is more difficult than that

of the black child in this country. The child often resents both parents, is unable to identify with either, and also resents siblings with characteristics that are racially different. However, data that might make this more than a suggestion is either lacking or too old to be meaningful today.

INTERCLASS MARRIAGES

Numerous studies show that adjustment rates are poor in marriages in which the partners come from widely separated social classes.

Men are more likely than women to have a successful marriage with a partner slightly below their own class. A female college professor may marry a colorful truck driver and get away with it, but it is more likely that they will find little in common once the initial romantic glow wears off. She may end by criticizing his dirty fingernails, and he will puzzle why she never noticed them before. Each will be right about, and wrong for, the other.

MONEY

In this nation, countless couples attribute their marriage failures to "money problems." Often it is not the amount but the manner of expenditures that is the major cause of marital friction. One wife told this story:

It's thirty years ago, but it's like yesterday. I was seven. I knew my father had just lost his job, but I pretended I didn't. He came out of the bedroom and told my mother, "I don't know. I just don't know where our next piece of bread is coming from." Sometimes, I can still hear him. His voice was quiet. In two years he was dead.

What's this got to do with my husband? He doesn't understand. He'll go out and spend three hundred dollars on a suit. Or he'll buy those expensive tires. He just doesn't know that being poor can kill a person like it killed my father. He doesn't know what it's like not to know where your next piece of bread is coming from.

It is true; he does not know. And the danger to their marriage is that he does not want to know. He has never known a day of financial want. His side of the story is typical:

We've been married eighteen years. I've never made less than thirty thousand a year. We've got money in the bank. Even if we didn't, my folks could help. They have always had more than they need. What's she so scared about?

The problems of this couple spring from their widely different economic pasts. Spending patterns are learned in childhood from family experience. She will forever tighten the purse strings that he will forever loosen.

Similar tensions overtake the rich girl-poor boy marriage. The woman who had almost everything she wanted as a girl may soon resent her husband's inability to provide anything but the bare necessities. The early fun of making up a household budget often becomes a weary trial when it comes to trying to make it work. She may soon see the sum of her expenditures as the dreary sum of her marriage.

How can these pitfalls be avoided? One should know not only the financial behavior pattern of the proposed mate, but also his or her ability to plan expenditures. How one fits finances into married life is often critical.

AGE

Teen-age marriages are particularly prone to failure. Numerous studies repeatedly emphasize the high divorce and poor adjustment rates of teen-age unions. In addition, teen-age marriages forced by pregnancy are the most unstable of all (see page 408).

How old should one be before getting married? Some students of marriage recommend twenty-nine for the man and twenty-four for the woman. Others suggest twenty-five and twenty-two, respectively. Setting the same age for everyone is pointless. Emotional stability and maturity are better indexes of marital success than is chronological age. One good way of deferring a possibly premature marriage while at the same time learning more about a potential partner is to have a reasonably long engagement: A year should tell the couple enough.

Marriage

Prologue

Next, when they had got them huts and skins and fire and woman was appropriately mated to one man, and the laws of wedlock became known and they saw offspring born of them, then first mankind begun to soften. For the fire saw to it that their shivering bodies were less able to endure cold under the canopy of heaven and Venus sapped their strength and children easily broke their parents' proud spirit by coaxing. Then also neighbors began eagerly to join in a league of friendship amongst themselves to do no hurt and suffer no violence, and asked protection for their chil-dren and womankind, signifying by voice and gesture, with stammering tongue, that it was right for all to pity the weak. Nevertheless concord could not altogether be established, but a good part, nay the most part, kept the covenant in good faith or else the race of mankind would even then have been completely destroyed, nor would birth and begetting have availed to prolong their posterity.[20]

So did the ancient Roman poet Lucretius describe the beginnings of families. People banded together and established protective rules. Those breaking the rules imperiled the group and were punished. Sexuality, love, and marriage, too, were controlled by group consensus. In that sense, the deepest intimacies between people became public business. In many ways, marriage has not changed much.

In every society, marriage and the family exist. All societies, moreover, have chosen marriage as the arrangement for having children.

It is marriage which is the basic social instrument of man's survival . . . for survival there must be an accommodation between the sexes . . . enduring enough to provide protection, care, and reasonable security for the offspring.[21]

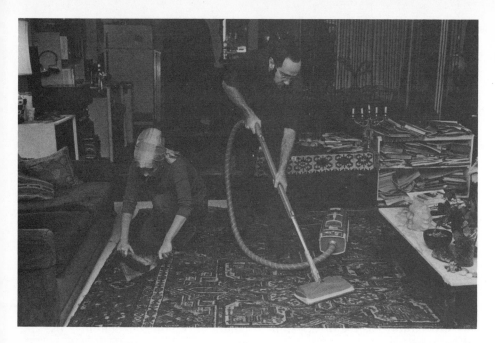

Today, the date of the marriage may not await the completion of education. And married college students share with all recently married people a new awareness of sexual relationships. No longer, for example, are woman's sexual needs regarded as incidental. Rapid social change, moreover, has added threats to the stability of marriage. The mobility of the family and the emancipation of women are but two of the factors contributing to fresh perspectives of this ancient institution. Consider some major aspects of marriage so characteristic of these times.

The Campus Marriage

It was not until World War II was over that married students were first seen in appreciable numbers on the nation's college campuses. Thousands of veterans used their benefits to obtain an education. Today's elderly professors remember them well. Those young veterans were not college boys. They were older, tougher. Some were filled with speechless anger. Most were intensely purposeful. They had no time to fool around. They had been through a war and knew something about time. Many were married. Their wives worked. In those days there was always pregnancy to think about. It was, for most vets, a difficult time. It was, for their wives, a time for marking time. Veterans were used to waiting. Their wives quickly learned.

One of the chief concerns of married students is money. Parents often pay for a considerable portion of students' expenses. Marriage changes that picture. Some married students want to make it on their own. Often parents are reluctant to help because of a sincere belief that such a prolonged dependency might harm the marriage. Others are more abrupt: "If you're old enough to get married, you're old enough to support yourself." Many parents do help. Nevertheless, married students receive much less parental cash than do single students. Many married students work. Not uncommonly, husband and wife take turns working while the other goes to school. Whatever the plan, it is beset with risks. That the vast majority of campus marriages succeed speaks well for the maturity of those who venture into them.

The possible problems of campus marriage must be dealt with early. Indeed, they are best discussed and planned for before the marriage takes place. Another aspect of marriage is rarely considered, even expected. So gradually does it develop that neither partner clearly sees it as a threat to their future. Too, for some it hardly exists. Others accept it. Still others resent it. It is the problem of monotony in marriage.

Marriage, Monotony, and the Appreciation of Both

> *And may her bride-groom bring*
> *her to a house*
> *Where all's accustomed,*
> *ceremonious;*
> *For arrogance and hatred are*
> *the wares*
> *Peddled in the thoroughfares.*
> *How but in custom and in*
> *ceremony*
> *Are innocence and beauty*
> *born?**

In the pattern of everyday married life, there is much that is honored

*Reprinted with permission of Macmillan Publishing Co., Inc., and M.B. Yeats, from "A Prayer for My Daughter" in *The Collected Poems of W.B. Yeats* by William Butler Yeats. Copyright 1924 by Macmillan Publishing Co., Inc.; renewed 1952 by Bertha Georgie Yeats.

by time. Custom and ceremony, no matter how subtle, add to the richness of the marital fabric. But mere repetition makes for a drab cloth. Individuality and custom can, however, be compatible. Indeed, customs provide an opportunity for sharing individuality. Her custom may be as simple as a best tablecloth for dinner. But unless he occasionally brings a bunch of flowers to decorate the table too, the time will come when neither sees the tablecloth. What is left? Monotony.

Many people find some marriage monotony a comfort, not a problem. They see it as a mark of their certainty about each other. Whether one can count on the other is a valid test of courtship. In marriage it is part of the loving. Life cannot be perpetual excitement, but enjoyment of each other can last a lifetime. There is surely some truth in this reasoning.

Others refuse to even recognize tedium as a possible part of marriage. They hark back to the "good old days," when people (meaning women) had no time for nonsense like boredom. "In the past," they say, "women knew their place; they never thought about being bored, and they never got a divorce either." Just how far back the good old days go for such philosophers is never clear. That Grandpa was a kindly soul, in whose beneficent light Grandma was ever content, may be true. Maybe.

In the early nineteenth century, *The Ladies' Book* quoted the following advice of a minister to a bride: "Your duty is submission.... Your husband is, by the Laws of God and of man, your superior; do not ever give him cause to remind you of it."[22] So wifely self-expression continued to be discouraged and total obedience to be expected. But the role of women changed. The shack-

ling notion of feminine obedience was discarded. Millions of women in this country have found work outside the home. And a great number of those who remain at home are bored. This is not to say that the working woman is never oppressed by monotony. Nor is homemaking a tedious occupation for many women. But many who choose to stay at home certainly find little opportunity to relieve the monotony of housekeeping. Sheer boredom then erodes the marriage. And her husband, tired and perhaps also bored with his work, joins her in an unrelieved tedium. What has happened? The individuality, the integrity, the inner sense of freedom of each marital partner is lost. Any loss of respect for these needs is erosive of marriage. Failure to show appreciation of each other's intellectual horizons can cause the ruin of any marriage.

Many marriages, then, die on the vine. Husband and wife simply stop noticing each other. True, the

arithmetic of living—the baby's allergy, the leaking roof, the clogged sink—does not add up to romance. But to keep a marriage alive takes work and planning. The couple must make time to do things together both at home and away from the home and office. Daily opportunities to share thoughts and feelings must be created. Privacy is not always easy to achieve. But no home needs to be the private preserve of a small child. Often a good babysitter will help. Timing is also crucial. A woman, exhausted by a toddler, may find it hard to end the day by concentrating on her husband's office difficulties. In turn, he may be too weary, at the moment, to be concerned about her problems. And so, at times, silence is the wisest and most appreciated course. Love in shared silence is, at times, a need of both partners.

In a marriage marred by boredom, a word of appreciation is usually long overdue. Sincere praise for accomplishment is a need of both

"Love in shared silence is, at times, a need of both partners."

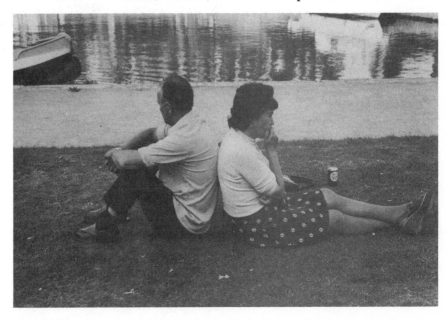

marital partners. There is the story of the unhappy man who ran around with other women, not because his wife did not understand him, but because she understood him only too well. To her, knowing him meant undermining him. The woman who cannot regard her husband without foil in hand, ready to pierce his ego, will destroy her marriage. Marriage is not a competition. One does not gain by the other's loss. Between the married, "one-upmanship" is a dangerous game. There is no victim in a good marriage. Moreover, the husband who does not accentuate his marriage with expressed appreciation may reap (and deserve) a bitter harvest. Both partners can express their appreciation for the other in many ways. Listening is essential. Another is by touching. Hugging and caressing are tender and gentle expressions. They should be an ongoing part of marriage and can help one endure the inevitable crises.

"It was a lot of little things," then, explains many a happy marriage as well as many a divorce. The difference is that the happily married couple, having worked at it, will know what happened to them. They will know why the customs and ceremonies of their marriage never lost freshness and meaning.

Alternatives to Marriage

There is little that is new about experimentation with alternatives to marriage. Some people still practice the polygamy of the ancient Hebrews. Indeed, there is some evidence that today polygamy is spreading in the western part of the United States.[23] A century ago, in New York State's large Oneida community, group marriage was practiced with rigidly prescribed rules for sexual sharing. There is another form of group marriage in which the community is held to a small size— perhaps two couples and three or four children. The number of such modern communities is not really known; reported impressions are that only a few young people are choosing to live in these communes.

Today, there are couples who "swing"—as did so many of the ancients—hoping to improve their marriage by sexual exchanges uncomplicated by deeper attachments. Reports have been published suggesting that some couples do not find swinging threatening to their marriage because it is a joint venture with the consent of both partners. Since initial data about the extent of modern swinging are at best unreliable, it does not appear possible to predict its increase or decrease in the 1980s. Ironically, it is the husband who most often discovers the possibilities of swinging and talks his wife into the practice; yet once begun, it is his fear of sexual inadequacy and his jealousy that are among the reasons that swinging seems to endure but briefly. Another stated reason for abandoning the practice is the fear of contracting sexually transmitted diseases.

Of all the alternatives to conventional marriage, perhaps the most common is the choice to live singly. People perceive loneliness differently both in themselves and in others. Being alone and being lonely are not the same thing. People can live alone and actively participate in community affairs, have a host of

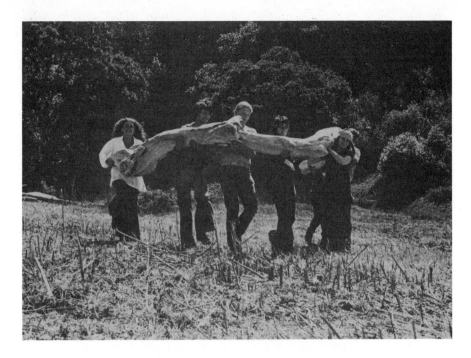

Building a gate for a commune.

friends, enjoy relatives, and generally lead rich and productive lives. And one can feel very lonely in a crowd or in a marriage that is not happy. Like other life styles that do not threaten society, it is a generally acceptable way of life. Here again, things have not changed much. In 1900 in this country a lower percentage of men and women were married than was the case in the 1970s.[24]

The greater availability of sexual partners, the high cost of raising children, the increased inability of the male to unquestioningly conduct his own household, the increasing economic and emotional independence of women, and the lessened desire to have children because of the population explosion are surely some of the reasons why some people are choosing the single life today. In the 1900s Benjamin Franklin's advice "First thrive, then wive" was doubtless a major cause of a high rate of unmarried people. Economics, then as now, had a marked influence on marriage rates.

Living Together (Cohabitation)

There have always been people who have lived together without marriage, and, as always, there will be those who will try hard to get them married, as the following story illustrates:

One day a couple who had horrified colonial New London, Connecticut, was met on the street by the town's outraged magistrate.

"John Rogers," the magistrate asked, "do you persist in calling this woman your wife?"

Yes, I do."

"And do you, Mary, wish such an old man to be your husband?"

"Indeed I do," was the reply.

"Then, by the laws of God and this commonwealth," said the magistrate, "I pronounce you man and wife."[25]

The results of an October 1977 *CBS News/New York Times* poll indicated that 82 percent of men and 69 percent of women between the ages of eighteen and twenty-nine said "living together" was either "O.K." or "doesn't matter." As expected, older people were less approving: Only 28 percent of the men and 12 percent of the women considered cohabitation acceptable. In that year, almost two million people in this country (957,000 couples) were indeed living together without being married. This represented an 83 percent increase in cohabitation in the United States since 1970. From 1960 to 1970 the increase had been much less startling—only 19 percent.

In many ways living together is similar to common-law marriage. Common-law marriages are also hardly new. In the past, they were prevalent in many European countries. The parties simply agreed that they were married, and for most purposes that seemed enough, although a ceremonial marriage was later required. In some countries sexual intercourse was supposed to be delayed until there was a religious ceremony.

Cohabitation is not entirely confined to the young. There is some evidence (but not much data) that it occurs more commonly among older people than used to be the case.

The number of couples cohabitating in 1977 represented only 2 percent of the country's forty-eight million couple-households. That, of course, is just another way of saying that 98 percent of all U.S. couples living together are married. However, it should be noted that the U.S. 1977 data showed an age difference when compared with data for all couples. In that year, among heterosexual couples in which the man was under 25, some 7.4 percent were living together unmarried. Thus, it is clear that young people during that time were both more liberal about living together and were trying this arrangement more often than their elders. Of course, the figures for this country are three years old. The trend to 1977 was an increasing form of this alternative. Whether it continues into the 1980s, and to what extent, will be interesting to watch. Considering the data as a whole, the United States has far to go before it reaches the 12 percent cohabitation rate that existed in Sweden in 1977.

The reasons people give for cohabitation are various. For some it is a more honest way of living that allows more freedom for personal development. Others, understandably influenced by the high divorce rate, consider it an easier way to discontinue a relationship. Still others consider it a trial marriage, just as did so many people in the medieval era. For others, cohabitation is believed to be a growing experience that can be had without the potential trauma of divorce. And many couples who live together before marriage believe it to be helpful to the success of their eventual marriage. For some people this may well be so.

There are other, less positive aspects to living together that must also be considered. A married couple might try harder than an unmarried couple to work out a difficulty, to compromise, rather than to terminate the relationship. Also, unmarried partners typically do not have the same legal rights as do their married counterparts. If one partner dies or leaves the other, any rights to an inheritance or a settlement often must be decided in an unpleasant and lengthy court battle. If there are children born out of wedlock, their rights, too, are not as well-defined as those of children whose parents are married. Finally, despite the opinion of many couples who cohabitate before marriage, there is no dependable evidence to show that people who have lived together have more successful marriages than those who have not done so.

Does the small 2 percent indicate at least a trend away from marriage? Nobody really knows. There have been extremely few reliable studies on the subject, and most of these are about college students. It is interesting to note that one study of men chosen at random from Selective Service records revealed that 18 percent had cohabitated with a woman at one time for six weeks or more, but that most had done so with only one partner. Also, at the time of the study interview, only 5 percent were cohabitating with anyone. Moreover, these cohabitations led to marriage in almost 40 percent of the cases. The authors of that study concluded that ". . . in terms of serious heterosexual relationships most young men in the United States are conventional."[26]

Saving the Marriage

Where can those with marital problems seek help? Family, friends, and relatives often must act as willing (or unwilling) family counselors. Doubtless, they are the ones most frequently asked for advice. Not enough are reluctant to give it. Some, however, are mindful that "marriage resembles a pair of shears, so joined that they cannot be separated; often moving in opposite directions, yet always punishing anyone who comes between them."[27] They are faced with the twin handicaps of involvement and lack of training—two serious shortcomings in an often explosive situation. In considering the intimate, interrelated complexity of the three elements of the ailing situation—the husband, the wife, and their marriage—one appreciates more clearly the need for professional objectivity and experience.

Family physicians or gynecologists often act as marriage counselors. Particularly if the problem is physical, they are in an invaluable position to promptly discover its source and to give practical advice. Many physicians are profoundly aware of the emotional needs of patients. They often suggest the services of a professional counselor.

Specialists in marriage counseling have organized the highly professional American Association of Marriage Counselors, composed of sociologists, psychologists, lawyers, physicians, and clergy. These counselors have both training and experience in a field requiring sensitivity and wisdom. Unfortunately, there are not enough of them. The more accessible Family Service Association of America comprises local Family Service agencies, which are found in most cities. Staffed by social caseworkers, these agencies charge fees based on ability to pay. Many such marriage counselors hope to explore the marital dilemma with both parties. Frequently, however, the tension between the two prevents this.

A basic first step is the acceptance by both partners that they need help. Sometimes "talking out" a problem, in the presence of an attentive third party, opens a road to its solution. Often, the marriage counselor can guide a degree of interaction between marital partners that is a revelation to both of them. Many married people simply do not talk enough to each other. As the years go by, they tend to confide less and less in each other. Some couples do not talk — they quarrel. Fear and pride and the sheer habit of quarreling have wrecked many a marriage.

Should the marriage counselor discover a deep emotional base to the marital problem, the couple may be urged to seek the help of a psychiatrist. One man may have been taught that sex is dirty. A woman may have had a hostile mother who taught her only of the baseness of men. Still another man may be frightened of giving or receiving love. "She can't give. I can't take." This tragic dialogue has been expressed in many ways to more than one therapist.

A marriage cannot be put on and taken off like a coat. It must be mended and refitted. But it can wear well. It can last a lifetime.

Many years ago the Lebanese poet Kahlil Gibran wrote a wise prescription for marriage. If more couples followed the advice contained in the following lines, there would doubtless be less need for marriage counselors.

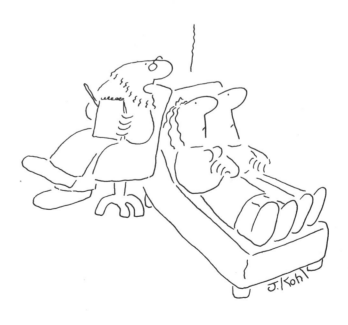

"You certainly seem compatible to me!"

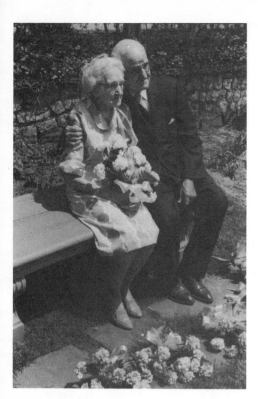

A rich old age is the reward of a lifetime of caring.

Then Almitra spoke again and said, And what of Marriage, master?

And he answered saying:

You were born together, and together you shall be forevermore.

You shall be together when the white wings of death scatter your days.

Ay, you shall be together even in the silent memory of God.

But let there be spaces in your togetherness,

And let the winds of the heavens dance between you.

Love one another, but make not a bond of love:

Let it rather be a moving sea between the shores of your souls.

Fill each other's cup but drink not from one cup.

Give one another of your bread but eat not from the same loaf.

Sing and dance together and be joyous, but let each one of you be alone,

Even as the strings of a lute are alone though they quiver with the same music.

Give your hearts but not into each other's keeping.

For only the hand of Life can contain your hearts.

And stand together yet not too near together:

For the pillars of the temple stand apart,

And the oak tree and the cypress grow not in each other's shadow.*

*From THE PROPHET, by Kahlil Gibran. Copyright 1923 by Kahlil Gibran and renewed 1951 by Administrators C.T.A. of Kahlil Gibran Estate, and Mary G. Gibran. Reprinted by permission of Alfred A. Knopf, Inc.

Divorce: Disruption and Rebuilding

On Dr. Holmes' list of stressful life events (Table 6–1, page 159), the inescapable trauma of divorce ranks second in severity only to the death of a spouse. And well it might. Gone are the high hopes that were the essence of the marriage. The expected happiness, commitment, sharing, and fulfillment all seem to be in ruins. That every year the U.S. divorce rate is increasing along with the marriage rate points to the need for a healing process after divorce. The stressful anxieties of divorce can be lessened by better planning. For example, one should not make the decision to divorce in haste. Divorce is a common cause of depression. If children are involved, their problems must be handled along with those of their parents. So divorce cannot be considered lightly.

But many people must consider it.

The causes of divorce may vary from one couple to another; however, it is often unavoidable, a last but only solution. The couple may have failed to realistically come to terms with their own and each other's expectation of marriage. Such failure of communication tends to breed hostility and, even worse, indifference. Or they may have failed to appreciate each other's potential for growth. Or they may have overlooked expressing their appreciation. One does not lose one's need for freedom of expression, for distant horizons, for being a person, because of marriage. Marriage should stimulate these needs. Contrary to some opinion, wedlock is not padlock.

There are those who compromise. If this is the case, it cannot be a one-sided compromise, or else it is doomed to fail. Chronic financial problems, adultery, alcoholism, insensibility to each other's emotional and physical needs, and seemingly endless monotony are but some of the causes of divorce. There are times when one of the partners grows while the other remains stagnant. For still others, there is a remaining affection, but it is no longer enough to hold the marriage together. The marriage rests on shifting sands; new roots cannot survive. Before divorcing, people would do well to be as certain as possible that they have given their marriage every chance. They would do well to seek the help of a marriage counselor. Yet even the efforts of such a skilled professional may fail to reestablish communication and open the door to a new view of the marriage. Staying together may then become destructive both for the married couple and, if there are any, for the children too. Centuries ago the conservative pre-colonial puritans recognized these possibilities. One of them wrote: "If it bee so, that they remayne styll together, what frowning . . . scolding, and chiding, is there between them, so that the whole house is filled up of those tragedies . . . unto the toppe."[28]

Is Divorce a Threat to the Institution of Marriage?

The divorce rate in the United States is the highest in the world. In 1977 the following calculations were made:

1. Of each 100 first marriages, 38 would end in divorce.
2. Of the 38 divorces, three-fourths would marry again.
3. Of those who did remarry, 44 percent would become redivorced.

TABLE 10–2 Number and Rate of Marriages and Divorces for Recent Years						
	NUMBER		RATE			
	1979	1978	1979	1978	1977	1976
Marriages	2,256,000	2,178,000	10.3	10.1	9.9	9.9
Divorces	1,129,000	1,087,000	5.2	5.0	5.0	4.8

SOURCE: National Center for Health Statistics, *Monthly Vital Statistics Report: Provisional Statistics*, DHEW Publication No. (PHS) 79-1120, Vol. 28 (April 10, 1979), p. 1.

4. Girls who married in their teens had a higher divorce rate than those who married later.

In 1976 and 1977 the rate of divorce in this country remained high but steady. There were speculations that the U.S. divorce rate was possibly leveling off. However, beginning in mid-1978 and continuing into 1979 the divorce rate started to increase again (see Table 10–2). In the past the traditional major events in human life have been birth, adulthood, marriage, and death. To these a great number of people have now added divorce. Over one-third of U.S. marriages end in divorce (see Figure 10–1). And if separations and desertions are included, some estimates of visibly failed marriages are one out of two.

Yet marriage remains popular and it, too, is increasing both in number and in rate. Table 10–2 gives ample evidence of that.

Some suggested reasons for the high and increasing rates of divorce are (1) readjustment problems due to the Vietnam War; (2) women's liberation; (3) increased acceptance (although not necessarily approval) of divorce among some religious denominations; and (4) the declining birthrate, which enables married women without children to return to singlehood more easily.

At Michigan State University, Professor of Management Eugene Jennings made a long-term study of various aspects of the nation's largest five hundred companies, as listed by *Fortune* magazine.[29] Reports from forty of these companies revealed that one-fifth of their executives nearing controlling positions are divorced. On this basis Jennings projected that by 1985 at least one-third of the chief executives in the five hundred companies would be divorced or legally separated. A 1978 article in *The Wall Street Journal* essentially supported Jennings' conclusions. Why are they of significance?

FIGURE 10–1
Chances of divorce for U.S. women now in their late twenties.

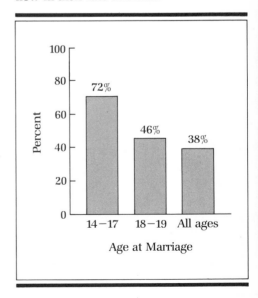

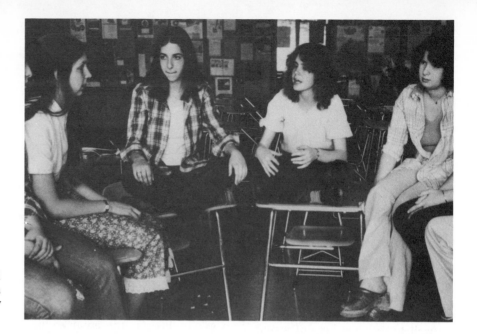

In this "Divorced Kids Group," one of about two dozen such groups throughout the country, high-school students whose parents have broken up discuss the special problems they face.

In the 1960s divorce meant an almost certain end to individual opportunities for career advancement. Today, that no longer seems to be the case. To be sure, a lasting marriage is hardly a handicap to promotion. But government regulations and fierce competition have enormously increased the complexity of administration. Since industry must operate on a profit margin, it cannot afford to discriminate against highly able executives because they are divorced. Divorce, Jennings further suggests, may well indicate that the executives choose the company over their spouses, are more able to move, give more attention to their tasks, and have rejected a marital life of sham. In terms of their attitude toward divorce, Jennings continues, the companies base their advancement decisions on the realities of corporate needs rather than on "human understanding."[30]

Although one might wish for more information about the actual number of executives in the studied forty corporations as compared with the total five hundred, there is certainly a suggested trend demonstrated by these figures.

Further evidence of the reality of divorce can be found in children's books. Before 1970 only two children's books on divorce had been published. By mid-1979 there were over three dozen.[31] Not all were good, but some were excellent.

Children and Divorce

By the time they are in school most children know about the possibilities of a divorce or divorce per se. Household stresses have usually become part of their daily existence. But the unavoidable stress need not become permanent emotional damage. The anxiety of children who are going through a divorce can be greatly relieved if it is explained to them that they are no more the cause of the divorce than they were the cause of the marriage. This should be honestly told the child. And with the wisdom of so many children, once they are relieved of their guilt, they may find that there is an advantage to living with one parent or the other rather than in a house wracked by dissension. Moreover, a child forced to live in the midst of marital turmoil will

surely grow to be an adult with a negative view of marriage. The child should not become the pawn of the divorcing parents. Parents do not own their children any more than they own one another. Children are not property to be divided like bank assets.

We have spoken repeatedly in this book of the need for self-esteem. The child's search for competence, the feeling of a worthy self, must not be destroyed during the divorce process. And the parents can help by making it clear that the child is still loved and needed by both. If the child is old enough, he or she should be given an opportunity to help make some of the decisions. Where shall I stay? What is best for me? What will become of me? Let the child who can do so take an active role in these decisions. There never was room for mystery between parent and child; there certainly is no room for it now.

Some children will use an impending divorce to act out resentment and poor behavior. Although this should be understood, it should not be allowed to become destructive. Parents who divorce have rights too, and the child who is old enough must understand this. Many problems can be averted by giving the child time to ask questions, to think about answers, and share them frankly with the divorcing parents. The questions are real. Will I have another Mommy? Another Daddy? Other brothers and sisters? Where do I get to eat? What school will I go to? Will I get to see my friends? By helping the child with such problems, the divorcing parents will be helping themselves all the more.

In Conclusion

After the divorce the parents may choose to remain single or they may decide to remarry. This means that the former marriage can best be used as a learning experience. Particularly is this true in courting and marriage. All the old mistakes need not be repeated. Many can be averted. And with some luck, with the help of good friends, and with one's self-esteem intact, another mate may be found. Second marriages can be happy marriages.

Summary

People are the only creatures on earth for whom the art of courtship and love is not instinctive but cultural. Among the ancient Hebrews, the family unit was established to provide stability and protection. Rigid sexual codes, supported even today by threat and guilt, began to develop from the earliest days of Christianity.

Love and courtship patterns vary greatly from culture to culture. Random dating, with little, if any, supervision or guidance, is the general practice in the United States. Courtship, or the time spent in preparation for marriage, has become more casual, and formal engagements are no longer considered necessary by some people.

People decide to marry for many reasons, including social pressure, sharing, sexual needs, and loneliness. But a successful marriage must provide a positive and creative opportunity for the self-realization of both individuals. Most importantly, the marriage must be based in love.

Love and self-respect must develop from the earliest years of a person's life if that person will be able to have a successful love relationship as an adult. Sexual intercourse without love will provide physical relief, but it probably will not give a person emotional satisfaction. Having learned to give love and to take it without exploitation, a person is ready for a permanent love relationship.

The courtship period should be a time when two people learn about each other and give serious thought to their compatibility. Before deciding to marry, the intelligent couple will consider many factors, such as personality, age, goals, money, and friends. Special consideration should be given if the two people planning to marry are of different faith, race, or class, because such marriages are subject to additional stresses and conflicts.

Marriage exists today for many of the same reasons it has survived over the centuries: It controls love and sexuality to the benefit of society, and it is the culturally chosen arrangement for having children. However, women's emancipation, a mobile population, and rapid social change have all added a new perspective to marriage. Yet another new aspect of marriage is the increase, starting after World War II, of the campus marriage, with its accompanying financial hardships for the couple.

As two people settle into the often monotonous pattern of daily living, they need to take special care to preserve the specialness of their marriage. Each must take the time to share with the other, to show appreciation and respect. There should be no competition between them. The customs and ceremonies of a marriage will never lose their freshness and meaning if the couple does not neglect them.

As has always been the case, there are people today who are unsatisfied with traditional marriage. Many alternatives exist: polygamy, group marriage (a form of communal living), and "swinging." One alternative that is frequently chosen is living singly. The greater availability of sexual partners, the increasing independence of women, and the lessened desire to have children are some of the factors that have contributed to the rising number of single persons. Another choice that has increased in popularity is cohabitation, or living together. This life style is more common among younger age groups, although it is certainly not restricted to them. Proponents of cohabitation consider it to provide more freedom for personal development, to be a growing experience, or to prepare the couple for marriage. However, it does have emotional and legal drawbacks.

If problems develop within a marriage, help is available if both partners agree it is necessary. The objectivity provided by a professional counselor can prove invaluable in identifying the harmful habits a couple often develops. Problems with a deep emotional base may require the help of a psychiatrist.

However, divorce is frequently the end result of marital problems, as is apparent from the rising divorce rate. Divorce has become so common that it no longer carries the stigma it did just twenty years ago. Some possible reasons for the increasing number of divorces are readjustment problems due to the Vietnam War, women's liberation, greater acceptance of divorce, and the increased likelihood that a woman will have no children and thus will find it easier to be single.

Children are an important consideration in a divorce. They will probably suffer less from the divorce than they will from the continued dissension between their parents if the parents take time to explain that they were not the cause of the divorce and if they do not become the pawns of the parents. Understanding on the part of the parents and frank discussions between parents and children will help all those involved to come through this disrupting experience without lasting emotional scars.

References

1. James Kemble, *Hero Dust* (London, 1936), p. xiii.
2. H. Smythe, *The Female of the Species* (London, 1960), p. 58.
3. Quoted in Willystine Goodsell, *A History of Marriage and the Family* (New York, 1934), p. 136.
4. Ibid., p. 152.
5. Edward Westermarck, *The History of Human Marriage*, 5th ed., Vol. 1 (New York, 1921), p. 49.
6. Ibid., p. 51.
7. Weston La Barre, "The Aymara Indians of the Lake Titicaca Plateau, Bolivia," *American Anthropologist*, Vol. 50 (January 1948), p. 129.
8. Quoted in Henry A. Bowman, *Marriage for Moderns* (New York, 1960), p. 129.
9. E.S. Turner, *A History of Courting* (London, 1954), p. 121.
10. Ibid., p. 195.
11. Thornton Wilder, *The Bridge of San Luis Rey* (New York, 1927), pp. 230–231.
12. Erich Fromm, *The Art of Loving* (New York, 1951), p. 54.
13. H.G. Wells, *Tono-Bungay*, quoted in Turner, *A History of Courting*, p. 15.
14. "More Than One-Third of U.S. Children Will Live in One-Parent Homes as Result of Broken Marriage," *Family Planning Perspectives*, Vol. 11 (March–April 1979), pp. 115, 119.
15. Quoted in Alan C. Valentine, ed., *Fathers to Sons: Advice Without Consent* (Oklahoma City, 1963), p. 16.
16. Szpilki (Warsaw, Poland), cited in *Atlas*, Vol. 16 (September 1968), p. 58.
17. Judson T. Landis, "Danger Signals in Courtship," *Medical Aspects of Human Sexuality*, Vol. 4 (November 1970), p. 40.
18. Patrick Ryan, "And the Last Word . . . On Divorce," *New Scientist and Science Journal*, Vol. 49 (March 18, 1971), p. 595.
19. Erasmus, "The Praise of Folly," in Louis Kronenberger, ed., *The Pleasure of Their Company* (New York, 1946), p. 564.
20. Lucretius, *On the Nature of Things*, quoted in Felding H. Garrison, *Contributions to the History of Medicine* (New York, 1966), p. 25.
21. William M. Kephart, *The Family, Society, and the Individual* (Boston, 1961), p. 64.
22. Cited in Vance Packard, *The Sexual Wilderness* (New York, 1967), p. 244.
23. Molly Ivins, "Polygamy, Growing in U.S. West, Is Encountering Little Opposition," *The New York Times*, Vol. 127 (October 9, 1977), pp. 1 and 80.
24. U.S. Bureau of the Census, *Statistical Abstract of the United States, 1971* (92nd edition), p. 33.
25. Donald Day, *The Evolution of Love* (New York, 1954), pp. 373–374.
26. "Marrying, Divorcing and Living Together," *Population Education Newsletter*, Vol. 7 (January 1978), p. 2.
27. Sydney Smith, *Lady Holland's Memoir*, Vol. 1 (London, 1885), Chap. 10.
28. Ivy Pinchbeck and Margaret Hewitt, *Children in English Society*, Vol. 1, quoted in *Tudor Times to the Eighteenth Century* (London, 1969), p. 54.
29. "Divorced Execs: It's Lonely at the Top," *Human Behavior*, Vol. 7 (December 1978), pp. 49–50.
30. Ibid.
31. Jane Merrill Filstrup, "Children's Books Confront Death and Divorce: A Reading Guide," *Harvard Magazine*, Vol. 81 (May–June 1974), pp. 64–68.

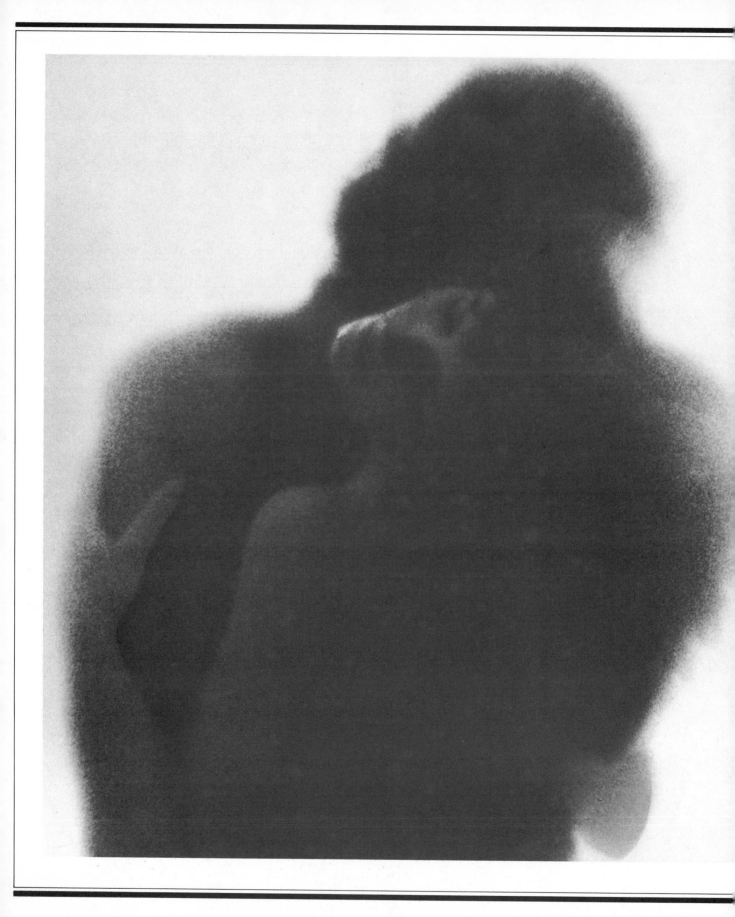

11
The Sexual Life

The Biological Logic of Mutuality

The First-Formed Female

"In the beginning, we were all created females; and if this were not so, we would not be here at all."[1] This remarkable statement is the result of years of biological research. In their first stage of development, the sex organs of the mammalian embryo (including the human) consist of two elevations of tissue. These are the *genital ridges*. Each ridge contains the primordial (or original) cells necessary for the development of either an *ovary* or a *testis*. Since it can develop in either direction—female ovary or male testis—each genital ridge must be considered an *undifferentiated* primitive **gonad**. (A gonad [Greek *gone*, meaning "seed"] is a gland producing *spermatozoa* or *ova*.) The outer rind of each undifferentiated gonad is capable of becoming an ovary; the inner core is capable of becoming a testis. However, although genetic sex is established at conception (when the sperm enters and fuses with the ovum), the sex genes do not exert their influence until the sixth to eighth week after fertilization. At that time, if the genetic instruction is to produce a male, the inner cores of the embryonic gonadal ridges develop into testes. For this to occur, some active secretory process is necessary. Once the primitive testes have been formed, they secrete both the male hormone *androgen* and a second substance. This second substance inhibits the development and causes the regression of those embryonic tissues that could become the organs of the female internal reproductive system (tubes, uterus, and vagina). The androgen causes the development of the male internal and external reproductive system. The male substances thus overcome the female pattern.

However, if the genetic instruction is to produce a female, the processes by which testes, androgen, and female-inhibiting substance are produced do not take place, nor do the subsequent events. The outer rinds of the genital ridges—the female cellular potentials—develop into ovaries. In the absence of androgen and the female-inhibiting substance, a female results from the already existing, and thus primordial, or original, tissue.

Clearly, then, the external female sex organs are not incomplete, imperfect, inadequate versions of the male sex organs, as many early scholars once believed. "Nature's prime disposition is to produce females; maleness only results from something added—androgens."[2] In other words, "only the male embryo is required to undergo a differentiating transformation of the sexual anatomy; and only one hormone, androgen, is necessary for the masculinization of the originally female genital tract."[3] The female genital tract develops independently, without cellular transformation by a hormone. Thus, it is the female whose tissue is primordial, and the sex organs of the male are an outgrowth of her original tissue. The penis develops from the primordia of the clitoris; the scrotum, from the primordia of the labia; the male, from the female.

These findings lend themselves to some further speculation. Is woman "superior," since she was em-

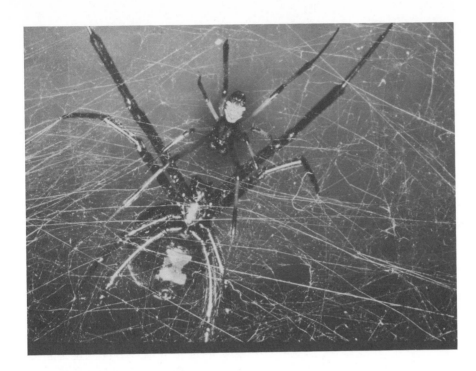

The much smaller male spider courts the female with justified caution.

bryologically first? Is man "superior," since he is "furthest along the evolutionary line"? Doubtless it is most sensible to put aside the notion of "superiority" and, instead, use this new information to gain a more mature, realistic, and therefore enjoyable appreciation of both sexes.

The Male Brain: An Androgenized Female Brain

Recent research has revealed some additional information about androgen. The results of experiments with laboratory animals support the following concept:

It does appear that one of the principle actions of androgen during development is to organize the immature central nervous system into that of the male. . . . We are talking about an active process; that is, the presence of androgen during development acts upon the brain to program, in effect, patterns of maleness. The absence of androgen permits the ongoing process of femaleness to pursue its natural course. The evidence to support this theory is now abundant.[4]

Thus "the brain makes do with one type of anatomic system. . . . The male brain is an androgenized female brain."[5]

What do some of these findings suggest? Modern biological knowledge does not support the sexual subordination of woman. In addition, these studies suggest an explanation for the greater prevalence of divergent sexual behavior among males. Most behavioral scientists agree that homosexual behavior (see pages 330–335), for example, is more prevalent among men than women. This difference is even more marked with other forms of divergent sexual behavior.

Elsewhere in this book, reference is made to the fragility of the male as compared with the female (see page 428). It has been speculated that man's comparative weakness is not limited to the more physical aspects of life. The male's "reproductive function and psycho-social development is much more easily tipped off-balance or derailed than that of the female."[6] It is the male embryo that is subject to the added chances for error caused by formidable anatomic changes. It is the male whose embryonic brain patterns must be radically altered. The female embryo is the original one; it develops independently. Furthermore, the changes necessary for the production of a male take place at a critical period in the development of the embryo.

The power of the critical period is so great that a single pulse of hormone in the laboratory may set for life the gender behavior as masculine or feminine (without there being any anatomic change in the body, for by this time the development of the reproductive anatomy is complete).[7]

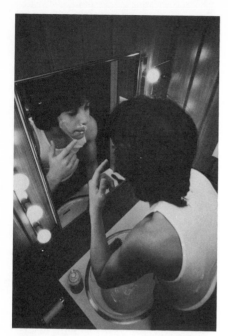

This adolescent boy probably does not need to shave yet, but what he has learned from the culture has a more powerful influence on his behavior than has his biological timetable.

The Roots of Sexual Behavior

The presence or absence of androgen does more than determine physical reproductive function. By its organizing effect on the hypothalamus and nearby nervous system tissue, it produces a change that predictably affects masculine or feminine sexual behavior. "Only if the fetal brain (hypothalamus) is organized by androgen does masculine behavior result. And, if normally occurring androgens are blocked in the male, then . . . femininity appears."[8] This has now been established beyond question by both clinical observation and laboratory experimentation with animals.*

The Role of Learning in Gender Identity

There are, however, more important factors influencing the child's gender (masculine or feminine) identity than the hormonal influences. These are the culturally learned patterns of behavior and thought that are instilled into the child from birth by the parents and by society as a whole. What the child is taught by the culture concerning gender identity is more important than the effects of chromosomes, hormones, and other physiological factors.

It is . . . clear that gender of assignment and rearing predictably take precedence over and over-

ride all contradictory determinants: chromosomes, hormones, gonads, internal and external sexual morphology [structure] and secondary pubertal changes. . . . The critical period for core formation of gender identity may be between 12 and 18 months . . . after about 2 to 2½ years of age, shift of core identity cannot take place, even when *all* sexual determinants are those of the other sex. Thus far in the literature there are no reported cases of successful shift after that age; there are, on the other hand, numerous case reports of psychological havoc and tragedy brought about by efforts to effect or enforce such a shift after the critical period."[9]

The overwhelming influence of learning on the child's sense of gender identity can be most clearly seen in the case of **hermaphrodites.**** There are various kinds of hermaphrodites; a *true* hermaphrodite, however, has both ovarian and testicular tissue either separately or in the same gonad.[10] Since the appearance of the external genitalia is inconclusive, the parents may be continuously uncertain about the sex to which their hermaphroditic child should be assigned. Faced with such uncertainty, the child will go through life believing that he or she is of neither sex or of both sexes. However, if the parents are certain of the child's gender (whether male or female), the child will also be certain. This is true even when the genitalia appear as both male and female.

Different interpretations of male-

*Significantly, moreover, it is the male hormone testosterone (see page 350) that most strongly influences sexual desire in both sexes. Females secrete most of their male hormones in the adrenal glands. Women who have had their adrenal glands surgically removed lose most of their sexual desire. Women who have had their ovaries removed, with subsequent loss of estrogens, rarely lose their sexual desire.

**"Hermaphrodite" derives from the names Hermes (the Greek god who served as messenger of the gods) and Aphrodite (the Greek goddess of love and beauty).

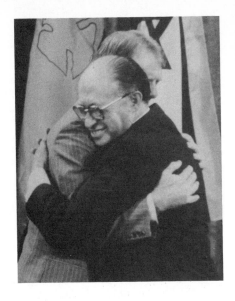

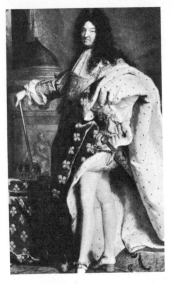

Ideas of acceptable male and female behavior and appearance vary with the culture, the time, and the circumstance. Left: Israeli Premier Begin and U.S. President Carter embrace warmly after the signing of the Middle East peace treaty in 1979. Right: King Louis XIV of France (1638–1715).

ness and femaleness have been made not only in various cultures but also during various periods of history. Is it the male who is always sexually aggressive? Not among all peoples. In many European countries, embracing men are a usual sight. In the United States such behavior in everyday encounters may be noticed with amused (and, one hopes, tolerant) doubts about gender identity, although embracing among women is acceptable. Men may, however, publicly embrace in this country under specific circumstances. Upon scoring a touchdown, football players not only embrace vigorously, but have been known to weep and to add an affectionate pat on the bottom to their expressions of affection.

Nor do clothes make the man—or woman. The colorful clothing and accessories worn by many young men in this country today were worn by many young men in this country years before them—the Navajo Indians. And the bejeweled, berouged, perfumed, powdered, curly-wigged, girdled, miniskirted, panty-hosed, high-heeled males of former days were not particularly noted for their indifference to women. Indeed, it was not until relatively recent times that women's legs replaced men's as objects of sexual admiration, and "unmentionables" were anything else but male garments.[11]

On the Physiology of the Human Sexual Response

William H. Masters and Virginia E. Johnson, of the Reproductive Biology Research Foundation at St. Louis, have written the most authoritative recent account of the physiology of the human sexual response.[12] Most of the discussion in this section is based on their work.

In their discussion Masters and Johnson divide the sexual responses of both sexes into four phases: the *excitement phase*, varying from a few minutes to hours; the intense, shorter (thirty seconds to three minutes) *plateau phase*; the three- to ten-second *orgasmic phase* (sometimes longer in women); and the *resolution phase*, lasting ten to fifteen minutes with an orgasm and, without orgasm, lasting as long as twelve to twenty-four hours.

Sexual expression is more than a total body experience. It is an experience of the whole personality. Keep in mind, though, that since there is no human equation, some individual variations are common and should be expected.

In the Female

Even the early feminine responses to adequate sexual stimulation (during the excitement phase) are not limited to the pelvis. They are widely distributed. From contracting great muscles of the thighs, abdomen, and back, to the tiny muscle fibers often erecting the nipples, the woman's sexual attention is total. The distention of the breast veins as they become engorged with blood, resulting in a marked increase in breast size, is called *tumescence*—swelling. (Tumescence occurs in all distensible parts of the body and is the major feature of the sexual response in both sexes. It results from the enormous increase of blood in the surface circulation. In these areas blood is forced in through the arteries faster than it can leave via the capillaries and veins. The presence of a special erectile tissue in some areas—the walls of the inner nose, the nipples, vaginal entrance, clitoris, and penis—makes them particularly susceptible to the swelling tensions of tumescence.)

During the late excitement phase, or early in the plateau phase, in perhaps three-fourths of women and one-fourth of men, there begins the *sex flush*. Much more noticeable in fair-skinned people, this temporary, measleslike rash first appears on the skin of the abdomen. As sexual excitement intensifies, the rash spreads, but it will disappear immediately after coitus. Often it does not occur. The clitoris also undergoes tumescence, and the vagina has already begun to secrete a lubricating fluid by a process not unlike sweating. This fluid aids penetration of the penis, thereby facilitating coitus. As sexual excitement continues, a sudden contraction of muscles encircling the vagina may cause some of this accumulated fluid to spurt out. This has led to the completely mistaken notion that women ejaculate as do men. In this first phase, the inner two-thirds of the vagina increases in size, and the uterus contracts rapidly and irregularly. The reaction of the labia depends on whether the woman has given birth. If she has not, the labia majora will thin and flatten; if she has, they will enlarge. In both instances the labia minora increase in size. Bartholin's glands may, in this stage or the next, and during pro-

longed coital activity, produce a slight secretion to ease the entrance of the penis. The heart rate quickens, and, as is to be expected with sexual excitement, the blood pressure rises.

In the second phase, the plateau phase, tumescence and the sex flush reach their peak. From head to toe, muscle tension reflects the physical and emotional absorption with the impending climax. Evidence of this is in the facial grimace, the flaring nostrils, rigid neck, arched back, and tensed thighs and buttocks. Now respiration increases, while the heart rate and blood pressure remain high. It is in the plateau phase that the clitoris withdraws from its normally overhanging position, pulling back deeply beneath its hood. Contraction of the encircling muscles of the vagina causes it to tighten about the penile shaft. Within these vaginal muscles, the veins become engorged with blood. Added to this venous congestion is that occurring in the veins of the irregularly contracting uterus as well as the other pelvic organs. And it is when the woman reaches the plateau phase of her sexual tension that her labia minora change color in a remarkable way. The color change of the labia minora with the woman who has never borne a child varies from a pink to a bright red. The labia minora of the woman who has borne a child varies from a bright red to a deep wine. So specific are these color changes of the labia minora that they have been termed the "sex skin." In the premenopausal woman, the sex skin is absolutely indicative of impending orgasm. The *pelvic congestion* is relieved during the third level of the sexual cycle, the orgasmic phase.

The orgasm is the pleasurable peak of the sexual experience. This explosive release of body-wide, pur-

posively developed, neuromuscular tension lasts from three to ten seconds. Hearing, vision, taste—all the senses are diminished or lost. It is during the excitement phase that this loss of sensory awareness begins. It has been said that only a sneeze is as physiologically all-absorbing as an orgasm. But a sneeze is mostly a local experience and an orgasm is not. Although the sensation of orgasm is centered in the pelvis, the whole body responds to it. Of all the widespread muscle responses, the contractions of the muscles in the floor of the pelvis that surround the lower third of the vagina cause the most unique phenomenon. These muscles contract against the engorged veins that surround that part of the vagina and force the blood out of them. This creates the orgasm. These contractions, in turn, cause the lower third of the vagina and the nearby upper labia minora to contract between three and fifteen times. The strength and number of these orgasmic contractions vary greatly and normally, as does the whole sexual experience.

The resolution phase of the woman's sexual response is marked by prompt disappearance of the sex flush, the fading of the sex-skin color, the decline of muscle tension and tumescence (*detumescence*), and a general return to the prestimulated condition.

In the Male

Masters and Johnson have emphasized the physiological similarities of the sexes in their sexual responses. All the phases and the general changes, such as muscle contractions and tumescence, also occur in the male. In the excitement phase, blood that is delivered to the

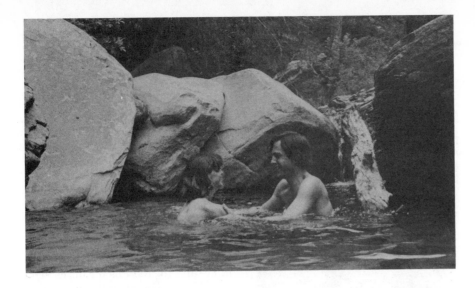

Actually, males and females are more alike than unalike in their responsiveness to sexual stimulation.

penis enters the spaces of its spongy erectile tissue. The structure within the penis efficiently prevents return of most of the blood from that organ into the general venous circulation. Penile enlargement and stiffening result. (There is no relationship whatsoever between the size of the penis and either virility or fertility.) During the male's plateau phase, the tumescent testes are elevated and become so congested with blood that they increase in size from 50 to 100 percent.

Orgasm and *ejaculation* occur simultaneously. The contractions of the epididymis, vas deferens, seminal vesicles, and prostate produce the sensation of imminent ejaculation. The force of perineal muscle contractions causes the seminal

fluid to squirt out from the penis. (See Figure 12–2 on page 351.) This ejaculation accompanying the male orgasm is the most definite difference in sexual response between the sexes.

In the resolution phase, general detumescence of the male is rapid. Penile detumescence usually occurs in two stages. After ejaculation the penis quickly returns to about half again the size of its prestimulated flaccid (soft and limp) state. Although complete erection increases the actual size of the penis considerably, it often seems that the initial stage of penile detumescence has not actually caused much decrease of the erection. Depending largely on the kind and duration of the stimuli of the excitement and

plateau stages, final detumescence requires a longer time. After orgasm, the male experiences a *refractory period*—a temporary resistance to sexual stimulation. During this period, the sexual stimulation that excited him earlier is no longer effective. It may even be distasteful. But restimulation of the woman after her orgasm may result in one or more additional orgasms. Nothing will help more in understanding this complex human difference than honest communication. The man, for example, may learn to delay his orgasm until the woman has been satisfied. Consistent premature ejaculation with loss of erection is a common problem that can be effectively helped (see pages 337–339).

Sexual Similarities Between Male and Female

Some essential similarities between the male and female sexual response may be noted from the preceding sections. The sexual response of each may be divided into four phases. Both sexes respond to touch and to a variety of other arousing stimuli (see pages 324–325). And,

contrary to popular belief, the female does not respond more slowly than the male to sexual stimuli. Her history of a tardy response is due to cultural repression. When the female is able to time her own responses (that is, when she herself regulates the rhythm and in-

tensity of the sexual stimuli, as occurs with masturbation), the time she requires to reach an orgasm is about the same as that required by the male. And, despite the male ejaculation, the physiology of orgasm has been found to be similar in both sexes.

Sexual Differences Between Male and Female

Differences in Adolescent Sexuality

Despite the similarities, there are some basic differences in the sexual responses of the male and female. These differences begin to be most noticeable at puberty. True puberty is marked by changes in the ovaries and testes and changes in their secretions. With the first ejaculation, or soon after, most boys produce living spermatozoa. In the female, however, puberty does not necessarily include the ability to become pregnant. And if pregnancy should occur, it does not follow that the child can be carried to term. Ancient physicians were aware of this distinction. *Puberty* (Latin *pubes*, meaning "hair") indicated the time that certain body parts became covered with hair. *Nubility* (Latin *nubis*, meaning "veil") meant the time that a girl was able to wear the nuptial veil and be married. A girl may experience a period of *adolescent sterility*. Although this is ordinary, there are exceptions. And the length of time that the adolescent female remains sterile varies greatly. Many adolescent menstrual cycles do not include ovulation. This developmental difference between the adolescent boy and girl may account for the subtle yet profound differences in sexual arousal and response. In addition, the dissimilar development of the sexual cells may explain why a physically mature adolescent girl usually is not strongly impelled to seek physical expressions of her sexuality, while a boy is.

When ova begin to mature completely, they do so singly and are discharged without accumulating.

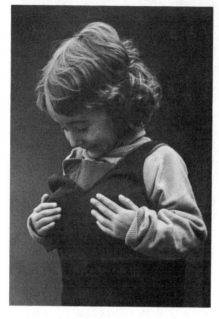

"What's it like to be grown up?"

Unlike the female, the male adolescent is vexed by accumulated and trapped sexual fluids, which must escape by ejaculation. In the young girl, sexual stimulation results in a rather diffuse reaction that is dominated by the cerebral cortex. Her increased adolescent sexuality is socially oriented. In the adolescent male, a similar amount of sexual stimulation results in the increased production of spermatozoa and the flow of secretions from the accessory sex glands. With this pressure the ejaculatory reflex is excited. His tensions can be relieved only by ejaculation. In the male this is not a diffuse, but a local reaction. It is not as cerebral as it is genital. His increased adolescent sexuality is genitally orientated. Although he is capable of great tenderness at this age, only later does his sexuality become social.

This contrast points to a basic distinction between the developmental processes for males and females: males move from privatized personal sexuality to sociosexuality; females do the reverse and at a later stage in the life cycle.[13]

Combine this with the ordinarily greater sexual imagery of the young male, and the reasons for his earlier interest in sexual relief becomes clear. However, despite his sexual urgencies, the young adolescent boy finds that girls his own age are quite indifferent to him. Indeed, they may be contemptuous of his clumsy shyness. The early sociosexual orientation of the young adolescent girl explains her interest in dating older boys. It is not sexual expression that she seeks; it is social expression. The awkward boys of her age lack the social sophistication that is necessary to gratify her needs.

Differences in Sexual and Cultural Conditioning

The sexes are not equally aroused by the same stimuli. It is believed that fewer women than men are sexually stimulated by nudity, erotic movies, or sexual stories. The fact that upper-class men seem to be more susceptible to stimulation by these than men of lower socioeconomic levels indicates that the response may be learned. Women seem to be more easily aroused by such stimuli as romantic movies and stories, although, again, cultural conditioning doubtless plays a major part in their response.

Sexual fantasies are much more common among men than women.

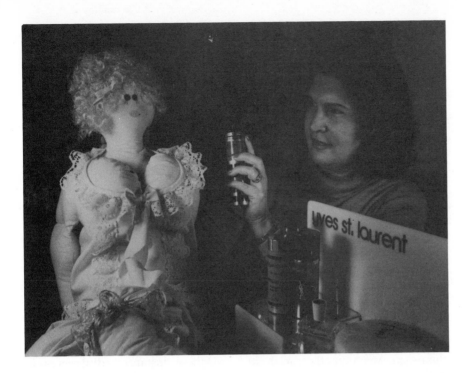

Sexuality is woven into the human personality both by nature and by a wide range of cultural stimuli.

During both masturbation and sexual intercourse, many more men than women are inclined to make use of sexual fantasies. Frequently the fantasy in which the man engages during these sexual expressions varies considerably from the actual expression. This is not usually the case with women.

Differences in Degree of Sexual Response

Among women, the variations in the degree of sexual response are much greater than among men. Some women, perhaps 10 percent, never reach an orgasm. Others do not have an orgasm until they are thirty or forty years old. Among men, this is exceedingly rare. At the other end of the scale, however, women far exceed men in the number of orgasms they can achieve in a given time period. Among a group of college students, for example, a few young women reported an average of twenty-five or more orgasms every week throughout their four-year college careers.[14] Moreover, women remain multiorgasmic far longer than do men (see page 326).

The sexes also vary in regard to the age at which they reach their peaks of sexual activity. When all kinds of sexual activity are considered, the average male of this culture reaches his peak before he is twenty years old. The average female increases her responses and activity more slowly, and she reaches her peak at about age thirty. From then until she is about fifty, and in many cases beyond that age, the average women's sexual drive and activity remain at a relatively even plateau. There are, of course, individual variations.

THE PERIODIC INCREASE IN THE WOMAN'S SEXUAL DESIRE

Still another difference between the sexes may be partly attributable to female physiology. Many women report increased sexual desire before the onset of menstruation. A lesser number experience this heightened sexual interest following menstruation or at the time of ovulation, which occurs at the midpoint of the menstrual cycle. Women whose sexual desire is greatest before the onset of menstrual bleeding may be stimulated by the pelvic congestion resulting from the increased amount of blood in that area. Thus, for many women there is a periodicity (or cyclicity) to their increased sexual desire. Again, however, individual variances are normal and numerous.

DIFFERENCES IN DESIRED FREQUENCY OF SEXUAL INTERCOURSE

How often do couples have sexual intercourse? The answer depends on a wide variety of factors, such as how old they were when they started and their individual needs.

There are no rules, just differences. There is evidence (some of which is derived from the work of Kinsey[15]) that the average male desires sexual intercourse more frequently than the average female. The word *average* is stressed here. Some women desire sexual intercourse more often than men, although many women report that they want it less often. It is noteworthy that the partners often may give significantly different estimates of the actual number of times they have sexual intercourse. This may be revealing of both their attitudes toward sexuality and their satisfaction with their relationship. For example, a woman who desires less intercourse may overestimate the number of times she has it, or a man who wants to have sexual intercourse more frequently might estimate the actual frequency to be closer to what he wants it to be, rather than to what it actually is. He may also report a greater frequency to emphasize his masculinity.[16]

The frequency of sexual intercourse is not as significant as is the frequency of rejection—and how the rejection is handled.

DIFFERENCES IN SEXUAL POTENCY

One of the most significant differences between the sexes lies in their relative potency. The fate of the comparatively frail male is considered on pages 319 and 428. Compared with women, men become ill much more often, and they die at a younger age. In addition, male psychosexual structure appears to be comparatively fragile. But there is yet another area in which the male is relatively feeble: He is not as sexually potent as the woman. While many young men are able to have several orgasms and ejaculations closely following the first, this capacity is generally lost by most males by the age of thirty.

Aside from ejaculation, there are two major areas of physiological difference between male and female orgasmic expression. First, the female is capable of rapid return to orgasm immediately following an orgasmic experience if restimulated before tensions have dropped below plateau-phase response levels. Second, the female is capable of maintaining an orgasmic experience for a relatively long period of time.[17]

Not only, then, are women able to be multiorgasmic, but they are also able to experience longer orgasms than men. Moreover, they need not undergo profound nervous system coordinations to prepare themselves anatomically for sexual intercourse, as men do. For the man an erection is a prerequisite to intercourse. He cannot submit; he must always perform. For countless people, the stress of constant submission or performance is not conducive to sexual competence. The striking difference between the sexes in their postorgasmic needs has been mentioned (page 323). During his refractory period, the man rejects further sexual stimulation; the woman may desire further stimulation in order to enjoy more orgasms. The man and woman who are experienced with each other are usually able to resolve this.

PROBLEMS ARISING FROM DIFFERENCES IN SEXUALITY

The differences in sexual expression between the sexes must be appreciated by both partners, otherwise lack of harmony may result. For example, the man may misinterpret the woman's lesser interest in sexual intercourse. Convinced that she is indifferent to him, he may look elsewhere for a seemingly more agreeable sexual partner. Better communication may help the man understand that the woman is more receptive than he had imagined.

The woman may attempt to meet the man's sexual demands by submitting to intercourse and pretending orgasm. This is essentially insignificant if it happens only occasionally. When it persists, a deep-seated emotional disturbance may be suspected. (This is no less true about the male who recognizes the pretense and accepts it.) Indeed, in these instances, differences in sexual desire may not be the basic problem. One woman may fear the abandon of orgasm. Another may be concerned that its very abandon makes her appear less attractive. By her pretense, a woman may express hostility toward her mate. Subconsciously, she dares her mate to notice the fraud. When the man fails to do so, the woman may then point to his deficiencies. A woman who has gone through a period of pretending orgasm may eventually begin to have and enjoy them. Then she may fear that her partner will notice the difference in her response. He may not. He might merely believe that "things are getting better and better."[18]

Not uncommonly, marital sexual dissension arises not from the woman's lesser interest in sexual intercourse but from her greater desire. This, coupled with her potential for more and longer orgasms and her later development of peak sexuality, may make her partner feel threatened. Fearing a loss of masculinity, he may begin to reject sexual-

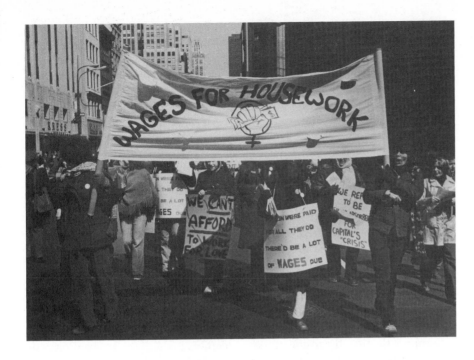

Many people feel that housework is a job like any other job, and, as such, it should command a salary.

ity. He may even become impotent (see page 337). What he must learn is that "the female's orgasm most plausibly represents nature's gift to femininity and not woman's bonus to masculinity."[19] If he can learn to accept this, he may also learn to enjoy it.

On Women's Release from Sexual Slavery

The modern obsession with the orgasm should surprise nobody. In this technological age, it is the technique rather than the art of love that sells marriage manuals. Yet, apparently technique alone does not suffice. Some college girls, who consider themselves sophisticated about sex, are often reduced to frustrated failure in achieving an orgasm.

Until recently in this culture the female half of the human species had much less experience with orgasm than the male. Not more than a hundred years ago, the opinion was held in Western cultures that only evil women ever admitted, even to themselves, that they enjoyed the sexual act. Sexual anesthesia was the price most women paid for the protection and support of their home and children. Society supported the male as ruler of the roost, and the double standard extended to the double bed. The male's sexual needs were gratified according to his, not the woman's wishes. He chose the time. He felt no need to give. Once satisfied, he rarely gave his docile mate a second sexual thought. Moreover, he had deeply founded memories of another woman who, presumably, had also been a wife. She had provided for other hungers. With affection he remembered his mother. For such various reasons, then, did the male find his married state agreeable. And this one-sided relationship doubtless helped lead to the justified (and remarkably patient) resentment felt by many married women.

The long overdue liberation of women changed all that. Enfranchised, and finding new employment and enjoyment opportunities open to them, women also, at last, expected equality in the marital bed. Many of their husbands then imposed upon themselves an unaccustomed husbandly duty—the sexual satisfaction of their wives. Many, but not all. One study has revealed that college-matriculated men are apparently more concerned with their wives' sexual gratification than are those with less education.

This concern of some men with the sexual satisfaction of women is to their credit; perhaps college is a civilizing influence after all.

Variations in Orgasmic Quality

"There is good evidence that the capacity for orgasm or sexual climax is a natural birthright of almost every healthy adult human being."[20] The quality of a human orgasm is to a great extent a matter of individual interpretation. Although an orgasm involves the same nervous pathways and the same total body responses in all humans, the degree of involvement varies with individuals and situations. This may be a factor causing subjective differences in the quality of different orgasms. On one occasion, for example, a woman may have sexual intercourse while she is depressed and tired. If her partner is matter-of-fact and pays no heed to her mood, she may have no orgasm or perhaps only a local clitoral sensation. But if her partner is sensitive to her mood, if he expresses his love and waits for her participation, her orgasmic experience, even if it is not intense, will more likely be satisfying.

Sexual Stimulation and Body Areas

In the discussion of the female and male reproductive systems in the next chapter, it will be pointed out that some body areas are especially sensitive to sexual stimuli, particularly to touch. These **erogenous zones**, however, are by no means limited to those areas. Nor is sexual desire stimulated by touch alone.

The most sexually sensitive areas are the head of the penis and its rim and underside, the clitoris, the mons pubis (or veneris), the labia minora, the vestibule (that is, the space between the labia minora into which the vagina and urethra open), and the opening of the vaginal canal. The vaginal canal, like the shaft of the penis, does not particularly respond to touch as an erotic area. However, the inner thighs, buttocks, the space between the genitalia, and the anus are all erogenous zones. Reportedly, King Louis XIV had two thousand enemas during his lifetime.[21] However, since he was provided with so many alternatives, it seems doubtful that this was his only source of erotic stimulation.

Certainly the lips, the inside of the mouth and tongue, fingertips, earlobes, and ear canals should be included in any list of erogenous zones. Generally, the genital areas are more sensitive to touch than other areas. But undoubtedly, the amount of nerve supply to an area is important. For many the breasts, nipples, throat, back and side of the neck, and the space between the side of the neck and shoulder are erogenous zones.

Erogenous zones are numerous enough to make generalizations risky. The possibility that any particular part of the body can be counted upon to be erogenous depends greatly on learning and experience. Added to this are the erotic stimuli that result from seeing, hearing, and even smelling sexually stimulating objects or materials. It has been said that men are more stimulated by seeing female genitalia than females are when seeing male genitalia. This, however, is likely a cultural result rather than a strictly functional phenomenon. Kinsey interviewed some women who could be brought to orgasm by having their eyebrows stroked or by having pressure applied to their teeth.[22]

The language of love is as complex as the individual. As two lovers seek to discover what pleasures the other, they may embark on a unique journey of intimacy. The explorations and discoveries, the givings and takings of love can bring about a transcendent and mystical enthrallment in which, as the English poet John Milton wrote, two people are "imparadis'd in one anothers arms."

Masturbation

When I was a schoolboy I thought a fair woman a pure Goddess; my mind was a soft nest in which some one of them slept, though she knew it not.[23]

At the age of about two or three, the child begins to explore and stimulate the genitalia. This gives the child pleasure but often creates anxiety in the parents. The parental anxiety is rooted in their own conditioning and culture.

The stigma attached to masturbation has ancient beginnings. Early Hebrews and Christians believed children should be sexless. In that period of constant external threat to both groups, it was thought necessary to forbid any practice that might become an internal threat. To strengthen the authority of the family and community, practical controls by adults, including strict sexual repression of the young, were thus deemed essential.

During the Dark Ages, fear of disease was added to sin as a deterrent to masturbation. This attitude died slowly. On August 10, 1897, Michael McCormick of San Francisco was granted patent number 587,994 for a male chastity belt. Fathers were to fit them on their adolescent sons to keep them from masturbating. It was a cruel device, but at least it was an improvement over those manufactured by Victorian engineers. In those days a padlock locked a metal cage that was fitted over the boy's genitals at bedtime. To make certain that he did not disturb himself while resting, the internal cage was outfitted with sharp spikes.

In those days the young were led to believe that masturbation would visit upon them every malady from sterility to stuttering. Even today, there are unfortunates who believe this. Others, who are fully aware that masturbation does not cause disease, still feel ashamed of masturbating. Thus, an aura of anxiety envelops practically all the males and perhaps three-fourths of the females in this culture.

"Don't do that!" This admonition, punctuated with a sharp slap, is often the two-year-old's introduction to a parent's lack of understanding about sexual development. The child is taught a crippling lesson: Part of the body is bad. What is worse, it is a part that feels good. This cruel lesson may never be unlearned. Faced with the catastrophe of losing parental love, the child learns early that masturbation is one pleasure that must be enjoyed in guilty secrecy. At age two or three, that is a harsh discovery, especially since the child loves the parent with all his or her dependent heart. Filled with a mournful sense of guilt, the child represses these feelings. But years later, they may be revived, cloaked in anxiety.

On the other hand, there are parents who are overly conscious of these possibilities. They certainly need not exercise excessive care to avoid disturbing the toddler during genital manipulations. The child should be interrupted if a diaper needs changing or for any other sensible reason. Some three- or four-year-olds masturbate publicly. They should firmly but gently be told why this practice is unacceptable. A

parent's instruction is better than a stranger's taunts.

Similarities and Differences Between Males and Females

"For most males of every social level masturbation provides the chief source of sexual outlet in early adolescence. It is in that period that the activity reaches its highest frequencies."[24] However, masturbatory activity may not reach its peak during the same age group for both sexes. The frequency of male masturbation usually declines after the teen years. With women, the frequency of masturbation often increases up to middle age. After that time the activity becomes more regular.

Why is it often more difficult for the male adolescent to divert his thoughts from masturbation than it is for the older male or the adolescent female? When he was quite old the ancient Greek thinker Sophocles thanked the gods that he was no longer ruled by the tyranny of sexual desire. In our society some believe that the repressed male adolescent lives with that tyranny and that it is a major cause of teen-age anxiety. Many students of the subject suggest that for the young adolescent boy, sexual stimulation results in an overpowering desire for release by sexual intercourse. Sex play, kissing, and petting all stimulate sperm and fluid production. Pressures are built up. The trapped sperm and fluids must be released. Ejaculation occurs. Some authorities also suggest that for the boy, sexual intercourse and love are quite unrelated. Unlike the girl, he usually does not romanticize his sexual tensions.

What is a local experience for the boy is more like a romantic experience for the young girl. Ova are not produced in great numbers, and unlike spermatozoa and their transporting fluids, there is no imprisonment to cause pressures that must be released. With the girl there is no ejaculatory reflex stimulation. In the young adolescent girl, therefore, nongenital sexual stimulation does not necessarily result in desire for sexual intercourse.

Secrecy about sexuality does not lead to emotional serenity. The young adolescent girl wants to know about menstruation and pregnancy and delivery, and she wants to know if sexual intercourse hurts. If she sees a magazine double-page spread of children with fins instead of arms, she wants to know all about that, too. She wants to know what kind of sexual activity boys have. And she should know that the majority of girls masturbate.

Before "wet dreams" occur, the boy should know about these entirely normal nighttime emissions; he will then realize that they are not "dirty." Almost all adolescent boys (over 95 percent) masturbate. The frequency varies from once or twice to several dozen times a month. This the boy needs to know, and he should be told. The realization that virtually all boys masturbate at his age dilutes his sense of guilt.

The senseless guilt and anxiety to which adolescents have been subjected because of masturbation has abated somewhat. There is considerable opinion among psychiatrists that masturbation is a valuable transition to mature sexual relations. One thing is certain: In this culture, no other activity indulged in by the great majority of males and females is looked upon with such intolerance.

Boys or girls who masturbate privately and without guilt or a sense of moral unworthiness will be able to give the best of themselves to a mate. Since they look upon themselves as people of worth, they give something valuable and good.

Those who find in masturbation their only source of gratification and consolation need help. But so does any disturbed person obsessed with one activity to the virtual exclusion of all else in a rich and varied world. From the point of view of body function, however, there is no scientific evidence whatsoever that masturbation can be excessively frequent.

Homosexual Behavior

She who superintended the wedding comes and clips the hair of the bride close around her head, dresses her up in man's clothes, and leaves her upon a mattress in the dark; afterwards comes the bridegroom, in his everyday clothes, sober and composed, as having supped at the common table, and, entering privately into the room where the bride lies, unties her virgin zone, and takes her to himself; and, after staying sometime together, he returns composedly to his own apartment, to sleep as usual with the other young men.[25]

In this way, did the ancient Greek writer Plutarch describe the wedding night of a Spartan girl. The groom had had a succession of male lovers since his twelfth year. Moreover, he had been taught that he owed love to neither his shorn wife nor to his child. The bridegroom dared not tarry long with his bride lest he suffer the jealous anger of his male lovers in the barracks. So casual was the marital relationship that the wife often bore a child without ever seeing the man who made her pregnant. Any children born of these unions were the property of the state. Male homosexual orientation was a cultural cornerstone of Spartan life. Its purpose was to perpetuate the state, as it was reasoned that love between young men increased their loyalty to one another and, therefore, to the state. Marriage to a female was expected but, again, only to provide warriors for Sparta.

A homosexual orientation, then, has an ancient history. In one society, at least, it was official policy. In ancient Rome it was tolerated, but considered unworthy of a Roman. And among the early Hebrews and Christians, it was regarded with disfavor.

The Hazards of Labeling

Almost twenty centuries later Kinsey and his coworkers wrote:

There are some persons whose sexual reactions and socio-sexual activities are directed only toward individuals of their own sex. There are others whose psychosexual reactions and socio-sexual activities are directed, throughout their lives, only toward individuals of the opposite sex. These are the extreme patterns which are labeled homosexuality and heterosexuality. There remain, however, among both females and males, a considerable number of persons who include both homosexual and heterosexual responses and/or activities in their histories. Sometimes their homosexual and heterosexual responses and contacts occur at different periods in their lives; sometimes they occur coincidentally.[26]

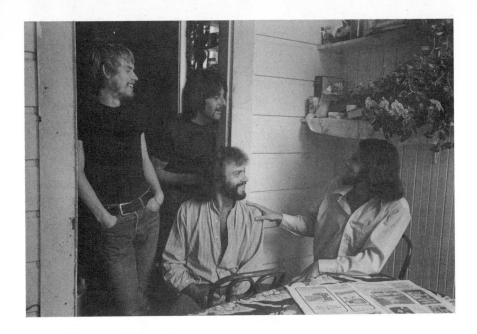

Gay men at home.

About male homosexual behavior they wrote further:

> Males do not represent two discrete populations, heterosexual and homosexual. The world is not to be divided into sheep and goats . . . nature rarely deals with discrete categories. Only the human mind invents categories and tries to force facts into separated pigeon-holes."[27]

Thus, homosexual behavior is not an all-or-none condition, and in evaluating it, considerations of time, place, and degree are especially important.

It is a mistake to associate body type or mannerisms or occupation with homosexual behavior. A brawny football player may prefer a homosexual behavior pattern; a graceful male ballet dancer may just as likely prefer a heterosexual pattern. Only a small percentage of people whose behavior is homosexual (fewer than one in twenty men and probably the same number of women) can be identified by such attributes as mannerisms or dress. There is a widespread belief that people whose behavior is homosexual are unusually artistic, based on

the observation that some professions demanding unusual creative ability seem to attract a large proportion of people who engage in homosexual behavior. However, this phenomenon is most likely due to the tolerance on the part of the members of those particular professions toward people whose homosexual behavior is known or apparent.

The Extent of Homosexual Behavior

How many individuals participate in homosexual behavior? Possibly millions. Kinsey estimated that the behavior of 4 percent of the adult white males in this country was exclusively homosexual after the onset of adolescence. Thirty-seven percent were estimated to have had at least some overt homosexual experience to the point of orgasm between adolescence and old age.[28] This estimate may be high. Since Kinsey had ready access to prisoners, he used them for many of his interviews. He thought that their experience was typical of the lower socioeconomic group. Such is not the case.[29]

The available data on the incidence of homosexual behavior among females is, at best, open to question. Female homosexual behavior seems to be treated with studious indifference. Unlike the male who is often hounded by the police, the female whose behavior is homosexual is rarely arrested. In this culture, such emotional and sexual involvements between women are more acceptable than those between men.

The Roots of Homosexual Behavior

VARYING INFLUENCES AT VARYING TIMES

Basically, human sexuality depends on three factors—*genetic, endocrine,* and *psychological*. Though all are involved in human sexuality, the degree of their influence on human development varies at different stages of growth. Genetic combinations are established during fertilization and subsequent cellular division. The cells contain the fundamental arrangement of chemical materials (DNA) necessary for the development of genital, nervous, and muscular structural patterns. Endocrine tissue has an early influence on the direction that the developing embryo will take. Its critical role in determining nervous and genital system structure was discussed earlier in this chapter (see pages 318–319). But this early activity of the endocrine hormones is not the only period during which their influence assumes primary importance. Puberty is marked by a second surge of endocrine activity. Androgens in the male and estrogens in the female, along with other hormones, stimulate further growth and development of the sexual organs. Hormones also increase the sensitivity of the sex structure to stimulation. Still other hormones, such as those from the thyroid gland and those growth hormones that affect vitality and strength, also have an influence on sexual development.

But neither the genes nor hormones alone determine the choice of the sex partner. It is cultural influences that teach most sexual behavior. Starting at birth, environmental influences begin to supersede and augment the now visible genetic-endocrine influences on the child. Not until puberty do the endocrine glands temporarily take over again and partly overcome the psychological influence of the environment. In the late teens or early twenties, when endocrine maturity is complete, the psychological factors in the environment again gain primary importance.

To summarize: Within the uterus, the genetic and endocrine factors exert their influence. In early childhood, the environment molds most of the sexual response. During puberty, the endocrine glands again assume primary importance. By the late teens or early twenties, psy-

chological influences again become supreme.

Although different influences are dominant at different times, they all operate to a certain extent all of the time. The seesaw effect resulting from the varying influences of genetic, endocrine, and psychological factors at different stages of human development can hardly be expected to guarantee one single form of sexual behavior. Considering the complexity of these relationships, it is not surprising that there is so much homosexual behavior. It is surprising that there is so little.

MASTERS AND JOHNSON REPORT ABOUT HOMOSEXUAL BEHAVIOR

In the spring of 1979 William E. Masters and his wife and co-worker, Virginia E. Johnson, published their results of ten years of research on homosexual behavior.[30] Following are some of their conclusions:

1. Homosexual behavior is learned.
2. Functionally, people with a homosexual orientation respond to the same sexual stimuli and experience the same physiological responses as do people whose sexual expression is heterosexual.
3. People can move in or out of patterns of homosexual behavior at any time in their lives.
4. There are no significant differences in fantasy patterns of free-floating thoughts between people of homosexual or heterosexual orientations.
5. People whose behavior is homosexual may be treated for sexual inadequacy with partners of their own choosing and with at least as much success as those whose behavior is heterosexual.
6. Perhaps because they need not decipher the sexual signals of the

opposite sex, people of a homosexual orientation are less hurried and more considerate during their sexual activities. In this respect they are thus more likely to enjoy their sexual expression than do people whose behavior is heterosexual. Moreover, those whose behavior is bisexual (equally attracted sexually to both males and females and termed "ambisexuals" by the authors) are more gentle, less hurried, and more considerate when they are with partners of the same sex. When they are with partners of the opposite sex they are more brusque, less considerate, and more preoccupied with orgasm.

7. Those whose sexual expression is homosexual but who *desire it to be heterosexual* could, with two weeks of help, achieve this goal about 65 percent of the time.

8. People with a homosexual orientation can and do enjoy their sexual expression as much as those whose behavior is heterosexual.

Like their book *Human Sexual Inadequacy* (Boston, 1970), Masters and Johnson's study on homosexual behavior has stimulated much professional criticism. Those who disagree with either book cannot be easily dismissed since these critics, too, are deservedly respected students of the subject. Doubts are being expressed about the methods and emphasis of various aspects of the study, the validity of some of the definitions, the results of treatment, the admitted failure to adequately follow treated patients, the belief that the patients were a biased small sample skewed in favor of success, the conclusion that homosexual behavior is primarily learned, and other factors. But as Dr. Masters has said about the

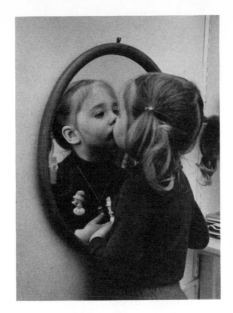

Sexual expression is learned.

study, "If it has any value, it will survive. If not, it should be rejected."[31]

In this he is certainly correct.

PREADOLESCENT SEXUAL BEHAVIOR

Before the onset of puberty there is much curiosity and, indeed, sexual play among both boys and girls. Both may masturbate and be capable of orgasm. Both are exceedingly curious, not only about their own genitalia, but also about the sexual organs of others. A few may even accomplish coitus. Occasionally small groups of children, usually of the same sex, participate in sexual play. Unless they are treated with senseless harshness by adults, they experience no particular anxiety as a result of this passing behavior.

EARLY ADOLESCENT NEEDS: HOMOSEXUAL-LIKE BEHAVIOR

The increased sexual drive that occurs at puberty can be a bewilder-

ing experience. Anxious young people are often unsure of what their relationship is to the opposite sex. They may retreat to more familiar ground—to members of the same sex. Many young people pass through a period of intense interest in the same sex before proceeding to a heterosexual adjustment. They share secrets and are comforted in the knowledge that they have similar problems. The variety of sexual expression during this ordinarily passing period may be considerable. Group exhibition and masturbation as well as mutual masturbation may occur. At this age homosexual behavior may be seen as a temporary defense against the fear associated with the move toward full heterosexual relationships. Again, overreactions by adults may lead to lasting personality problems for the adolescents.

No single behavioral clue is, by itself, an absolute indicator of an eventual orientation to an active preference for same-sex sexual partners. When several clues do appear to suggest a primarily homosexual orientation on the part of the adolescent and are causing parental concern, the advice of a trained psychologist should be promptly sought. It is wise for the parents to be initially interviewed by the psychologist without the child. The concern may be groundless, but the hurt to the child may be lasting. And, indeed, it may be the parents rather than the child that need help.

POSSIBLE PARENTAL FACTORS IN HOMOSEXUAL BEHAVIOR

Studies of adolescent girls whose behavior pattern is homosexual have identified a disruptive and unstable family background as a major contributing factor to the girls' homosexual behavior. In such cases a wide variety of emotionally traumatic experiences seem to lead to a deep sense of insecurity that is at least minimally relieved by another woman. This leads to the seeking of female relationships.[31]

However, it should be emphasized that parental attitudes are by no means the only (and often not the major) factor in the development of a homosexual behavior pattern. This is not to deny the profound effect of parental attitudes on children. However, it must be pointed out that a simple cause-and-effect relationship between parental behavior and a homosexual orientation in their children has not been established.

Nevertheless, there are cases of homosexual behavior that would seem to be strongly associated with parental actions. With his son, a father is harsh, unforgiving, punitive. With his daughter, he is gentle and understanding. Will not the son then contemplate the advantages of being a girl? An overbearing, domineering mother constantly ridicules the father, who is but a shadow in the home. How can the son then perceive the advantages of manhood? So may it have been with the female whose behavior is homosexual. Possibly the girl's mother gave her reason to fear womanhood. Or the mother may compete with the daughter. She defeminizes her by repeatedly telling her that she is gawky and unladylike. The father may be too submissive to help his daughter. Or, uneasy about the girl's budding sexuality, he is only too glad to avoid her. Perhaps, however, he subtly seduces his daughter. He ruthlessly criticizes both her male and female

friends. Feeling guilt because of his interest in the girl's body, he forbids her every expression of femininity common to our culture—playing with dolls, using cosmetics, shopping for pretty dresses. "This image of a close-binding overly intimate father [is] a counterpart to the close-binding, intimate mother found in studies of male homosexuality."[33]

Is Homosexual Behavior an Illness?

By the mid-1930s, Sigmund Freud was known as the greatest living physician of the human mind. His name had become a household word, and a bewildered mother had written him imploring his help. Freud's answer is now part of psychiatric literature. "Homosexuality," he wrote her, "is assuredly no advantage, but it is nothing to be ashamed of, no vice, no degradation, it cannot be classified as an illness."[34] However, this statement hardly settled the issue. Many psychiatrists consider homosexual behavior a disease that should be treated. The majority do not. In December 1973, the Board of Trustees of the American Psychiatric Association announced their unanimous decision to no longer consider homosexual behavior per se a disease. In this they were supported by a majority of the membership. The tendency among many is to help the homosexually oriented person adjust to his or her sexual situation.

Whether the homosexually oriented person is sick or merely different, being treated as a criminal and a social outcast when he or she is not predatory and does not bother children is unwarranted. Harassment only creates or increases emo-

tional distress. Recent evidence suggests that there is growing understanding and tolerance of this form of sexual behavior.

A recently published study[35] of people of homosexual orientation by present members of the original Kinsey Institute has several shortcomings. First, its 1970 picture of "gay life" does not reflect events and feelings since the rise of the homosexual rights movement. Second, the study was made in a city probably more tolerant of people of a homosexual orientation (San Francisco) than most. Indeed, so large is the homosexual community in San Francisco that the group wields considerable political power.*

The 1970 findings revealed little that was new. The best-adjusted people of homosexual orientation were those who had close, long-lasting relationships. Most of the women reported ten or fewer partners during their lives. The average male had engaged in sex acts with several hundred men, and 25 percent reported that, as adults, they had engaged in sexual activities with boys under the age of sixteen. In both sexes, 25 percent believed homosexual behavior to be an emotional disorder, and a higher percent

---

*In November 1978, eight years after the study was made, Californians resoundingly rejected a statewide ballot that would have banned people of a homosexual orientation from teaching in schools. Many of the most conservative politicians in the state rejected the proposal, pointing out that existing laws already protected children from "immoral" teachers, whether homosexual or heterosexual. In addition, there was little if any evidence that teachers who have a homosexual orientation had affected California children. Lastly, the suggested law could, it was believed, be a gross invasion of privacy. For an interesting description of San Francisco's homosexual community, see Herbert Gold, "A Walk on San Francisco's Gay Side," *The New York Times Magazine*, November 6, 1977, p. 67.

had considered discontinuing their activities at least once in their lives.

Sexually transmitted diseases among women of a homosexual orientation were almost unknown. However, over 60 percent of the men had had a sexually transmitted disease at least once.

About 16 percent of the males had little or no interest in sexual activity; they were apathetic people of low self-esteem. Compared with men of a heterosexual orientation, the homosexual exhibited signs of greater emotional damage in selected areas, such as depression and paranoia. Twenty percent of homosexually oriented men had tried suicide compared with 4 percent of the heterosexual men interviewed. Thirteen percent suffered severe psychosocial and sexual problems. On the other hand, homosexual women were almost as well adjusted as the studied heterosexual women.

The report has classified homosexually oriented people into five groups. Two of these, the "close-coupled" and "functional" enjoyed a higher sense of self-worth and self-confidence. Their psychological test scores were almost equal to those of heterosexually oriented people. A third category, "open-coupled" —those living with a partner and looking outside the home for fulfillment—scored well also. Categories four and five—termed "asexuals" and "dysfunctionals"—comprise 40 percent of male gays; they suffered the greatest proportion of psychosocial and sexual disturbances.

The classification, although original, may have limited usefulness. The researchers were unable to classify about one-third of the people interviewed because they did not match any category. Perhaps that is to be expected of all people.

TREATMENT FOR THOSE WHO WANT IT

Several studies have been designed to prove that homosexual behavior can be changed through psychiatric treatment. Moreover, it is claimed that many (although not all) of those who seek treatment want to develop a heterosexual behavior pattern. Both men and women have successfully changed their homosexual orientation.

One study, extending over eighteen years, included 710 patients drawn both from clinics and from private practice. Including partially and fully heterosexual adjustments, the reported "change rate" was about 45 percent.[36] One professional made these observations:

Most lesbians are bisexual. Some will have had heterosexual experiences before their homosexual debut, some move back and forth pendulum style from heterosexual to homosexual affairs. . . . Interest in heterosexuality is never completely abandoned by homosexuals of either sex—if not consciously, then on a subconscious level. The dreams of even confirmed homosexuals continue to reveal conflicts about their sexual direction. Since women need not concern themselves with problems of potency and erection on purely functional grounds, it is easier for them than for male homosexuals to satisfy heterosexual curiosity and yearnings. However, a firmly established heterosexual adaptation is rarely if ever achieved without psychiatric intervention. Today lesbianism is a treatable condition. About 50 percent who undertake psychotherapy, and stay with it, shift to heterosexuality, although the younger the patient the more favorable the outlook.[37]

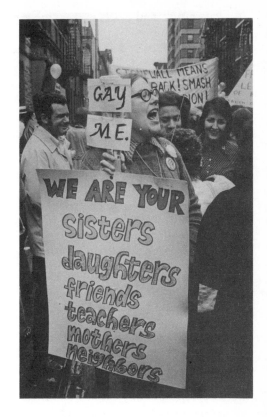

Masters and Johnson
on Inadequate Sexual Response

Among the contributions of Masters and Johnson is their clarification of the definitions of various human sexual problems. For example, because of the vagueness of the word "frigidity," they reject its use as a diagnostic term. They regard "inadequate sexual response" as a more satisfactory general term to describe such problems in both men and women.

In the Female

All aspects of both female and male inadequate sexual response require careful individual evaluation. Three aspects of inadequate female sexual response have been studied by Masters and Johnson.

DYSPAREUNIA

Dyspareunia (painful coitus) may result from physical causes, such as vaginal infection, an irritating collection of *smegma* (an oily secretion of the glands around the clitoris, or a chemical irritation (as occurs with some douches or inserted chemical contraceptives). Older women may experience dyspareunia as a result of thinning of the vaginal mucous membrane. This condition is easily treated.

Dyspareunia may also be caused by psychological problems that result in insufficient vaginal lubrication. Among these emotional impediments may be the woman's fear of injury or pregnancy, hostility toward her mate, or conflict over her sexual role (as may result from a highly repressive childhood).

ORGASMIC DYSFUNCTION

As recently as the nineteenth century, the famed London physician William Acton wrote that "most women happily for them [or, in a later edition, "happily for society"] are not troubled with sexual feeling of any kind."[38] Today, happily for both society and its men and women, Acton's pronouncement is considered nonsense. Nevertheless, it did contribute to the social acceptance of the notion that decent women were not supposed to have orgasms. *Orgasmic dysfunction*, which refers to difficulties encountered by women in reaching orgasm, is even today often rooted in a mid-Victorian-type rejection of one's own natural sexual desires.

The treatment of orgasmic dysfunction requires the couple's understanding of each other's past sexual experiences and sexually tinged memories. Those factors that sexually stimulate or depress the woman should be discussed. The nonorgasmic* woman is often one whose partner ejaculates prematurely.[39] Should this be a chronic experience, the male will need professional help. If successful, that help will increase the man's awareness of the woman's needs. Heedless of the woman's needs, he may have succeeded in having an orgasm, but failed to help her have one. A fear of inadequacy may make the woman unable to achieve the sexual tension necessary for orgasm.

*Lately the word "nonorgasmic" has been replaced by some experts with the word "preorgasmic," suggesting the correctable nature of the problem.

Whether there is dysfunction or not, every couple must be willing to discover and resolve their individual and mutual needs in order to enjoy a rich and satisfying sexual life together.

VAGINISMUS

Vaginismus is a spasm of the vagina that results in a constriction of the vaginal outlet. The spasm is in no way under the control of the woman who experiences it. It is brought about by "imagined, anticipated, or real attempts at vaginal penetration. Thus, vaginismus is a classic example of a psychosomatic illness."[40] Psychosomatic disorders originate in the mind and are manifested as physical symptoms.** One of the causes of vaginismus is repressive sex education from which the child learns that sex is dirty and sinful. The psychic trauma of rape or a painful initial coital experience may also result in vaginismus.

Since penile penetration is impossible or, at best, extremely difficult with this condition, vaginismus is commonly the cause of unconsummated marriages or ones in which coitus is very infrequent. Male sexual inadequacies, such as impotence, are not uncommonly associated with vaginismus. This

**The term psychosomatic is from the Greek *psychikos*, "mind," + *soma*, "body." Emotional stimuli are referred by the brain to body organs, resulting in effects ranging from goose flesh to vaginismus. The ancients were well aware of psychosomatic influences. "Diseases of the mind impair the powers of the body," wrote Ovid. Nor did the seventeenth-century English writer John Donne contradict Ovid when he wrote that "the body makes the minde."

emphasizes the importance of a diagnostic and treatment approach that involves both partners.

In the Male

DYSPAREUNIA

The causes of male dyspareunia are generally physical in nature. Poor personal hygiene may lead to an infection beneath the prepuce (foreskin). The resultant inflammation may be painful even without the stimulation of sexual intercourse. Old scars within the urethra from a subsided gonorrheal infection may cause a stricture of the urethral passage, which not only may result in painful coitus but, indeed, may interfere with the passage of the urine through the penis. Many, but by no means all, strictures are due to untreated gonorrhea. Early and adequate treatment of gonorrheal infection is the best prevention for gonorrheal strictures.

A third cause of male dyspareunia is *phimosis* (from the Greek *phimosis*, meaning "muzzling" or "closure"). Men with phimosis have an unusually long prepuce that is so tight that it cannot be drawn back from over the glans penis. As with many other penile problems, the condition may be painful even when the man is not attempting sexual intercourse. Phimosis can become quite complicated if it is not treated. Fibrous tissue may grow between the prepuce and the glans. These fibrous adhesions make the prepuce even less retractable. Smegma may collect and cause infection, inflammation, and even ulceration, all of which may be very painful. Fortunately, these problems are easily corrected — usually by circumcision and administration of medication to relieve the infection.

Still another cause of male dyspareunia may be found within the environment of the vagina. Not uncommonly, contraceptive chemicals and douche preparations may cause allergic manifestations in sensitive penile tissue.

IMPOTENCE

"It is the heaviest stone that Melancholy can throw at a man, to tell him he is at the end of his nature." So did the seventeenth-century English physician and writer Sir Thomas Browne describe the despair of impotence. Men who suffer from *primary impotence* have either never had an erection or have been unable to maintain an erection long enough to have sexual intercourse. Those who suffer from *secondary impotence* were once sexually capable but have lost the ability to have an erection and maintain it long enough to enjoy coitus.

Primary impotence usually is the result of a deep-seated psychological problem. A boy may grow up to be impotent if he is taught that sex is sinful and dirty, or if he is so overwhelmingly impressed by his mother that her sex is preferable to his.

Secondary impotence has a wide range of causes. Biological-physical causes include disease, injury, and impotency-inducing medication. Among the psychosocial factors are rigidity during childhood training, an affiliation with an orthodox religious group with highly restrictive sexual mores, and an orientation toward homosexual behavior. The major cause of secondary impotence in the Masters and Johnson study population was premature ejaculation (see the next section). This type of impotence may take years to develop. Drinking too much alcohol is the second major cause of secondary

impotence. Sometimes excessive alcohol consumption can lead to a single episode of impotence. In most cases this is no cause for undue concern. However, to be convivial or to build up his courage, a man may consistently drink a small amount of alcohol before engaging in sexual intercourse. If this becomes habitual, he may increase his intake. Then he experiences an episode of impotence. Anxiety about the next performance may result in another failure. He may try to drown his fear of failure in more alcohol. Soon fear of failure to have an erection haunts the afflicted man. Like an angry bystander, he observes himself with anxiety. No longer does an erection occur as naturally to him as does breathing. He watches to see if he will perform, and he cannot. He hopes that by his very frustration he can will his penis erect. But no man can will an erection. If he seeks treatment, this is one of the first facts that he must learn.

PREMATURE EJACULATION

With this condition, the male loses much of his erection as soon as he ejaculates. He is thus unable to continue intravaginal intercourse. Should the ejaculation occur before his partner is sexually satisfied, it may be considered premature. A variety of reasons may account for premature ejaculation. By no means are all of them unusual. The time between his sexual contacts may have been too long. Or he may have enjoyed too prolonged a period of foreplay. An occasional premature ejaculation should not concern either partner. When it becomes a chronic part of the sexual pattern, serious problems arise.

Many men in this culture regard the ability to satisfy their sexual

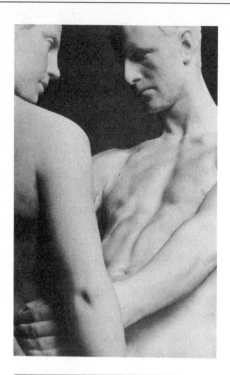

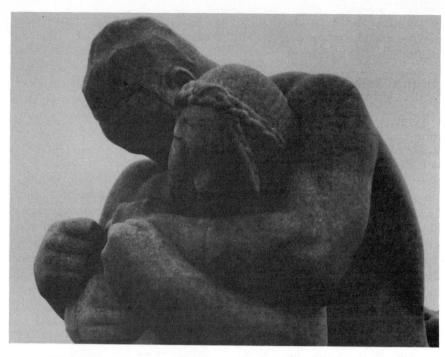

PHOTO ESSAY
The embrace of life.
These sculptures are by the Norwegian artist Gustav Vigeland (1869–1943).

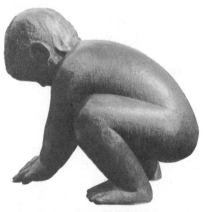

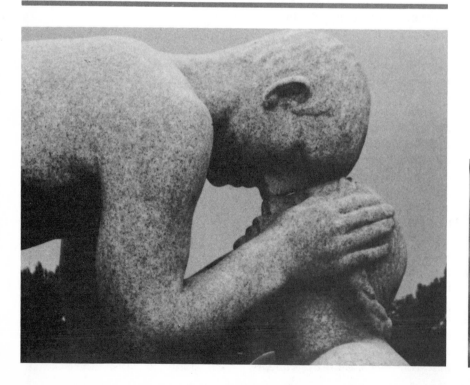

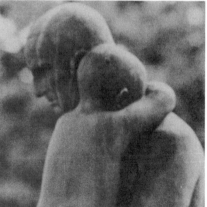

partner as one measure of masculinity. Persistent failure to do so causes the man to lose confidence in his masculinity. Even a few failures may make him feel that he is on trial. This makes him anxious, and his mounting anxiety causes him to ejaculate prematurely—often even before his penis enters the vagina. At first the woman may be patient with him. She avoids stimulating him before coitus. If this fails, she may resort to self-pity. "You're just using me," she may tell him angrily. Now their sexual experience is out of its context of love. It is no longer an expression of understanding and caring. It is surrounded by embarrassment, anxiety, failure—even hate.

Masters and Johnson consider premature ejaculation a problem if the male cannot control his ejaculation during vaginal containment long enough to satisfy his partner for at least 50 percent of their coital exposures. Of all the male dysfunctions, they find premature ejaculation the easiest to cure.

EJACULATORY INCOMPETENCE

The man with *ejaculatory incompetence* usually has no difficulty in having an erection. However, he cannot ejaculate in the vagina. This disability is "the clinical opposite of premature ejaculation . . . separate from impotence."[41] Fortunately, it is rare. A severely restrictive upbringing, a fear of causing pregnancy, or a shocking emotional upset may cause ejaculatory incompetence. Sometimes a single traumatic event may cause the problem. It has been noted that wives of husbands with this condition may feel rejected. Despite this, they may frequently experience multiple orgasms.

Today, careful studies have revealed new ways of helping those with many of these sexual inadequacies —not only the young but also the elderly. It is as if scientific investigators, respectful of human significance and dignity, have helped bring to pass these wistful lines from the *Rubáiyát*:

> *Ah Love! could you and I with Him conspire*
> *To grasp this sorry Scheme of Things entire,*
> *Would not we shatter it to bits— and then*
> *Remold it nearer to the Heart's desire!*[42]

Exploring Some Myths and Misconceptions about Human Sexuality

Open-minded and frank discussions about sexual matters is a recent phenomenon. Unfortunately, much of the content of these discussions is based on past misinformation. What are some of the more common of these misconceptions?

1 To have a satisfactory sexual experience, the woman and man must have an orgasm each time they have intercourse.

This often unrealized ideal has been a hazard to many relationships. The difference in the degree of sexual interest between the sexes has already been mentioned. As a relationship matures and intimacy deepens, the frequency of orgasms may increase.

However, both the young man and the young woman often approach their new sexuality with some guilt and anxiety. They do not suddenly awaken to maturity after a long period of sexual somnolence. Nevertheless, instead of preparing adolescents for their future sexual function, much of society merely tries to control them. This sexual control is matched by a conspiracy of parental silence about the subject. The growing boy is not helped by the slick magazines, nor by the refusal of his parents to talk about sexuality, nor by the embarrassment of his teachers. Too often, his education is a compound of the sniggering anxieties of his contemporaries and furtive, short-lived, basically uncomfortable liaisons. He drifts alone on the murky waters of opinionated misinformation. Sexuality is associated with something dirty.* It may then be loaded with guilt and anxiety.

The young woman may be similarly ill-equipped. Her secret anxiety may be increased by the unspoken message that she equal the alluringly abandoned creatures her mate sees in some magazine centerfolds. And the slick magazines designed for her offer hundreds of mixed messages about how to be a "real woman." Confusion is inevitable.

Marriage poses special anxieties that require patience, enormous

*This association may have begun before adolescence—on the day the small child was punished for examining the genitalia.

understanding, and a sense of humor about oneself and one's mate. No matter what their previous experience has been, the couple is ceremoniously thrust into new, often threatening roles. They must prove themselves. Right now. Every time. It will relax the couple to know that orgasm with each intercourse is not necessary to a happy marriage. Research by Masters and Johnson suggests that the intensity and duration of a woman's orgasm is not necessarily related to her sense of sexual gratification. An orgasm of relatively low intensity and short duration, during a sexual experience with the man she loves, may indeed be evaluated by the wife as a complete and fulfilling sexual experience.[43] The consistent sexual competency of the wife or husband is not as important to marital happiness as understanding and patient communication. Feeling safe and feeling a sense of trust are no less profoundly involved with marital happiness than the orgasm.

2 Simultaneous orgasm is absolutely essential for ultimate and satisfactory sexual expression.

This nonsense, a favorite of some manuals about sexuality, is another anxiety producer. The woman must, after all, either begin to have, or have, an orgasm before the man. If the former is true, simultaneous orgasms are possible. These are delightful experiences. However, many couples never have them, nor do they miss them. To insist on a simultaneous orgasm is another way of putting oneself on trial. The man who is on constant trial does not relax. He may become unable to have an erection. This failure may, in turn, make him fear that he has lost his sexual prowess. Shame torments

him. Sometimes a man may become impotent with a woman with whom he feels on trial. Instead he finds himself potent with "another woman." Or, with his mate, he may have premature ejaculations, with attendant guilt feelings and anxiety. Again the male doubts his potency.

Male sexual activity is circumscribed by a basic requirement. He must feel certain of his active role and that role requires an erect penis. He cannot, like his mate, simply submit to sexual intercourse. Also, although constant submission may relieve the women of some of the stress of performance, it will not afford her a full and satisfying expression of her sexuality. Both partners should feel comfortable with the woman taking an active role whenever the mood strikes her. For her, too, coitus should be neither a test nor a contest. Some marriage manuals make effective chaperones.

3 Direct clitoral stimulation during sexual intercourse is essential.

There are some misguided writers who detail the crucial importance of direct clitoral stimulation to arouse sexual desire. Research disputes this advice. For a great number of women the difference between clitoral excitement and irritation is slight. Many lovers discover that manual clitoral stimulation is distinctly disagreeable, if not painful. Many, instead, prefer manual stimulation of the general mons area. There is only one best way to find out. A man should feel free to ask his mate what she finds pleasurable.

Effective manual stimulation of the general mons area results in a clitoral retraction reaction (see page 322). The clitoris normally retracts upward.

This physiological reaction to high levels of female sexual tension creates a problem for the sexually inexperienced male. The clitoral-body retraction reaction frequently causes even an experienced male to lose manual contact with the organ. Having lost contact, the male partner usually ceases active stimulation of the general mons area and attempts manually to relocate the clitoral body. During this "textbook" approach, marked sexual frustration may develop in a highly excited female partner. . . . Once . . . clitoral retraction has been established, manipulation of the general mons area is all that is necessary for effective clitoral-body stimulation.[44]

4 Vaginal orgasm, which is mature, is distinct from clitoral orgasm, which is immature.

This mistaken notion dates back to the outmoded idea that female sexual organs are incomplete male organs, nothing more than a perpetual case of arrested genital development. It was thought impossible, if not indecent, for women, who were thus hopelessly sexually retarded, to enjoy, much less desire, sexual intercourse. Freud did not fall into this trap, but he did fall for the idea of the female as an incomplete, hence inferior, male. He considered woman biologically dependent on man. He thought that lacking a penis, she was passively envious. "Freud's theories buttressed all the prevailing prejudices and promoted the notion that the female was a deficient male and a second-class citizen."[45] Reflecting the patriarchal culture of his time, he attributed to biology what was, in reality, culturally prescribed. To this was added another error. Girls who masturbated usually did so by manual clitoral stimulation. This, it was decreed by many early writers, was immature. Hence, manual clitoral stimulation to orgasm by adults was also immature. Although clitoral stimulation during intercourse was considered acceptable, only vaginal orgasm was the mark of the normal and sexually mature woman.

The trouble with all this is that it is wrong. What are the facts?

Among the sexually sensitive areas of the female genitalia are the clitoris and the labia minora (see page 361). As a source of erotic arousal, the mons area ranks with the clitoris and the labia minora; it is, however, not strictly a part of the genitalia. Although there are many variations, the labia minora are not as sensitive as the clitoris and the mons area.

The upper two-thirds of the vagina has a different embryological origin than the lower third; that is, it arises from a different group of cells. The lower third of the vagina and the labia minora have the same embryological origin; they arise from the same group of cells. The clitoris and the lower third of the vagina are inseparable structures.

The upper two-thirds of the vagina plays no part in the orgasm. Nor does it play a part in the development of erotic feelings.

With one exception, there are no nerve or muscle or blood vessel connections between the clitoris and the vagina. The exception is a network of veins from the clitoris that merges into a network of veins lying along the walls of the vagina. During sexual excitement, these veins are engorged with blood, causing tumescence. Within ten to thirty seconds after sexual excitement, a lubricating fluid appears on the vaginal walls. This fluid seeps onto the vaginal walls directly from the plexus of veins surrounding the vaginal barrel.

Like the penis, the clitoris is generously endowed with nerves and is capable of tumescence, spasmodic contraction, and detumescence.

During coitus, the penis rarely comes in direct contact with the clitoris. This is because of the above-mentioned retraction reaction. The traction of the penis on the sensitive labia minora stimulates the shortened, hidden clitoris. The thrusting movements of the penis

create simultaneous stimulation of the lower third of the vagina, labia minora, and clitoral shaft and glans as an integrated, inseparable functioning unit with the glans being the most important and, in by far the majority of instances, the indispensable initiator of the orgasmic reaction. . . . it is a physical impossibility to separate the clitoral from the vaginal orgasm.[46]

During the female orgasm, the male often feels contractions on the shaft of his penis. What are they? The vagina itself does not produce these contractions of orgasm. Then what does contract? The orgasmic contractions are of the muscles located in the floor of the pelvis that surround the lower third of the vagina. With female orgasm, these muscles contract, not directly against the vaginal wall, but against the network of engorged chambers of veins and blood channels about that part of the vagina. In this way the venous passages are emptied of blood (detumescence). These muscle contractions about the vaginal veins cause the lower vaginal walls to be passively pushed in and out. Moreover, these muscle contractions cause the upper labia minora to contract. That is what the male feels. "Therefore there is no such thing as an orgasm of the vagina.

What exists is an orgasm of the circumvaginal venous chambers."[47]

Thus, one cannot distinguish between vaginal and clitoral orgasm. Regardless of how it happens, the nature of the orgasm is the same.

Present knowledge of the origin, anatomy, and function of the female genitalia should help to dispel many female fears. Long depressed by the idea of the inferiority of the clitoral orgasm, many women blamed either themselves or their mates for their failure to achieve "vaginal orgasm." The whole notion, however, of a vaginal orgasm separate from clitoral orgasm is biologically impossible and, therefore, utterly invalid. And to consider clitoral orgasm immature and vaginal orgasm mature is senseless. "The tendency to reduce clitoral eroticism to a level of psychopathology or immaturity because of its supposed masculine origin is a travesty of the facts and a misleading psychologic deduction."[48]

5 **The size of the genital organs (penis or vagina) is related to sexual prowess.**

This error is based on myths that have been dispelled by considerable research, most recently by that of Masters and Johnson.[49]

First, the size of the penis is in no way related to the size of the man. In a group of 312 men ranging from twenty-one to eighty-nine years, it was found that the longest penis in the flaccid (soft) state belonged to a man five feet seven inches tall who weighed 152 pounds; the smallest penis was that of a man four inches taller and twenty-six pounds heavier.

Second, upon erection, a larger penis does not necessarily increase to a greater size than does a smaller penis. For example, one man's penile measurement in the flaccid state was 7.5 cm. (2.95 in.); in the erect its length increased to more than double its flaccid state—it lengthened 9 cm. (3.5 in.) to equal 16.5 cm. (6.5 in.). Another man's flaccid penis was 11 cm. (4.3 in.) long; it increased only 5.5 cm. (2.2 in.) as a result of erection; erect, its length also totaled 16.5 cm.* The ex-

*Does the penis ever decrease in size from the flaccid (soft) stage? Yes. Cold, severe exhaustion resulting from undue and prolonged physical strain, advanced age, surgical castration are among the reasons that the size of the penis diminishes from that of its usual flaccid state in an individual. Prolonged impotence of over two years may also have this effect. In addition, this may occur immediately after a man has attempted but failed to have sexual intercourse. This last cause fortifies the belief that lessening of penile size, like erection, is not only the result of a spinal reflex, but is also profoundly influenced by stimuli from the higher brain centers. (Masters and Johnson, *Human Sexual Response*, pp. 180–181.)

tent to which misinformation about penile length can concern some individuals is demonstrated by the young man who reportedly tied weights of increasing size to his penis every day in an attempt to lengthen the organ. He failed.[50]

Third, during the late excitement or early plateau phases, the vagina lengthens and also expands in its upper (deeper) area of the cervix. This creates a receptacle to receive the seminal pool that is about to be deposited. This overdistention of that upper part of the vagina makes some women feel that the penis is "lost in the vagina." This sensation has nothing to do with penile size. It is more apparent in the woman whose vagina has been traumatized during childbirth and then inadequately repaired. However, under ordinary circumstances, it is most unusual for the vagina to be so

large as to interfere with coital pleasure. Unless the woman is highly aroused, accommodation of the penis may be difficult if her vagina is unusually small, or if the lining of the woman's vagina has shrunken somewhat as a result of prolonged restraint from intercourse or post-menopausal changes. In summary,

penile size usually is a minor factor in sexual stimulation of the female partner. The normal or large vagina accommodates a penis of any size without difficulty. If the vagina is exceptionally small, or if a long period of continence or of involution [shriveling] intervenes, a penis of any size can distress rather than stimulate, if mounting is attempted before advanced stages of female sexual tension have been experienced.[51]

Summary

The developing human embryo has two elevations of tissue, the genital ridges. If the embryo is to become a female, the primordial tissue of the outer ridge develops into ovaries, and the rest of the reproductive system follows. However, if it is to become a male, a hormone must cause the transformation of the inner ridge into testes. The testes then secrete androgen, which causes the male reproductive system to develop, and a second substance, which is necessary to inhibit the development of the internal organs of the female reproductive system. Androgen must also act upon the brain to program "patterns of maleness." The fact that there are more chances for mistakes during development of the male is believed to explain the greater prevalence of divergent sexual behavior among males.

The roots of sexual behavior are varied. The action of androgen is only one cause. Culturally learned patterns are instilled in the child from birth by both parents and the society. These patterns are set by age 2½.

The work of Masters and Johnson has established the physiology of the human sexual response. In both sexes, they have identified four phases: the excitement phase, the plateau phase, the orgasmic phase, and the resolution phase. Although the organs involved obviously differ, the physiology of the sexual response is very similar in both sexes.

This is not to say that sexual differences do not exist. Differences become apparent at puberty. Sexual stimulation causes in boys a mostly genital reaction, whereby accumulated sexual fluids are released by ejaculation, while in girls the reaction is diffuse, dominantly cerebral and socially directed. In general, men and women are aroused by different stimuli and have different sexual fantasies, probably due to cultural conditioning. There are many differences in degree of sexual response. For instance, after orgasm the male experiences a refractory period, in which he is temporarily resistant to sexual stimulation. Women, on the other hand, are multiorgasmic. Also, women achieve their sexual peak later than men, but they maintain that peak for a greater number of years. These and many other differences will not create a problem if they are understood by a couple, and if the couple also accepts that individuals, whether men or women, vary greatly in their sexual responses.

Masturbation is very common among both men and women. Although people are often made to feel guilty about masturbation, such feelings are senseless. Many psychiatrists believe that this activity is a valuable transition to mature sexual relations.

Although parents often become concerned, same-sex preadolescent sexual play and adolescent homosexual behavior is common and generally only a part of the development of heterosexual behavior patterns. A lasting homosexual orientation usually has other causes. The complex interaction of genetic, endocrine, and psychological factors is one. Possible parental factors is another. It is wrong to associate particular body types, mannerisms, or occupations with homosexuality. Despite a recent report by Masters and Johnson on the subject, much about homosexuality remains to be studied.

The American Psychiatric Association unanimously decided in 1973 that homosexual behavior per se is not an illness or a disease. One classification of homosexually oriented people revealed that the majority of those who could be matched to a category were about as well adjusted as those who were heterosexually oriented. However, psychiatric treatment is available and has been successful for some of those who desire to change their homosexual behavior.

Another contribution made by Masters and Johnson is their study of the causes of *inadequade sexual response* (a term that they introduced to replace the vaguer and more limited term *frigidity*). In the woman, the dysfunction may be dispareunia (painful coitus), orgasmic dysfunction (inability to have an orgasm), and vaginismus (spasm of the vagina, which prevents intercourse). The male may also experience dyspareunia, as well as impotence, premature ejaculation, and ejaculatory incompetence. The causes of these dysfunctions may be psychic or physical or a combination of the two.

There are many common misconceptions about human sexuality. It is not necessary to have an orgasm every time one has intercourse, nor is simultaneous orgasm essential. Direct clitoral stimulation is not necessary. A vaginal orgasm is not distinct from, or more mature than, a clitoral orgasm. Finally, the size of the genital organ (penis or vagina) is unrelated to sexual prowess.

References

1. Mary Jane Sherfey, "The Evolution and Nature of Female Sexuality in Relation to Psychoanalytic Theory," *Journal of the American Psychoanalytic Association*, Vol. 14 (January 1966), p. 43.

2. Warren J. Gadpaille, "Research Into the Physiology of Maleness and Femaleness," *Archives of General Psychiatry*, Vol. 26 (March 1972), p. 19.

3. Sherfey, "The Evolution and Nature of Female Sexuality in Relation to Psychoanalytic Theory," p. 45.

4. Seymour Levine, "Sexual Differentiation: The Development of Maleness and Femaleness," *California Medicine*, Vol. 114 (January 1971), p. 13.

5. Robert J. Stoller, "The 'Bedrock' of Masculinity and Femininity: Bisexuality," *Archives of General Psychiatry*, Vol. 26 (March 1972), p. 209.

6. Gadpaille, "Research Into the Physiology of Maleness and Femaleness," p. 203.

7. Stoller, "The 'Bedrock' of Masculinity and Femininity: Bisexuality," p. 210.

8. Ibid., p. 209. See also Gadpaille, "Research Into the Physiology of Maleness and Femaleness," p. 194.

9. Gadpaille, "Research Into the Physiology of Maleness and Femaleness," p. 200.

10. John W. Money, *Sex Errors of the Body* (Baltimore, 1968), pp. 42–43. (This wise and authoritative little book is highly recommended to anyone interested in this field.)

11. Uno Stannard, "Clothing and Sexuality," *Sexual Behavior*, Vol. 1 (May 1971), p. 30.

12. William H. Masters and Virginia E. Johnson, *Human Sexual Response* (Boston, 1966).

13. William Simon and John Gagnon, "Psychosexual Development," *Trans-action*, Vol. 6 (March 5, 1969), p. 13.

14. *Sexuality and Man*, compiled and edited by the Sex Information and Education Council of the United States (New York, 1970), p. 28, citing Alfred C. Kinsey et al., *Sexual Behavior in the Human Female*, pp. 537–543.

15. Kinsey et al., *Sexual Behavior in the Human Female*, pp. 348–349.

16. George Levinger, "Husbands' and Wives' Estimates of Coital Frequency," *Medical Aspects of Human Sexuality*, Vol. 4 (September 1970), pp. 42–43ff.

17. Masters and Johnson, *Human Sexual Response*, p. 131.

18. Salo Rosenbaum, "Pretended Orgasm," *Medical Aspects of Human Sexuality*, Vol. 4 (April 1970), p. 84.

19. Ibid.

20. *Sexuality and Man*, p. 25.

21. Felix Martini-Ibanez, "Two Windows on Medical History," *M.D.*, Vol. 14 (February 1970), p. 16.

22. Kinsey et al., *Sexual Behavior in the Human Female*, p. 590.

23. John Keats, from a letter dated July 18, 1818.

24. Alfred C. Kinsey, Wardell B. Pomeroy, and Clyde E. Martin, *Sexual Behavior in the Human Male* (Philadelphia, 1948), p. 506.

25. Plutarch, quoted in Stanley E. Pacion, "Sparta: An Experiment in State-Fostered Homosexuality," *Medical Aspects of Human Sexuality*, Vol. 4 (August 1970), p. 31.

26. Kinsey et al., *Sexual Behavior in the Human Female*, p. 468.

27. Kinsey, Pomeroy, and Martin, *Sexual Behavior in the Human Male*, p. 639.

28. Ibid., pp. 650–651.

29. "In the News," *Medical Aspects of Human Sexuality*, Vol. 3 (July 1969), p. 104.

30. William H. Masters and Virginia E. Johnson, *Homosexuality in Perspective* (Boston, 1979).

31. Quoted in Hara Marano, "New Light on Homosexuality," *Medical World News*, Vol. 20 (April 30, 1979), p. 14.
32. "Research with Adolescents Sheds New Light on Early Lesbianism," *Science News*, Vol. 96 (July 19, 1969), p. 45.
33. Harvey E. Kaye, "Lesbian Relationships," *Sexual Behavior*, Vol. 1 (April 1971), p. 83.
34. Ernst L. Freud, ed., *Letters of Sigmund Freud* (New York, 1960), p. 423.
35. Alan Bell and Martin Weinberg, *Homosexualities* (New York, 1978).
36. Lawrence J. Hatterer, *Changing Homosexuality in the Male: Treatment for Men Troubled with Homosexuality* (New York, 1970), p. 492.
37. Tony Bieber, "The Lesbian Patient," *Medical Aspects of Human Sexuality*, Vol. 3 (January 1969), p. 12.
38. Quoted in Melva Weber, "Sexual Inadequacy: How Masters and Johnson Treat It," *Medical World News*, Vol. 11 (May 1, 1970), p. 47.
39. William H. Masters and Virginia E. Johnson, *Human Sexual Inadequacy* (Boston, 1970), pp. 228–229.
40. Ibid., p. 250.
41. Ibid., p. 126.
42. *Rubáiyát of Omar Khayyám*, tr. by Edward FitzGerald.
43. Warren R. Johnson, *Human Sexual Behavior and Sex Education* (Philadelphia, 1968), pp. 50–51.
44. Masters and Johnson, *Human Sexual Response*, p. 202.
45. Leon Salzman, "Psychology of the Female," *Archives of General Psychiatry*, Vol. 17 (August 1967), p. 195.
46. Sherfey, "The Evolution and Nature of Female Sexuality in Relation to Psychoanalytic Theory," p. 78.
47. Ibid., p. 84.
48. Salzman, "Psychology of the Female," p. 196.
49. Masters and Johnson, *Human Sexual Response*, pp. 191–195.
50. Eugene Schoenfeld, *Dear Doctor Hip Pocrates* (New York, 1968), p. 19.
51. Masters and Johnson, *Human Sexual Response*, p. 195.

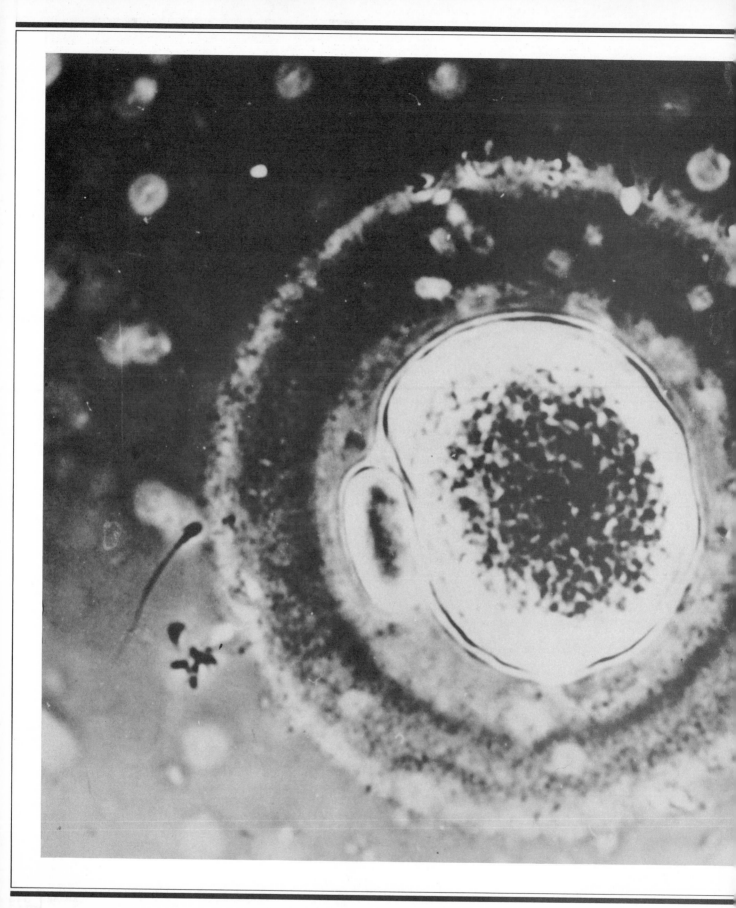

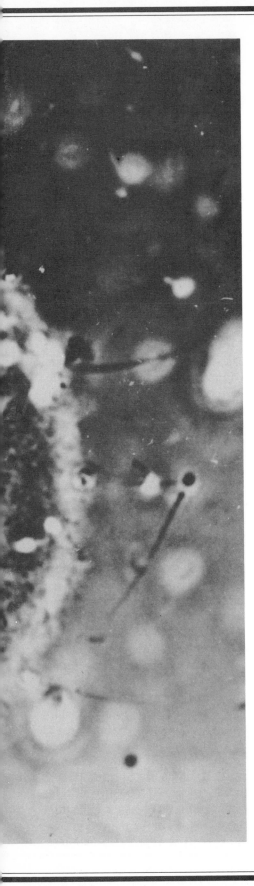

12

Reproduction, Overreproduction, and Birth Control

Reproduction, overreproduction, and birth control are intimately related to glandular function. For this reason a general knowledge of the ways the glands work is essential to a good understanding of much of the material in this chapter.

About Glands

A **gland** is a cell, a tissue, or an organ that produces a chemical substance that either is used elsewhere in the body (by secretion) or is eliminated from the body (by excretion). Glands are either exocrine or endocrine. **Exocrine glands** secrete their chemicals into outlet tubes called **ducts; endocrine glands**, on the other hand, secrete their products directly into the bloodstream. Among the exocrine glands are the *sweat*, *tear*, *salivary*, and *mammary (breast)* glands.

Unlike the exocrine glands, the endocrine glands do not have ducts (see Body Chart 15). From the many chemicals carried in the blood of the arteries, the endocrine glands make their own powerful chemical secretions or **hormones.** Hormones are normally released directly into the veins at definitely timed periods and in perfectly accurate doses, greatly influencing many body processes.

A gland can contain *both* exocrine and endocrine tissue. The *pancreas* has insulin-producing cells that are endocrine and that are important in the disease *diabetes mellitus*. It also has a duct leading to the upper small intestine that carries fluid essential to digestion.

Table 12–1 lists some of the effects of the endocrine glands. Notice that some endocrine gland hormones have a general effect on the body. For example, too much growth hormone from the anterior (front) pituitary gland will result in a giant; too little, in a dwarf. Other hormones produced in one gland travel by way of the blood to other glands, on which they will have an influence. For instance, hormones from the front, or anterior, lobe of the pituitary (such as *luteinizing hormone*) go to their target organs (in this case, the ovaries or testes). The target organs or glands are then stimulated to produce powerful hormones of their own. Endocrine gland cells are in a part of the brain called the *hypothalamus* (see Body Chart 15), the nearby anterior part of the *pituitary gland*, the *thyroid gland*, the *thymus gland*, the *parathyroid glands*, part of the *pancreas* (which is both endocrine and exocrine), the *adrenal glands*, and tissues within the *gonads* (ovaries and testes).

A gonad, then, is an endocrine gland or organ capable of producing **gametes.** What are gametes? They are either male (sperm) or female (ova) reproductive cells, which are able to enter into union with one another in the process of *fertilization*. The glands influencing reproduction are of particular interest here.

The endocrine reproductive hormones are outlined in Table 12–2. Note that their action is stimulated by hormones made in the hypothalamus. The hypothalamus is only a small fraction (1/300th) of the whole brain. Yet it is naturally influenced by the rest of the brain, and its own activity is great. Its action as

The photograph on pages 346–347 shows human spermatozoa surrounding an ovum just before the moment of fertilization.

TABLE 12–1
Some Human Endocrine Glands and Hormones and Some of Their Effects

ENDOCRINE GLAND	HORMONE	PROCESSES AFFECTED OR CONTROLLED	RESULTS OF EXCESS	RESULTS OF DEFICIENCY
Thyroid	Thyroxin	Level of metabolism, oxidation rate, etc.	Irritability, nervous activity, exophthalmos	Cretinism when severe in infancy; lethargy; myxedema
Parathyroids	Parathyroid hormone	Calcium balance	Bone deformation	Spasms; death if severe[1]
Adrenal medulla[2]	Epinephrine	Stimulation similar to that of sympathetic nervous system	Increased blood pressure, pulse rate, and blood glucose[3]	None
Adrenal cortex	Aldosterone	Salt balance	Accumulation of body fluid[4]	Addison's disease[5]
	Hydrocortisone	Carbohydrate metabolism, etc.	Abnormality of sugar and protein metabolism	None
Pancreas[6]	Insulin	Glucose metabolism	Shock, coma	Diabetes
Ovary[7]	Estrogen	Female sex development and menstrual cycle	None	Interference with menstrual cycle and sexual activity
	Progesterone	Control of ovary and uterus during pregnancy	None	Sterility or miscarriage
Testis[8]	Testosterone	Male sex development and activity	None	Lessened development of male characteristics and lessened sexual activity
Pituitary Anterior lobe	Adrenocorticotropic hormone (ACTH)	Control of adrenal cortex	Symptoms related to glands controlled.	
	Thyrotropic hormone	Control of thyroid		
	Gonadotropic hormones	Control of sex glands, etc.		
	Growth hormone	Growth	Gigantism	Dwarfism
Posterior lobe	Vasopressin	Kidney action	Excessive water in body	Excessive loss of water
	Oxytocin	Milk production and contraction of uterine muscle	None	Lessened or no milk production

1. Parathyroid deficiency used to follow the surgical removal of thyroid tissue when part or all of the parathyroids were accidentally removed at the same time. Surgeons are now aware of this danger and avoid it.
2. The medulla is the inner part of the adrenal gland. The hormone epinephrine is also known as adrenalin.
3. The symptoms noted are apparently normal results of increased adrenal secretion, but they may result from other causes not involving excessive epinephrine secretion.
4. Aldosterone causes the kidney to retain sodium. Excessive sodium retention causes the retention of an osmotically equivalent amount of water.
5. Addison's disease, fortunately rare, has among its symptoms coloration (bronzing) of the skin, low blood pressure, general weakness, loss of water from the body, and upset carbohydrate metabolism.
6. The pancreas as a whole is not an endocrine gland, but it contains clusters of cells, the islets of Langerhans, that have an endocrine function and secrete insulin.
7. The ovary as a whole is not an endocrine gland, but some of the cells around the developing eggs produce estrogen. After an egg leaves the ovary, *corpus luteum* develops, and this secretes progesterone.
8. Like the ovary, the testis is not exclusively an endocrine gland but does contain hormone-producing tissue.

SOURCE: From LIFE: AN INTRODUCTION TO BIOLOGY, Second Edition, by George Gaylord Simpson and William S. Beck, Copyright ©1965 by Harcourt Brace Jovanovich, Inc. Reprinted by permission of the publisher.

TABLE 12-2
Reproductive Hormones of the
Brain's Hypothalamus and Anterior Part of the Pituitary Gland

BRAIN'S HYPOTHALAMIC HORMONE	ANTERIOR (FRONT LOBE) PITUITARY HORMONE REGULATED	TARGET ENDOCRINE GLAND AFFECTED	SOME FUNCTIONS AFFECTED OR CONTROLLED
Follicle stimulating hormone releasing hormone (FSHRH)[1]	Follicle stimulating hormone (FSH)[2]	Female ovary	Promotes (1) process of development of ovarian follicles and (2) Formation of ovarian hormones
		Male testes	Promotes sperm development (*spermatogenesis*)
Luteinizing hormone releasing hormone (LHRH)[1]	Luteinizing hormone (LH)[2]	Female ovary	Promotes (1) formation of *corpus luteum* in the ovary after ovulation has taken place and (2) formation of ovarian hormones
		Male testes	Stimulates the formation of the hormone testosterone by specific cells in the testes

1. In 1979 FSHRH and LHRH were generally believed to have the same chemical structure and both were called gonadotropic releasing hormone (GNRH).
2. FSH and LH have different chemical structures.

NOTE: When enough FSH or LH is available for the target gland's function, it sends chemical messages back to the anterior lobe of the pituitary. From there the chemical message is relayed to the hypothalamus to stop the production of more unneeded hormone.

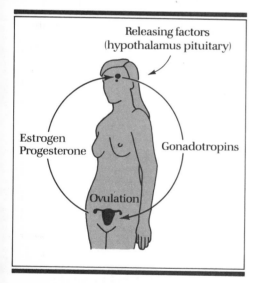

FIGURE 12-1
How the hypothalamus affects the female reproductive system. Hormones from the hypothalamus stimulate the anterior lobe of the pituitary to produce and release other hormones, which go to the target glands—the ovaries. Gonadotropins are then sent back from the ovaries to the anterior pituitary. From there chemical messages tell the hypothalamus to stop producing hormones. Thus, a complete feedback loop is created.

a gland is basic, but it is also involved in the regulation of all of the following: the body's temperature, the way water is handled in the body, appetite, thirst, blood sugar levels, sleeping, waking, pain, pleasure, and more. Control of the reproductive system is but one of the many duties of this very important brain structure. (See Figure 12-1.)

Now consider the organs of reproduction.

The Male Reproductive System

The male reproductive system (Figure 12-2) is made up of external visible parts and internal invisible parts. The only visible external parts are the *penis* and the wrinkled bag of skin behind it, the *scrotum*. Among the invisible internal parts are the pair of *testes* (singular, *testis*) within the scrotum. Cells within the testes develop into **sperm** (the male reproductive cells). Other cells produce the hormone **testosterone**.

Also internal is a system of ducts that store and transport sperm. These ducts are the paired *epididy-mides* (singular, *epididymis*), *vasa deferentia* (singular, *vas deferens*), *ejaculatory ducts*, and the single *urethra*. There are also contributing or accessory structures to the male reproductive system. They are the two *seminal vesicles*, the single chestnut-sized *prostate gland*, and the two *bulbo-urethral glands* (also called Cowper's glands).

The **penis** is the male organ of sexual union. At the tip of its smooth highly sensitive head (or **glans**) is the slit-like opening of the *urethra*. The male urethra is a canal eight to nine inches long that extends from the neck of the urinary bladder and passes through the length of the penis. Through it, by different mechanisms, pass both urine and semen. From the back of the head of the penis to its body is a thin strip of skin. It is also very sensitive to the touch. So is the rim, or *crown*, of the penile head. The crown of the penis dips slightly into the *neck* that leads to the *body* of the organ. Except for the glans, the skin of the nonerect penis is loose. It is not nearly so sensitive to touch as is the skin of the glans. However, this looseness of the skin of the body of the penis allows the organ to expand when an erection occurs.

In uncircumcised males, the **prepuce** or **foreskin** of the penis can be seen as a fold of skin covering the glans. Beneath the prepuce and in the rim and neck are tiny glands that produce a cheesy material called *smegma*. Nobody knows its purpose. With poor personal hygiene smegma will collect and become foul-smelling. The prepuce can be surgically removed by circumcision. Aside from its very important religious meanings to some people, there is no strictly medical reason for *routine* circumcision. However, some suggest that circumcision is associated with a decrease of cancer of the penis. There is, moreover, some evidence that cancer of the cervix (the lower portion of the uterus) is less common among wives of circumcised men. Some physicians believe that cancer of the penis and cervix may, in some cases, be caused by the collection of irritating smegma under the prepuce of uncircumcised men. There is no disagreement that circumcision is generally necessary when the foreskin is very tight and cannot easily be drawn back over the head of the penis.

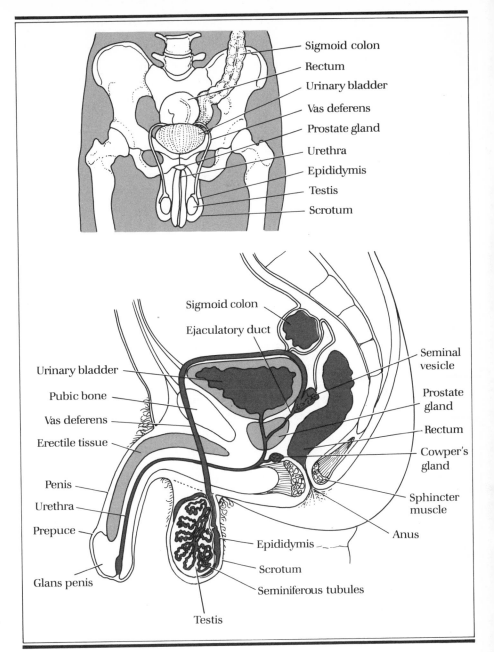

FIGURE 12–2
The male reproductive system.

Unlike other flesh-eating animals, such as the dog and cat, a human's penis does not have a bone in it nor does it contain muscles. Throughout history the penis has been both worshipped and cursed. Much nonsense about it is accepted as truth. A few of these fallacies were discussed in the previous chapter.

Unlike the penis, the **scrotum** does contain muscle fibers. These contract with sexual stimuli or exposure to cold. Each **testis** within the scrotal pouch is about two inches long, one inch wide and one inch thick. Its external side (away from the body's midline) is free. However, attached to the border of each testis nearest the body's midline is the crescent or C-shaped epididymis. A testis and its attached epididymis are usually called a *testicle.*

The testes contain a complicated system of tiny lobes or lobules. It is within these numerous lobules that **spermatozoa** develop. For this reason they are called the **seminiferous** (semen-producing) **tubules.** The network of seminiferous tubules eventually joins into a system of collecting ducts, which empty into the epididymis.

The epididymis coils and folds upon itself and is actually eighteen to twenty feet long. In it are stored some spermatozoa previously manufactured in the seminiferous tubules. In it, too, spermatozoa continue to mature. The epididymis continues on as the vas deferens. It is here that most of the spermatozoa are stored.

The vas deferens on each side leads into the abdominal cavity via the *inguinal canal* of its side. Then the vas deferens extends backward over the urinary bladder. Finally the end of each vas deferens joins the **seminal vesicle** of its side. The seminal vesicles are glands that secrete a mucuslike material.

The place at which the end of each vas deferens joins the duct of each seminal vesicle becomes an *ejaculatory duct.* Each ejaculatory duct enters the *prostate gland.* The single prostate gland lies at the base of the urinary bladder. It is made up of both muscle and glandular tissue and is surrounded by a capsule. The capsule plays a part during **ejaculation** of semen because it, as well as the prostatic muscle fibers, contracts along with other organs involved in the process. The fluid of the prostate is what gives semen its milky appearance. The urethra runs through the entire length of the

prostate and all the way down to the opening at the head of the penis. The ejaculatory ducts also run into the prostate gland but empty into the urethra as it passes through that gland.

The bulbo-urethral (or Cowper's) glands look like tiny yellow peas and are internally located at the base of the penis. They secrete a variable amount of thin fluid that enters the penile urethra. This fluid may contain thousands of spermatozoa before actual ejaculation occurs. For this reason, pregnancy may result even when ejaculation does not occur and when there is only partial or no actual penetration of the vagina by the penis.

Erection and Ejaculation

Not every penile erection is the result of sexual stimulation. For example, partial erection may result from lifting heavy loads or from straining while having a bowel movement. This is due to stress on the muscles of the perineum. Newborn males may have a penile erection, which is probably related to the infant's increased muscle and nerve irritability, such as may be caused by crying. When a penile erection is caused by sexual excitement, the stimuli responsible for the erection originate in the higher brain centers; the erection itself is the result of a spinal reflex. Cerebral influence is apparently not always necessary for an erection; indeed, it may inhibit an erection. Man does not have voluntary control of an erection; he cannot will it. To understand how the spinal nerve reflex causes erection, consider first the internal structure of the penis.

The penis contains three cylindrical bodies of erectile tissue (see Fig-

ure 12–2). They run the length of the penis to its head. These cylindrical bodies contain many small vascular spaces; they are thus a spongy erectile tissue. For an erection to occur, nerve stimuli cause dilatation of the little penile arteries (arterioles). At the places where the arterioles and the vascular spaces join are valvelike structures. When the penis is flaccid these structures (called *polsters*) cause blood to be shunted away from the vascular spaces and fed directly into the veins. With adequate nerve stimuli these polsters relax. This permits rapid inflow of blood into the spaces of the cylindrical erectile tissue of the penis. The rate of the inflow of blood from the arterioles is then temporarily greater than the rate of the outflow from the veins, causing an increase of blood volume in the penis. When a steady state is reached, in which blood inflow equals outflow, penile enlargement ceases, and the penis is stiff.

The ejaculatory process begins with contractions of the ducts leading away from the seminiferous tubules in the testes. These contractions continue along the epididymis to the vas deferens. The vas deferens then contracts along with the seminal vesicles. The contents of the vas deferens, as well as those of the seminal vesicles, are expelled into the part of the urethra that passes through the prostate. The prostatic capsule and muscles have also been contracting rhythmically to add fluid to the ejaculatory content. At the onset of the ejaculatory process, the ringlike band of muscle fibers (the sphincter) surrounding the exit from the urinary bladder contracts. Semen is thus prevented from entering the urinary bladder; semen and urine are not ordinarily expelled together. After ejaculation, nerve stimuli cause constriction of

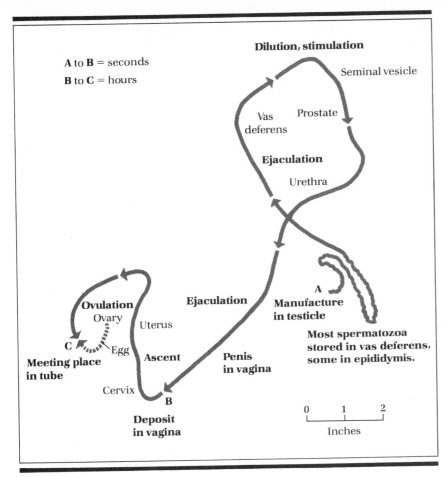

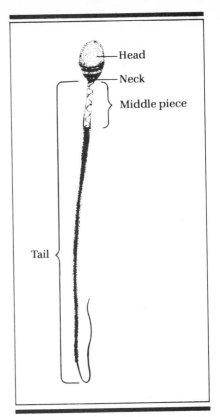

FIGURE 12-3
The route of a spermatozoon from its origin to its fertilization of an ovum.

the penile arterioles, and the erection is gradually lost.

Semen

The ejaculated fluid containing the sperm is a thick, whitish material. It is about a teaspoonful in amount. However, the consistency and amount of the seminal fluid may vary, for example with the age of the male. During ejaculation, the entire transit from testes to vagina occupies but a few seconds. Although sperm can remain motile (able to move) in the vagina for as long as two hours, some can reach the cervix in seconds. Indeed, ejaculation may well take place directly on the cervix. However, hours may be required for ascent of the sperm through the uterus and part of the Fallopian tube in order to fertilize an ovum (a distance of about six inches). On an average, the journey probably requires about an hour (see Figure 12-3). Each spermatozoon has a bulbous head. Its long mobile tail propels it to its destination (see Figure 12-4). When one compares the size of a spermatozoon with the relatively enormous distance it must travel to fertilize an ovum, one cannot help but be struck by its vigor. Of the millions of spermatozoa emitted in each ejaculum, many are able to reach the ovum, but usually only one manages the task of fertilization.

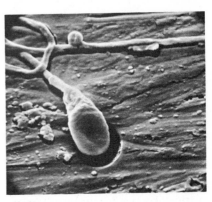

FIGURE 12-4
A spermatozoon in diagram (top) and as seen through a scanning electron microscope (bottom), showing the head, neck, middle piece, and part of the tail.

The Female Reproductive System

The essential glands of the female reproductive system (Figure 12–5) are the internal pair of female gonads, the ovaries. The female reproductive duct system is also internal. It is composed of the *Fallopian tubes* (named after the Italian anatomist Gabriello Fallopio), the *uterus* (or *womb*), and the *vagina*. The associated structures—the external genitalia—are called the **vulva**. The vulva includes the *mons pubis*, the *major labia* (or lips), the *minor labia*, the *clitoris*, and the opening of the vagina. For convenience, the *mammary glands* (breasts) may also be considered as part of the female reproductive duct system (see Figure 12–9 on page 362).

The Ovaries and Ova

The two **ovaries** (egg containers) are the fundamental organs of femininity. About the size and shape of a shelled almond, one ovary is situated on each side of the *uterus*, attached to it by ligaments. Just as the organs of masculinity (the testes) produce male sperm and male hormone, so do the ovaries produce mature **ova** (singular, **ovum**) and female hormone. When the female child is born, each of her ovaries contains about 200,000 tiny sacs, or *follicles*. In each follicle lies a microscopically small beginning (primordial) sex cell (or *oogonium*). Each female is born with all the primordial sex cells she will ever have. At this primitive, unripened stage, no sex cell is capable of fertilization. The ripening process whereby a primordial sex cell becomes a mature ovum must await puberty. This usually occurs be-

tween the ninth and seventeenth year (12½ years is the average). During a woman's lifetime, only about 400 (perhaps 1 in 1,000) mature ova leave either of the ovaries.

Every month the mature human female experiences a series of changes basically involving the hypothalamus of the brain, the anterior lobe of the pituitary gland, the ovaries, and the *endometrium* (the lining of the uterus). The purpose of these changes is to prepare for possible pregnancy. For pregnancy to occur, an egg must leave the ovary, be fertilized, and then be firmly implanted in the endometrium of the prepared uterus.*

What happens to the ovary (ovarian cycle) is related to what happens to the uterus (menstrual cycle). *Ovulation* and *menstruation* are different events, happening at different times, to different organs. But each intimately affects the other.

Ovulation

To follow the events leading to **ovulation**, or the release of a mature egg from the ovary, let's start with a landmark, say day 1, the beginning of the menstrual period. Why day 1? Because the woman can observe the first day of her period more easily than her last. She can thus count from that day more reliably. Also assume that every twenty-eight days the average female menstruates for a period of five days. With different

*The Roman Catholic Church teaches that conception occurs with fertilization. Other bodies, such as the American College of Obstetrics and Gynecology, consider biological life to begin with implantation.

people these time periods vary normally. The time periods used here are only examples. Note, however, that the ovarian and menstrual cycles are correlated here on the basis of this average schedule.

1. Menstruation begins on day 1 and continues through day 5 (see Figures 12–6 and 12–7). Chemicals from the hypothalamus stimulate the anterior lobe of the pituitary gland to produce and release the **follicle-stimulating hormone** (**FSH**) directly into the venous bloodstream.
2. The FSH reaches and activates the ovaries. Not one but several (of the many thousands) of immature ovarian follicles in one or both ovaries respond to the FSH and begin to ripen. Which ovary is more affected is unpredictable. Estimates of the number of immature follicles that respond to the FSH usually vary from two to thirty-two.
3. The cells of those ovarian follicles that are ripening multiply greatly, and the single maturing ovum within each follicle increases in size. The increased layers of follicular cells secrete a *follicular fluid*. This fluid forms tiny pools, which first separate groups of cells but which then run together to form a little lake within each follicle (see Figure 12–7). The follicles mature at different rates of speed, so some are at earlier stages of development than others. By about day 10, a few of the most mature follicles look like fluid-filled rounded sacks. The developing ovum is in the wall of the sack and is surrounded by follicular cells, which separate it

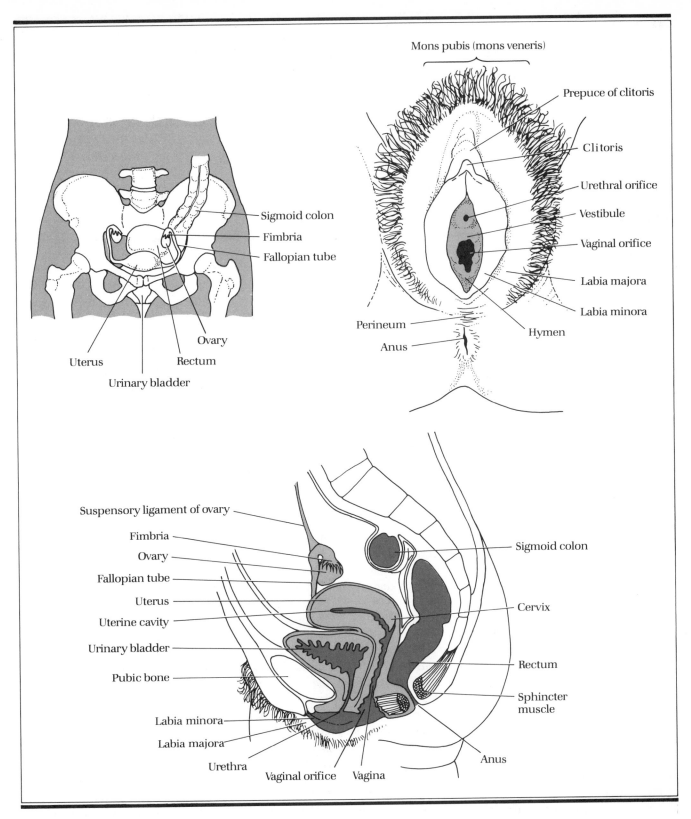

FIGURE 12–5
The female reproductive system.

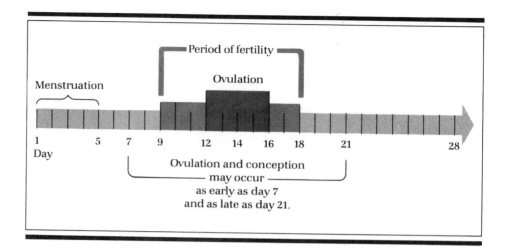

FIGURE 12–6
The menstrual cycle.

The figure shows a horizontal bar representing days 1 through 28. Labels on the bar read "Menstruation" (days 1 to 5), "Period of fertility," "Ovulation" (around days 12–16), with day markings at 1, 5, 7, 9, 12, 14, 16, 18, 21, and 28. Below: "Ovulation and conception may occur as early as day 7 and as late as day 21."

from the lake. The follicle is now called a **Graafian follicle**, after a seventeenth-century Dutch anatomist, Regner de Graaf, who first described it.

4. As they ripen, the cells of maturing follicles also produce a hormone, called **estrogen**. Its function at this stage is to begin the preparation of the uterus for implantation of a fertilized ovum.

5. On about day 10, one (or, very rarely, two) of the follicles undergoes a sudden spurt of growth. In three or four days it is completely mature. As a rule only one follicle and ovum matures, and only one ovum leaves the ovary. (If a woman has a tendency for multiple births, there may be more than one.) No one knows what determines which follicle and ovum will be selected. The other follicles, and their contained ova that are not destined to leave the ovary, develop to varying extents, only to regress, die, and be replaced by small scars. No other trace of them remains.

6. A few hours before the ovum is ready to leave, the follicle that contains it migrates to the sur-

face of the ovary. By day 13 or 14 the ovum is ready to go. It has been seen, during surgery, as a tiny protrusion from the ovarian surface.

7. A few days before, the anterior lobe of the pituitary gland had begun the release of a second hormone, the **luteinizing hormone** (LH), directly into the venous blood. Like the FSH, the release of LH is governed by hypothalamic chemicals from the brain. Moreover, it is believed that the same hypothalamic chemical governs the manufacture and release of both the FSH and LH hormones in the front lobe of the pituitary gland.

8. Along with the FSH, the LH causes the follicle to continue to mature and, finally, to rupture. Together, then, the increase in FSH and LH results in the release of the ovum from the ovary (see Figure 12–7). This release is called ovulation. On the average, ovulation occurs on day 14. Ovulation, then, takes place at about the middle of the menstrual cycle. In 1972, it was reported that the ovary contracts slightly to gently squeeze the ovum loose

and send it on its way.[2] Apparently, just a few nerve-supplied muscle cells are responsible for one of the most significant squeezes in biology.

To this point it has been seen that, influenced by released chemicals from the brain's hypothalamus, the anterior lobe of the pituitary gland produces and releases two hormones. One, FSH, stimulates the growth of follicles that, as they develop, cause the ovary to produce estrogens. The second pituitary hormone, LH, helped by the increased FSH, causes rupture of the follicle, which releases the egg.

Three parenthetical observations are noteworthy. First, **conception**, the fertilization of an ovum by a sperm, cannot occur unless both mature sex cells are viable (living). Upon being released from the ovary, the ovum usually survives for twenty-four to thirty-six hours. For the ovum, assume a maximum survival time of two days. Upon being deposited in the vagina, sperm usually survives for one to three days. (This would include the several hours of survival in the vagina and the two or three days in the cervix and above.) For sperm, assume a maximum survival time of three days. Usually ovulation occurs, in the average woman, about fourteen days before the onset of the next menstrual period, give or take two days. Keeping in mind the average maximum survival times of the ovum and of sperm, as well as the average day of occurrence of ovulation (with its two-day leeway), refer to Figure 12–7 for an illustration of the average period of fertility of the woman who menstruates every twenty-eight days. Counting from day 1 of the menstrual period, she will ovulate between day 12 and day 16. However, her ovum will survive for about two days. A viable ovum may thus be available for fertilization until approximately day 18 of the menstrual cycle. The woman may have ovulated as early as day 12. For about three days a sperm can survive to fertilize an ovum. It then follows that conception can occur if a sperm is deposited in the vagina as early as three days before ovulation. If the woman menstruates regularly every twenty-eight days (and many normal women do not), she will, on the average, be most likely to become pregnant if sperm is deposited in the vagina between day 9 and day 18 of her menstrual cycle. Throughout this book human individuality is stressed. Menstruation and ovulation are hardly exceptions. Some women menstruate every twenty-one days, others, every thirty-five days. They should calculate their periods of maximum fertility accordingly. For example, the woman who menstruates every twenty-one days can set an ovulation date on day 7 of the menstrual cycle. The woman who menstruates every thirty-fifth day will usually ovulate on day 21. In either case her calculations of maximum fertility must make allowances for a two-day lee-

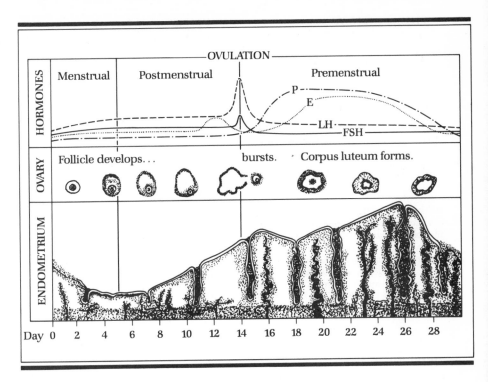

FIGURE 12–7
The menstrual and ovulatory cycles. (FSH = the follicle-stimulating hormone; E = estrogen; LH = the luteinizing hormone; P = progesterone.) Note that the progesterone level is detectably higher within twenty-four hours after ovulation occurs.

way for ovulation and the viability of both ovum and sperm. There are many women whose menstrual cycles are irregular from month to month. Without obtaining a reliable average over a year, they cannot calculate a reasonably reliable period of maximum fertility. This information becomes particularly important when the rhythm method of birth control is used (see pages 375–376).

Second, when ovulation occurs, the rupture is accompanied by a small amount of ovarian bleeding. This blood may be irritating and may cause brief abdominal discomfort. With right-side middle-of-the-month pain, the woman may

worry that she has appendicitis. Only the physician is equipped to differentiate between the two.

Third, as the follicle develops, its estrogen (point 4 above) affects the uterus. In preparation for implantation of the developing product of the fertilized egg (the embryo), the lining (endometrium) of this organ thickens, as does the muscle layer. Estrogens also affect the cervical secretions, making them more receptive for the sperm if it is there. They also cause the Fallopian tubes to contract more rapidly. (Estrogens, the basic group of female sex hormones, are responsible for many of the female sex characteristics, such as growth of breast tissue.)

THE DESTINY OF THE RELEASED OVUM

Where does the ovum go? It enters the **Fallopian tube*** nearest the ovary from which the egg came (see Figure 12–8). At its lower end, each of these three- to five-inch tubes opens into the upper uterine cavity. At its upper end, each Fallopian tube lies close but not directly

*Obstruction of these tubes by inflammation is one of the most common causes of sterility, for the egg cannot reach the uterus. Sometimes, with a partially blocked tube, the sperm does reach the egg to fertilize it. But then the larger fertilized egg cannot get through the tubes to the uterus. A tubal pregnancy results, which can be terminated surgically.

attached to its corresponding ovary. This free end of the Fallopian tube ends in fingerlike projections called *fimbria*. And it is the fimbria that draw the escaped ovum into the Fallopian tube. Now the ovum is ready to be fertilized, to make the journey to the uterus. Unlike spermatozoa, however, it cannot move alone. By the gentle sweeping motions of hairlike cilia lining the Fallopian tube, and by waves of contractions passing along the tube itself, the ovum is helped along its way.

As the ovum begins its journey down the Fallopian tube, what goes on in the emptied follicle that remains behind in the ovary? Under the influence of FSH and LH it

closes, grows to the size of a lima bean, and takes on a yellowish tint. Now it is called the **corpus luteum** (Latin *corporis*, "body" + *leuteum*, "yellow"). Its future function depends on whether the ovum is fertilized.

If the ovum is not fertilized within forty-eight hours, it continues down the Fallopian tube to the uterus. There it disintegrates. Any remnant of it is eliminated through the vagina with the menstrual flow. In the ovary the corpus luteum produces the hormone **progesterone**, which means "to promote pregnancy." Indeed, this is its function. Acting upon the uterine endometrium, progesterone causes it to mature in preparation for a fertilized ovum. In the absence of fertilization, the corpus luteum continues to produce progesterone until late in the menstrual cycle. Not until about day 25 does the corpus luteum begin to degenerate into a small depressed scar in the ovarian tissue. Progesterone is then diminished. Fragments of the uterine endometrium and mucus from the uterine glands slough off with an average of one to three ounces of menstrual blood. A new ovarian cycle is ready to begin.

If the ovum is fertilized (usually in the upper part of a Fallopian tube), the sequence is entirely different. The fertilized ovum (*zygote*) divides, becoming a tiny mass of cells (*blastocyst*) during its two- to four-day trip down the tube to the uterus. Once there, it is not immediately implanted in the uterine wall. Several days may go by before the uterine endometrium is entirely ready. So it is about five to seven days following ovulation that implantation occurs. The elaborately prepared uterine endometrium receives the new life. The zygote is now an embryo. Implantation usually happens between day 18 and

FIGURE 12–8
An ovum leaving the ovary. The same ovum is shown later being fertilized in the upper Fallopian tube. The fertilized ovum (zygote) will cleave daily (becoming a blastocyst) as it continues down the Fallopian tube to the uterus. After floating in the uterus for several days, it will be implanted in the uterine wall. It should be noted that this is a highly schematic representation.

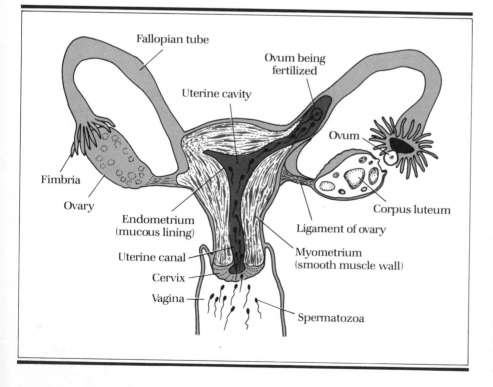

day 22. It may, however, occur as late as day 23 of the menstrual cycle.* After implantation, the membranes of the embryo produce a **gonadotropic hormone**. This hormone also stimulates the corpus luteum to produce progestèrone.

Indeed, with pregnancy the corpus luteum in the ovary continues its activity for twelve weeks before some of its functions are taken over by the placenta (afterbirth). By its timely continued production of estrogens, such as progesterone, it promotes persistent endometrial growth, which is essential in sustaining the intrauterine being. It also prevents the maturation of new follicles. And this last fact makes possible one type of contraceptive pill—a chemical combination of progesterone and estrogen. Properly taken, the pill prevents ovulation (see pages 371–372).

The Uterus and Menstruation

The hollow **uterus**, about the size and shape of a pear, is a muscular pelvic organ. Nourished and sheltered in this abode, the developing child is an *embryo* for two months, then a *fetus*, and, upon birth, an *infant*. The upper part of the uterus, its *body*, is mostly muscle. During pregnancy, the uterus enlarges to about sixteen times its normal size. Its muscle enlarges enough to produce contractions adequate to help expel the baby. The smaller lower end of the uterus, the **cervix**, points downward and tilts slightly toward

*This assumes ovulation occurs on about day 14. Add approximately two to four days in the Fallopian tube and about another two to four days in the uterus.

the back into the vagina. It can be felt by the woman and has the consistency of the tip of the nose. Its identification is important to the woman who uses a diaphragm for birth control. The physician can both see and feel the cervix with ease. This is fortunate, for it affords early diagnosis of cancer of the womb, which most commonly begins at this site. There are small mucous glands in the cervix that may become infected. Sometimes they become clogged, causing a mucoid discharge.

The uterus is loosely moored to the bony pelvis by tough fibrous bands called *ligaments*. It is thus suspended in the pelvic cavity between the bladder, in front, and the rectum, behind. The stretching of these ligaments during pregnancy may cause a pulling sensation in the groin. The enlarging pregnant uterus diminishes the space for the bladder and rectum (see Figure 12–5). This explains the frequent urinary dribbling that occurs during late pregnancy and the importance of emptying both bladder and rectum to ease delivery of the child.

As has been mentioned, the endometrium (the lining of the uterine cavity) is elaborately prepared in anticipation of a viable fertilized egg. Hospitality for the fertilized egg is the basic function of the uterus. Under the influence of estrogens from the ovary and its maturing ovarian follicle, the endometrium thickens. Fluid accumulates. Blood engorges the tissue. However, when these preparations are met with nothing but an unfertilized and, therefore, degenerating egg, the uterus bleeds. With **menstruation**, the excess endometrium loosens and is discharged, with the mucus from the uterine glands, as blood-filled tissue through the cervical opening and vagina.

SOME UNTRUTHS ABOUT MENSTRUATION

The Greeks, wrongly considering menstruation to be a cleansing process, called it *katharsis*. In the first century, a Roman historian wrote that menstrual blood dulled razors, and Aristotle thought menstruating women ruined mirrors. The early Hebrews punished those who had intercourse during menstruation. During medieval times, menstruating women were excluded from churches and wine cellars alike. In the latter case it was believed they would spoil the wine. Menstruating women are still segregated in "blood huts" by some African tribes. Child marriage developed among the Hindus because they incorrectly believed that the menstrual blood is essential for the embryo. To lose menstrual blood before pregnancy is still considered irreligious by many Hindus. Not long ago, in rural Russia, menstrual blood was collected in flasks by unmarried girls from as many village women as possible. It was then used by the village witch to determine fertility. Elsewhere in Europe a drop of menstrual blood used to be placed in a suitor's wine to help him win the love of the donor.

SOME TRUTHS ABOUT MENSTRUATION

During menstruation an absorbent pad is used to absorb the *menses*, or menstrual flow. It may be worn externally, although many women prefer an internal tampon. Tampons may be worn by girls who have just begun to menstruate. That they cannot or should not be used by virgins is a myth. To lessen chances of infection, tampons should be changed at least twice daily. There is no reason whatsoever to limit activity during menstruation. The menstruating woman may engage in any normal activity that she enjoys when she is not menstruating. Bathing, swimming, horseback riding, hairwashing, bicycling, dancing, gym classes—all these are perfectly permissible. Some couples enjoy sexual intercourse during menstruation, and there is usually no contraindication to this. The mild abdominal cramping that sometimes occurs during menstruation may require an aspirin or two, but usually even this is not necessary. Douching at the end of menstruation is neither necessary nor recommended. The action of normal vaginal bacteria maintains vaginal cleanliness and health. Because of fluid retention some women may gain a pound or two during the week before the onset of menstruation. This does not call for a change in diet; with the onset, the weight is lost, as is an occasional heavy feeling in the pelvis and legs. *Premenstrual tension*, manifested by increased moodiness and irritability, even mild depression, is not uncommonly experienced during the few days prior to the onset of menstruation. These are not usually significant symptoms. In a very few cases, the mild physical discomfort and increased emotional sensitivity combine to make a woman a trial both to herself and to others. Occasionally a woman will even use this situation to gain sympathy. The very rare personality change associated with menstruation usually indicates other deeply rooted problems. The vast majority of women handle their monthly menstrual periods as what they are—an entirely normal indication of femininity during the reproductive years.

Dysmenorrhea, or painful menstruation, does not refer to the ordinary discomfort mentioned above; it is more severe. It may have a wide variety of causes, either physical, psychological, or both. *Menorrhagia* refers to excessive and usually prolonged uterine bleeding occurring at regular intervals. *Metrorrhagia* is uterine bleeding at completely irregular intervals. The amount may be normal, but the flow may be prolonged. *Amenorrhea* refers to the absence of menstruation. Before a girl is old enough to menstruate, after the menopause (see below), and during pregnancy and lactation (the formation and secretion of breast milk), amenorrhea is normal. Sudden changes in climate or emotional distress, such as depression, are among the variables that may cause a change in the amount of menstrual flow. A period may be delayed or may even be skipped because of such factors. Amenorrhea of longer duration is, of course, most commonly due to pregnancy. However, endocrine gland disorders or severe malnutrition and anemia may cause amenorrhea. Dysmenorrhea, menorrhagia, metrorrhagia, and prolonged amenorrhea all indicate prompt consultation with a physician.

NORMAL DIFFERENCES AMONG WOMEN

Women who desire to be different from other women surely accomplish this with their menstrual histories. The normal onset of menstruation (**menarche**) varies. On the average, as noted above, it occurs at about 12½ years of age. First menstruations are usually irregular. They may not be associated with ovulation. Some girls menstruate for months or even years without ovulating; so the onset of menstruation does not always mean

fertility has begun. Abnormally early onsets of menstruation and ovulation are rare. Lena Medina, a classic case in medical history, was delivered of a healthy child when she was only five years and nine months old. An ovarian tumor had accelerated her sexual maturity. Her pregnancy had been caused by rape.

Women normally differ as to the duration (one to six days, with an average of four or five days) and the amount (one to eight ounces, with an average of about two or three ounces) of menstrual bleeding. Individual women also vary from month to month in their onsets of bleeding. For women who calculate "safe periods" for sexual intercourse based on the first day of menstruation, it is essential to keep an accurate record of monthly onsets for at least a year.

An important note: *It is vital for a particular individual to know what is ordinary for her. Any marked departure is the signal for an immediate visit to a physician.* A gross change in menstruation, such as excessive bleeding or spotting between periods, may be of minor significance. It may, however, signify disease, such as cancer, that, treated early, is easily curable. The diagnosis of such cancers by means of the Papanicolaou test is a painless procedure.

THE MENOPAUSE

The age of the cessation of menstruation (**menopause**) also varies widely. Today, the U.S. average is about forty-nine. Some women may cease menstruating even before forty, though this is rare. Many women menstruate in their fifties. It is possible that the better general health of the woman of today is responsible for the later occurrence of menopause.

Although both ovulation and menstruation may stop abruptly, the menopause is usually not a sudden event. With most women, ovulation and menstruation taper off gradually; failure to realize this may result in pregnancy. Because of the irregularity of ovulation at this time, the "change of life" baby is not a common event. Nevertheless, many physicians advise that family planning be continued until no menses have occurred for six months. Just as puberty is accompanied by body changes and the beginning of menstruation, so is the menopause accompanied by body changes and the cessation of the function. The **climacteric** refers to those phenomena, both physical and psychological, which are associated with the end of menstruation in women and, in both sexes, with a diminution in the production of certain chemical compounds, including sex hormones. In the woman, it is the period that is begun by the menopause and during which she enters her postreproductive years. In the man, it is generally marked by some lessening of sexual activity.

Several grossly cruel and senseless untruths should be dismissed. First, the menopause heralds neither old age nor obesity. Second, it is not a common cause of insanity. By far the greatest majority of menopausal women need no extensive medical treatment. As a rule, sexual activity continues. Frequently, it improves. For many women, the feeling of warmth and flushing of the face, neck, and upper body ("hot flashes") and the sweating are mere annoyances. For an unknown reason, they seem to occur most often at night. Some women suffer embarrassment because they believe their hot flashes are noticed by others. This is not so. There are no outward indications of hot flashes.

With a considerable number of women they do not occur. For a few, other symptoms include headaches, irritability, insomnia, and depression. In such cases, overeating results in overweight. Results of the treatment of these symptoms are generally excellent.

An important note: *A heavier menstrual flow, or "flooding," is not a usual characteristic of the menopause. Excessive bleeding and bleeding between periods (regardless of the time of life) always indicate immediate consultation with a physician. Delay has cost many women their lives.*

The Vagina

The **vagina** is a tube about 3½ inches long. The vaginal walls are composed of muscle. The inner surface of the vagina is lined with transverse folds of mucous membrane. During childbirth both muscle and folds expand tremendously. Cells from vaginal fluid are useful in determining not only the time of ovulation but also whether there is cancer of the uterus. In both instances the cells characteristically reflect these changes. In the virgin, the sexually sensitive external opening of the vagina may be partially closed by a fold of mucous membrane called the **hymen** (see Figure 12–5). However, the hymen is commonly absent in females who have never had sexual intercourse. Rarely, the hymen interferes with the passage of menstrual blood, a condition that is easily corrected by the physician.

The normal reaction of the vagina is acid. A bacillus is involved in maintaining this normal reaction. If this acid reaction is not maintained, the vagina is prone to infection.

Douching may be advised by a physician to encourage the acidity of the vagina. However, a woman should not douche unless advised to do so by her physician. Some popular douches not only harm delicate tissues but remove beneficial bacteria.

The External Genitalia

The sexually sensitive *mons pubis* is a rounded fatty pad above the labia majora and over the front pubic region (see Figure 12–5). The *labia majora* are skin folds that pass backward from the mons pubis. Like the mons they are fatty pads covered, in the adult, with hair. The *clitoris*, at the upper end of the labia minora, is extremely sensitive. Its sole purpose is to stimulate sexual desire. The *labia minora* (also sexually sensitive) are about as thick as a large rubber band. They arise from the clitoris and then pass backward, enclosing a sensitive area called the *vestibule*. The mons, vestibule, the opening of the vagina, labia minora, and clitoris, then, are all sexually sensitive.

The *urethra* (leading from the urinary bladder) and vagina open into the vestibule, as do the **Bartholin's glands** (or *vulvovaginal glands*). During prolonged sexual excitement, the Bartholin's glands secrete a small amount of lubricating material, which should not be confused with the vaginal lubrication that occurs early (within seconds) in the woman's sexual response (see page 322). On either side of the opening of the female urethra are the several small *Skene's ducts*. These and the Bartholin's glands may easily become infected, particularly by the gonococcus.

FIGURE 12-9
The mature female breast.

*The significance of Cooper's ligaments has recently been reemphasized by two consultant surgeons. These fibrous attachments help to support the breasts. Without adequate brassiere support the ligaments stretch, as does the intrinsic connective tissue. This causes the breasts to droop. No amount of exercise will restore the ligaments. However, exercise may embellish breast contour (sagging or otherwise) by improving posture and increasing the thickness of the underlying pectoral muscle. Modern surgery can restore severely pendulous breasts. Patients who have had such surgery may find that they do not need brassieres as consistently as do other women. (John H. Wulsin and Milton T. Edgerton, "Cooper's Droop: Mystique of the Bra-Less Mamma Maligned," *Journal of the American Medical Association*, Vol. 219, No. 5 [January 31, 1972], p. 625. The term "Cooper's Droop" is credited to Dr. Carl Manion of the University of Kansas Medical Center.]

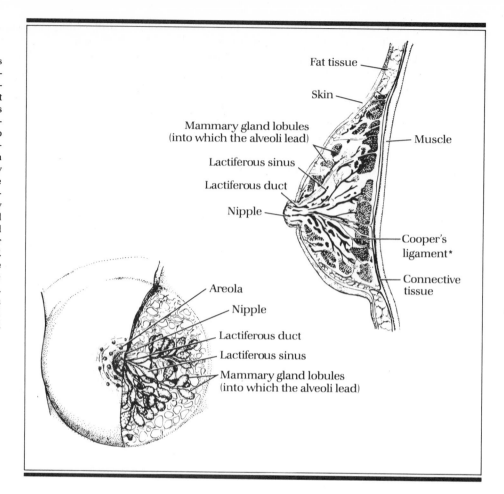

The Mammary Glands

Before puberty there is little difference between the male and female breasts. In normal adult males they remain rudimentary. However, with the onset of puberty in the girl and the production of certain hormones by the ovaries, the breasts begin to develop. With each menstrual cycle the breasts enlarge slightly; they feel heavier, and the nipples are more sensitive.

Just below the center of the adult female mammary gland is the raised *nipple*, surrounded by the circular pigmented *areola* (see Figure 12–9). Small openings on the surface of the nipple mark the openings of the ducts of the underlying glandular structures. With pregnancy, these are quite visible during the time milk is secreted (*lactation*). The numerous small elevations on the areolar area are caused by sebaceous glands. The breast structure is composed of about twenty distinct tubular glands, or *lobes*, which, in turn, are composed of many *lobules*. The lobes are embedded in loose connective tissue and fat, which give the breast its shape. Each lobe eventually drains into the *lactiferous duct* of the nipple. Just before the duct terminates into the nipple, it is dilated as a *lactiferous sinus*.

During pregnancy the nipples and areolae darken. Around the areola a secondary, lighter areola usually develops. The sebaceous glands of the areola enlarge. They are then called *Montgomery's glands*. They secrete an oily material that keeps the nipple supple and prevents the skin from cracking. Early in pregnancy a thin, scanty, yellow-white precursor of milk is secreted. This continues throughout the entire pregnancy. This secretion is called *colostrum*. During the first days of the baby's life, colostrum is a good food. Before the milk is produced, colostrum may be drawn off to stimulate milk flow. The sense of fullness and the tingling of the breasts sometimes felt in the early months of pregnancy soon lessen.

Overreproduction

Some years ago the following item appeared in *The New York Times:*

The Japan National Railways has hired 470 more sturdy "pushers" to help cram long-suffering Tokyo commuters into trains already crowded far beyond capacity at the height of the winter crush hour.

The new "oshiya-san" (honorable pushers), mostly students hired on a part-time basis, bring to 2,500 the number stationed at key Tokyo rail points to help move an average of nearly four million commuters daily between their homes and places of work. . . .

The "oshiya-san" double as "hagitoriya-san"—pullers or peelers—with the frequently vital job of snatching surplus passengers out of the cars to permit the doors to close and the tight two-minute operating schedules to be maintained.[3]

With this quotation, a central problem of this era is approached: overpopulation. Long ago the Biblical prophet Isaiah warned against overcrowding. Today the "pushers" and "peelers" of the elegant Japanese symbolize a world threat.

Why is a book on health concerned with the problem? The answer is that better health is one cause of the population explosion. In the past, famine, war, and pestilence limited the human population. Aided by these three, birth and death rates were equated. Methods of birth control were primitive, but "death control," though tragic, was effective. Today, things have changed. Communicable disease, for one, is under increasing control. The twentieth-century plague in Los Angeles killed fewer than forty people. In the fourteenth century,

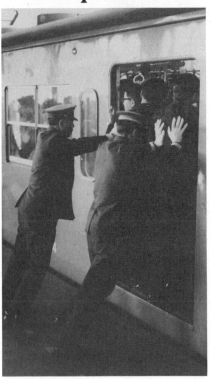

Oshiya-san ("honorable pushers") in a Tokyo subway station.

the same microorganism cost over forty million lives. Famine and war still threaten, but there can be only conjecture about their total future effect. Those spared today live to reproduce tomorrow. Better health promises too large a population and, ironically, threatens health. There is no better evidence of this than the increasing pollutions of our ecosystems. People busily organize societies to save nonhuman creatures whose existence is endangered by pollution. They would do well to include themselves as an endangered species.

It is in the crowded and threatening ecosystems on the scale of life that people compete with other living beings. And only to the extent that humans can best the nonhuman competitors in their mutual environmental prison can they hope to prevail. People are not lacking in the capacity to reproduce. With all our sophistication, we are not able to escape the biological laws. Nature ensures our multiplication by providing superabundant numbers of reproductive cells. Each human ovary contains more than 200,000 primitive, undeveloped eggs, while only one is needed for conception. Each ejaculation of human semen contains 250 to 500 *million* spermatozoa, while, again, only one is needed for fertilization.

In its abundance, human seed is not unique. If all the offspring to one April mating of houseflies were to live, they would, by August, cover the entire earth with a layer of houseflies forty-seven feet deep. Ruthlessly, and fortunately, nature provides for no such endurance. It does so by limiting the space and food that would be necessary for their existence. So for the fly, the wages of overcrowding are death.

More complex species have more complex methods of population limitation. For example, the number of Minnesota jack rabbits rises and falls cyclically. After a rise, episodes of mass dying occur. Neither food shortages nor their natural enemies account for the rabbits' deaths. Examinations of the dead jack rabbits have shown their livers and other glands to be diseased. In addition, they have signs of high blood pressure, and their arteries are hardened. Their deaths resulted from "stress sickness" (see pages 156–162). Similar episodes of crowding have produced similar illnesses in many other animals.

How does overcrowding contribute to human stress? Does it directly

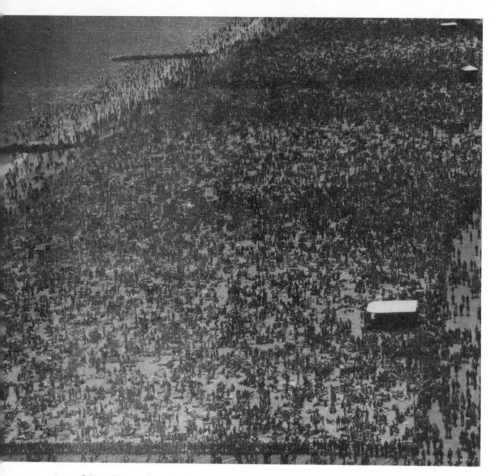

Searching for a place in the sun.

landscapes, contains the world's coldest areas. They offer little hope for the production of food. Russia has issued glowing reports about the successes obtained at the agricultural stations located in its coldest climates. However, few Russians willingly go to them. Finland, Sweden, and Greenland have grown food on previously unused Arctic areas. But these advances remain experimental, and mass hunger cannot await the results of even the most potentially valuable experiments.

Is the Solution Out of This World?

Less than two decades ago one expert given to projections stated:

> It is possible to demonstrate mathematically that at present rates of increase we will have standing room only by 2500 A.D. or that in 5,000 years the human race will be expanding so fast that it will form a solid ball of flesh growing out into space at the speed of light."[4]

Of course, such projections assume a sustained increase in population at our current rate of growth, which is impossible, since the planet cannot support such growth. But they do reflect the concern of scientists about overpopulation and point out the need to seek solutions. Apprehensive of uncontrolled population growth, some scientists think of the possibilities of building human-designed planets that could eventually become self-sustaining. But money and a disagreeing Congress would have to be dealt with as well as people who do not care to live outside of this world. One senator has decreed "not a penny for this nutty phantasy."[5] True, there may be a kernel of truth in every

cause sickness and death? Further research will provide more complete answers. Yet no research is necessary to know that too little food for too many people is overwhelmingly stressful. That overcrowding contributes to social sickness is undeniable. That it can be an indirect cause of death is a matter of record. In Java, for example, in a desperate search for living space, people move into craters of dormant (temporarily inactive) volcanoes. In Bangladesh thousands are driven into flood-prone lowlands. The Javanese may die if the volcanoes erupt. Thousands of Bangladesh people have been killed by numerous tidal waves. For people, too, then, the wages of overcrowding may be death.

Our Limited Land

The total land area of the earth is about fifty-eight million square miles. However, only 25 percent of the earth's total surface is suitable for farming. Impossible climates or unyielding soil force people to let millions of acres go unused. Only 5 percent of the earth's mountainous terrain is usable for farming. Over a third of the earth's land is desert or semidesert, and this is increasing (see page 24).

Cold lands take up about 29 percent of the planet's surface. Antarctica is almost twice the size of the United States. Not one single human being lives there permanently. And the Arctic, covering millions of square miles of frozen, treeless

nut. But consideration of the expense, much less the paperwork, does boggle the human mind. One scientist has summed it up this way: "Technically the idea would work fine if money grew on trees."[6]

Are there better, more natural frontiers to explore? There is talk of people settling on other planets someday. First stop, the moon. Perhaps someday a scientific laboratory will be built there. Yet visits to this ancient cinder show little about its ecosystems to invite human colonization. But cannot the moon be a bus-stop to other, more inviting planets in our solar system? Depending on the planet, people would meet with vast fogs, violent dust storms, poisonous gases, heat that would melt lead, and cold that would freeze it.

Countless planets whirl outside the earth's own solar system. Could not some be a paradise? For human beings, no nearby known planet could be anything but a hell without a sun to warm it. And the nearest sun to earth's would require more than one ordinary long lifetime to reach. Even then, the trip would have been in vain. For human needs, its warmth is too weak. One would not even shiver to death, for to shiver one must first be warm. And so people seeking a nourishing home outside of this world would have to go on and on, careening past endless, lonely emptiness, occasionally passing faintly glimmering suns that would fail to keep any planet decently warm. Sometimes twin suns would be seen. They maintain deadly heat. After over a century of travel, one constellation (about ninety-four million million miles from earth) might be reached. Maybe it maintains a kindly planet or two for human comfort. Perhaps even a vacation spot. Perhaps not. Nobody knows. In any case, it would be a long journey, and there is always the return trip to be considered.

So, it is on earth that we must seek solutions to our overpopulation problems. And we must always remain aware of our own environmental limitations, of the limits of our world's ecosystems.

Population Growth Is "Built-In"

Of the billions of people born on this earth up to the year 1980, over 95 percent are dead. Furthermore, it took hundreds of thousands of years before the world's total population reached its first billion (about 1830). A brief consideration of these two statements might lead one to believe that no true population problem exists. Not so. The one billion people of 1830 doubled to two billion in just one hundred years (1930). And a mere forty-five years later (in 1975) the world's population had doubled still again. The four billion people of 1975 increased to about four and a half billion in only about five years (1980). This was so despite the fact that in 1978 the world's *birthrate* (the number of live births per one thousand population) was the lowest in modern recorded times.

Why, then, is there a continued increase of people? It is because there is a *built-in momentum* for population growth. What does this mean? First, there has been a relatively recent worldwide decline in death rates, particularly in the developing countries. Worldwide, more people are living longer, which increases the total number of people. And, upon that fact is added yet another. Although the *percentage rate* of population growth has remained constant (or even decreased slightly), the *numbers* of people

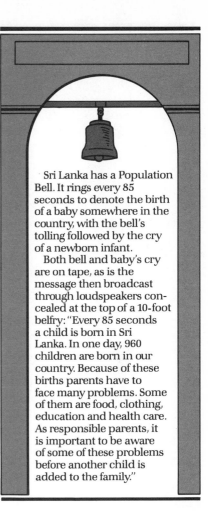

Sri Lanka has a Population Bell. It rings every 85 seconds to denote the birth of a baby somewhere in the country, with the bell's tolling followed by the cry of a newborn infant.

Both bell and baby's cry are on tape, as is the message then broadcast through loudspeakers concealed at the top of a 10-foot belfry: "Every 85 seconds a child is born in Sri Lanka. In one day, 960 children are born in our country. Because of these births parents have to face many problems. Some of them are food, clothing, education and health care. As responsible parents, it is important to be aware of some of these problems before another child is added to the family."

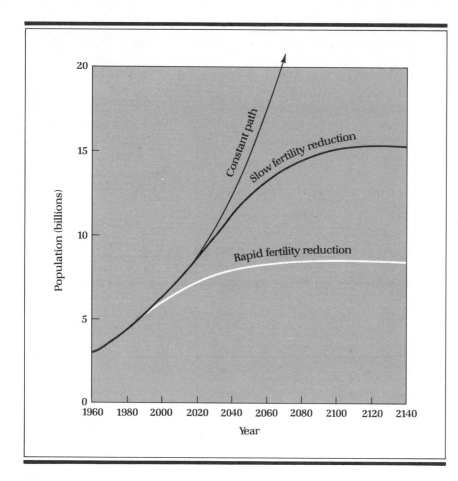

FIGURE 12-10
World population: three alternative futures.

population finally peak? This will depend on the success of economic development and family planning in the developing world.

How Did People Increase Their Numbers?

People began to significantly increase in number when they succeeded in better controlling their ecosystems. One of the first triumphs that led to better environmental control was the invention of the microscope. With it, scientists first identified some of their most dangerous enemies. Previously invisible, these competitors of humanity could at last be attacked (refer back to the discussion on page 54 in Chapter 3).

The scientific experiments that followed this discovery quickened a series of great revolutions in human history. Scientists sought to increase life—and to decrease death. Such leading investigators as Pasteur, Freud, Koch, Ehrlich, Lister, Nightingale, Semmelweiss, the Curies, and many others helped build the scientific structure for the twentieth century. From the back of humankind they lifted a load of sickness and death, but by so doing, they undermined a major form of population control—a high death rate. The lack of both death control and birth control quickly resulted in vast overpopulation. (For a projection of U.S. population expansion, including that of persons sixty-five and older, see Figure 12-11.)

Also, along with the scientific revolution came an agricultural revolution. Improvements in plant breeding, crop rotation, cultivation, and farm machinery brought more food from the earth. In ancient times people ate whatever was

have increased exponentially. In other words, at a growth rate of 10 percent, a population of 1,000 people will increase by 100 people per year, but a population of 1,000,000 people will increase by 100,000 people a year.

What can be done? First, let's look more closely at the figures. The *fertility rate* is a better measure of population growth than the birthrate because it relates births more nearly to the age group most likely to add to the population—those between fifteen and forty-four.

Figure 12-10 shows three possible paths of future world population growth. The *constant path* assumes that the 1978 growth rate will continue unchanged into the future. This predicts uncontrolled population growth and eventual disaster. The *slow fertility reduction* curve suggests that the world's population would stabilize at about fifteen billion by 2100 A.D. The *rapid fertility reduction path* assumes that the world's population could stabilize at about eight billion sometime during the twenty-first century. That is about twice the population of today's overcrowded world. At what dangerously high level (from eight to fifteen billion) will the world's

available. With the advent of tools and scientific farming methods, however, they could make available the food that they needed. In time, humanity's most powerful tool became the mind. Even today, though, ways to prevent hunger are still unknown throughout much of the world.

Areas of Crisis

Countless people in developing countries of Latin America, Asia, and Africa do not have enough to eat. Most of the malnourished pre-school children in the world live in these countries. Hundreds of millions of children in those countries suffer brain damage because of poor nutrition. With one hand, progress gives them life; with the other, it takes it away. And if they are not robbed of life, they are deprived of its quality.

Technical knowledge exists to meet the world's food shortage for some years to come. Yet at present in the Western industrialized nations, less than one-third of the total world population consumes as much protein as does the rest of humanity combined. That ratio cannot be expected to promote friendly feelings on the part of those with the least toward those with the most.

Nor can the world's poor be any more hopeful of soon solving their housing problems. Millions in Africa, Asia, and Latin America live in dwellings of mud, straw, or cardboard. Their housing is dilapidated beyond belief. Toilets and clean water are luxuries. It is in such facilities that the population will double in less than a generation. Countless others, with no place to go, swarm in the streets of crowded cities. They beg; they prostitute; they hold out a skinny hand to a heedless world.

What are the realistic financial opportunities of these malnourished, inadequately housed people of the developing countries? The future of any nation rests with its children. Millions of children under the age of fifteen live in countries with a national per capita income of less than $500 per year. What hope do these youngsters have of earning incomes higher than those of their parents? A major obstacle is the increasing population. In some countries the annual population increase is so great that it outstrips all attempts to improve the standard of living.

FIGURE 12–11
Growth chart. The bars show the number of persons age sixty-five and older compared with the total population from 1900. The chart extends to the year 2030.

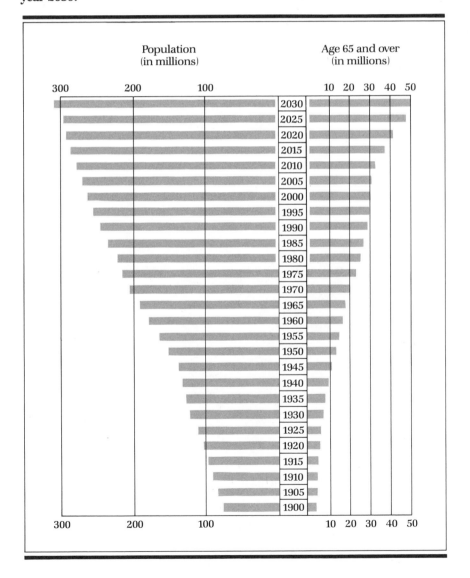

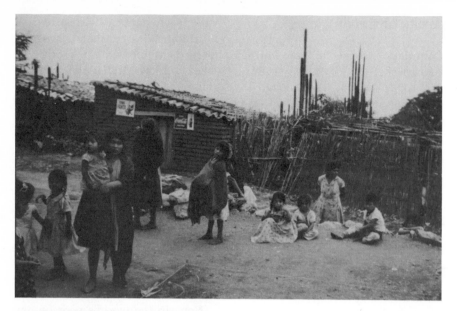

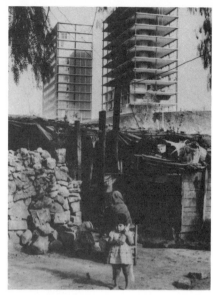

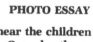

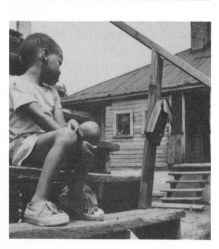

PHOTO ESSAY

**"Do ye hear the children weeping
O my brothers,
Ere the sorrow comes with years?"**
ELIZABETH BARRETT BROWNING

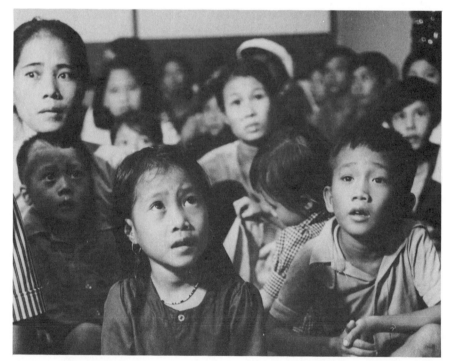

Watch Us Grow

In the closing months of 1979, the United States population was estimated to have passed 220 million. Will that figure reach 300 million before the turn of the century? That depends on the number of children per family. If the average number of children per family is three, the population will reach 300 million in 1996. If the average is two, that day will be postponed another twenty-five years, to the year 2021. If the average continues as it is at present, between two and three children per family, there will be 300 million people in the United States by about 2008.

In this century, a continuous replacement rate is a possibility. However, *zero population growth* (ZPG) will not happen in the near future. ZPG means no population increase or decrease. But, as has been seen, population growth is a product of past events. It cannot be brought to an abrupt halt. To achieve ZPG would take at least seventy years. Why?

Not until 1958, after eight years of steady rise, did the United States birthrate begin to descend from its 1957 historic peak of 25.3 per 1,000 people. But now the babies born during the "boom" years are beginning to have babies of their own. Today, the number of persons moving into childbearing age is much larger than it was in their parents' childbearing years. In 1975, there were about 5.5 million more people in the prime childbearing age group (twenty to twenty-nine) than there were in 1971. By 1985, that number will have increased another 5.5 million.

Despite these projections, there is growing evidence that the baby boom of former times has become a birth dearth. In 1960, the United

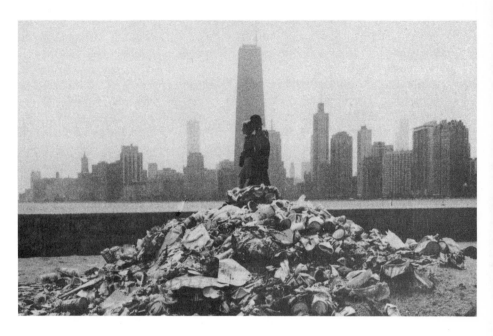

"Where can people today find a Walden Pond?"

States birthrate was 23.7.* In 1976 it was 14.7, the lowest annual rate ever observed in this country. The birthrate in 1978 was up slightly to 14.9. Nevertheless, for reasons explained above, the "built-in" population growth assures a massive increase in the U.S. population during the next generation.

"Watch us grow!" was once the challenge of little cities to the big. Los Angeles grew. And now an astronaut can get around the world in less time than the average suburban commuter can get home from work on the Los Angeles freeways. Manhattan grew. Now at day's end, people flee the island. Rather than live in the congested city, many commuters choose to travel two or more hours a day to get to and from their jobs. Another price of overpopulation in this country is a serious shortage of energy. Creating sources of power is very costly, but

the price of distributing it is even greater. Schools are overcrowded; air is polluted; water is scanty (millions now drink safely treated sewage); noise is deafening; housing is in short supply. George Washington headed a nation of 4 million people. Today, the president worries about over 220 million; each senator courts an average of 2.5 million; and each representative, an average of about three-quarters of a million people. As population increases, taxes increase, but representation per person decreases.

But perhaps the most subtle evil of overpopulation is the loss of personal significance. In his essay "Civil Disobedience," the nineteenth century U.S. author Henry David Thoreau wrote of his night in jail for refusal to pay a poll tax. At least in prison Thoreau felt free because he felt significant. This lover of solitude found his true significance in a cabin near Walden Pond in Massachusetts. Now Walden Pond is a polluted watery receptacle for various wastes.

*Crude birth rate = $\dfrac{\text{Number of live births}}{\text{Total population}} \times 1,000$

Where can people today find a Walden Pond? Every year many thousands of acres of lush countryside are bulldozed. Cities stream noisily into one another and form a monstrous megalopolis. Today, a majority of the U.S. population lives in three great megalopolitan areas. These are the Great Northeastern megalopolis (including the Atlantic seaboard and the Great Lakes region), the California region, and the Florida region. These three major areas presently contain about 150 million people. Even at the currently low birthrates and fertility rates, they will, by about 1990, be the home of the majority of the nation's people.

At present, 130 million polluting vehicles, traveling more than one thousand billion miles yearly, slay thousands of people a year. The roads on which these vehicles operate are built at a cost of millions of dollars a mile. For each road mile, about forty acres of agricultural land is sacrificed. Add to this a further decrease in agricultural land for the purposes of homes, shopping centers, parking garages, resort communities, reservoirs, flood control areas, and countless other increasing needs.

Well, Thoreau, at least, found a quiet spot.

If Not War, Then What Solution?

Is war the inevitable "solution" to the overpopulation problem? It has been suggested that human aggression has helped limit population. Overpopulation also promotes war. For example, this generation finds more than 900 million restless Chinese seeking more real estate. Will the next generation find more than one billion Chinese any less restless? Eighty-five percent of the Chinese now are forced to live on but one-third of their land (much of China's territory is uninhabitable desert or high mountains). China is making an enormous effort to educate its population about birth control. This is combined with a relatively late age of marriage and a general acceptance of premarital chastity among young people. Nevertheless, China's vast population will increase for the same built-in reasons that the population of other nations will increase. Where will the Chinese go? Or the billion people that will inhabit India by 2000 A.D? Humankind cannot accept war as a solution. The threats of all-out modern warfare are too inhuman to consider.

Some recommend *abortion* (see pages 376–377). Japan practices it with remarkable success. In 1947 Japan's birthrate was 34.3. The death rate was 14.6. The natural increase (the difference between the two) was 19.7. In 1948 a law authorized individual physicians, on their own responsibility, to induce abortion for physical or financial reasons upon request of the pregnant woman. By 1957, ten years after the abortion law, the birthrate had dropped to 17.2. The death rate was 8.3. The rate of natural increase was 8.9, less than half that of 1947. Every year more than 1.25 million abortions are performed in Japan. Since these are done only by physicians, no unusual number of deaths is noted from the procedure.[7]

Abortion, however, is not the only cause of the low Japanese birthrate. Birth control is widely practiced in Japan. In this country, too, abortion has been gaining in popularity among many women who have failed to use available birth control methods (see pages 371–382) or whose method of control has failed. It has also met with widespread resistance. Abortion has become a nationwide debate.

An *economic* solution to the population problem also has been recommended—that of greater efficiency in food production. However, as long as population numbers outstrip ability to meet needs, this concept remains unrealistic. Today, hundreds of millions starve in miserable housing. Despair is their constant companion. What realistic reason is there to think that the next generation will have solved the overwhelming problem of poverty for twice the number of today's poverty-stricken people?

Some experts fear that the battle to feed the world's population may already be lost. They believe that only a vast crash program of population control can prevent a global calamity. There is no doubt that the need for such a "crash" program is great and urgent.

A continuous worldwide *educational* approach has been suggested. Directing such programs toward the area of family planning is wise. Of special importance is the education of the mother who has already borne a child, for it is she who is most likely to increase the population. There is, moreover, expert opinion that instruction in population problems and family planning should begin in high school. Indeed, in Baltimore, detailed information on family planning and family growth is given to the high-school student. The material, incorporated into the social studies and biology courses, has been found to be valuable both to students and to their parents.

Since population control depends, first of all, on reduction of the birthrate, let's consider now some methods of birth control.

Birth Control

Ancient writings often gave prescriptions for birth control. In one old Egyptian document (1850 B.C.), crocodile dung is recommended. Twenty-seven hundred years later, a famed Arabian physician substituted elephant dung for that of the crocodile. Few if any prescriptions, contraceptive or otherwise, persisted for as many years as did dung.

Coitus interruptus (the withdrawal of the penis from the vagina before ejaculation) is described in the Bible. Although one of the least reliable and most sexually frustrating methods of birth control, it is still widely practiced. *Infanticide*, the murder of infants, is also mentioned in the Bible,[8] although it was condemned by Hebrews and Christians alike. Nevertheless, even though it is much less common today than formerly, infanticide still occurs. In eighteenth- and nineteenth-century Europe, infanticide was not uncommon. Corpses of newborn infants lying in the streets or on the garbage heaps of London and other large European cities were a common sight.

The views of the great Catholic theologian Saint Thomas Aquinas have been vastly influential. In the *Summa Theologica*, he wrote: "In so far as the generation of offspring is impeded, it is a vice against nature which happens in every carnal act from which generation cannot follow."

Nevertheless, by 1970, two-thirds of all Catholic women were using contraceptive methods disapproved by their Church; this figure reached three-quarters for women under age thirty. The change between 1965 and 1970 was especially striking for Catholic women who had attended college.... Perhaps the most significant finding is that the defection has been most pronounced among the women who receive Communion at least once a month. Even among this group, the majority now deviates from Church teaching on birth control; among the younger women in this group the proportion not conforming reaches two-thirds.[9]

Five years after this report, with the exception of sterilization, U.S. Catholic and non-Catholic contraceptive practices were found to be essentially similar.[10]

Birth control involves the use of a contraceptive or it may be tried without a contraceptive. The contraceptive methods are much more likely to control birth.

A **contraceptive** is any agent that prevents **conception**—the fertilization of an ovum by a spermatozoon. Contraceptives may be *hormonal*, such as the pill; they may be *chemical* (but not hormonal), such as vaginal foams, jellies, and creams, and douches containing various chemical substances; or they may be *mechanical*, such as the diaphragm, condom, and IUD. Noncontraceptive methods of birth control are the *rhythm method* and *coitus interruptus*, as well as *surgical methods*.

Oral Contraceptives

Most of the currently marketed oral contraceptives ("the pill") are composed of synthetic (artificial, laboratory-prepared) estrogens and synthetic progesterone (progestin). It was explained earlier that ovulation depends on a delicate balance of hormones. The pill slightly changes normal hormone levels to prevent ovulation. The pill also causes the cervix to produce a thick mucus, making it difficult for sperm to enter the uterus. In addition, the lining of the uterus is affected so that a fertilized ovum cannot become implanted in it.

The pill has several advantages: It is almost 100 percent effective and does not interfere with lovemaking. Some women find that their menstrual cycles become more regular, and it may relieve acne. Moreover, since a woman must obtain a prescription refill, she visits her physician, who can then examine her regularly.

Since pills are prescribed for individuals who may react differently to them, they should not be borrowed. In case of loss, an extra month's supply should be kept. The pill should be taken at the same time every day. If one is missed, it should be taken as soon as possible and the next one taken at the ordinary time. If two are missed, then two should be taken for the next two days; however, for extra protection an additional contraceptive (a condom or diaphragm) should be used for at least a week.

There are over three dozen brands of birth control pills made. Some contain a low dosage of estrogen along with the progesterone because it is believed that higher doses of estrogen may be the cause of blood clots. These pills are slightly less effective than the ordinary combination estrogen-progesterone pills.

Minipills contain progesterone only. These may cause nonmenstrual bleeding, or they may cause menstruation to cease. Their major action is believed to be on the rate at which the egg travels down the Fallopian tube, on the quality of the mucus at the cervical opening necessary for sperm passage, and on the inner lining of the uterus. Mini-pills have a somewhat higher failure rate than the combination (estrogen and progesterone) type.

An injection called *Depo-Provera* contains progesterone. It is injected every three months and can cause menstrual irregularity. Apparently it may cause sterility although this does not happen often. The sterility may be temporary or permanent. After the injections have been stopped for some months, some women are again able to become pregnant. Its use in this country is in dispute and so is limited.

SIDE EFFECTS

Millions of women in this and other countries use the pill. However, despite its almost 100 percent effectiveness when used properly, the pill is losing some popularity because of its side effects, which will be discussed shortly. It is true that the death rates of U.S. women taking the pill are much lower than the already decreasing deaths from pregnancy. However, statistics are of little comfort to the individual woman who has a serious complication from the pill. Moreover, there are completely safe methods of birth control with only slightly less effectiveness when used intelligently. The pill should not be prescribed carelessly. Its use should be an individual matter decided by the woman and her physician, both of whom are fully aware of its risks. To determine the risk to the particular individual, the physician will need to take a thorough history. For example, has the patient a history of clots, cardiovascular disease, diabetes, overweight, high blood pressure, liver disease, high cholesterol levels, migraine headaches, or any other illness that increases her risk? What is her physical condition? Should the pill be prescribed, the woman will need to be checked about every six months.

The side effects of oral contraceptives, some of which are serious, are described below.

BLOOD ABNORMALITIES Recall from Chapter 4 that a *thrombus* is a clot of blood and, in this context, an *embolus* is a clot or a piece of a thrombus that has broken loose and is carried by the bloodstream until it plugs a blood vessel. One study suggested that the blood of women who take the pill clots faster and more firmly than the blood of women who do not use oral contraceptives. Still another study showed that oral contraceptives were associated with a four-fold increase in the risk of clots that result in stroke. The risk of clots is lower with lower amounts of estrogen in the pill. However, there is no evidence that any dose of estrogens presently used in contraceptive pills is totally free of this risk. Yet another long-term study, begun in 1968, comparing thousands of women who did and did not take oral contraceptives, pointed to a marked increase in venous clots among those who did. These included more than five times as many deep vein clots in the legs and four times as many in the vessels of the brain.

MYOCARDIAL INFARCTIONS Oral contraceptives affect the way the body handles fats. As a result, they have a tendency to increase the level of serum *triglycerides* (page 97). Such an increase is associated with myocardial infarctions, or heart attacks involving damage to the heart muscle (see pages 96–97). One British study found that the risk of death from heart attacks was almost three times greater among users of oral contraceptives who were between the ages of thirty and thirty-nine than among nonusers. In the forty to forty-four age group, the risk was almost five times greater. Moreover, the use of oral contraceptives by women already at risk from being overweight or having high blood pressure or diabetes significantly increases their chances of having a heart attack. The risk goes up markedly with women who take oral contraceptives and also smoke.

It should be noted, however, that two recent U.S. studies consider the British reports of pill-cardiovascular disease correlations highly exaggerated. One U.S. statistician, after careful analysis, rejects reports by the Royal College of General Practitioners that all women who had ever taken the pill increase their risk of dying from heart attacks, strokes, and other cardiovascular disease by more than four times.[11] Moreover, another study by a U.S. statistician,[12] refutes the conclusions by one of the authors of the Royal College report, which asserted that there is a severe risk of cardiovascular disease among pill users in twenty-one countries in Europe, Asia, and North America. Neither U.S. study claims that the pill does not increase the risk to women of death from cardiovascular disease to some extent, or that the risk is not increased with women in the older age groups with such predisposing factors as heavy cigarette smoking. Yet there are relatively few older women who smoke heavily and who also use the pill; therefore, much of the risk might be concentrated among this small group.

LIVER TUMORS   These tumors are not malignant, but they are dangerous. At one time they were extremely rare, and though still uncommon, a number of studies have reported a sharp increase in their occurrence among women who use the pill. Why are these tumors dangerous? Because they may cause internal bleeding. Several cases of death from such hemorrhages have been reported.

HIGH BLOOD PRESSURE   In some women, oral contraceptives seem to cause high blood pressure. One study estimates that the risk is increased 2½ times.

GALLBLADDER DISEASE   Oral contraceptive users run about twice the risk of developing gallbladder disease than do nonusers.

BACTERIAL INFECTIONS   Infections of the urinary bladder and of the vagina are more frequent among users than nonusers. Indeed, one of the most common causes of an increased vaginal discharge is the use of oral contraceptives.

DES

Diethylstilbesterol (DES) or "the morning after pill" is an estrogen used as a contraceptive pill *following* intercourse. Its major danger, and it is small, is the development of cancer of the vagina in some female children of women who received the drug early in pregnancy. Nevertheless, noncancerous vaginal changes appear more often. Second, there is an excess of abnormalities in the genitals and possibly in the lower urinary tract of males born to mothers who took DES during pregnancy. Third, women who have taken DES during pregnancy *may* have a greater tendency to develop

cancer of the breast and reproductive organs, although this has not been proved. There is, in addition, some disagreement over whether it does prevent pregnancy. And it may have such side effects as nausea, vomiting, and headache. A prescription is required.

DES is not a substitute for the ordinary contraceptive pill. It should be considered only when a fully informed patient and her physician are aware of no other alternatives to it. When used, thorough birth control counseling should be part of the physician-patient relationship. Women who have previously used DES or other estrogens, or who have been exposed to these drugs before birth, should avoid DES. Also, DES should not be used to suppress lactation.[13]

THE PILL: NOT THE BEST WAY OF BIRTH CONTROL FOR MOST TEEN-AGERS

A comprehensive nationwide study published in 1977 revealed that in this country slightly over 40 percent of unmarried women between the ages of fifteen and nineteen had experienced sexual intercourse at least once.[14] Other studies published before 1977 produced only slightly different results. Thus, total *abstinence* (refraining from sexual intercourse) serves— either directly or indirectly—as a method of birth control for the majority of the nation's single teenagers. Partial abstinence serves the same purpose among many of the more sexually active members of that age group. Among teen-age nonvirgins, about half reported no sexual intercourse in the month before the interview, and only one-third had had sexual intercourse as often as three times in that month.

In addition, as a rule, most sexual contacts were limited to one partner. Moreover, oral contraceptives have a high discontinuance rate among sexually active teen-agers.

Therefore, considering the relatively low frequency of regular sexual intercourse among most teen-agers, the high rate of discontinuance of the pill, and its possible serious complications, one can conclude that the pill is not the best choice of contraception for teenagers. Given the alternatives, it would appear that the condom (see page 374) might well be the preferred choice.

Nonhormonal Chemical Contraceptives

DOUCHES

Some douches are merely water. Others contain chemicals. As a form of birth control, both are entirely ineffective. The belief that the douche will wash out the sperm in the vagina is merely wishful thinking, since the sperm have already reached the uterus seconds after ejaculation. In addition, many douches may easily irritate sensitive vaginal tissue and change the ecology of the vagina from a normal to an abnormal state. Unless prescribed by physicians, they are a waste of time and money. Some women douche regularly without a physician's advice because it is supposed to clean the vagina. This is not only nonsense, but it is often unhealthy. Vaginal deodorants are similarly needless. They do nothing that a good shower cannot do except often cause harmful irritations.

SPERMICIDES

These chemicals are inserted into the vagina. They coat vaginal surfaces and the cervical opening and kill sperm. They may also act as a mechanical barrier. They provide protection for about an hour.

Used alone, the effectiveness of these vaginal chemical contraceptives is much lower than if they are used with a diaphragm or a condom. Nevertheless, pregnancy may be avoided by the use of these simple methods, although the failure rate is high.

VAGINAL FOAMS The foam is packed under pressure (like foaming shaving cream) and is inserted into the vagina with an applicator. Among this type of contraceptives, vaginal foams are the most effective. Foaming tablets and suppositories are the least effective. Failures with the best of these methods, are about 28 per 100 women per year.

VAGINAL JELLIES AND CREAMS These are also inserted into the vagina with an applicator. Used alone, these preparations may drain from the vagina. They should be used with a diaphragm or a condom.

VAGINAL SUPPOSITORIES These small cone-shaped objects melt in the vagina. They must be inserted in sufficient time to melt before sexual intercourse.

VAGINAL TABLETS The tablets are moistened slightly and inserted into the vagina; foam is produced. They must be inserted in sufficient time for the tablets to disintegrate before sexual intercourse.

Foaming tablets may cause a temporary burning sensation. This method is acceptable to many women primarily because it is available to them without a prescription.

Mechanical Contraceptives

THE CONDOM

The condom is a very thin, strong sheath made of rubber or animal skin, to be worn once (never reused) over the erect penis to prevent spermatozoa from entering the vagina. All condoms must meet high federal standards, but the more expensive ones are probably more reliable. (The woman may also use a sperm-killing, or spermatocidal, vaginal foam, cream, or jelly to provide added protection.) The condom should have a small nipple at the end to hold the ejaculate and a rubber ring at the top to hold it in place. If the condom has no end nipple, at least a half inch of space should be left at its end. The condom itself may be lubricated with a spermatocidal jelly as an added protection. As soon as the ejaculation is over and while the penis is still erect, the penis should be withdrawn from the vagina. During withdrawal, the top of the condom should be held to prevent leakage of semen into the vagina.

A high degree of protection (about 97 percent or better) is offered if the condom is used correctly and consistently. Although the penis does not experience as much sensation, this may prove beneficial in that it slows the male's excitation, thus helping to prevent premature ejaculation. This fact and having the female put the condom on as part of foreplay easily make up for the slight loss of sensation. Failures are due to tearing of the sheath or its slipping off after climax. The condom should not be lubricated with petroleum jelly, since petroleum products dissolve rubber. KY jelly or prelubricated condoms are acceptable. A condom cannot long withstand months in the hot glove compartment of a car or of pressure in a wallet. The condom is also one of the best preventives against some kinds of sexually transmitted diseases, such as gonorrhea, genital herpes, and trichomonas infections (see pages 78–84). It can be purchased without a prescription.

INTRAUTERINE DEVICES (IUDs)

Intrauterine devices (IUDs) are objects of different shapes usually made of plastic. They are inserted into the uterus by a physician most often during menstruation, when there is some dilatation of the cervical opening. IUDs may be left in place indefinitely. The IUD has a nylon thread that protrudes into the vagina from the opening of the cervix. It should be checked regularly, particularly after menstruation. New designs are causing less complications and are retained better.

How the IUD prevents pregnancy is not completely understood. It does not prevent the ovary from releasing eggs. Evidence suggests that it probably speeds descent of the egg in the Fallopian tube, or the egg may reach the uterus at a time when it cannot nest there. There is also a theory that it stimulates the production of white cells, which attack and destroy spermatozoa.

Some women cannot satisfactorily use the IUD because of expulsion, excessive bleeding, or discomfort such as backache and cramps. Among the contraindications to the use of the IUD are pregnancy or suspected pregnancy, abnormalities that distort the uterine cavity, infection or inflammation of the uterus or adjoining tissues, a history of infection with abortion within the past three months, and endometrial disease. Serious problems reported to be associated with the IUD are

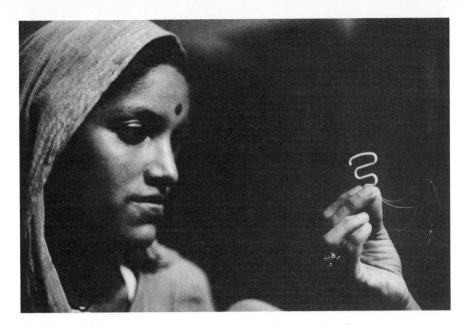

Will this Indian woman use the intrauterine device? Many factors, among them tradition and belief, will influence her decision.

pelvic inflammatory disease and perforation of the uterus. Pregnancy can occur with the device in place.

IUDs are very acceptable when sustained motivation is lacking, when the user is fearful of using the pill, or when other methods cannot be used successfully. For the women who has never borne a child, the small copper wire type may be ideal. The Progestasert is an IUD that releases a specific amount of progesterone into the uterine cavity. It will need further study before a decision can be reached concerning its desirability.

THE DIAPHRAGM

The diaphragm is a flexible hemispherical rubber dome attached to a rubber-covered metal ring. It is used in combination with spermatocidal cream or jelly. The spermatocidal material is spread over the inside of the diaphragm, which covers the cervix when it is in place. The outside and rim of the diaphragm should also be covered with a spermatocidal product. The lubricated diaphragm is inserted into the vagina so that it covers the cervix. It thus provides a barrier to spermatozoa. It must be left in place at least eight hours after intercourse and may be left in place as long as twenty-four hours. If a second intercourse occurs within the eight-hour period, more spermatocide should be inserted into the vagina. The diaphragm must be fitted by a physician and refitted every two years and after each pregnancy. It should be washed after use. The arcing spring type stays in place better. This is important since the upper vagina enlarges during sexual excitement.

The diaphragm offers a high level of protection, particularly when used with a spermatocide. Failures are about 17.5 per 100 women per year. A rate of two to three pregnancies per 100 women per year would seem to be a fair estimate for careful and consistent users. If motivation or self-control is weak, much higher pregnancy rates must be expected. Failures may be due to improper insertion or displacement of the diaphragm during sexual intercourse. The diaphragm is the method of choice among the wives of obstetricians. Many physicians will not dispense the diaphragm until the woman has shown she knows how to use it. There is no medical risk, but the diaphragm cannot be used by some women with certain uterine variations, such as a uterus that is not in proper position.

The Rhythm Methods

The rhythm methods are the only forms of birth control approved by the Roman Catholic Church. They may be practiced in two ways: by computing the safe, or nonfertile, period, or by taking the temperature to determine the time of ovulation.

The safe, or nonfertile, period is the time during which a mature ovum is not available for fertilization (see Figure 12–6, page 356). The rationale on which this method is based is discussed on pages 356–357.

The major drawback to this method is that most women do not menstruate as regularly as they think they do. An accurate record of the length of each menstrual cycle must be kept for one year in order to obtain any degree of success with this method. On this record, the shortest and longest menstrual cycles are noted. By subtracting nineteen from the number of days in the shortest cycle, the number of safe days during the first half of the cycle is obtained. By subtracting eleven from the number of days in the longest cycle, the number of safe days during the second half of the cycle is found. For example, if the shortest cycle is twenty-four days, the five days following the first day of the menstrual flow are safe. If the longest cycle is twenty-eight days, the seventeenth day of the cycle to the beginning of the next menstrual period is safe. Between the fifth and the seventeenth day of the menstrual cycle fertilization of the ovum (conception) is possible.

It will be noted that the unsafe period of fertility, in Figure 12–6 on page 356, is from the ninth to the eighteenth day of the menstrual cycle. This is because the calculations for that illustration are based on one regular twenty-eight-day cycle. Few women menstruate regularly every twenty-eight days. Even then, long periods of abstinence each month are required. Such problems account for at least a 20 to 30 percent failure rate.

The temperature method is based on the fact that the temperature of most women is relatively low during their menstrual period and for the eight days that follow it. When they ovulate, there is first a decline in temperature and then a sharp increase of between 0.5 to 0.7 of a degree. This is the unsafe period. This rise in temperature continues until about two days before the next menstrual period. The woman who wishes to use the temperature method must first practice by taking her temperature upon awakening for six months to a year. She may not leave her bed, eat, or indulge in any other activity before computing her temperature reading. In this way she learns to predict her safe period.

This method is complicated by inaccuracies in reading a thermometer, by ordinary variations in human temperature, and by minor colds or other illnesses. In addition, the correlation between the temperature rise and ovulation is not dependable. It can vary by as many as four days. Also, the average woman cannot spare the time in the morning to remain in bed and take her temperature.

Surgical Methods of Birth Control

VASECTOMY

A vasectomy is a relatively simple operation to prevent spermatozoa from entering the ejaculate through the vas deferens. Cutting and tying the vas deferens can be done in the doctor's office or hospital under local anesthesia and usually in less than thirty minutes. This operation must be considered permanent. Attempts to reconnect the vas deferens are very expensive and, in many cases, are unsuccessful.

After a vasectomy, the male is considered sterile. However, after the operation has been performed, several laboratory tests are necessary before this conclusion is a certainty. Vasectomy decreases neither the desire nor the ability for sexual intercourse, nor the amount of ejaculate. Some men, however, experience psychological effects, such as fear of lost manhood, after this surgical procedure. Many respond to assurance that there is no reason for this fear.

TUBAL LIGATION

Cutting and tying (ligation) of the Fallopian tubes prevent the egg from reaching the uterus. This procedure can be done through the abdominal wall or sometimes through the vagina. Often it is done just after childbirth. New surgical methods have greatly increased the chances of reversing the operation to about 75 percent.

A tubal ligation is virtually 100 percent effective. A very few failures with this method have been reported. It is more complicated than a vasectomy, so it is usually performed in a hospital. However, recent techniques have made tubal ligation possible on an outpatient basis. It has become an acceptable method for women who desire permanent sterilization.

Abortion

A *viable* fetus is one that has reached the stage of development at which it can live outside the uterus. The premature expulsion from the uterus of a nonviable fetus or an embryo is considered an *abortion*. Abortions are not just *elective* or *therapeutic* (medically indicated). For a variety of reasons, many occur *spontaneously*. Lay people refer to a spontaneous abortion as a "miscarriage."

Spontaneous abortions end 10 to 15 percent of pregnancies. Most occur before the eighth week of pregnancy. Vaginal bleeding ("spotting") and cramps are early signs of a possible spontaneous abortion. The causes of spontaneous abortions are numerous and often unclear. Trauma, maternal illnesses, and malnourishment are often causative. In most spontaneous abortions the cause remains unknown.

To many physicians, chronic hypertension, kidney disease, and breast and uterine cancers are examples of indications for therapeutic abortion. In addition, there can be little doubt that elective abortions are today being widely done as a "back-up" for women who have not used an adequate birth control method or who have ignored such methods altogether. In 1976 the United States reported the highest number of legal abortions in the world. Of those countries reporting abortions by the woman's age, the United States had the highest number (32 percent) of teen-agers who obtained legal abortions.[15]

With the exception of cases involving cancer of the uterus and ectopic pregnancy (pregnancy outside of the uterus), abortions are generally not done in Catholic hospitals.[16] Ethical and theological problems arise when people attempt to define indications for abortion. Complicating the issue even more is the present gulf between some scientists and some theologians.

Opponents of abortion place a sacred and infinite value on each separate beginning, on each potential life. Many consider that this value must be protected even beyond the mother's life. Threats to this concept are often considered to be selfish, irresponsible, and promiscuous, and they are especially condemned.

COMMON METHODS OF INDUCING ABORTION

VACUUM ASPIRATION (OR SUCTION) This method is particularly suited for abortions during the first three months of pregnancy. It is relatively inexpensive, can be done on an outpatient basis, and requires but a few minutes. Within the first two months of pregnancy, it may not be necessary to dilate the opening of the cervix. Little or no anesthesia may be necessary. One end of a suction tube is inserted through the cervical opening of the uterus; the other end is connected to a suction pump. Although complications such as hemorrhage, cervical tearing, and infection of the uterus do occur, they are not common. By 1980, close to 90 percent of all U.S. abortions were done by this method.

DILATATION AND CURETTAGE (D AND C) In this procedure, the opening of the cervix is dilated. A hand instrument called a *curette* (a metal spoon or scoop on the end of a long, thin handle) is inserted into the uterus through the cervical opening. With hand manipulation of the curette, the physician gently scrapes the pregnancy tissue from the inner surface wall of the uterus and then removes it. Most physicians prefer to limit dilatation and curettage to about the ninth week of pregnancy. Beyond this time complications occur more frequently.

SALINE INJECTION INTO THE AMNIOTIC SAC In this procedure, a hypodermic needle approximately six to eight inches long is inserted through the abdominal wall into the amniotic sac, and some of the amniotic fluid is withdrawn. This fluid is then replaced by a strong salt solution. The salt solution upsets the delicate water and chemical balance within the sac, placenta, and fetus. Fetal death is quick and hastened by placental damage, which results in sharply lessened oxygen and food supplies to the fetus. In addition, the hormonal balance, so necessary to maintaining the pregnancy, is disrupted. The hormone oxytocin is released from the pituitary gland, thus stimulating contraction of uterine musculature. Usually from twelve to twenty-four hours after receiving the salt injection the uterus begins to contract. The placenta and fetus are expelled from thirty-six to forty-eight hours after the injection.

Most physicians prefer the technique of introducing the saline solution into the amnion for pregnancies that have already progressed from sixteen to twenty weeks because, before that time, the amniotic sac is small and difficult to locate. Complications are more common with this method than the other two that were discussed.

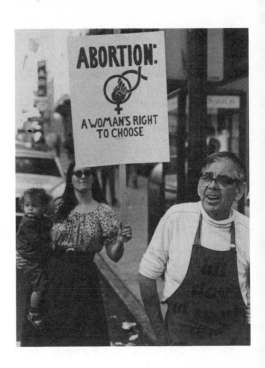

Contraception:
Comparing the Options

A number of methods of contraception are available today. Some can be obtained by anyone without a doctor's prescription or advice; others require a prescription and medical consultation and followup.

When choosing a method there are several factors to consider, among them personal preferences, psychological or religious attitudes, and individual medical history. But many people looking for a suitable means of contraception know very little about the available methods—how they work, how effective they are, what side effects they may have, what health problems may be related to their use.

Here, in chart form, is basic information on the contraceptive methods most widely used today. It is beginning information only, to help the individual understand the choices. Discussion with a physician can help an individual make an intelligent selection.

No method of contraception is 100 percent effective. Correct use of a method is essential in making sure it will be as effective as possible. Other factors, however, also contribute to failure: diaphragms have been improperly fitted, intrauterine devices (IUD's) can be expelled without the woman being aware of it, a foam or jelly might be used too long before intercourse.

Effectiveness figures in the following chart are expressed in terms of pregnancies per 100 woman years, which means the number of women out of 100 who would become pregnant in one year when using the method. If no contraceptive method were used 60 to 80 women out of 100 would become pregnant.

A wide range of effectiveness is shown for some methods because people differ in how well they use them. For example, a method may be more effective when used by 30-year-old college graduates but less effective when used by teenagers in high school.

SOURCE: U.S. Department of Health, Education, and Welfare, Public Health Service, and Food and Drug Administration, Office of Public Affairs, HEW Publication No. (FDA) 78-3069.

THE PILL   Prescription Required

"The Pill" refers to any of the oral contraceptives. The most widely used contains two female hormones, estrogen and progestin, and is taken 21 days each month. Another (sometimes called the "mini-pill") contains progestin only and is taken continuously. A woman should be sure to receive from the druggist, doctor, or person who gives her the pills an FDA-required brochure that explains the use, benefits, and risks of the product in greater detail.

Effectiveness   Effectiveness depends on how correctly the method is used. Of 100 women who use the combination estrogen and progestin pill for one year, less than 1 will become pregnant. Of 100 women who use the progestin-only pill (mini-pill) for one year, 2 to 3 will become pregnant.

Advantages   The combination pill is the most effective of the popular methods for preventing pregnancy. No inconvenient devices to bother with at time of intercourse.

Disadvantages   Must be taken regularly and exactly as instructed by the prescribing physician.

Side Effects   Side effects may include tender breasts, nausea or vomiting, gain or loss of weight, unexpected vaginal bleeding, higher levels of sugar and fat in the blood. Although it happens infrequently, use of The Pill can cause blood clots (in the legs, and less frequently in the lungs, brain, and heart). A clot that reaches the lungs or forms in the brain or heart can be fatal. Pill users have a greater risk of heart attack and stroke than non-users. This risk increases with age and is greater if the Pill user smokes. Some Pill users tend to develop high blood pressure, but it usually is mild and may be reversed by discontinuing use. Pill users have a greater risk than non-users of having gallbladder disease requiring surgery. There is no evidence that taking The Pill increases the risk of cancer. Benign liver tumors occur very rarely in women on The Pill. Sometimes they rupture, causing fatal hemorrhage.

Health Factors to Consider   Women who smoke should not use The Pill because smoking increases the risk of heart attack or stroke. Other women who should not take The Pill are those who have had a heart attack, stroke, angina pectoris, blood clots, cancer of the breast or uterus, or scanty or irregular periods. A woman who believes she may be pregnant should not take The Pill because it increases the risk of defect in the fetus. Health problems such as migraine headaches, mental depression, fibroids of the uterus, heart or kidney disease, asthma, high blood pressure, diabetes, or epilepsy may be made worse by use of The Pill. Risks associated with The Pill increase with age, and as a women enters her late 30's it is generally advisable to seek another method of contraception.

Long-Term Effect on Ability to Have Children   There is no evidence that using The Pill will prevent a woman from becoming pregnant after she stops taking it, although there may be a delay before she is able to become pregnant. Women should wait a short time after stopping The Pill before becoming pregnant. During this time another method of contraception should be used. After childbirth the woman should consult her doctor before resuming use of The Pill. This is especially true for nursing mothers because the drugs in The Pill appear in the milk and the long-range effect on the infant is not known.

DOUCHING

Use of a vaginal douche immediately after sexual intercourse to wash out or inactivate sperm is completely ineffective for preventing pregnancy.

FOAM, CREAM, OR JELLY ALONE   No Prescription Required

Several brands of vaginal foam, cream, or jelly can be used without a diaphragm. They form a chemical barrier at the opening of the uterus that prevents sperm from reaching an egg in the uterus; they also destroy sperm.

Effectiveness   Effectiveness depends on how correctly the method is used. Of 100 women who use aerosol foams alone for one year, 2 to 29 will become pregnant. Of 100 women who use jellies and creams alone for one year, 4 to 36 will become pregnant.

Advantages   Easy to obtain and use.

Disadvantages   Must be used one hour or less before intercourse. If douching is desired, must wait 6 to 8 hours after intercourse.

Side Effects   No serious side effects. Burning or irritation of the vagina or penis may occur. Allergic reaction may be corrected by changing brands.

Health Factors to Consider   None.

Long-Term Effect on Ability to Have Children   None.

VAGINAL SUPPOSITORIES   No Prescription Required

Vaginal suppositories are small waxy "tablets" that are placed at the opening of the uterus just before intercourse.
Note: Very few vaginal suppositories are intended for birth control. Ask before you buy.

Effectiveness   No figures available, considered fair to poor.

Advantages   No devices needed.

Disadvantages   Must be inserted 15 minutes before intercourse. If placed earlier, they may become ineffective. If placed later (too close to intercourse) the suppository will not have time to melt and will be ineffective.

Side Effects   No adverse side effects.

Health Factors to Consider   None.

Long-Term Effect on Ability to Have Children   None.

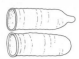

CONDOM (RUBBER)

No Prescription Required

The condom is a thin sheath of rubber or processed lamb cecum that fits over the penis.

Effectiveness   Effectiveness depends on how correctly the method is used. Of 100 women whose partner uses a condom for one year, 3 to 36 women will become pregnant.

Advantages   In addition to contraception, may afford some protection against venereal disease. Easily available. Requires no "long-term" planning before intercourse.

Disadvantages   Some people feel the condom reduces pleasure in the sex act. The male must interrupt foreplay and fit the condom in place before sexual entry into the woman. The condom can slip or tear during use or spill during removal from the vagina.

Side Effects   No serious side effects. Occasionally an individual will be allergic to the rubber, causing burning, irritation, itching, rash, or swelling, but this can easily be treated. Switching to the natural skin condom may be a solution.

Health Factors to Consider   None.

Long-Term Effect on Ability to Have Children   None.

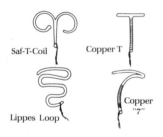

Saf-T-Coil   Copper T

Lippes Loop   Copper "7"

INTRAUTERINE DEVICE (IUD)

Prescription Required

The IUD is a small plastic or metal device that is placed in the uterus (womb) through the cervical canal (opening into the uterus). As long as the IUD stays in place pregnancy is prevented. How the IUD prevents pregnancy is not completely understood. IUD's seem to interfere in some manner with implantation of the fertilized egg in the wall of the uterus. There are 5 kinds of IUD's currently available—Copper-7, Copper-T, Progestasert, Lippes Loop, and Saf-T-Coil. IUD's containing copper (Copper-7 and Copper-T) should be replaced every three years; those containing progesterone (Progestasert) should be replaced every year.

Effectiveness   Effectiveness depends on proper insertion by the physician and whether the IUD remains in place. Of 100 women who use an IUD for one year, 1 to 6 will become pregnant.

Advantages   Insertion by a physician then no further care needed, except to see that the IUD remains in place (the user can check it herself but should be checked once a year by her doctor).

Disadvantages   May cause pain or discomfort when inserted; afterward may cause cramps and a heavier menstrual flow. Some women will experience adverse effects that require removal of the IUD. The IUD can be expelled, sometimes without the woman being aware of it, leaving her unprotected.

Side Effects   Major complications, which are infrequent, include anemia, pregnancy outside the uterus, pelvic infection, perforation of the uterus or cervix, and septic abortion. A woman with heavy or irregular bleeding while using an IUD should consult her physician. Removal of the IUD may be necessary to prevent anemia. Women susceptible to pelvic infection are more prone to infection when using an IUD. Serious complications can occur if a woman becomes pregnant while using an IUD. Though rare, cases of blood poisoning, miscarriage, and even death have been reported. An IUD user who believes she may be pregnant should consult her doctor immediately. If pregnancy is confirmed, the IUD should be removed. Although it rarely happens, the IUD can pierce the wall of the uterus when it is being inserted. Surgery is required to remove it.

Health Factors to Consider   Before having an IUD inserted, a woman should tell her doctor if she has had any of the following: cancer or other abnormalities of the uterus or cervix; bleeding between periods or heavy menstrual flow; infection of the uterus, cervix, or pelvis (pus in Fallopian tubes); prior IUD use; recent pregnancy, abortion, or miscarriage; uterine surgery; venereal disease; severe menstrual cramps; allergy to copper; anemia; fainting attacks; unexplained genital bleeding or vaginal discharge; suspicious or abnormal "Pap" smear.

Long-Term Effect on Ability to Have Children   Pelvic infection in some IUD users may result in their future inability to have children.

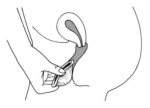

DIAPHRAGM (WITH CREAM, JELLY, OR FOAM)

Prescription Required

A diaphragm is a shallow cup of thin rubber stretched over a flexible ring. A sperm-killing cream, jelly, or foam is put on both sides of the diaphragm, which is then placed by the woman inside the vagina before intercourse. The device covers the opening of the uterus, thus preventing the sperm from entering the uterus.

Effectiveness   Effectiveness depends on how correctly the method is used. Of 100 women who use the diaphragm with a spermicidal product for one year, 2 to 20 will become pregnant.

Advantages   No routine schedule to be kept as with The Pill. The diaphragm with a spermicidal product is inserted by the user. Can be inserted up to two hours before intercourse. No discomfort or cramping, as with the IUD. No effect on the chemical or physical processes of the body, as with The Pill or the IUD.

Disadvantages   Must be inserted before each intercorse and stay in place at least six hours afterwards. Size and fit require yearly checkup, and should be checked if woman gains or loses more than 10 pounds. Should be refitted after childbirth or abortion. Requires instruction on insertion technique. Some women find it difficult to insert and inconvenient to use. Some women in whom the vagina is greatly relaxed, or in whom the uterus has "fallen," cannot use a diaphragm successfully.

Side Effects   No serious side effects. Possible allergic reaction to the rubber or the spermicidal jelly. Condition easily corrected.

Health Factors to Consider   None.

Long-Term Effect on Ability to Have Children   None.

RHYTHM METHOD

The woman must refrain from sexual intercourse on days surrounding the predicted time of monthly ovulation or, for a higher degree of effectiveness, until a few days after the predicted time of ovulation. Ways to determine the approximate time of ovulation include a calendar method, a method based on body temperature, and a mucus method. Using the calendar method requires careful recordkeeping of the time of the menstrual period, and calculation of the time in the month when the woman is fertile and must not have intercourse. To use the temperature method, the woman must use a special type of thermometer and keep an accurate daily record of her body temperature (body temperature rises after ovulation). To use the mucus method the woman must keep an accurate daily record of the type of vaginal secretions present. The temperature method and the mucus method used alone or concurrently with the calendar method are more effective than the calendar method alone.

Effectiveness   Effectiveness depends on how correctly the method is used. Of 100 women who use the calendar method for one year, 14 to 47 will become pregnant. Of 100 women who use the temperature method for one year, 1 to 20 will become pregnant. Of 100 women who use the mucus method for one year, 1 to 25 will become pregnant. Of 100 women who use for one year the temperature or mucus method with intercourse only after ovulation, less than 1 to 7 will become pregnant.

Advantages   No drugs or devices needed.

Disadvantages   Requires careful record keeping and estimation of the time each month when there can be no intercourse. To use any of the three methods properly a physician's guidance may be needed, at least at the outset. If menstrual cycles are irregular, it is especially difficult to use this method effectively. Dissatisfaction because of extended time each month when sexual intercourse must be avoided.

Side Effects   No physical effects, but because the couple must refrain from having intercourse except on certain days of the month, using this method can create pressures on the couple's relationship.

Health Factors to Consider   None.

Long-Term Effect on Ability to Have Children   None.

WITHDRAWAL (COITUS INTERRUPTUS)

This method of contraception requires withdrawal of the male organ (penis) from the vagina before the man ejaculates so the male sperm are not deposited at or near the birth canal. The failure rate with this method is high and it should not be considered effective for preventing pregnancy.

FEMALE STERILIZATION

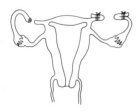

The primary method of sterilization for women is tubal sterilization, commonly referred to as "tying the tubes." A surgeon cuts, ties, or seals the Fallopian tubes to prevent passage of eggs between the ovaries and the uterus. Several techniques are available. With one new technique the operation can be performed in a hospital out-patient surgical clinic with either a local or general anesthetic. Using this method, the doctor makes a tiny incision in the abdomen or vagina and blocks the tubes by cutting, sealing with an electric current, or applying a small band or clip. Hysterectomy, a surgical procedure involving removal of all or part of the uterus, also prevents pregnancy, but is performed for other medical reasons and is not considered primarily a method of sterilization.

Effectiveness   Virtually 100 percent.

Advantages   A one-time procedure—never any more bother with devices or preparations of any kind.

Disadvantages   Surgery is required. Although in some cases a sterilization procedure has been reversed through surgery, the procedure should be considered permanent.

Side Effects   As with any surgery, occasionally there are complications such as severe bleeding, infection, or injury to other organs which may require additional surgery to correct.

Health Factors to Consider   There is some risk associated with any surgical procedure, which varies with the general health of the patient.

Long-Term Effect on Ability to Have Children   Procedure should be considered nonreversible. Once the surgery is performed successfully, the woman cannot become pregnant. There have been exceptions, but they are very uncommon.

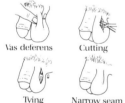

Vas deferens   Cutting

Tying   Narrow seam

MALE STERILIZATION

Sterilization of men involves severing the tubes through which the sperm travel to become part of the semen. The man continues to produce sperm but they are absorbed by the body rather than being released into the semen. This operation, called a vasectomy, takes about half an hour and may be performed in a doctor's office under local anesthetic. A vasectomy does not affect a man's physical ability to have intercourse.

Effectiveness   Virtually 100 percent.

Advantages   A one-time procedure that does not require hospitalization and permits the man to resume normal activity almost immediately.

Disadvantages   Although in some cases a vasectomy may be reversed, it should be considered permanent. The man is not sterile immediately after the operation—usually it takes a few months. Other means of contraception must be used during that time.

Side Effects   Complications occur in 2 to 4 percent of cases, including infection, hematoma (trapped mass of clotted blood), granuloma (an inflammatory reaction to sperm that is absorbed by the body), and swelling and tenderness near the testes. Most such complications are minor and are treatable without surgery. Studies by the National Institutes of Health show that vasectomy does not affect a man's sexual desire or ability.

Health Factors to Consider   None.

Long-Term Effect on Ability to Have Children   Procedure is considered nonreversible. Once surgery is performed successfully, the man cannot father children. There have been exceptions, but they are very uncommon.

Summary

A gland is a cell, a tissue, or an organ that produces a chemical substance that is either used elsewhere in the body or that is eliminated from the body. *Exocrine glands* secrete their chemicals into *ducts; endocrine glands* secrete their products, *hormones*, directly into the bloodstream. Several of the endocrine glands influence reproduction.

The visible parts of the male reproductive system are the penis and the scrotum. The head of the penis, or glans, and the rim, or crown, are very sensitive to touch. In uncircumcised males, a prepuce or foreskin covers the glans. Along the length of the penis runs the urethra, through which both urine and semen can pass (though at different times). A spinal nerve reflex causes the blood volume in the penis to increase, resulting in erection. Held by the scrotum are the testes, where spermatozoa develop in seminiferous tubules and testosterone is produced. A testis and an attached duct called the epididymis make up a testicle. Spermatozoa travel through the epididymis to the vas deferens, where they are stored. During ejaculation, contractions force the spermatozoa and the contents of the seminal vesicle into the ejaculatory duct, and then into the urethra. The prostate gland adds a milky-white fluid to the semen.

In the female reproductive system, the ovaries produce mature ova and female hormones. From birth, the ovaries contain about 200,000 tiny sacs, or follicles, and within each of these is a primordial sex cell, or oogonium. At puberty, a woman begins a monthly cycle during which some oogonia ripen into mature ova. This process is initiated by hormones in the hypothalamus that stimulate the production and release of an anterior pituitary hormone called follicle-stimulating hormone (FSH). Several follicles within the uterus mature into Graafian follicles. These produce the hormone estrogen, which begins to prepare the uterus for implantation of a fertilized ovum. Now the FSH is joined by another anterior pituitary hormone, luteinizing hormone (LH), to cause the final maturation of usually only one follicle and ovum (the others disintegrate). The follicle ruptures to release its ovum, a process known as ovulation. This ovum is gathered by fingerlike projections, or fimbria, into the Fallopian tubes. The follicle from which the ovum burst now becomes a corpus luteum, producing the hormone progesterone, which further prepares the uterine endometrium for a fertilized ovum. If the ovum is fertilized, it will begin to develop and become implanted in the prepared uterus. The embryonic membranes will produce gonadotropic hormone, which causes the corpus luteum to continue producing progesterone. If fertilization does not occur, the ovum and the corpus luteum degenerate. As the progesterone supply diminishes, the uterine endometrium sloughs off in the process of menstruation. This process will be repeated monthly until the cessation of menstruation, or menopause, which occurs at the average age of forty-nine.

The vagina receives the penis during sexual intercourse. In the virgin, the vaginal entrance may be blocked by a fold of skin, the hymen. The vagina is normally acidic. The external genitalia include the mons pubis, the labia majora, the vestibule, the labia minora, and the clitoris. Except for the labia majora, all of these are sexually sensitive, as is the opening of the vagina. Lubrication to ease the passage of the penis is provided by the vagina and the Bartholin's glands.

On the surface of the mammary glands is the nipple, which has small openings, and the surrounding pigmented areola. Each breast is composed of tubular glands, or lobes, embedded in tissue and fat. During pregnancy, colostrum, and later milk, that is produced in the lobes drains into the nipple's lactiferous duct.

Since human reproduction has not been effectively controlled, and since the death rate (which once balanced out the birthrate) has been declining, overpopulation has been the result. Though there has been a recent decline in the birthrate, a built-in momentum is causing exponential growth of the population. This growth has dramatically increased in modern times due to scientific advancements that have allowed people to fight sickness and premature death. But now hundreds of millions of people are malnourished, overcrowded, and inadequately housed. An intensive program to educate the world's people to the necessities of family planning and the use of birth control is desperately needed.

Birth control may or may not involve the use of a *contraceptive*. There are three types of contraceptives: hormonal, mechanical, and chemical (nonhormonal). In addition, conception may be prevented by surgery.

The hormonal oral contraceptives (birth control pills) slightly change the woman's normal hormone levels to prevent ovulation. They are almost 100 percent effective and do not interfere with lovemaking. There are many brands of pills, with different combinations of progesterone and estrogen that may be more acceptable to individual women in terms of the side effects that result. Among the side effects of oral contraceptives are blood clotting that can result in strokes, myocardial infarctions (particularly among older women and smokers), liver tumors, high blood pressure, gallbladder disease, and urinary and vaginal infections. The pill must be used under the close supervision of a doctor.

Diethylstilbesterol (DES) is an estrogen used as a contraceptive following intercourse. Its use requires careful counseling. If it fails to prevent pregnancy, it may cause abnormalities or an increased risk of cancer in the offspring.

Douches are completely ineffective as a contraceptive measure. Several chemical nonhormonal contraceptives can be used, though they are often difficult to use correctly and have a high rate of failure. These include vaginal foams, jellies and creams, suppositories, and tablets.

There are three mechanical contraceptives that have a very high rate of success when properly used. The condom is a sheath made of rubber or animal skin that fits over the erect penis, preventing spermatozoa from entering the vagina. Intrauterine devices, or IUDs, are plastic objects that are inserted into the uterus. It is not known exactly how they prevent pregnancy. The diaphragm is a rubber dome that fits over the cervix as a barrier to spermatozoa. It must be used with a spermatocide.

The rhythm methods of birth control are the only forms approved by the Roman Catholic Church. They can be practiced either by computing the safe, nonfertile period of the woman's cycle or by taking the temperature to determine the time of ovulation. (Ovulation is accompanied by a slight increase in body temperature.) These methods require a year of accurate record-keeping before they can be used with any success. The irregularity of most menstrual cycles and the long periods of abstinence required each month result in very high rates of failure.

Two very effective surgical methods exist to prevent pregnancy. In the male, the vas deferens is cut and tied in a simple operation known as a vasectomy. This prevents spermatozoa from entering the ejaculate, but it has no effect on sexual performance. The operation should be considered permanent. In the woman, tubal ligation is used to prevent the egg from reaching the uterus. This operation can possibly be reversed.

The controversial choice of abortion is used as a "back-up" when a contraceptive fails or when none at all was used. The most common legal methods of inducing abortion are (1) vacuum aspiration, used during the first three months of pregnancy; (2) dilatation and curettage (D and C), used to about the ninth week of pregnancy; and (3) saline injection into the amniotic sac, preferred for the sixteenth to twentieth week of pregnancy.

References

1. Adapted from a quotation by Malcolm K. Jeffrey, in Laurence J. Peter, *Peter's Quotations* (New York, 1977), p. 363.
2. "The Gentle Squeeze That Sent You on Your Way," *New Scientist*, Vol. 53 (February 17, 1972).
3. *The New York Times* (January 16, 1966), Section 1, p. 8.
4. Carl E. Taylor, "Crosscurrents of Opinion," *Medical Tribune* (December 18–19, 1965), p. 7.
5. Arthur Haupt, "Births, Deaths, and Population Changes of the Third Kind: Migration to Outer Space," Intercom, Vol. 6 (August 1978), p. 6.
6. Ibid.
7. Kitaoka Juitso, "How Japan Halved Her Birth Rate in Ten Years," in *The Sixth International Conference on Planned Parenthood* (London, 1959), pp. 27–36.
8. See, for example, Leviticus 18:21; Deuteronomy 12:31; II Kings 3:27, 16:3; II Chronicles 28:3, 33:6; Psalms 106:38; Isaiah 57:5; Jeremiah 19:5; and Ezekiel 16:21.
9. Charles F. Westhoff and Larry Bumpass, "The Revolution in Birth Control Practices of U.S. Roman Catholics," *Science*, Vol. 179 (January 5, 1973), p. 44.
10. Charles F. Westhoff and Elsie F. Jones, "The Secularization of U.S. Catholic Birth Control Practices," *Family Planning Perspectives*, Vol. 9 (October 1977).
11. Christopher Tretze, "The Pill and Mortality from Cardiovascular Disease: Another Look," *Family Planning Perspectives*, Vol. 11 (March–April 1979), pp. 80–84.
12. Mark A. Belsey, Yvonne Russell, and Kay Kinnear, "Cardiovascular Disease and Oral Contraceptives: A Reappraisal of Vital Statistics Data," *Family Planning Perspectives*, Vol. 11 (March–April 1979), pp. 84–89.
13. "HEW Recommends Follow-up on DES Patients," *FDA Drug Bulletin*, Vol. 8 (October 1978), p. 31.
14. E. James Lieberman, "Teenage Sex and Birth Control," *Journal of the American Medical Association*, Vol. 240 (July 21, 1978), p. 275, citing M. Zelnik and J. F. Kantner, "Sexual and Contraceptive Experience of Young Married Women in the U.S., 1976 and 1971," *Family Planning Perspectives*, Vol. 9 (1977), pp. 55–65.
15. U.S. Department of Health, Education, and Welfare, Public Health Service, Center for Disease Control, *Abortion Surveillance 1976* (August 1978), p. 12.
16. Herant A. Katchadourian and Donald T. Lunde, *Fundamentals of Human Sexuality*, 2nd ed. (New York, 1975), p. 552.

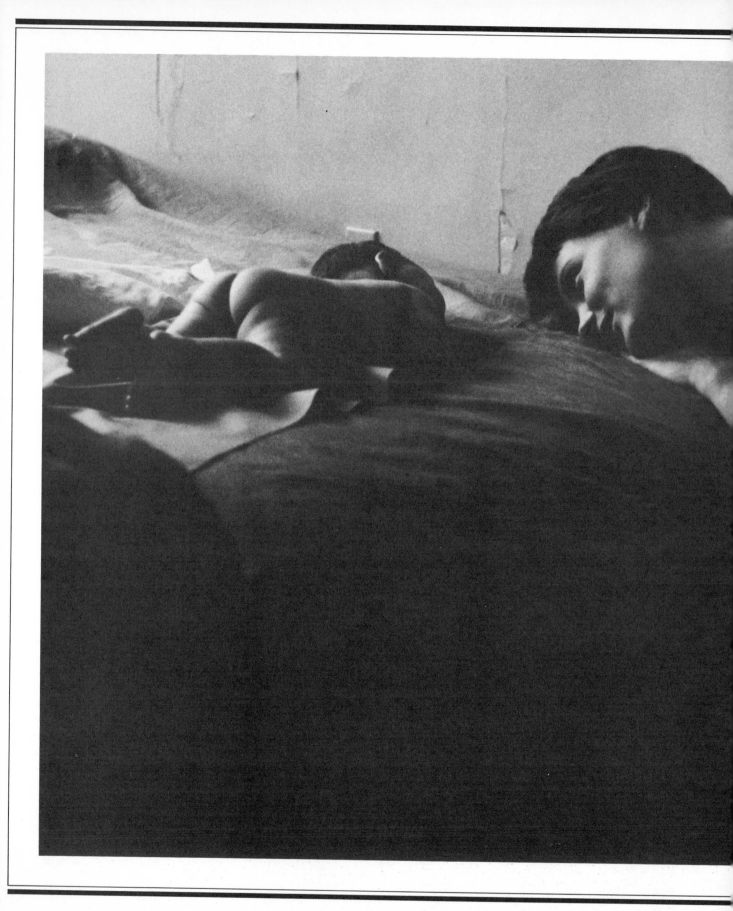

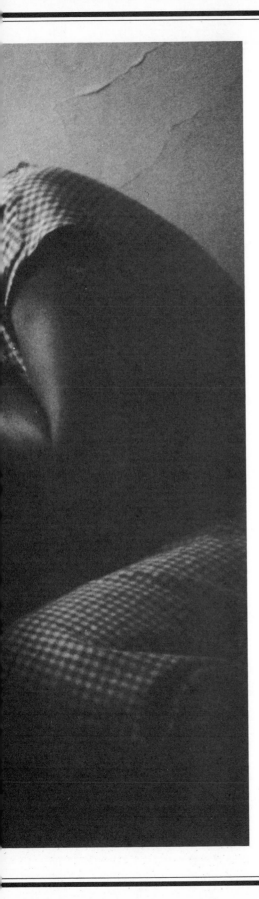

13
Human Beginnings: Part I

Pregnancy: A Process

Now is that sweet unwritten moment when all things are possible, are just begun.[1]

The ovum is one of the body's largest cells; the sperm, the smallest. Alone, they are just potential. Together, they can fuse, and the product of their fusion can multiply to form a creature that can wonder. But even in the earliest phases this product is already remarkable. "Every child starts as an invisible unit with a weight of only 5/1000 of a milligram and gains during the first weeks of life more than a million percent in weight. Which industry, whatever direction or planning boards there may be, can claim such an increase in output?"[2]

The Duration of Pregnancy

Counting from the time of fertilization of the egg by the sperm (*conception*), the duration of the pregnancy is 9½ lunar months (38 weeks, or 266 days). A "lunar" month is 28 days because there is a full moon every 28 days. Counting from the first day of the last menstrual period, the average pregnancy lasts 10 lunar months (40 weeks, or 280 days).

In calculating the expected date of birth, three months are subtracted from the date of the beginning of the last normal menstrual period. Then seven days are added. For example, if the first day of the last normal period was June 17, the expected date of birth would be March 24.

But these calculations are only based on averages. Perhaps 10 percent of all pregnancies end 280 days after the beginning of the last menstrual period; less than 50 percent end within one week of the 280th day. The time required for the fetus in the uterus is individual. Extreme but normal variances of 240 days to 300 days in the uterus occur. The calculated expected date of birth is not often exact. There is less than a 50 percent chance that the child will be born within a week of that date and a 10 percent chance that labor will occur about two weeks later.

The Child Within the Uterus

Before pregnancy the uterus weighs one ounce. At the end of pregnancy, the empty uterus weighs 2.2 pounds and its capacity has increased more than five hundred times. (A short time after delivery, it returns to almost its original size.) The remarkable events occurring during the development of the child in the uterus are described in the science of *embryology*—the study of the development of a new creature.

THE FIRM ESTABLISHMENT OF THE NEW LIFE

As was pointed out on page 358, the new individual begins as a fertilized egg—a *zygote*. This tiny life, no larger than a speck of sand, does not wait long in the Fallopian tube. While on its two-to-four-day, four-to-five-inch journey to the uterus, the zygote divides daily. When the minute mass of cells arrives in the uterus, the lining of that organ is not ready for it. About two to four days pass as the small, continuously

388   CHAPTER THIRTEEN ▪ HUMAN BEGINNINGS: PART I

multiplying cell mass floats in the uterus. As it does so it soaks up nourishing fluid that is in that organ. Meanwhile, the uterine lining continues to prepare for the new life.

At last, as much as ten or eleven days after fertilization, the little cell mass, now called an **embryo**, becomes embedded in the uterine lining (or **endometrium**). During these beginning days of attachment, nourishment seeps from the mother's blood to the developing cells. The process by which the embryo becomes embedded in the lining of the uterus is known as *implantation*. Should implantation fail to occur, there would be menstruation. However, if the embryo remains embedded and continues to develop for two months, it will be known as a **fetus**.

TWINS

Sometimes two ova instead of one leave the ovaries to be fertilized by separate spermatozoa. During the pregnancy they develop at the same time. Such twins are born no more or less alike than ordinary brothers and sisters. They are improperly called **fraternal twins** (brother relationship), although both may be girls. A more appropriate term would be *biovular* (developed from two fertilized ova) or *dizygotic* (developed from two zygotes) twins.

Identical twins develop from one fertilized ovum and are, of course, the same gender. The embryo is the stage of development lasting from fertilization of the ovum to the end of the eighth week of pregnancy. What happens is that early in embryonic cellular division, before the cells have become differentiated into what tissues they will become (perhaps by about the tenth day after fertilization), the cellular mass splits in half. Nobody knows why. The two separate cellular masses then go on to differentiate and, thus, to become twins. And although they look remarkably similar, because they share all the same hereditary material, they may be different emotionally. This difference is the result of the powerful influence of the environment. Twins occur more commonly among black people in the United States (one birth in about seventy) than among whites (one in about ninety). Only about one-third of all twins are identical. There is a familial tendency to produce dizygotic (fraternal) twins but not identical twins. Again, nobody knows why.

NOURISHING THE UNBORN BABY

Not all of the zygote, or fertilized egg, becomes an embryo. Some of the dividing cells become nonembryonic structures. Almost all of these accessory additional structures are designed to support the life of the unborn child. Among these is the **placenta,** or **afterbirth**. It begins to develop shortly after implantation. One side of the placenta becomes deeply attached to the inner lining of the mother's uterus. In fact, cells from the lining contribute to that side of the placenta. The other side of the placenta will be connected to the developing baby by means of a cablelike **umbilical cord**. Within the umbilical cord are two arteries and one vein. Through these vessels, oxygen and nourishment are brought to the unborn child from the mother's blood, and the baby's wastes are carried away to the mother's blood. The mother then rids herself of her baby's wastes in the same way she gets rid of her own. At no time during the pregnancy will there normally be a

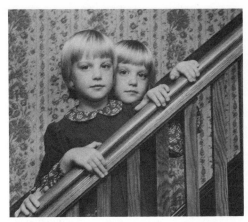

Identical twins.

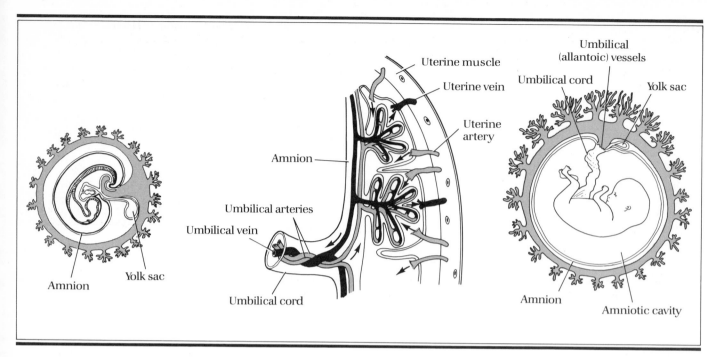

Uterine muscle

Uterine vein

Uterine artery

Umbilical (allantoic) vessels

Umbilical cord

Yolk sac

Amnion

Umbilical arteries

Umbilical vein

Umbilical cord

Amnion

Yolk sac

Amnion

Amniotic cavity

FIGURE 13–1
The development of human embryonic membranes. Two stages of embryonic development are shown. The drawings at left and right depict the interrelationship of the embryo and membranes; at center is a cross section of the placenta.

direct connection between the blood of the mother and the fetus.

The placenta is delivered shortly after the baby is born. Since it does not remain in the body, it is but a temporary organ. Nevertheless, it has another function aside from bringing oxygen and food to the baby and removing wastes. The placenta also produces chemical substances—hormones—that help maintain the pregnancy. For this reason the placenta must also be thought of as a gland.

The Amnion

Aside from the placenta, other non-embryonic equipment is also formed (see Figure 13–1). One of these is a sac—the **amnion**. At the age of about two weeks the embryo is tucked beneath the surface of the uterine lining. A hollow beneath the embryo enlarges to become a fluid-filled cavity. This cavity becomes surrounded by the amnion. The

amniotic sac is filled with **amniotic fluid**. By the fifth month the fetus is swallowing some amniotic fluid.

As long as the fetus remains within the amniotic sac in the uterus, it lives the watery life of a fish. Like an astronaut in a space capsule, the fetus within the amniotic sac is in a state of weightlessness. Therefore, the child is able to move about without expending energy that is needed for growth and development. In addition, the fluid protects the delicate tissues and provides a stable temperature for the child. When the time for birth is reached, the amnion is of some help in dilating the cervix. This happens during the early stage of labor. Usually the amniotic sac ruptures during labor. If this does not happen the doctor will rupture the membranes of the amniotic sac. This enables the baby to breathe immediately at birth.

Let's consider now the month-by-month changes that take place in the human being during its residence in the uterus.

Stages
of Fetal Development

END OF THE FIRST
LUNAR MONTH

About twenty-eight days after conception, the embryo is about one-quarter of an inch long (about the size of a pea) and resembles a sea urchin. About one-third of the embryo is the head, which almost touches the tail. The bulging, beating heart propels blood through primitive vessels. From a developing mouth leads a tube that will become the digestive tract. The beginnings of eyes, ears, and nose appear, and buds that will become extremities are all visible. Soon the umbilical cord will develop, not as an outgrowth from the baby's body but from accessory tissue.

END OF THE SECOND
LUNAR MONTH

Every week the embryo has grown one-quarter of an inch, and it is now a fetus weighing one-thirtieth of an ounce. Sex organs are apparent, but the sex of the fetus is difficult to determine. The developing brain causes the head to be disproportionately large. Pawlike hands have appeared. The half-closed eyes will soon close completely; they remain closed until the end of the seventh month. A few muscles are developing, and the feet may kick a few times (but much too feebly to be felt by the mother). The tail begins to get smaller. At the end of two months, almost all the internal organs have begun to develop. The changes now are mostly related to growth and tissue differentiation.

END OF THE THIRD
LUNAR MONTH

The three-inch fetus weighs about an ounce, but the placenta weighs more. The ears rise to the level of the eyes, and the eyelids are fused. Soft nails appear on the stubby fingers and toes. Gender sex can now be determined. From beginning kidneys, small amounts of urine are excreted into the amniotic fluid. Tooth sockets and buds are apparent. Now the mother's enlarging uterus can be felt below the umbilicus.

END OF THE FOURTH
LUNAR MONTH

The four-ounce fetus is not quite seven inches long. On the scalp a few hairs may sprout. Soon there will be a fine, downy, whorled growth of hair called *lanugo* covering the whole body. The mother may feel the first subtle movements of the fetus (*quickening*) at the end of this period. Usually, however, these do not occur until the following month.

END OF THE FIFTH
LUNAR MONTH

The ten-inch fetus weighs about eight ounces. The heart can be heard through a stethoscope. The baby moves actively. Later in pregnancy movements may become quite vigorous, but they do not hurt. Since the lungs are not sufficiently developed, babies born prematurely at this time do not survive; they may live but a few minutes.

END OF THE SIXTH
LUNAR MONTH

Now the fetus weighs a pound and one-half and is about a foot

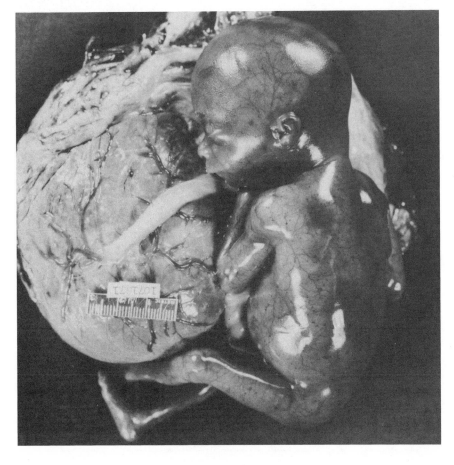

Human fetus at five months.

PHOTO ESSAY
The development of a human.

1. **Human blastocyst sixty hours after conception.**
2. **Human blastocyst four days after conception.**
3. **Human embryo at twenty-two days.**
4. **Human embryo at six weeks.**
5. **Human embryo at eight weeks.**
6. **Human fetus at twelve weeks.**

4.
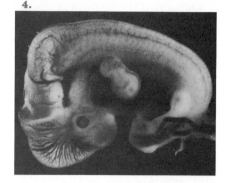

5.
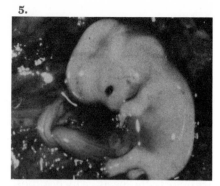

1.
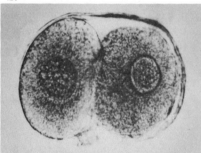

2.
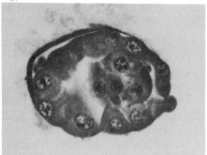

3.
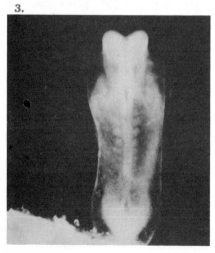

6.
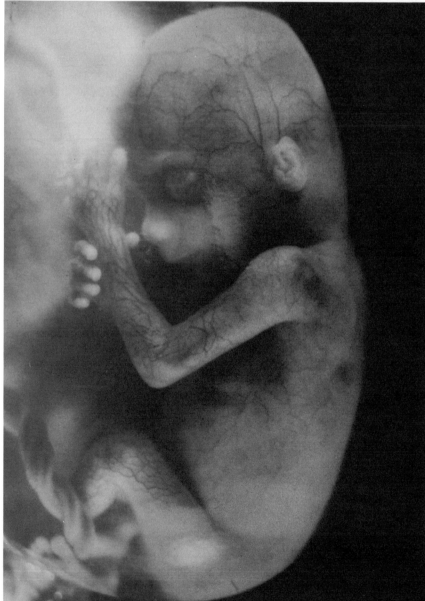

long. The fetus is not idle, sucking an available thumb, swallowing amniotic fluid, exercising developing muscles, even managing an occasional spasmodic chest movement. Noise startles the child in the uterus. When the mother rocks, the child may go to sleep. The child's activity may waken the mother. Intrauterine quarters are crowded, and some children are more restless than others. The skin glands and cells that are shed from the wrinkled skin combine to provide a protective *vernix caseosa*, or "cheesy varnish." At birth this may be one-eighth of an inch thick. At the end of this month, the eyelids separate and eyelashes form. If born at this stage, the child is still too undeveloped to survive.

END OF THE SEVENTH LUNAR MONTH

The two-and-one-half-pound fetus is about fifteen inches long. The eyes are open, and if the child were born at this time, seeing light would be possible. In the male fetus the testicles are usually in the scrotum. Fat begins to flatten out a few wrinkles. Every day in the uterus at this stage is vital. A baby born at this time has only a fair chance of survival because the lungs and intestinal canal are incompletely developed.

END OF THE EIGHTH LUNAR MONTH

The fetus now weighs about four pounds and measures some sixteen and one-half inches. The bones of the head are soft. The fetus looks like a little old man. If provided with good nursing and medical care, a baby born now has a much better chance of surviving than one born in the previous month.

END OF THE NINTH LUNAR MONTH

The fetus, weighing about six pounds and measuring about nineteen inches, begins to make ready to leave the weightless watery ecosystem within the uterus. As if to prepare for the new environment, the fetus gains half a pound a week and wrinkles now disappear. The fingernails need cutting, and the fetus may be born with harmless scratch marks. If born prematurely during this month, the chances for survival are good.

THE TENTH LUNAR MONTH

By about the middle of the tenth lunar month, the full-term twenty-inch fetus is born, weighing about seven pounds (girls) or about seven and one-half pounds (boys). The umbilical cord is about as long as the baby. The placenta weighs about one and one-quarter pounds; it is a disc that is about six to eight inches in diameter. There is from one-half to two quarts of amniotic fluid. Most of the lanugo is gone, although some may remain about the shoulders. The vernix caseosa remains and has to be wiped away. The hormones that cause the mother's breasts to enlarge cause the unborn child's breasts to protrude a little. The newborn may secrete milk ("witch's milk"). Within a few days after birth, the breast enlargement subsides, and there is no further secretion of milk. The final hue of the slate-colored eyes cannot be predicted.

The Mother

Some pregnant women eagerly await a first child. Many others want a baby, but not at the moment. Some feel a trifle taken in by their pregnancy. Frequently, a first-time mother may need time to accept the idea. She has about three months to do so. During that time, she weighs herself often, but the scales say little. Her pregnancy is not very real. Nothing much changes.

In the second three months, she grows, and not just physically. The emotional preparations may be more profound than the physical ones.

For many women, the last three months of pregnancy drag. A dozen discomforts plague her. This ordeal, she thinks, will be capped by still another. She may wish to be rid of her pregnancy. Yet, she may fear its end. She is weary of glossy magazine pictures of overjoyed women hurrying to the hospital without a care in the world. She wishes she could control her urinary bladder better. And she may worry that her husband, too, is tiring of her pregnant condition.

During pregnancy, some women (not all) are somewhat less interested in sexual intercourse. The sensitive husband will understand that his wife's pregnancy profoundly affects her emotional state and will not feel rejected. It is here that his responsibility is so considerable. As never before, she needs his love, patience, and confidence.

NUTRITION DURING PREGNANCY: CHANGED CONCEPTS

Pregnant women are often confused by a barrage of conflicting advice about their nutrition. Some of this conflict is the result of the changed opinions on the part of experts in the field who, through careful research and years of experience, have developed new concepts about the subject.[3]

It is known that the weight of the newborn child is the most important single factor affecting his or her health. And the basic influences deciding the newborn's weight are the length of the mother's pregnancy, the mother's weight before pregnancy, and her weight gain during pregnancy. It used to be thought that if a mother gained too much weight she was more likely to develop *toxemia of pregnancy*, a serious and rare disorder marked by swelling of body tissues and increased blood pressure. Rarely, toxemia can lead to the more serious and fortunately even more rare *eclampsia*, which may be accompanied by coma, convulsions, kidney failure, and even death. Nowadays most specialists no longer believe that the toxemia of pregnancy or eclampsia are caused by a marked increase in weight. On the contrary, it now seems that *restriction* of weight gain during pregnancy is more dangerous than gaining too much weight. A woman of normal weight should gain at least twenty-two to twenty-six pounds during pregnancy, with most of this gain occurring during the last six months. Obese pregnant women may not need to gain quite as much; however, they should not be on a reducing diet during pregnancy.

Other changes in the physician's nutritional advice to pregnant women include a reversal of the earlier admonitions to restrict salt intake and to use vitamin supplements. There is no proof that toxemia of pregnancy is caused by a normal or even a high intake of salt. Most pregnant women normally experience some excessive fluid in the tissue (*edema*) and retain somewhat more sodium than in the nonpregnant state. Moreover, women who eat an adequate diet do not need calcium supplementation. Also, the

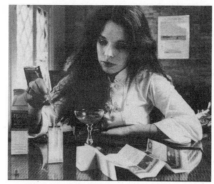

Home pregnancy tests. Manufacturers' claims for accuracy vary. Most state that if the result is positive, accuracy is over 95 percent, and if the result is negative, accuracy is about 80 percent.

use of vitamins must be under the physician's control. Enough vitamin A is found in a diet rich in green or yellow vegetables. Should a woman take too many vitamin A capsules she may give birth to a severely damaged child. A pregnant woman will have enough vitamin D if she is adequately exposed to the sunshine of the seasons, or if she drinks four

cups of vitamin-D-fortified whole or skim milk daily. But too much vitamin D can cause serious abnormalities in the child. During pregnancy, large doses of vitamin C should be particularly avoided. Why? Because such doses condition the unborn child to a high vitamin C environment. Then, as a newborn, scurvy may result. The vitamin folic acid should be added to the diet as a supplement during pregnancy, as should iron. Table 13–1 provides a recommended daily food guide for pregnant, nonpregnant, and breast-feeding women.

ABOUT SOME CHANGES, PREGNANCY TESTS, AND RULES

A regularly menstruating woman's first, and most common, sign of pregnancy is a missed menstrual period. In addition, the breasts are sensitive, and the nipples become enlarged and pigmented. More than one-half of all pregnant women ex-

	DAILY SERVINGS[1]		
FOOD GROUP	Nonpregnant	Pregnant	Breast Feeding
Protein Foods	4	4	4
Milk and Milk Products	2	4	5
Breads and Cereals	4	4	4
Vitamin C Rich Fruits and Vegetables	1	1	1
Dark Green Vegetables	1	1	1
Other Fruits and Vegetables	1	1	1

TABLE 13–1
Daily Food Guide

1. See Figure 9–2 on page 271 for examples of the size of a serving of representative foods from within each food group. For example, one slice of bread constitutes one serving from the bread and cereal group.

SOURCE: California Department of Health Services, Maternal and Child Health, "Eating Right for Your Baby," Nutrition for Pregnancy and Breast Feeding series.

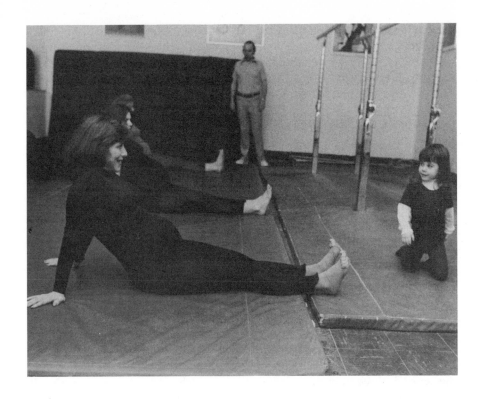

It is not too early for the little girl to share with her pregnant mother the benefits of good exercise habits.

perience nausea. Vomiting is infrequent. This is not necessarily "morning sickness." It may occur at any time of the day. It may hardly occur at all. It is much less frequent than formerly. Serious vomiting during pregnancy rarely occurs anymore.

Within days after the first missed menstrual period, laboratory tests indicating pregnancy are over 95 percent accurate. Injection of urine into immature female mice or rabbits that causes ovarian changes in these animals is no longer used. With a male frog, the hormone causes spermatozoa to occur in the urine. Other such biological pregnancy tests are constantly under study. Several nonanimal chemical tests are also being used to diagnose pregnancy. One of these involves an antigen-antibody reaction. The urine hormones are the antigen; these react with a prepared antibody. When performed by properly trained technicians, this test is

highly accurate about two weeks after a missed menstrual period. A third kind of test requires giving progesterone to a woman who has missed a menstrual period. If the woman is not pregnant, a normal menstruation usually begins in four to five days. Recently developed is a test capable of determining twins born as a result of sexual intercourse with two different fathers.[4] This is the result of "the fertilization in one woman of two separate ova within a short time as a result of separate coital [sexual intercourse] acts. . . ."[5] This test is important in that it establishes paternity (fatherhood).

Pregnancy also has some cosmetic effects. Skin blemishes often disappear. The complexion glows. But pink stretch marks (*striae*) may appear, mostly on the abdomen. Neither massage nor costly oils prevent them. Most (but not all) will disappear. There also may be, temporarily, increased pigment on the abdominal midline, around the

nipples, and on the face. The breasts fill. By three months, *colostrum*, the precursor to milk, is secreted.

Pregnant women with good eating and exercising habits, and who continue these habits under a physician's direction during and after pregnancy, have the best chance of keeping their figures. Walking is also good. During the first four months, women who play golf may continue doing so. Swimming may be permitted in the early months. Some physicians also allow swimming in later months. However, surf bathing, horseback riding, and tennis are not advisable because they involve bumping and compression. Long trips should be avoided unless absolutely necessary. Nonfatiguing employment is acceptable. In considering the amount and kind of activity that is best for the patient, the physician always considers the individual. Some pregnant women seem able to do more than others. One recent Olympic swimmer was not much handicapped by her three-and-one-half-month pregnancy; she placed third in her class. It has been reported that of the twenty-six female Soviet Olympic champions of the Sixteenth Olympiad, in Melbourne, Australia, ten were pregnant.[6]

Extra rest is essential. Although showers are preferable in the last month, a daily tepid bath adds to comfort. It is not true that bath water enters the vagina or that vaginal secretions contaminate bath water. Thus, the fear that bath water may infect a pregnant woman is a myth. The teeth, although more vulnerable, are not demineralized. "For every pregnancy a tooth" is an untrue old wives' tale. The kidneys need special attention. The doctor will examine the urine often. Constipation may be relieved by fruits and vegetables; prunes, dates, and figs help.

Prenatal Care

Two or three weeks after the first missed period, a doctor should be consulted. This marks the beginning of a relationship that, as much as any other single factor, has made pregnancy so safe. Compared with just a generation ago, decreased maternal (and infant) mortality rates in this country have been spectacular.

The pregnant woman must visit her doctor regularly. This *prenatal* (before birth) *care* is essential to her well-being. The whole complex of physical examinations—laboratory examination of the blood (for syphilis, blood types, Rh factor, and anemia), urine tests, and more—create a constancy of communication between patient and doctor that has brought security to mother and child. Problems can be pre-

vented. If trouble threatens, the doctor is better prepared to avert it.

Unless special problems arise, visits to the doctor are scheduled every three or four weeks during the first six months. In the next two months, these are usually increased to every two or three weeks. Visits after six months are usually weekly.

SEXUAL INTERCOURSE DURING PREGNANCY[7]

As has been noted, some women respond to the complex physical, hormonal, and psychological changes of pregnancy with a decreased desire for sexual activity. Some, on the other hand, experience an increased desire for sexual activity. There are women whose sexual desire increases particularly during the second three months of their pregnancies. During the last three months, sexual interest may wane. (The same may be true of husbands.) An increasing number of physicians permit their pregnant patients who have no complications to have sexual intercourse throughout the entire period of pregnancy, up to the time of the rupture of the membranes. However, not all cases are alike, and there are valid reasons for exceptions. The decision must be made by each physician on an individual basis. Three potential hazards are of concern to the physician: uterine contractions, infection, and mechanical injury.[8] Let's consider these separately.

Some physicians are legitimately concerned that the contractions of the uterus resulting from orgasm might initiate premature labor. Others disagree. They believe that the harm done by forbidding intercourse during the last three months of pregnancy is greater than that done by the unproved risk of uterine contractions resulting from orgasm.

Of course, orgasm resulting from masturbation also causes uterine contractions, and these contractions are often more intense than those resulting from sexual intercourse. Therefore, concern about uterine contractions would also logically indicate the prohibition of masturbation during the last three months of pregnancy.

There is still some concern that sexual intercourse may cause infection. This may occur at the opening of the cervix, in the intact membranes, and—despite the intact membranes—in the amniotic fluid. This last is associated with some fetal damage. The first two are easily treated. Whether intercouse should be avoided during the last three months of pregnancy is a medical decision.

There are times during pregnancy in which sexual intercourse should be avoided. Abdominal or vaginal discomfort or pain is always a reason to avoid coitus during pregnancy and at any other time. These may be due to a vaginal or cervical wound that coincides with the pregnancy; the penis can mechanically interfere with the healing process. (When the discomfort can be relieved by the physician's care, coitus may sometimes be resumed.) Uterine bleeding during pregnancy is also a valid reason to abstain from coitus. In addition, the pregnant woman should avoid all genital play as well as sexual intercourse after the membranes have ruptured. Inattention to this is dangerous. When the membranes are ruptured, the hazard of infection from coitus is greater than at any other time during pregnancy. Infection that occurs from sexual intercourse after the membranes rupture may harm both the mother and the child. There is general agreement among physicians that these three conditions are definite contraindications of sexual intercourse during pregnancy: abdominal or vaginal discomfort, vaginal bleeding, and ruptured membranes. As noted, other hazards also may be defined. These are always the concern of the physician in charge.

It is of importance to note that the fetus is adequately protected in the amniotic sac and that the position of sexual intercourse up to the onset of labor should be determined by the comfort of the husband and wife rather than by fear that the unborn child will be hurt.

Labor

A few days before the onset of true labor, "false labor" may occur. It is the onset of regular, rhythmic contractions that heralds true labor. Discomfort, beginning in the lower abdomen, spreads to the back and thighs. The "bag of water" (amniotic sac) may break. (A "dry birth," or one in which the water breaks before delivery, does not prolong labor. Indeed, it may shorten it.) The "show" is another common sign of early labor. This pink vaginal discharge occurs with the onset of cervical dilation. Most first-time mothers may start for the hospital when contractions occur every ten minutes. Others should pay no attention to timing. When contractions are regular, they should go to the hospital. Long before, several reliable ways of transportation should have been arranged.

The Stages of Labor

There are three stages of labor. The first stage is the longest. The upper part of the uterus contracts. The lower cervix dilates. To allow passage of the infant into the vagina, dilation of the cervix to four inches must be complete. In this stage the baby, assisted by uterine contractions, does the work. Both mother and doctor must await dilation of the cervix and the descent of the baby into the proper position. To minimize the possibility of infection,

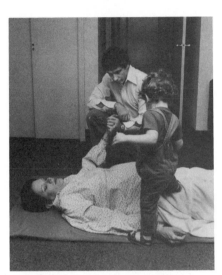

Practicing the Lamaze method should be a family affair, but stepping on mother's abdomen is definitely not a recommended part of the procedure.

the pubic hair may be shaved, and to increase the space in the pelvic cavity, an enema may be given. As the first stage progresses, the uterine contractions become more frequent and of longer duration. When the cervix is fully dilated, the mother is taken from the labor room to the delivery room. If for any reason the fetus cannot do its job, if it cannot adequately act as a wedge, the doctor will perform a **Caesarean section**. By this safe surgical procedure, the infant is removed through an incision in the abdomen and uterus.

It is in the second stage of labor that the mother works. By bearing down only with each contraction, she adds her fifteen pounds of pressure to the twenty-five pound pressure of the uterine contraction. Very occasionally, for special medical reasons, such as a premature baby, the physician will shorten this stage. For the mother who desires to see her baby born, a mirror can be arranged.

After the birth of the baby, the afterbirth (placenta) is delivered. This is the third stage. A drug is then given to further contract the uterus.

Dr. Grantly Dick-Read, an English obstetrician, correctly taught that ignorance breeds fear and fear impedes labor. Although fear is not responsible for all the pain of childbirth, it can cause much of it. The pregnant woman is not helped by those who exaggerate those pains, which, in any case, vary greatly with the individual. Read's concepts of natural childbirth include education plus exercise in relaxation and breathing. All this is commendable. For many couples, there is much in favor of natural childbirth. Not only the mother but also the expectant father may derive considerable psychological benefit from the experience. There is a long overdue, growing awareness of the father's opportunities to participate in the birth experience.

There has been an increasing acceptance of the Lamaze method of

A child is born.

1. A full-term baby, ready to be born.

2. Early first stage. Strong uterine contractions cause the cervix to dilate.

3. Early second stage. Pains every two minutes; membranes rupture; cervix completely dilated; head has begun to extend.

4. End of second stage. Head is born; shoulders have rotated in birth canal.

5. Third stage. Uterus expels placenta and cord.

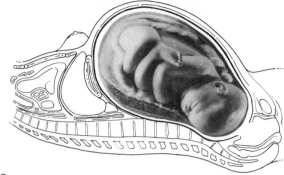

2.

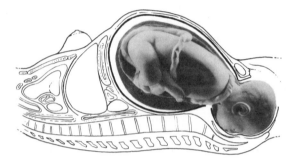

3.

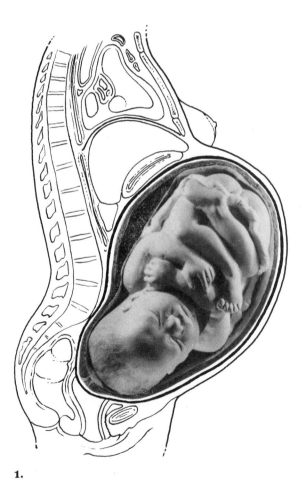

1.

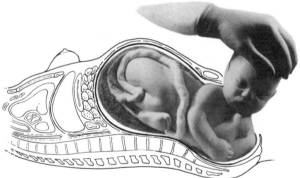

4.

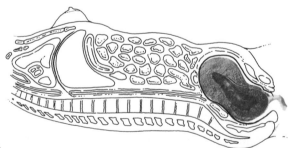

5.

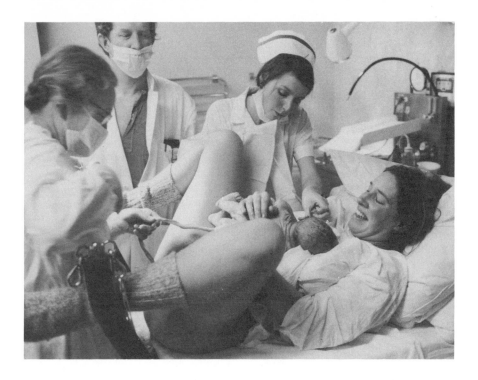

childbirth, commonly referred to as natural childbirth. Both the pregnancy and the actual childbirth process become a family affair. Together, husband and wife attend prenatal classes to learn the facts about pregnancy, labor, and delivery. The mother-to-be is given breathing and muscle exercises that are useful during labor and delivery. The husband is taught to monitor them correctly. The husband is with his wife during labor and in the delivery room, and he puts his knowledge to good use.

With severe pain, drugs may be used judiciously. The decision should be made on individual need by those most competent to make it. The wise use of appropriate drugs prescribed by a properly trained physician is by no means necessarily harmful to the baby.

At the present time a long-term study is being made of the childbirth medical practices in the United States. This study is sup-ported by the National Institutes of Health. Incomplete data suggest that some drugs, such as inhalant anaesthetics, the narcotic Demerol, and possibly other widely used medications may harm the about-to-be-born child. The ability to sit up, hold the head erect, and manipulate a bell, and the child's gait, *may* be among the activities affected. How lasting these and other nervous system effects are remains to be seen.[9]

THE LEBOYER METHOD OF DELIVERING BABIES

It is now thought by many physicians that the trauma of birth to the child can be reduced by creating, as much as possible, an immediate postbirth environment that duplicates the environment within the uterus. In 1975 Frederick Leboyer published his theory on the im-portance of easing the transition from the ecosystem of the uterus to the external environment and his method for accomplishing this.

A small night light replaces the usual ultrabright light of the operating room. (A special source provides light for the working physician.) Those in the delivery room whisper. The umbilical cord is not cut immediately upon delivery; five minutes are allowed so that the newborn continues to receive oxygen until the lungs become accustomed to breathing. The child is laid on the mother's belly and gently massaged. This is intended to duplicate the feeling of warmth within the uterus. After cutting the umbilical cord the physician places the child into a relaxing, warm body-temperature bath. Finally, the child is returned to the warmth of the mother's waiting arms. It is hoped that this gentle and considerate treatment of the newborn is a better introduction to life outside the uterus.

Helping Mothers and High-Risk Babies

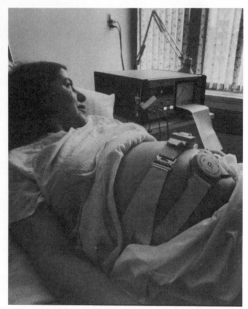

Between contractions, a woman in labor watches the patterns of her baby's heartbeat on a fetal-heart monitor. There is some disagreement that electrofetal monitoring is of any benefit to low-risk babies.

But what am I?
An infant crying in the night:
An infant crying for the light:
And with no language but a cry.
ALFRED LORD TENNYSON
"In Memoriam"

Many changes that benefit both mother and unborn have been introduced into the labor rooms of some hospitals. For example, a pair of belts fitted around the laboring woman's abdomen each contain a small electronic sensor. On a monitor that looks like a small television set, these record the heartbeat of the unborn child during labor and the contractions of the uterus. On the "screen" of the box the professional people caring for the mother can see lines moving up and down across a graph. Watching the relationship between the two lines gives them information about what is happening to the baby. For example, if the cord gets too tightly wound around the neck of the child— a common event—the baby's oxygen supply is jeopardized. Usually this problem is not lasting, but it can persist. If so, the result can be cerebral palsy, a damaged brain resulting in mental retardation, or even a dead baby. Need the mother *always* be rushed to the operating room? No. Sometimes changing the mother's position or giving her oxygen or fluids in a vein may relieve the problem. The parents-to-be should always be told about the monitor before labor so that it does not cause them concern.

Many parents ask about home delivery and whether a mother need always be delivered in a hospital. The answer is that she does. No physician can always predict when a serious emergency will arise during a delivery.

Postnatal Concerns

Before leaving the hospital the mother is examined, and then in six to eight weeks she should be examined again. Of particular interest to the physician are her weight, blood pressure, and the condition of her breasts, uterus, cervix, vagina, and genitalia. She should be advised that her first menstruation may normally be somewhat profuse. Some women are troubled by a vaginal discharge, which is easily treated. The busy mother may forget or defer the examination. This is unwise. She cannot adequately take care of anyone else unless she also takes care of herself.

Mother Love: Not Always at First Sight

It is widely believed that the moment the mother beholds her baby for the first time she feels an immediate love for the child. For many women this is not true. Some mothers apparently love their new babies immediately, but many good mothers do not. During labor the woman usually limits her thoughts to completing the job entailed in the birth process. After the birth many mothers want to see their babies to make certain they are healthy, or simply out of curiosity. A study of fifty-four mothers from the middle and upper socioeconomic levels of Washington, D.C., revealed some interesting information in this regard. Thirty-three percent of the mothers reported having no particular feelings upon seeing their babies for the first time. Seven percent had negative feelings. Fifty-nine percent reported positive feelings that were, nevertheless, quite impersonal. Most of the mothers did not note the beginnings of positive feelings until the third week following childbirth. With the return of her strength, a growing sense of competence, and a reciprocating baby, the mother's attachment to her child grew. By the end of the third month the attachment had become powerful. Although there is no data, it must be assumed that love for the child evolves at least as slowly in the father as in the mother. For most parents, then, mother love and father love grows slowly; it is not mature upon the birth of the baby. Many parents feel a totally unwarranted sense of guilt for not loving their babies immediately.

Sexual Intercourse Following Childbirth

Most women do not desire sexual intercourse for some days following childbirth. This is understandable. The new mother may experience fatigue resulting from delivery. A new baby, moreover, means adjustments for both parents, especially if the child is the first born. During the first month or so following childbirth, the stresses of motherhood may cause the woman to be less interested in coitus. Her desire for sexual intercourse may be further lessened by postpartum depression. The cause of this ordinarily temporary depression is not clear. It may be associated with the

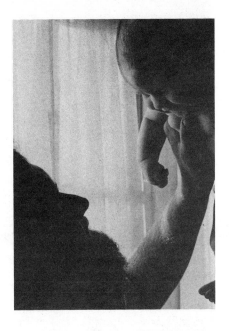

return of the menstrual cycle following pregnancy. A profound series of endocrine gland readjustments occur. It would be surprising if the woman did not experience some emotional changes.

Added to all these new stresses is a certain amount of discomfort about the anus and vagina. Incisions and small tears must heal. There may be some vaginal bleeding. When healing has occurred and the bleeding has stopped, sexual intercourse may be resumed. A small amount of brown vaginal discharge may persist for a while, but this is no reason to defer coitus. After the birth of a baby, a woman usually wants to resume sexual intercourse as soon as possible. There is no reason to discourage her if she is comfortable with it; by that time the bleeding usually has stopped.

Conception During Breast-Feeding

Contrary to popular notions, sexual intercourse during the time a woman is a nursing mother *can* re-

sult in pregnancy. Breast-feeding tends to prolong the period following childbirth during which the woman does not menstruate (*postpartum amenorrhea*). During this period, conception usually will not occur. But the extent of the prolonged amenorrhea and the delayed conception cannot be accurately estimated in individual women. As soon as ovulation occurs, conception can take place, and a woman may ovulate before her first menstrual period following childbirth.

ABOUT BREAST-FEEDING

Pediatrics, the speciality of medicine that deals with children, is organized in North America into two major organizations—the American Academy of Pediatrics (AAP) and the Canadian Paediatric Society (CPS). In a 1978 joint statement, both groups emphasized that mother's milk is best for human infant nutrition. First, mother's milk provides more immunity for the infant. This is important because babies are born with their immune systems not yet fully developed. Thus, the mother's milk provides antibodies that the baby needs. Second, mother's milk is better than cow's milk because it provides superior nutrition. The fats of mother's milk that are so necessary for energy are much more easily absorbed by the baby than are the fats contained in cow's milk. Also, since 50 percent of the iron in human milk is absorbed, breast-fed infants are less likely to lack iron than are babies fed cow's milk. Third, early and long-time contact between mother and infant is healthful. "Bonding" is a sensitive period for the newborn. Contact between mother and child is necessary for the process of bonding.

What can the mother do who is

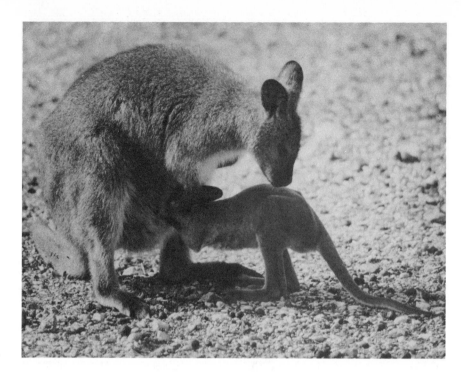

All mammals breast-feed their young.

employed? Although there is some medical opinion that one year of breast-feeding is best, there is also reliable advice that a six months minimum provides an excellent start for the newborn. For the working mother, bottle-fed, hand-expressed milk, refrigerated daily for a period of not longer than twenty-four hours, is the best substitute. All this means a change in the practice of some hospitals. Babies should not be routinely formula-fed to convenience the hospital staff. Breast-feeding requires free access of mother to child, good instruction, and encouragement. Studies indicated that over 95 percent of mothers were able to breast-feed successfully when circumstances were favorable.[10]

There are instances in which breast-feeding should be avoided. Breast infections and drugs that are prescribed for the mother may pass to the child via breast milk and harm the child. In such cases, the production of milk (*lactation*)

should be suppressed. This is accomplished by lessening fluid intake, wearing a breast-binder or well-fitting brassiere, applying ice packs, taking a limited amount of medication to relieve pain, and, sometimes, receiving an injection of a glandular (androgen-estrogen) preparation toward the end of labor or immediately after delivery. A woman who had a spontaneous or therapeutic abortion after the sixteenth week of pregnancy, or whose child was stillborn, will usually require help to suppress lactation.[11]

The Sudden Infant Death Syndrome

Each year, some 25,000 to 30,000 U.S. babies are put to bed at night and unexpectedly found dead in the morning. Typically, the child is between two and four months old (90 percent are between one and nine months; the average age is 2.8 months).[12] The child had previously

been in good health and had given no warning of the tragedy, although there may have been some minor symptoms of an upper respiratory infection. This situation is now known as the Sudden Infant Death Syndrome (SIDS). It is also called "cot death" and "crib death."

The agonized parents ask why this has happened.* Research has proved the following about the SIDS: (1) It is in no way related to the adequacy of parental care and occurs among the best loved and cared-for babies; (2) It is not hereditary; (3) It does not cause the

*Oftentimes, parents mistakenly blame themselves for the sudden death of their child. To increase public education about the problem, the National Foundation for Sudden Infant Death, Inc. (NFSID) was formed. The address of its national headquarters is 1501 Broadway, New York, New York, 10036. Chapter members, themselves SIDS parents, devote many hours talking to and helping other parents learn to cope with the sudden death of their infant. Recent SIDS families are also often referred to professional help. See "The National Foundation for Sudden Infant Death, Inc.," *Clinical Pediatrics*, Vol. 11 (February 1972), p. 83.

afflicted child to suffer; (4) It cannot yet be predicted by the ordinarily watchful parent; (5) It is not caused by vomiting, nor by regurgitating and choking from the last feeding; and (6) It often occurs under conditions in which there is no possibility of smothering.

What, then, causes the Sudden Infant Death Syndrome? Two English scientists have attempted to establish "risk factors." Their studies revealed no less than forty risk factors for sudden infant death. Among these were younger mothers rather than older; mothers whose blood groups were O, B, or AB, rather than A; mothers who had urinary tract infections during pregnancy; babies who were bottle-fed rather than breast-fed; and babies who were born prematurely. Applying these risk factors to some six thousand newborns, the researchers found that those babies with the highest scores tended to die at a rate six times as high as babies with lower scores. They further discovered that their scoring of risk factors could be applied to a program of increased watchfulness that could result in a decreased number of sudden infant deaths. The British researchers believe that newborns with an increased risk of sudden death can be identified at birth and that many such deaths can be prevented by increased watchfulness by doctors beginning at that time.[13] Other research reveals that during normal sleep the infant does not breathe 5 to 10 percent of the time. During a hardly noticeable virus infection the spells during which a child does not breathe may increase to 25 and 30 percent of the time. In addition, it has been shown that the ability of the nervous system to react varies among infants. An immature nervous system to which is added an easily missed viral infection plus the already mentioned numerous risks may well add up to the cause of the Sudden Infant Death Syndrome.

One physician suggests that not all reported crib deaths actually occur in the crib. A considerable number occur in the parents' bed. Smothering occurs when a parent accidentally lies over the child. Such a tragedy was first reported in the Bible by the woman who tells King Solomon that "this woman's child died in the night; because she overlaid it." Today, this accident is called "overlying." "Parents must be informed that to sleep in the same bed with an infant is to invite disaster which is as ancient as the Temple of Solomon."[14]

Hyaline Membrane Disease

This condition of the newborn is marked by breathing difficulties. Within the uterus, the child obtained oxygen via the placenta. At birth, oxygen is obtained through the lungs. This dramatic accomplishment depends partly on the mature development of certain lung cells. Ordinarily, these cells mature adequately shortly before birth. If they do not, the lung air spaces collapse and the immature lung cannot retain air, making each baby breath as difficult as the first gasp. Soon, plasma (the fluid portion of the blood) leaks out into the lung tissue, coating the air spaces. "This glassy pink coating gives respiratory distress in the newborn the name hyaline membrane disease"[15] ("hyaline" is from the Greek word *hyalos*, meaning glass).

Just a few years ago, hyaline membrane disease killed some 25,000 babies in this country every year. Today, intensive care, including assistance in breathing, is saving most of them. Research regarding this condition also promises much success.

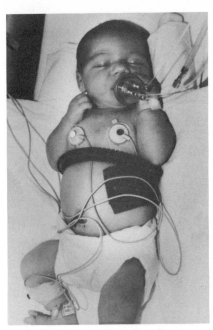

One of the many theories about Sudden Infant Death Syndrome is that the baby has not learned how to cope with respiratory difficulties. In the photograph above, the baby's respiration is being measured by a pneumobelt, the heart rate by electrodes, sucking behavior by an automatic nipple, and general body movements by a stabilimeter (on which the baby is lying). The object of these tests is to learn more about what causes the breathing problems and, eventually, to devise methods for teaching infants how to develop "appropriate defensive behavior."

Subfertility

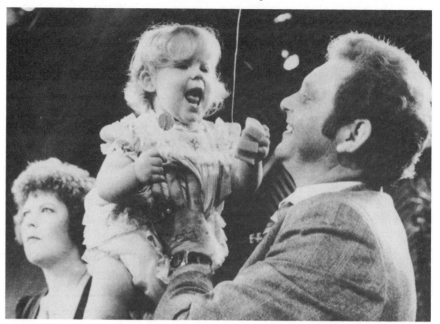

Louise Brown, now almost two years old, was the world's first "test tube" baby. Her father's spermatozoa and her mother's ovum were mixed in a laboratory Petri dish, and the resulting embryo that formed was then inserted into Mrs. Brown's uterus, where it continued to develop normally. This method of artificial insemination may turn out to be a solution to certain cases of infertility.

A couple wants a baby. How long should it take before they may expect conception to occur? Usually six months of coition without birth control results in pregnancy. If conception does not occur within a year, the couple would do well to seek the advice of the family doctor.

Subfertility refers to a state of being less than normally fertile. It is relative sterility. **Infertility,** or **sterility,** refers to the inability to conceive or to induce conception. It is estimated that about 15 percent of married couples are unwillingly childless; another 10 percent have fewer children than they desire. In this culture, many people incorrectly consider subfertility to be primarily a fault within women. But, of course, the problem occurs about as often within men.

The cause of subfertility may be easily discovered, or it may require a long investigation. Sometimes it is necessary to consult various medical specialists.

Severe nutritional deficiencies have been known to cause reduced fertility. Both ovulation and menstruation may be impaired in this way. Alcoholism (alcohol may act directly as a poison to the testes), other drug abuse, and chronic infections all may contribute to subfertility. Physical problems may range from excess obesity of one or both marital partners (interfering with penetration) to a blocked Fallopian tube. Obstruction of the Fallopian tube and failure to ovulate are the two major causes of female infertility. A kinked tube, or one blocked as a result of an infection, may be unable to receive the ovum and permit its passage to the uterus. Or it may stop the sperm's ascent to the ovum. Many women fail to ovulate because they secrete too much of a hormone called prolactin (see pages 354–359).[16] Early reports of the use of a drug called bromocriptine to treat this condition appear promising.[17]

The physician must investigate the couple. After a thorough physical examination, there are various tests to be done. In the case of the male, spermatozoa are examined for number, motility, appearance, and other features. A varicose vein of the testes can cause infertility and may be corrected by surgery. Some men produce many sperm that lack the ability to move. In this case, taking the first part of an ejaculation and injecting it directly into the cervix may result in pregnancy. Some men may be subfertile because of a zinc deficiency. Although how zinc affects sperm function is unclear, treatment with zinc sometimes restores the life to sperm.[18] A recently discovered cause for male infertility is an insensitivity to the male hormone androgen.[19]

The search for the cause of female subfertility is also complex. It may be a persistent, simply treated vaginal inflammation. Or the physician may find that the couple has intercourse too infrequently to permit a good chance for conception. Some doctors feel that *coitus interruptus* (page 382), if practiced over a sustained period of time, sets up a reflex resulting in withdrawal before ejaculation.

The causes of inability to conceive may be multiple and complex, and patience is needed in investigating them. Only with the discovery of the cause of the problem may a rational approach to its solution be taken. When the cause is failure of the

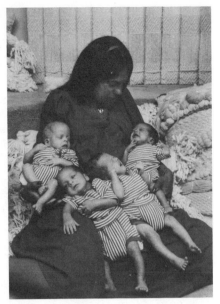

A personal population explosion. The mother of these quadruplets took fertility drugs to increase her chances of becoming pregnant.

woman to ovulate, "fertility drugs" (discussed below) may be considered.

The Sometimes Overefficient "Fertility Drugs"

Gonadotropins are substances that have an affinity for, or stimulate, the gonads (ovaries and testes). In recent years several of these substances have been used to stimulate the ovary to ovulate. Among these is the luteinizing hormone, or LH (see page 356). These substances are the so-called "fertility drugs."

A major problem with their use has been the difficulty in controlling them. Some women become pregnant with more than they bargained for. One twenty-nine-year-old Australian woman who had been given a fertility drug gave birth to nine in-

fants. They were twelve weeks premature. None survived. However, the possibility of multiple births should not condemn the use of fertility drugs. Often they do exactly what they are meant to do. For example, one New Jersey woman became pregnant twice with the aid of fertility drugs, and both were single pregnancies. To prevent excessive ovulation, fertility specialists are developing new techniques to regulate dosage. Moreover, the recent discovery of the chemical structure and the synthesis of the luteinizing hormone-releasing factor of the hypothalamus (LHRH) may well revolutionize infertility therapy. (It will be remembered that the luteinizing hormone controls the release of the ovum from the ovary.) Its laboratory production may result in safe and inexpensive fertility stimulators.

Already some success has been reported in this area. In one woman, egg production was induced by an injection of follicle-stimulating hormone, or FSH (see page 354) followed by an injection of natural LHRH. Not only did she ovulate, but she also had a healthy baby. Single ovulations have also been induced in two women by giving each of them two injections of LHRH ten days apart. In these two cases, no FSH was used beforehand.

A wide variety of procedures that stimulate ovulation but that do not involve drugs are being perfected. Among these are the correction of uterine defects, surgical procedures to reconstruct the Fallopian tubes, and the increased use of artificial insemination. This last procedure offers some hope. Within present limits, improved freezing techniques may make it more possible for newly established semen banks to help solve problems caused by male infertility.

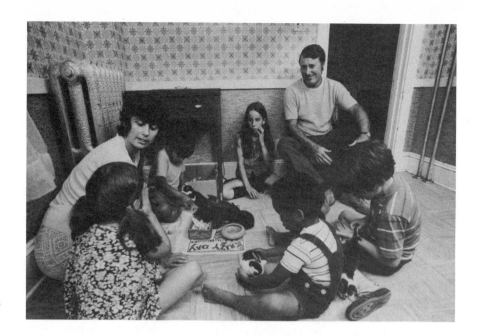

A happy family of adopted children and their parents.

Adoption

The ancient Greeks and Romans adopted children to assure continuance of the family line, thereby protecting their property. The child was secondary. Today, the child is primary. A secure home and love are needed. Adopting parents must be able to give both.

The depth of relationship between adopted child and parents is no less profound than that with the biological parents. The risk is mutual.

Unfortunately, many women who seek homes for their babies are unaware of the strict privacy available at social welfare agencies. Fearing exposure, they place their children through "black market" agencies. In this way, they put both themselves and their babies at a disadvantage because there is no assurance whatsoever that proper homes and parents will be found for the children. There is yet another problem. There are twice as many nonwhite illegitimate children as white. Yet, most

couples who want to adopt are white and thus desire a white child. Moreover, adoption is becoming more difficult because most unmarried pregnant teen-agers are now keeping their babies.

A couple considering adoption should seek help from the social welfare agency in their community. They will further profit from conferences with a good attorney and physician.

It has been observed that adopted children are brought for psychiatric treatment with considerable frequency. This may be due to the greater anxiety of the adopting parents or to their increased awareness of the psychological problems of an adopted child. Some psychiatrists believe that such problems are somewhat more frequent among adopted children.[20]

Before the adoption takes place, the parents are frequently under stress. During the nine months of

pregnancy, natural parents have time in which to build a basic beginning and basic emotional structure for parenthood. For adopting parents, however, the waiting period may be long and filled with anxiety, rather than with pleasurable anticipation. Most adopting parents are, moreover, older than natural parents; they are more set in their ways and may find a new personality in their midst a demanding trial. For some parents, the adopted child may even be a symbol of their infertility, which creates an unconscious hostility toward the child. In addition, an errant adopted child may be too severely judged by the parents. Childish transgressions may stimulate the parents into unconscious or even conscious condemning thoughts, such as "bad blood will tell."

The adopted child also has problems. The need of all children to answer the question "Who am I?" and the difficulties inherent in the search for self-identity have already been discussed (see pages 131–133). For the adopted child this search is even more difficult. To the natural child, for example, the parents are powerful and beautiful—for a while at least. During this time (when such a child, as Erik Erikson has written, "hitches his wagon to nothing less than a star"), fantasies about parents help to establish one's own uniqueness as a person. For the adopted child, however, the fantasy has a measure of reality. Indeed, the child does not know who the real parents are. The child's inability to fuse his or her image of the unknown parents with that of the adopted parents may cause much anxiety. In an effort to establish continuity in life, as well as some identity, the adopted child may even run away in search of the real parents. However, this is not common.

Authorities generally agree that the child should be told of the adoption. There is some disagreement as to when. There is no exact time for all children; it should be individualized. There are those who insist that the child should be told as soon as possible and that the information should be affectionately, but consistently, reiterated in a variety of ways. For example, the child could routinely be introduced as one's adopted child. The theory to support this advice is that, in this way, the adopted child becomes desensitized to the knowledge. Later, the theory holds, when the child learns the meaning of adoption, it is more acceptable. Others dispute this; they believe that the concept of adoption means little to the very young child. The period between six and ten years of age has been suggested as the best time to tell the child about the adoption; during those years most children are usually less beset by emotional difficulties.[21] To develop a sense of identity, the adopted child will need the opportunity to develop a strong sense of self-esteem. Then, together, child and parents can come to see how they have helped one another while meeting one another's needs.[22] In this, they are like all parents and children. And that they succeed is borne out by the hundreds of thousands of well-adjusted adopted children in the United States.

Children Having Children

She took the crying baby out of his crib and held him close to her thin chest. "Mustn't cry, Peter," she murmured. "Mommy loves you. Mommy will take care of everything."

"Let me hold him," her mother said, not unkindly. "Practice some of your shorthand and typing." She paused. "You're lucky I get this day off every week," she said.

"I don't want to be a secretary," the girl said above the baby's crying.

"Well, what can you be?" said the mother. "You'll be fifteen next month."

"I dunno. I just want to take care of Peter." The baby stopped crying. "See," she said to her mother, "he needs me."

"You're lucky your father doesn't live here," the mother said, "else there wouldn't be any room."

"Yeah," the girl said dreamily. She smoothed her baby's hair. "I'm all luck."

In 1979, almost a million U.S. teen-age girls were pregnant. Over 80 percent were unmarried. More than 300,000—half of them seventeen years old or younger—sought abortions. More than 600,000 gave birth to a baby. About a quarter of a million of these births were to girls seventeen years old or younger. And more and more girls between ten and fourteen are giving birth to babies. Despite the number of abortions, the number of U.S. teen-age pregnancies ranks high compared with other nations. Between the ages of fifteen and nineteen, the rates are about three times those of the Netherlands and Switzerland, and twice those of France, Belgium, and Denmark.

Of considerable importance is the case that began this section. She is only one of the 95 percent of unmarried teen-age girls who keep their babies. Why? Some experts write that the girls are seeking love and dependency, which a baby gives them. Others note that the girls are pressured by their mothers. Their daughters' babies, it is theorized, make them feel younger or perhaps needed again. But whatever the reason, many teen-agers are taking on the role of parents, for which they are generally not ready. And their babies are not ready to be born. For both mother and child, and for the father too, a teen-age pregnancy is usually the beginning of handicaps and risks that can beset them for the rest of their lives.

Disadvantages to the Parents and to Society

Long-term studies have shown that for both sexes, teen-age pregnancy

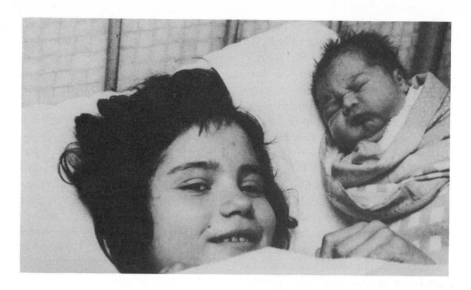

A child and her child.

has a very negative effect on educational, occupational, and economic satisfaction and success. Eight of ten teen-age girls who become mothers at seventeen or younger never finish high school. Four of ten who have a baby by the age of fifteen never finish the eighth grade. These child-parents begin and usually must stay with rock-bottom jobs. The United States has the world's highest divorce rate. Teen-age marriages end in divorce at twice the rate of the general U.S. population. And, as problems beget problems, statistics show that at least 50 percent of out-of-wedlock children receive welfare. Federal Aid to Families with Dependent Children given to teen-age mothers amounts to almost half a billion dollars a year. In 1979 the Stanford Research Institute International reported that teen-age pregnancies in this country cost the taxpayers about $8.3 billion a year in welfare and related outlays. This is more than the entire budgets of some countries, such as New Zealand and Portugal, and higher than the total budgets of such federal agencies as the Departments of Commerce, Interior, and State.[23]

Health Risks to the Mother

Compared with twenty- to twenty-four-year-old mothers, those fifteen to nineteen years of age endure a greater risk of anemia, abnormal bleeding, toxemia, difficult labor, and other complications. Worse, a little more than half of pregnant adolescents receive no medical care during the first three months of their pregnancies. Moreover, adolescents delay abortion longer than older pregnant women, and late abortions are more dangerous than those done in the early months of pregnancy.

Health Risks to the Children

Children born to adolescents, compared with those born to twenty- to twenty-four-year-old mothers, are more likely to be underweight and premature. For mothers under fifteen, the risk to their babies is more than double. Children of adolescents are also more prone to die in the first year of life than are those

born to twenty- to twenty-four-year-old mothers.

The Prevention of Teen-age Pregnancies

The incidence of teen-age pregnancy has not been reduced by the development of birth control methods. Pregnancy prevention is often learned by teen-agers the hard way. Female adolescents seek family planning only after a year or more of sexual activity, after an abortion, or when getting a pregnancy test. Male adolescents rarely go to family planning clinics.

Various suggestions have been made to reduce pregnancies among teen-agers. Sex education, including a better knowledge of the risks of pregnancy, contraceptive information and availability without parental consent, knowledge of the consequences of early parenthood, and teachers who have experienced the consequences, are among the recommendations. All these efforts will, it is hoped, help U.S. teen-agers learn a better sense of responsibility toward their own sexuality.

Summary

Conception takes place when an ovum is fertilized by a sperm. The fertilized egg is a zygote. Even before implantation in the uterine *endometrium*, the zygote begins to divide to become an *embryo*. After two months, it is considered a *fetus*. If two eggs are released by the ovaries and fertilized, *fraternal twins* will result. If a single zygote splits during division, the resulting cell masses will develop into *identical twins*. Some of the zygotic cells become nonembryonic structures, which serve to support the developing life. The *placenta*, or *afterbirth*, is attached on one side deep within the mother's uterine lining, and on the other side to the baby by means of the *umbilical cord*. The placenta is derived from the zygote, but the mother contributes to it, too. However, there is no direct connection between the blood of the mother and that of the infant. Oxygen and nourishment reach the baby through the umbilical arteries, and wastes are carried away through the umbilical vein. Another nonembryonic structure is the *amnion*, a fluid-filled sac that surrounds the developing child, protecting it and providing it with a stable temperature. Fetal development requires ten lunar months, or forty weeks.

During pregnancy, the mother should gain at least twenty-two to twenty-six pounds. As a result of new ideas about nutrition during pregnancy, women no longer need to restrict their salt intake. The only vitamin supplement that probably will be needed is folic acid. Iron should also be taken.

Signs of pregnancy are a missed menstrual cycle, sensitive breasts, and nausea. Accurate testing for pregnancy can be done within days of the first missed menstrual period. A pregnant woman should visit her doctor regularly for prenatal care. The woman may have sexual intercourse unless there is abdominal or vaginal pain, discomfort, uterine bleeding or ruptured membranes, or for other reasons determined by her doctor.

Labor occurs in three stages. During the first, the upper part of the uterus contracts and the lower part, the cervix, dilates to allow for the passage of the baby. If any problems exist during this stage, the baby can be delivered surgically through the abdomen and uterus by means of a *Caesarean section*. In the next stage, the pressure of the contractions expel the baby from the mother's body. The third stage involves delivery of the afterbirth.

There has been a recent trend toward natural childbirth and away from the use of drugs, such as inhalant anaesthetics and Demerol. The Lamaze method, which involves the father in the birth process, has seen increasing acceptance. The Leboyer method of delivering babies emphasizes easing the transition from the uterus into the external environment. While interest in home delivery is increasing, it is safest for both the mother and child for delivery to take place in the hospital, where medical emergencies can be handled effectively.

Six to eight weeks after delivery the woman should be sure to have a physical examination. Breast-feeding will prolong postpartum amenorrhea, but the woman can ovulate, and thus become pregnant again, before menstruation resumes.

Recent medical opinion states that breast-feeding is best for most babies. Mother's milk is nutritionally superior to cow's milk; it provides antibodies that give the baby temporary immunity to disease; and the contact between mother and child is emotionally healthful. However, since drugs and infection in the breast can pass to the child through the mother's milk, breast-feeding may need to be avoided in some instances.

Sudden Infant Death Syndrome ("cot death" or "crib death") occurs unexpectedly to many infants during sleep. Research has identified risk factors for this syndrome, and it is hoped that the incidence of SIDS will decrease. Another cause of death in newborns is hyaline membrane disease, caused by immaturely developed lung cells.

Subfertility is a state of being less than normally fertile. *Infertility*, or *sterility*, is the inability to conceive or to induce conception. In the male, subfertility can be caused by immotile sperm, zinc deficiency, or a varicose vein of the testes. In the female, it can result from blocked Fallopian tubes or vaginal inflammation. Other causes in both sexes are infrequent intercourse, alcoholism, drug abuse, nutritional deficiency, chronic infection, or obesity. If pregnancy does not result after a year, a physician should be consulted for the cause and possible treatment of the subfertility. One problem, failure to ovulate, can be treated with fertility drugs containing the gonadotropin luteinizing hormone. The use of these drugs is being perfected to prevent multiple births.

An alternative to having one's own children is adoption. This is often a long and difficult process, and the adoption may cause psychological problems in both the parents and the child. There is some uncertainty as to when the child should be told that he or she was adopted, though it is agreed that this information should be given. However, despite these problems, successful adoption is common.

The United States has an exceptionally high occurrence of teen-age pregnancies. Eighty percent of these young mothers are unmarried. Pregnancy at this age results in educational, occupational, and economic disadvantages. The health risks to both mother and child are high. The cost to society in welfare payments is staggering. Suggestions to reduce teen-age pregnancies include sex education, contraceptive information and availability without parental consent, and education about the risks of pregnancy and the consequences of early parenthood.

References

1. Donald Culross Peattie, *An Almanac for Moderns* (New York, 1935), as quoted in Louise B. Young, *Population in Perspective* (New York, 1968), p. 314.
2. G.M.H. Veeneklass, cited in *Physicians Bulletin*, Vol. 24 (November 15, 1959), p. B8.
3. "Nutrition in Pregnancy," *The Medical Letter*, Vol. 20 (July 28, 1978), pp. 1–2.
4. Paul I. Terasaki et al., "Twins with Two Different Fathers Identified by HLA," *The New England Journal of Medicine*, Vol. 299 (September 14, 1978), pp. 590–592.

5. Kenneth J. Ryan, "Paternity and Pedigree, from Superfecundation to 'Test Tube' Babies," *The New England Journal of Medicine*, Vol. 299 (September 14, 1978), p. 603.

6. Michael Bruser, "Sporting Activities During Pregnancy," cited in "Sports and Pregnancy," *Briefs: Footnotes on Maternity Care*, Vol. 33 (April 1969), pp. 51–53.

7. Much of the material in this section is based on Chapter 4, "Sexual Relations During Pregnancy and the Post-Delivery Period," in *Sexuality and Man*, compiled and edited by the Sex Information and Education Council of the United States (New York, 1970).

8. Selig Neubardt, "Coitus During Pregnancy," *Medical Aspects of Human Sexuality*, Vol. 7 (September 1973), p. 197.

9. Robin Marantz Henig, "Perils of Painless Childbirth," *Human Behavior*, Vol. 7 (October 1978), pp. 50–51.

10. May Annexton, "Breast-Feeding Lauded by Pediatricians," *Journal of the American Medical Association*, Vol. 240 (December 8, 1978), p. 2612.

11. Helmuth Vorherr, "Suppression of Postpartum Lactation," *Postgraduate Medicine*, Vol. 52 (July 1972), p. 145.

12. Frederick B. Hodges, "Sudden Infant Death Syndrome," *California Medicine*, Vol. 116 (January 1972), p. 85.

13. "Preventing Sudden Infant Deaths," *Science News*, Vol. 110 (September 10, 1977), p. 167.

14. J. J. Francisco, "Smothering in Infancy: Its Relationship to the 'Crib Death Syndrome,'" *Southern Medical Journal*, Vol. 63 (October 1970), p. 1114.

15. Mary Ellen Avery, Nai-San Wang, and H. William Taeusch, Jr., "The Lung of the Newborn Infant," *Scientific American*, Vol. 228 (April 1973), p. 75. This article is particularly recommended for its lucid explanation of hyaline membrane disease.

16. Gina Bari Kolata, "Infertility: Promising New Treatments," *Science*, Vol. 202 (October 1978), pp. 200–203.

17. "Bromocriptine for Infertility," *Medical World News*, Vol. 20 (June 11, 1979), p. 52.

18. John H. Douglas, "New Hope for Infertile Men," *Science News*, Vol. 114 (November 4, 1978), p. 311.

19. James Aiman et al., "Androgen Insensitivity As a Cause of Infertility in Otherwise Normal Men," *The New England Journal of Medicine*, Vol. 300 (February 1, 1979), pp. 223–227.

20. Henry H. Work and Hans Anderson, "Studies in Adoption: Requests for Psychiatric Treatment," *American Journal of Psychiatry*, Vol. 127 (January 1971), pp. 124–125.

21. Marshall D. Schechter, "Is Adoption a Handicapping Condition?" *Medical Insight*, Vol. 3 (August 1971), p. 21.

22. American Academy of Pediatrics, Committee on Adoptions, "Identity Development in Adopted Children," *Pediatrics*, Vol. 47 (May 1971), pp. 948–949.

23. "Pregnant Teens Cost $8 Billion in Taxes," *Health Care Horizons*, Vol. 11 (June 3, 1979), pp. 1 and 16.

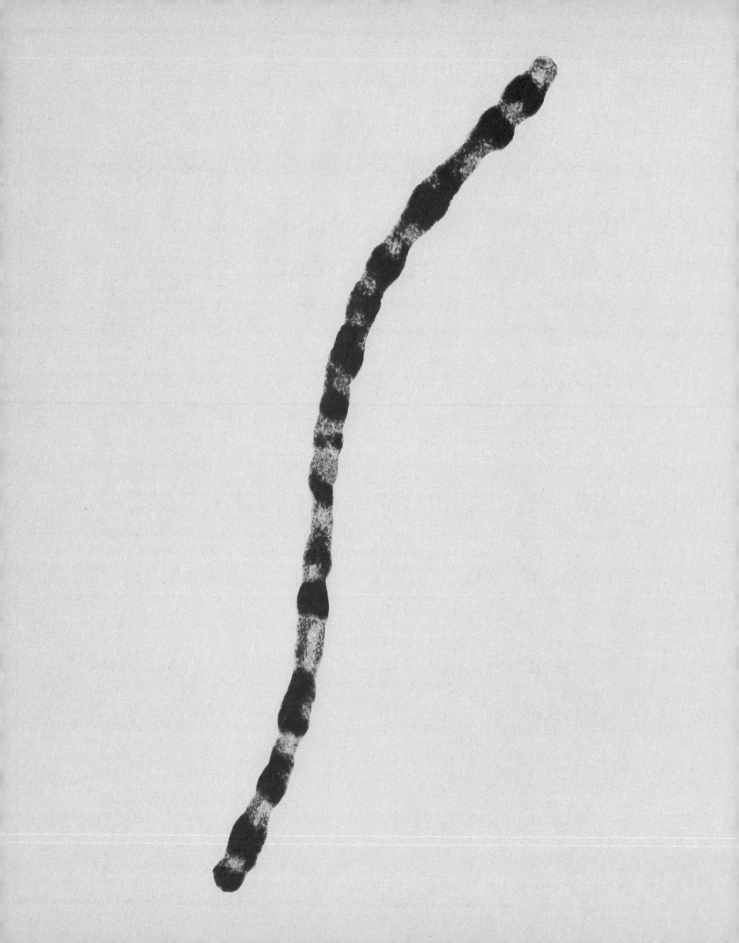

14

Human Beginnings: Part II

Before I was born out of my mother generations guided me.

WALT WHITMAN
"Song of Myself"

Many thousands of years ago there was no life in the world. Then, in a particular right time and environment, certain chemicals combined and were sparked into living fragments. That is, they reproduced themselves exactly. Sometimes they failed to do this and reproduced themselves inexactly. This accident was then duplicated exactly.

In time the living fragments became cells. Cells became tissue. Tissues were formed into creatures. Countless trillions of different individuals were born into a million species, and died. Some, like the dinosaur, perished forever. Others, like people, endured and became more complex. Even so, the "gills" we have as embryos may serve to remind us that our genes continue to send ancestral messages, although our needs have modified the outcome of those messages. Our "gills" now become glands and major blood vessels. This transformation occurs as a result of genetic instruction and the process of evolution.

Genetics: Molding a New Person

The reasons for interest in heredity are several. First, the *chromosomes* within the *nucleus* of the human cell give directions that help decide the characteristics of humanity. Change those directions and humanity can be changed. Many people are apprehensive that scientists will "tamper with heredity." To better understand and control human destiny, every generation must understand some genetics.

A generation ago, the British novelist and critic C.S. Lewis wrote these warning words:

What we call Man's power over Nature turns out to be a power exercised by some men over other men with Nature as its instrument. . . . And all long-term exercises of power, especially in breeding, must mean the power of earlier generations over later ones. . . . If any age really attains . . . the power to make its descendants what it pleases, all men who live after it are the patients of that power.[1]

By late 1973, scientists had synthesized the first gene that had the potential to function in a living cell. Moreover, its product could also be detected in a living cell. By 1978 they had successfully transferred a functioning gene from one mammalian species to another (monkey to rabbit).[2] This was accomplished by using *recombinant DNA techniques*. What are these techniques? In 1972 scientists discovered certain **enzymes** (chemicals that can start or continue a chemical reaction without becoming part of the reaction) that could slice off a piece of the hereditary chemicals—the DNA of genes. These cut-off portions of genes could be joined with pieces of DNA in the cells of a different organism. In 1975, scientists from sixteen countries advised that strict controls of recombinant DNA research be established. Why? Such research might develop a new bacterium dangerous to people, for which science has no cure. Knowledge is not wisdom, as human history has amply shown. It is the unwise use of knowledge—knowledge without judgment—that today imperils humankind. Thus we have

The photograph on page 412 is a human chromosome magnified 12,500 times.

a second basic reason for understanding heredity.

Atomic energy provides a third reason for concern with genetics. The fallout from atomic testing may produce an effect, most likely harmful, on the human hereditary material—the *genes*. But more than bombs are involved. Future generations will see a greatly expanded industrial use of atomic energy. The effect of possible atomic radiation on future generations is urgent

health business, and only an informed public can influence government policymakers to safeguard health. Everything must be done so that future generations do not inherit the ill winds of this atomic age.

The involvement of genetics with illness is yet a fourth reason the subject demands study. About three thousand varieties of birth defects perplex scientists. Some, like flat feet, are minor. Others, like Down's

syndrome, are more serious. In all such disorders, genes play a varying role. Sometimes it is the gene that is basically at fault. In other cases it is the environment that disturbs genetic processes. And there are conditions for which the primary cause is unclear. But one concept is clear: All genetic processes must be considered within their ecosystems. Every gene interacts with its environment and is in turn influenced by it.

The Cell: Unit of Life

The *cell* (Figure 14–1) is the basic unit of life. Its **protoplasm** is made mainly of cellular proteins, fats, carbohydrates, and inorganic salts in a watery medium. It contains thousands of enzymes (see page 421). Enzymes are eventually used up and must continuously be created anew by the cell from available nutrients. Cells also contain special materials that are needed to carry out the cell's particular activity, such as the *glycogen* seen as granules in the liver cell.

The ministructures in the cell's protoplasm, the little organs, or *organelles*, function in concert with their intracellular environment. The membrane-encircled **nucleus**, the largest of the cell's organelles, contains and is surrounded by protoplasm. Protoplasm outside the nucleus is called **cytoplasm**. Thus, the two major parts of most cells are the nucleus and the cytoplasm. The events that occur in the cytoplasm, such as digestion, respiration, secre-

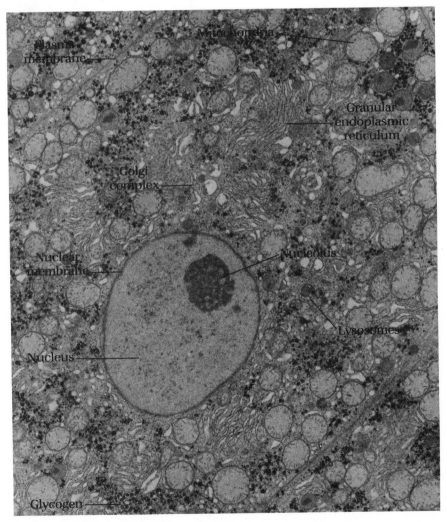

FIGURE 14–1
A mammalian cell. Visible in this liver cell are granules of glycogen.

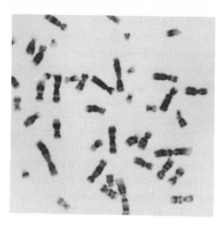

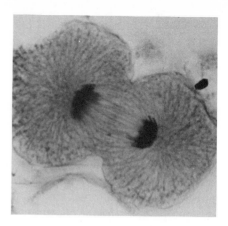

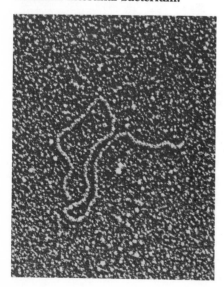

FIGURE 14-2
Chromosomes of a normal human male (left) and of a whitefish (right). The chromosomes of this whitefish cell have duplicated themselves, and the cell itself is dividing into two cells.

FIGURE 14-3
A single gene, isolated from a common intestinal bacterium.

tion, and excretion, depend on the activity within the nucleus. The nucleus is also essential for the reproduction of the cell.

The Nucleus

Within the nucleus are the **chromosomes** (Figure 14-2), and within the chromosomes are the **genes** (Figure 14-3). Genes are the units of heredity, but they are even more. Because each gene is composed of DNA, the gene governs the life of the cell. And because DNA can reproduce itself during cell division, the DNA code is thus transmitted to subsequent cells.

In the cell community, red blood cells are unique. During their maturation in the bone marrow they lose their nuclei. Bereft of DNA, these cells cannot synthesize protein. Red blood cells live only as long as their enzymes last—about 120 days. Every second some 2.5 million red blood cells must be released into the circulation.

The Cytoplasm, the Plasma Membrane, and the Endoplasmic Reticulum

Policing the kind and amount of material entering the cell is its

enveloping, porous **plasma membrane**. The plasma membrane, made up of fats, proteins, carbohydrates, and other components, does more than merely mark the cell's boundaries. It is a complex structure performing a wide range of tasks that are essential to health and life. It admits some molecules that seek to enter the cell; it rebuffs others. It also permits the escape of waste materials from the cell but holds in essential substances.

All chemical and electrical information that reaches the cell does so through its membrane. Hormones, insulin for example, initiate their effects through interactions with receptor sites on cell surfaces. . . . Many drugs act through cell-surface contacts, muscle contractions are triggered by electrical stimuli acting on membranes, and a host of enzymatic activities are carried out on the cell surface.[3]

When cancer occurs, disorders of the plasma membrane are common. A better understanding of the plasma membrane has a high priority in the science of the 1980s.

At various places the plasma membrane appears to fold inward, extending into the cytoplasm of the cell as the **endoplasmic reticulum**. Thus is created a membranous system of canals along which needed materials are transported deep into the cell's cytoplasm. The endoplasmic reticulum communicates with the surrounding nuclear membrane. By this route nutrients for the nucleus are delivered. Wastes can be carried out via these canals too. Guiding the transport of materials within the cell and helping the cell to maintain its shape, then, is this system of tiny tubules.

Some of the Organelles Within the Cytoplasm

On part of the endoplasmic reticulum are clustered granules called **ribosomes**—the sites of protein synthesis. In the cytoplasm of most cells are the *mitochondria* and *lysosomes*. **Mitochondria** are the cell's energy sources. Like tiny fuel furnaces distributed throughout the cellular cytoplasm, mitochondria convert the chemical energy of cellular nutrients into a high-energy compound called **adenosine triphosphate** (**ATP**). ATP is released as needed for the cell's work. Mitochondria are enclosed by a membrane. So are the **lysosomes**, the cell's digestive organelles. Each lysosome contains enzymes that break down complex nutrients into simpler substances. Another duty of the lysosome is to act as a minute garbage disposal, helping to rid the cell of bacteria or worn-out materials.

Consider the treasure of past and future generations contained within the cell: the nucleus, the power-packed mitochondria, the digesting lysosomes, the membranous network of endoplasmic reticulum that provides a transportation system for cellular nutrients and wastes, and a ribosomal site for protein synthesis. All these and other active islands are surrounded by a small sea of protoplasm, which, in turn, is enveloped by the meticulously selective plasma membrane.

Scientists speak of the balanced organization within the cellular ecosystem. But scientific investigation of the cell is not limited to ultramicroscopic searches for its ministructures. Studies are being made of the chemical mechanisms that enable these cellular ministructures to operate so that health and life occur. In recent years an increasing amount of attention has been drawn to chemical substances of enormous importance to cell (and body) function and dysfunction.

Meiosis and Mitosis

There are two basic kinds of cells in the human body: *germ cells* (gametes) and *somatic cells* (Greek *soma*, "body"). A **germ cell** of an organism is a cell whose function it is to reproduce the species; these are the ova (eggs) and the spermatozoa.* All other body cells are **somatic**.

When a mature sperm fertilizes a mature ovum, the resultant fusion is a cell called the **zygote**. To achieve the maturity necessary to participate in zygote formation, the germ cells, starting from primordial (beginning) sex cells, must go through

---

*Women are born with their total supply of primitive eggs, which nestle immature in the ovary until puberty. Beginning at puberty, men continually replenish their supply of sperm cells.

a special process of cell division called **meiosis**. Primordial sex cells of a human have forty-six chromosomes, but when meiosis of a primordial sex cell is complete, the mature gamete has only twenty-three chromosomes. Twenty-two of these are single, nonsex chromosomes and are called **autosomes**. The remaining chromosome is either an **X** or a **Y sex chromosome**. At the end of meiosis, the mature ovum carries a single X chromosome, and the mature sperm either an X chromosome or a Y chromosome (see Figure 14–4). It is a basic (although not the only) function of the Y chromosome to direct the production of the male sex glands (testes).

When fertilization of the mature ovum by the mature sperm occurs, each parent contributes twenty-three chromosomes to the resultant zygote—twenty-two autosomes and one sex chromosome. A normal ovum always contains an X chromosome. Referring to Figure 14–5, you can see that if an ovum is fertilized by a normal sperm containing an X chromosome, the result is XX (female):

X (ovum) + X (sperm) = XX (female)

If an ovum is fertilized by a sperm containing a Y chromosome, the result is XY (male):

X (ovum) + Y (sperm) = XY (male)

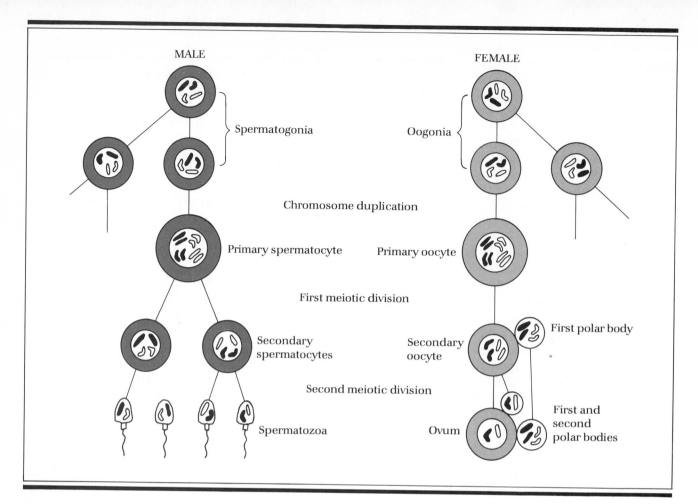

MALE

Spermatogonia

Chromosome duplication

Primary spermatocyte

First meiotic division

Secondary spermatocytes

Second meiotic division

Spermatozoa

FEMALE

Oogonia

Primary oocyte

First polar body

Secondary oocyte

First and second polar bodies

Ovum

FIGURE 14–4
Meiosis. The mature gametes (spermatozoa or ova) have half the number of chromosomes that the primordial sex cells (spermatogonia or oogonia) had. During the maturation process, polar bodies simply degenerate. For simplicity, cells shown here have only four chromosomes.

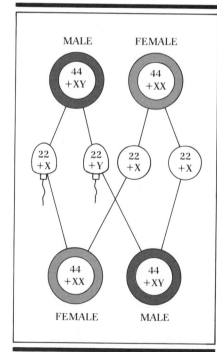

MALE   FEMALE

44 +XY   44 +XX

22 +X   22 +Y   22 +X   22 +X

44 +XX   44 +XY

FEMALE   MALE

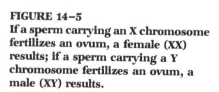

FIGURE 14–5
If a sperm carrying an X chromosome fertilizes an ovum, a female (XX) results; if a sperm carrying a Y chromosome fertilizes an ovum, a male (XY) results.

FIGURE 14–6
Karyotype (chromosomal chart) of a
normal human male. The karyotype
of a female has two X chromosomes
where the X and Y chromosomes
appear here.

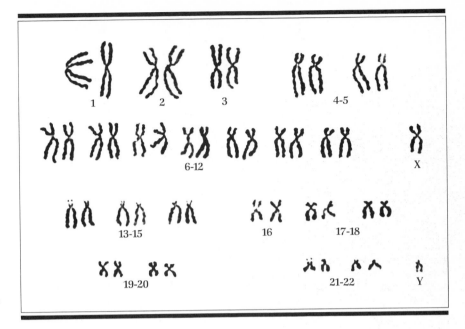

So the zygote and all subsequent somatic cells normally contain twenty-three *pairs* of chromosomes (a total of forty-six chromosomes), of which twenty-two pairs are autosomes and one pair are sex chromosomes. Each autosomal pair is different in genetic content and usually in appearance from all other pairs. Figure 14–6 shows the chromosomes arranged in pairs to form a chromosomal chart called a **karyotype**. Note that each autosomal pair is numbered from 1 to 22 and that the sex chromosomes are appropriately labeled either X or Y.

As noted above, only the primordial sex cells increase in number by meiosis. The zygote and all subsequent somatic cells multiply by **mitosis**. In the process of mitosis, the threadlike chromosomes in the nucleus of a cell duplicate themselves; the duplicate sets are separated, with one set going to each of the two "daughter" cells produced by the division of the original cell. Thus in *mitosis* each of the two cells produced by the division of a single cell has a *full* set of chromosomes, whereas in *meiosis* each of the cells has *half* the number of chromosomes the original cell had. By mitosis the body grows and replaces discarded cells. In both meiosis and mitosis there are plenty of chances for errors. Should a cell, be it germ or somatic, fail to receive its proper share or composition of chromosomes, abnormality results.

Genetic Order

By their union in the Fallopian tube, the mature sperm and egg contribute their twenty-three single chromosomes to the fertilized egg to form a zygote with its full normal complement of forty-six. Mitosis begins. The zygote prepares to divide. Each of the forty-six chromosomes splits into two parts, which are exact replicas of each other. The cell divides. Now there are two body cells. Normally, each has its full share of forty-six chromosomes. Several hours later the two somatic cells cleave again. There are then four body cells. Normally, each still contains forty-six chromosomes. And so cell multiplication continues. Every day the somatic cell cluster continues to divide as it travels down the Fallopian tube toward the uterus. With each division these cells double in number. Normally, they never have fewer or more than forty-six chromosomes.

At last, the tiny, multiplying cellular mass is implanted in the uterine endometrium. Membranes begin to form. Within two or three weeks after fertilization, the embryo is being fed via these membranes. In another week there is a heart. A week later the heart begins to beat. Now cell differentiation continues rapidly, and so does organ development. Each cell must multiply in the limited space allotted to it and under pressure from every other cell. And, as will be seen, each cell is instructed as to its future function. This is the nature of cellular ecosystems.

The cells of various organs are specific for those organs. In other words, the cells of the heart are different from those of the gut, which, in turn, are different from those of the nerves, and so on. By birth, roughly fifty successive cell divisions have taken place, resulting in trillions of marvelously organized cells. With normal cell division, every one of those trillions of cells contains the identical number of chromosomes

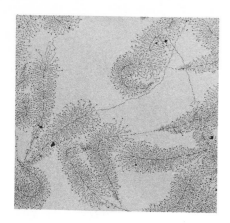

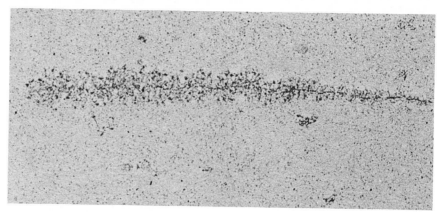

FIGURE 14-7
This electron photomicrograph of a salamander oocyte is one of the first to show genes (the spine of the spindle-shaped structure) in the process of producing molecules of ribosomal ribonucleic acid (rRNA), seen as hairlike fibers extending from the genes (× 25,000). Right: The only electron photomicrograph that shows what are presumed to be ribosomal RNA genes of a human cell (× 36,000).

as the original individual single zygote contained. How did this happen? How does one kind of cell end up as part of a bladder muscle, another kind in the eye, still another in a toenail, and yet a fourth in a mole on the left cheek? How does each cell get the message telling it what to become? The answer lies within the nucleus of the cell, in the DNA making up the genes of the chromosomes.

DNA, the Master Plan; RNA, the Obedient Worker

Chemically, a chromosome consists mostly of proteins combined with a substance called **deoxyribonucleic acid (DNA)**. The chromosomal DNA is the material of the gene. Within it is stored the genetic information. Chromosomal DNA cannot leave the nucleus.* It appears imprisoned within it, capable of duplicating itself with each cell division and serving as a blueprint for the formation of **ribonucleic acid (RNA)** molecules. Thus, chromosomes incidentally contain RNA. As will be seen,

*DNA has been demonstrated outside the nucleus, both in mitochondria and in the cytoplasm. Whether these DNA molecules originate from the nuclear chromosomes has yet to be determined, and scientists have not yet clarified the function of DNA outside the nucleus.

three kinds of RNA are made: *ribosomal RNA, messenger RNA,* and transfer RNA. Each plays a definite role in the building of cell proteins.

Outside the nucleus, as part of the cell's cytoplasm, there are still other proteins. Like all body proteins they are originally derived from food and are composed of *amino acids*. It is from this nutrient pool in the cytoplasm that amino acids are taken and brought to the ribosomes.

How the Ribosomal Factory Is Made

Peering through the electron microscope at an amphibian oocyte** (Figure 14-7), biologists believe they have discovered how ribosomes originate. A gene is spindle-shaped. Each gene is linked with every other gene like the beads of a necklace. Running from the broad base of the spindle to its tip is a thread. This thread is DNA—a tiny segment of a chromosome. The DNA of the gene directs the production of molecules of ribonucleic acid (RNA). These hairlike molecules, extending from the gene, spiral about the DNA

**An *amphibian* is a vertebrate animal (a frog or a toad, for example) able to live both on land and in water. An *oocyte* is a female gamete that has not reached full development; mature, it is an ovum.

thread and decrease in size from the base to the tip of the spindle. (The RNA is not an actual part of DNA; the DNA merely governs the manufacture, or synthesis, of RNA according to its present code.) The length of the RNA fiber and its structure are dictated by the DNA, which directs its manufacture from cytoplasmic amino acids. As it is synthesized, the RNA molecules place themselves next to a part of the DNA pattern in such a way as to reflect specific chemical configurations. RNA is thus instructed by the DNA. According to DNA instructions, each RNA fiber breaks off and, when free in the nucleus, is broken up into segments, probably by an enzyme.* First one, and then a second part of the original RNA fiber leaves the nucleus, deserting the nuclear DNA, which may not leave. Bearing the specific instructions of the DNA, these segments of the RNA fiber meet in the cellular cytoplasm to form a single ribosome. John Lear has described this remarkable process:

According to the biochemical evidence, the opening event in the sequence of the spindle's operation is the extrusion of the RNA fiber from the main thread of DNA. As the extrusion proceeds, the fiber is strung with a protein coat according to coded instructions from the DNA. This process goes on until each fiber reaches a predetermined length . . . , after which that particular RNA fiber separates from the DNA thread like a quill from a porcupine's back. The fibers depart individually after attaining individual maturity. En route they pass under an unidentified biological

*An enzyme is frequently a protein and has the power to initiate or accelerate certain chemical reactions in plant or animal metabolism.

knife (presumably an enzyme) that chops each fiber into segments. The first segment to be severed is about one-sixth the length of the whole fiber. This segment moves into the cytoplasm very quickly and at once coils into a tiny sphere. The coiling apparently occurs in response to instructions the DNA thread imprinted on the RNA fiber before setting the fiber loose. That part of the fiber that remains in the nucleus is subsequently chopped several times, until the surviving segment is about one-third as long as the original fiber had been. The final segment then moves out through the nuclear membrane into the cytoplasm, finds a tiny sphere formed by an earlier segment of fiber, and coils into a larger sphere alongside the tiny sphere. The two spheres together make a ribosome.[4]

How Body Protein Is Made

With the understanding of how ribosomes are created from RNA, consider now what happens at the site of a single ribosome.

First, an amino acid is brought and attached to it. Then a second amino acid is brought to it. With the assistance of an enzyme, the second amino acid is linked to the first. But only in a predetermined way. A third amino acid is brought to the ribosome and linked to the second —again in a manner previously decided, and helped by an enzyme. A fourth amino acid then reaches the assembly line at the ribosomal factory. It is linked to its predecessor. Still another follows it. Then another and another. To all the ribosomal depots, in all the somatic cells, whether in a developing embryo or in an aging adult, amino acids, derived from the nutrient

pool of cytoplasmic proteins, are brought and linked one to the other. At each ribosome, then, a series of linked amino acids, a chain, is formed. Bonds between these amino acid chains form complex proteins. The manner of arrangement of the amino acids determines protein structure. And protein structure decides body structure and, therefore, function. So the chemical arrangement of the amino acids at the ribosomes results in proteins that will become blue eyes or brown eyes, liver or heart, a short or tall person. The variations in the arrangement of amino acids at the ribosomal workbench are no less endless than the variations of hereditary characteristics.

How do the amino acids get selected out of the cytoplasmic protein? How is their sequence determined? How are they brought to the ribosome? And, once at the ribosome, how does it happen that amino acids are so properly arranged? It is the nuclear DNA that governs all this. Only that DNA contains the genetic formula, so only that DNA can impart the genetic code, the hereditary instructions. But how can these DNA instructions reach the ribosome? It has been seen that the DNA may not itself leave the nucleus to direct protein structure at the ribosome. It seems imprisoned within the nucleus, locked within the chromosomal pattern. It appears fixed, a template, a mold of chemicals. Since that DNA is unable to carry its own message outside the nucleus, a messenger is needed.

That messenger must somehow obtain the exact complex message, the specific instructions, of the DNA. Like the ribosomal RNA before it, that messenger must, therefore, in turn become a template, a mold of part of the DNA code. And unlike that DNA, the messenger

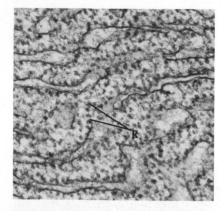

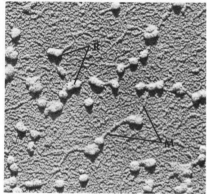

FIGURE 14–8
Ribosomes: the sites of protein synthesis. The top photo shows granular endoplasmic reticulum (× 60,000), on which ribosomes (R) are located. The bottom photo shows ribosomes (R) at a higher magnification (× 88,000). Numbers of ribosomes are connected by filaments (M), which are believed to be messenger RNA.

must be able to leave the nucleus. Obediently that messenger must make its way to the waiting ribosome, bringing to it the DNA message of instructions. A special kind of RNA is that messenger. Somehow, **messenger RNA** (as it is called) must obtain the patterned message, established by the coded position of certain chemical elements in the DNA. (As will be seen, the message obtained by the messenger RNA is for a different purpose than that obtained by ribosomal RNA.) Figure 14–8 shows two high-magnification photographs of ribosomes and messenger RNA.

Within the cell's nucleus, messenger RNA places itself alongside part of the DNA code. It arranges its chemical structure to exactly match that of a definite part of the DNA. The RNA transcription (or copy) of that part of the DNA template is thus formed.* In this way the messenger RNA has itself become a template, a mold, a mirror copy of part of the DNA chemical structure. Having incorporated within itself the instruction of the DNA, having acquired within its very structure the position of the coded chemical elements of the DNA, the messenger RNA deserts the DNA. It passes through the nuclear membrane. It enters into the midst of the cellular cytoplasm. There the DNA-code-carrying messenger RNA heads for a waiting ribosome. For, as has been stated, it is at the ribosomal workbench that protein is manufactured. And these synthesized proteins contribute to the specific characteristics of the creature-to-be.

Upon finding a ribosome, the messenger RNA is associated with

it. Thus is established, at the ribosome, the copy of the DNA code of instructions. Now amino acids, the building material of proteins, must be taken from the surrounding cytoplasmic protein and brought to the ribosome. And, with the instructions awaiting their arrival, the amino acids must be properly arranged at the ribosome. This can be done only as instructed by the nuclear DNA. For although that DNA seems imprisoned, it remains the master. The traveling messenger RNA, associated with a ribosome, remains but a mirror copy. And now the readied ribosomal workbench (the synthesis of which was also specifically directed by the DNA) awaits amino acid delivery. To construct specific proteins, to create specific tissue as instructed, amino acid building blocks must be brought to the ribosomal factory from the nutrient cytoplasmic protein pool.

How is this accomplished?

While the ribosome was receiving its instructing messenger RNA, the DNA in the nucleus was not idle. It kept busy directing the production of still another, smaller type of RNA. This third RNA is called **transfer RNA.** Also instructed by the nuclear DNA, in a fixed sequence, transfer RNA leaves the nucleus and enters the cytoplasmic protein pool of amino acids. For each separate amino acid there is a separate transfer RNA. On its way to the ribosome the transfer RNA picks up its selected amino acid from the protein pool. On reaching the ribosome, the amino acid leaves the transfer RNA and, helped by enzymes, attaches itself to the ribosome. One after another, in assembly-line fashion, and as instructed by the messenger RNA, the amino acids are linked one to the other.

*The rate at which messenger RNA is transcribed from the DNA is determined by the arrangement or sequence of the chemicals of the DNA. In some manner light affects this rate. It sets the biological clock.

So transfer RNA keeps leaving the nucleus, picking up selected amino acids from the cytoplasmic protein pool, and delivering them to be linked to the growing amino acid chain at the ribosomal protein factory. But recent work suggests that this factory, this ribosomal RNA, is not merely an inert organelle; it is more than a passive building site. It is believed that the ribosome moves. The message brought to the ribosome from the nuclear DNA by the messenger RNA is in the form of a string of chemicals arranged in a specific sequence. Along this messenger RNA these chemicals are arranged in groups of three, and each group is called a **codon**. Each codon specifies a particular amino acid. So the messenger RNA associated with a ribosome is like a string of beads; each bead is a codon, which is composed of an exact sequence of three chemicals. And each codon waits for transfer RNA to bring it to an allocated amino acid. It is the codon, then, that the transfer RNA must recognize in order to know at what point at the ribosome to bring its amino acid. Imagine such a string of messenger RNA beads or codons (see Figure 14–9) and, for the sake of explanation, give each codon a number from 1 through 10. (There are actually many more.) Also for convenience, number each molecule of transfer RNA carrying its particular amino acid. Transfer RNA number 1 brings its specific amino acid, number 1, from the cytoplasmic pool to the ribosome, which is now located at codon number 1 of the messenger RNA. There, amino acid number 1 is attached to the ribosome. Transfer RNA number 1 is then released to seek another of its specific amino acids. Carrying its first amino acid, the ribosome moves on to codon number 2. There another transfer

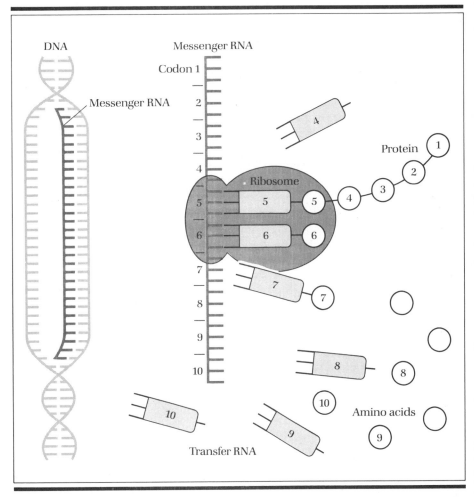

FIGURE 14–9
The synthesis of proteins. The diagram at the left represents the transcription of genetic information from DNA to messenger RNA. The rest of the illustration schematizes the process by which transfer RNA brings its specified amino acid to the ribosome, which is situated at the codon specifying that particular amino acid. Here amino acid number 6, specified by codon number 6, has just been bound to its site on the ribosome by the corresponding transfer RNA. Amino acid number 6 will bond to amino acid number 5, adding to the growing chain. Then the ribosome will move along the messenger RNA to codon number 7. In this example, the chain will be complete when amino acid number 10 has been bonded to it. (Most proteins, however, consist of two or more chains of amino acids.)

RNA (number 2) waits with its amino acid number 2. Amino acid number 2 is then bound to amino acid number 1. The ribosome moves on to the third bead (or codon) of the string of messenger RNA. The process is repeated, and amino acid number 3 is bound to amino acid number 2. In this way one after another specific amino acids are bound to one another, as shown in Figure 14–9. In this sense the ribosome makes its own string of beads, and each bead is an amino acid. The completed amino acid chains are the components of complex proteins. Thus, the ribosome conducts the synthesis of proteins. Finally and, as always, according to DNA instructions, the ribosome has had enough. There are no more codons for it to move along. The ribosome then rids itself of its linked chain of amino acids—of its protein component. What becomes of the complete protein? It contributes to the body structure and function. It will contribute to the eye, or to the heart, or to an enzyme. Multiplied billions of times, this process accounts for the creation of a unique person.* The wonder is not that an occasional error or defect occurs. The wonder is that it occurs so rarely.

How extensive is all this activity?

If it were possible to assemble the DNA in a single human cell into one continuous thread, it would be about a yard long. This three-foot set of instructions for each individual cell is produced by the fusion of egg and sperm at conception and must be precisely replicated billions of times as the embryo develops.[5]

After birth, too, and as long as the individual grows, develops, and ages, the genetic process by which cellular proteins are manufactured is repeated still more billions of times. As long as the person lives, it goes on.

The New Person: Product of Genetics, Environment, or Both?

DNA instructions are many and they are related one to the other. And the whole genetic process takes place in, and is affected by, an all-encompassing environment. Each cell, each nucleus within the cell, each strand of DNA within the nucleus, each chemical component within the DNA, functions within the context of its environment. So there are genetic ecosystems.

If the whole genetic process operates in an environment, it is unavoidably influenced by it. An individual is not merely the result of the *genotype*.**

The genotype is the sum total of the [heredity material] the individual has received, mainly . . . in the form of DNA in the chromosomes of the sex cells. The cytoplasm may also contain some heredity determinants; if so, they are likewise constituents of the genotype.[6]

But with cell division and the resultant increase in the number of cells, with the growth of the organism, the constituents of the genotype must continuously reproduce themselves (replication). The material for this replication is taken from the environment. Consider just the change in size that occurs from our beginning as a fertilized ovum to the time we reach full adulthood.

A human egg cell weighs roughly one twenty-millionth of an ounce; a spermatozoon weighs much less; an adult [male] weighs, let us say, 160 pounds, or some fifty billion times more than an egg cell. . . . The phenotype is, then, a result of interactions between the genotype and the sequence of the environments in which the individual lives. . . .

The "environments" include, of course, everything that can influence [humans] in any way. They include the physical environment —climate, soil, nutrition—and, most important in human development, the cultural environment—all that a person learns, gains, or suffers in his [or her] relations with other people in the family, community, and society to which he [or she] belongs.[7]

Thus, to say that an individual is entirely genetically predetermined is more than an unjustified limitation on human potential. It is also scientifically invalid. And there is an element of absurdity to the "heredity versus environment" argument. For whatever happens in the genetic system is an occurrence within an environment. Genes are not fateful. By themselves, they may decide relatively little.

Nevertheless, practicality does require an answer to the question, "To what extent can genes predispose an individual to develop certain illnesses?" Some disorders are dependent on the presence of a particular genetic error (though not all individuals who carry such errors will necessarily manifest the disorders). Then what is the role of the surrounding environment? This varies. In some instances, such as hemophilia (a disease in which blood fails to clot properly), the environmental influence, compared with the genetic, is surely small. With other conditions, the environment plays a more distinct role. Coronary artery disease, as an example, is greatly influenced by both genetic instruction and environment. Men with a history of heart attacks in their families are more prone to coronary heart disease than men without such a history. But diet (environment) plays

---

*Here one can best comprehend the individuality of the single being. Within each new zygote formed by the union of sperm and ovum is a completely new organization of DNA, a new master plan, a new set of instructions. Never before has there been a zygote with exactly the same DNA code.

The **genotype is the genetic basis of the trait; the **phenotype** is the physical appearance of the individual that results from the interaction of the genotype and the environment.

an important role too. How long the condition remains latent and, when revealed, how severely it is manifested may be profoundly influenced by the environment. Another example: Much has been written of the relationship between an XYY chromosomal pattern and aggressive behavior. The association may have some truth. However, most aggressive behavior is unrelated to the XYY chromosome. Moreover, a gentle, well-adjusted person may carry an XYY chromosomal aberration and harm nobody. Another with the same genetic disorder will be a violent, homicidal menace. The difference may be in the environment.

Genetic Disorder

Human genetic problems are related either to (1) an error in the physical or chemical *structure* of a chromosome or (2) an error in the *amount* of chromosomal material in the cell. This second error is generally expressed in terms of the *number* of chromosomes in the cell.

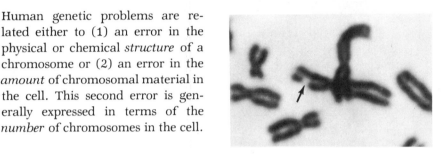

FIGURE 14–10
A chromosomal break (arrow) due to radiation.

ketonuria or PKU (see page 434) are examples. Or disease of the blood or blood-forming organs may result. Hemophilia is one of these. By no means are all mutations spontaneous, however. Some are plainly *induced* by an external environmental stimulus. An example is genetic disorder caused by radiation (see Figure 14–10).

Disorders of Chromosomal Structure

SPONTANEOUS MUTATIONS

Our ancestors were once fishlike, and within the uterus we still live submerged in water like a fish. Slowly, over millions of years, our ancestors left the sea and, over still more millions of years, adapted to a new environment. All these adaptive changes were made possible by infinitely gradual gene changes, or **mutations** (Latin *mutare*, "to change"). But there are many more rapid changes that happen as a result of environmental factors, such as occurs when the German measles virus attacks the embryo. However, some genetic changes, although occurring in the environment, do not seem to be primarily caused by it. These are called *spontaneous*, meaning that for some reason a spontaneous change of some part of the chemical structure of the DNA takes place. So a change of structure in the DNA string of chemicals just

happens without any known influence on it by anything in the environment. If the change is not basically molded by the surrounding environment, how, then, may one account for the existence of a mutation in chromosomal structure? What causes a spontaneous change in DNA? The answer to this question remains unknown. But it is known that even one spontaneously mutant gene can result in profound developmental changes and hereditary health problems. Anatomical and, therefore, functional deviations from the norm result. There may be inborn errors of metabolism. Disorders of carbohydrate metabolism (the way the body handles sugars), such as diabetes mellitus, and of amino acid metabolism such as phenyl-

CHROMOSOMAL TRANSLOCATION AND DELETION

Sometimes a chromosome breaks, causing DNA structure to be disrupted. The chromosome may heal into a new and different structure. Or it may remain in fragments. Or it may be just partly repaired, leaving a piece out of its structure. Or two chromosomes may exchange pieces. *Translocation* occurs when a segment or a fragment of one chromosome shifts into another part of a noncorresponding chromosome. Sometimes, one of the products of such an exchange is so small it gets lost. This is called *deletion*. Whatever occurs, the chromosome is changed for the worse. Genetic instruction by the DNA of the affected chromosomes is awry. Usually a fertilized egg that contains a broken or wrongly formed chromosome dies. Occasionally, the zygote lives. The individual develops to suffer various deficiencies.

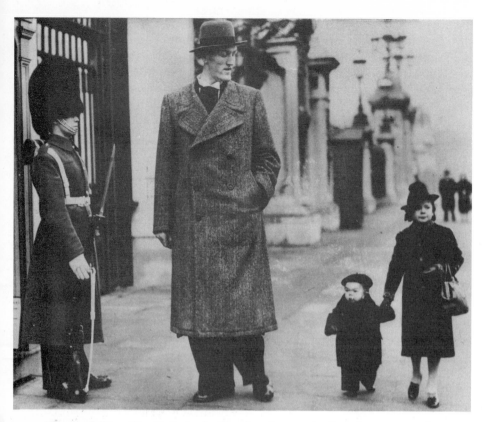

Three adults with pituitary dysfunction (a genetic disorder) walk past a sentry at Buckingham Palace. Olaf Petursson, 25, is eight feet six inches tall; Prince Daumling, 33, is eighteen inches; and Helga, 29 is three feet six inches.

Disorders of Chromosome Number During Meiosis or Early Mitosis

Sometimes it is not a changed chromosomal structure that results in disease. Rather it is an error in the total number of chromosomes that find their way into the cells. Normally, there are forty-six. With genetically related sickness, there may be too many or too few. How can this happen?

ERRORS DURING MEIOSIS

Study again Figure 14–4 illustrating meiosis. This shows how the chromosomes, having duplicated themselves, separate. Consequently, after the first cell division, when two cells are formed, each cell normally has duplicates of only a single member of each original pair of chromosomes. Sometimes, though, something goes wrong, and during meiosis, the chromosomes of a pair do not separate. Then, one cell receives both chromosomes of the pair, while the other gamete receives none. This is called *meiotic nondisjunction*. Nobody really knows why it happens.

It will be further noted in Figure 14–4 that there are two meiotic divisions. Meiotic nondisjunction can also occur during the second meiotic division after a normal first division. Upon fertilization, should a gamete with a missing chromosome unite with a normal gamete, the zygote and all the cells consequent to its multiplication by mitosis will have forty-five chromosomes instead of the normal forty-six. This condition is called *monosomy.* Should a gamete with an extra chromosome unite with a normal gamete, the zygote will have forty-seven chromosomes. This is *trisomy.* The trisomy and monosomy of meiotic nondisjunction can affect both the autosomal chromosomes and the sex chromosomes.

TRISOMY 21   The most common trisomy affects the twenty-first autosome. **Trisomy 21** is one cause of **Down's syndrome,*** in which nondisjunction occurs with chromosomes other than the X and Y. As a result of this autosomal aberration, the individual has forty-seven instead of forty-six chromosomes. Much more rarely, an extra 21 chromosome may in some way join with another chromosome. Although the total number of chromosomes is forty-six, the Down's syndrome still occurs. This is called the *translocation type* of Down's syndrome. Children with Down's syndrome (named after a nineteenth-century English physician, John Down) are physically and mentally retarded. Muscle tone is poor. The tongue is large. The eyes appear slanted, which accounts for the former name of the condition— Mongolism. Palm-prints and foot-prints are abnormal. The age of the mother is a factor in Down's syndrome. After about the age of thirty-five, the older she is at the time of her pregnancy, the greater her chances of giving birth to a child with this condition. Nevertheless,

*A *syndrome* refers to a set of signs and symptoms occurring together, as a group, in a disease state.

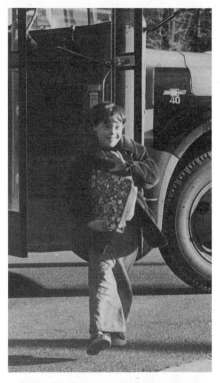

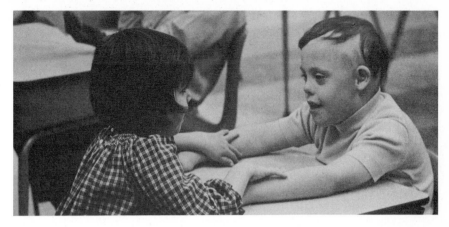

PHOTO ESSAY

These pictures show some moments in a day of ten-year-old David Roberts' life. David has Down's syndrome (Trisomy 21). A loving and generous boy, his I.Q. is only 52, but expressed in terms of emotional development it is a superior 115. David is more fortunate than most children with Down's syndrome. He has understanding parents. His father, a professional photographer, took these pictures; his mother, a writer, collaborated with her husband on a moving book urging that children like David be kept in a warm family environment if possible. David also has an informed physician, and he leads a rich social life.

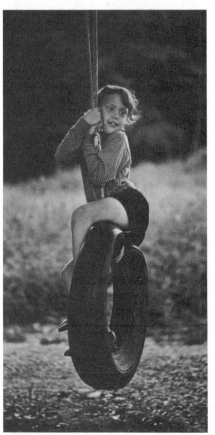

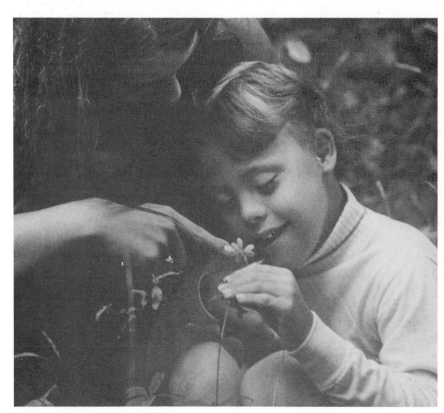

more of these babies are born to younger women than was formerly thought. Also, it should not be thought that the mother's age is a *deciding* factor in Down's syndrome. In a fourth of the cases, the extra chromosome comes from the father.[8]

ERRORS DURING MITOSIS

Most abnormalities from nondisjunction occur during meiosis, but nondisjunction can also occur during mitosis. This is how. A normal sperm fertilizes a normal ovum. But during the early mitotic cellular multiplication following fertilization, two chromosomes may fail to separate. In this way, half the body cells of the affected individual have three rather than two of a particular chromosome (forty-seven total), and the other half of the body cells have one instead of the normal two (forty-five total). This condition is called *mosaicism*. Sometimes three types of cells may occur in one person's body: normal (forty-six chromosomes), trisomic (forty-seven), and monosomic (forty-five). Mosaicism can also result not from failure of chromosomes to separate, but from the loss of a chromosome during the cell division of mitosis. In all these mitotic variables there is the potential for grave illness.

Illness and the Genes of Sex and Race

Illness patterns are profoundly influenced by such genetic factors as sex and race.

Sex

Fortunately, the union of the human sperm and egg results in about 140 males for every 100 females. Fortunately, because the male's hold on life is relatively feeble compared with that of the female. Even within the safety of the uterus, 50 percent more males than females perish. In all age groups up to the age of eighty, there is a consistent excess of male over female deaths. In 1977 almost three times as many males between the ages of fifteen and twenty-four died as did females in the same age group (refer back to Table 5–1 on page 148). Neither U.S. civilians nor members of the armed forces who died outside this country were included in these data. Moreover, the ratios were similar in 1960, a year in which the United States was not engaged in hostilities. Long-time U.S. statistics show that male death rates are greater than female death rates in every five-year age group from birth to the eightieth year. And, in the fifteen-to-twenty-four age group the difference usually is almost three times as great.

For the fragile male, almost all disease categories are more lethal. Death rates from the major heart and blood vessel diseases, as well as those from cancers, accidents, and the more common infections, are considerably higher for males. Aside from the complications of childbirth, it is only in a relatively few disease categories that females die more frequently. Syphilis has been called "the chivalric disease." It surely shows special consideration for the female. For her, the disease is milder and less likely to involve the heart and central nervous system. Syphilis kills less than half as many females as males. When suitable antibiotics are given to a male child with bacterial meningitis, his chances for survival are less than those of a female child of about the same age and in the same circumstances. Adverse effects of atomic radiation are more frequent in boys than girls.

Why the difference? There is a good theory. As has been stated, of the forty-six chromosomes in the primordial sex cell of the ovum or sperm, two are sex chromosomes. The female has two X chromosomes. These are equal. The male, however, has one X chromosome and one Y chromosome. Thus, the arrangement of the chromosomes is possibly to the advantage of the female. If something goes wrong with one of her X chromosomes, perhaps she can rely on the other. The male is denied such possible insurance. There is evidence, at present inconclusive, that this biological inequality may be gradually equalizing because of the inactivation of one of the female X chromosomes. Nonetheless, the male is indeed the weaker sex.

Race

Sickle-cell anemia (discussed below) is much more frequent among Negroes than Caucasians. In the United States, tooth decay is more common among Caucasians than Negroes. Among women in Japan, cancer of the breast is rare. One should, however, view with caution the varying frequency of diseases in races. True, heredity helps decide body reactions to disease. But social and economic opportunity, rather than genes, accounts for the comparatively greater frequency of such illnesses as tuberculosis and syphilis among blacks in this country. Moreover, recent studies emphasize the association between the malnutrition of poverty and mental retardation.

SICKLE CELL DISEASE

Sickle cell disease is a genetically transmitted abnormality in the chemical structure of the hemoglobin molecules within the red blood cells. As a result, the hemoglobin molecules can link together to distort the cell. Thus, the ordinarily doughnut-shaped red blood cell is forced into the shape of a sickle (see Figure 14–11). The molecular change is minute; the human suffering caused by it is immense. In this country, sickle cell disease largely affects the Negro population. However, the disease can occur among Caucasians from the Mediterranean area and among people of the Middle East and certain parts of India. More than two million U.S. Negroes carry the relatively benign *sickle-cell trait*; that is, they have the capacity to pass the disease on to their children. Over fifty thousand U.S. Negroes have the much more serious **sickle-cell anemia**.

With sickle-cell anemia, all the red blood cells contain the abnormally structured hemoglobin molecules; all the red blood cells are potential candidates for sickling. A child with this disease can become desperately ill even without the occurrence of a special set of circumstances. Normally, the oxygen tension in the capillaries and small veins is low. In these tiny blood vessels, red blood cells containing abnormally structured hemoglobin will tend to sickle. Worse, the misshapen red blood cells clump together. In this way, they plug the small blood vessels and thus partly or wholly deprive needy tissues of blood and oxygen. Cells die, as do the tissues of which they are a part. Pain, loss of appetite, joint swellings, and ulcers all can plague the afflicted child. (The pain is similar to the pain of an acute heart attack and occurs for the same reason—lack of oxygen to the tissues.) Normally, red blood cells live more than one hundred days. Sickled, they are destroyed, mostly in the spleen, in ten to twenty-five days. The patient is exhausted, wan, often desperately anemic. There is constant risk from infections, such as pneumonia. Periodically, crises of intense sickness imperil life.

Those who suffer from sickle-cell anemia can find hope in renewed research and treatments. And it has been recently reported that it is possible to have sickle cell disease in a mild form. One study of a small group of adults with mild sickle cell disease revealed that they had few or no crises of pain, were actively employed, and led normal lives. How often this mild form of the illness occurs is undetermined. Those who find that they carry the trait must make their own decision as to whether to risk passing on a tragic genetic legacy to future generations. However, early diagnosis remains essential. It not only makes possible early treatment but also affords the time necessary to make thoughtful decisions about having children. Someday, genetic surgery may be possible to replace the gene responsible for the abnormal hemoglobin with a gene that codes for normal hemoglobin.

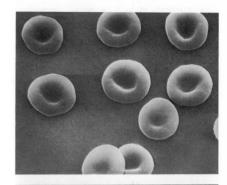

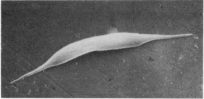

FIGURE 14–11
The round objects in the top photograph are normal human red blood cells; at bottom is a typical sickle-shaped red blood cell.

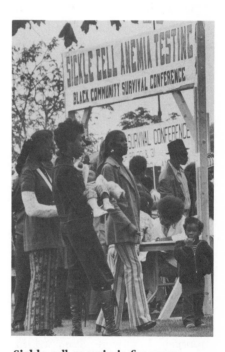

Sickle-cell anemia is far more common among blacks than whites. A carrier of the sickle-cell trait must often make his or her own difficult decision about having children. Physicians and counselors trained in this area of medicine can be of great help.

The Genetic Ecosystem:
Environmental Influences on the Fertilized Ovum

Within the nucleus of the cell, the basic genetic chemicals are arranged in relation to one another. And they are dependent on one another. So, inside the very nucleus there is an environment with ecological balance or imbalance.

The genes contain a pattern set to direct development, but no amount of healthy genetic instruction can bid cytoplasm sickened by an abnormal environment to be normal. Nor can a healthy cytoplasm receive beneficial patterns of instruction from a gene made deviant by its environment. Normal genetic action, then, depends on a normal environment inside and outside the cell. The internal drama of the cell will be disarranged not only when the chromosomal players unaccountably neglect their proper parts but also when they are surrounded by destructive microorganisms or hostile drugs or searing radiation. That is why German measles (rubella) and thalidomide and atomic radiation kill and cripple the unborn. Let's consider these and other influences now.

Nutrition

The importance of good nutrition, and the consequences to the child of improper diet, were discussed in detail in Chapter 9. In summary, women who eat a balanced diet and who take the vitamin folic acid and iron as supplements are giving their unborn children the best chance for successful development.

Infection

Women who develop *German measles* (rubella) during the first three months of pregnancy are over five times (15 percent) more likely to give birth to a defective child than are women who do not have the disease (2.8 percent). The heart, hearing, and vision (cataracts) are most commonly affected. There is some medical opinion that a woman who contracts *regular measles* (rubeola) also has a greater chance of having a defective child. But many physicians think that this is unproved. Effective vaccines are now available to prevent both regular measles and German measles (page 66).

There is some limited evidence that *infectious hepatitis*, a third viral illness, can affect chromosomes. Because *smallpox vaccine* is composed of a living virus, it may affect the unborn child. Consequently, pregnant women are not usually vaccinated against smallpox. *Syphilis* can also be transmitted from mother to unborn child. Adequate treatment of the mother can prevent tragedy for both. Another major infection that may be transmitted from the pregnant woman to the fetus is *cytomegalic inclusion disease* (page 73). This illness, usually noted during the first month of life, is caused by a viral infection. It is revealed by a wide variety and degree of malformations in the child. As with German measles, children with the disease may be contagious for months after delivery. They should, therefore, be isolated, particularly from pregnant women.

Direct Radiation

Excessive exposure of a pregnant woman to X-rays can result in either fetal death or a malformed child. Women should, therefore, always advise a doctor who plans to X-ray them of a possible, still unapparent, pregnancy.

There have been large-scale experiences with radiation. Seven out of eleven Hiroshima children were born retarded if, within the first twenty weeks of conception, their mothers stood within 1,200 meters of absolute center of the atomic bomb blast. Others, whose mothers were at a greater distance, had malformed hips, eyes, and hearts. Some, symptomless at birth, developed poorly.

In 1954 the United States made a test explosion of a nuclear device at Bikini. An unpredictable wind deposited significant amounts of radioactive material on the residents of four nearby islands as well as on twenty-three Japanese fishermen. Years later, children of the islands who were less than five years old at the time of exposure were found to be retarded in physical growth.

Why does radiation cause abnormal babies? The baby is a triumph of recent cellular multiplication. And radiation has a preference for multiplying cells. It requires more radiation to kill a fly than a mouse. Why? As a maggot, the fly passes through all its phases of growth and development. As an adult, it has few dividing cells. Adult mice and humans have many dividing cells. It is these that are sensitive to radiation.

Radiation reaching the testes or ovaries, and thereby the reproductive cells, can cause changes in the structure of the DNA (genes). Mutation rates are increased by radiation. Since over 99 percent of mutations are harmful, and since they do accumulate in humans, the threat to future generations is apparent. Depending on the amount, moreover, radiation may cause chromosomal breaks and translocations. So another danger of radiation, more recently recognized, is related to chromosomal damage. Thus, radiation may be one of the causes of a wide variety of genetic disorders.

Chemical Pollution

The placenta is no longer considered an effective barrier against environmental pollutants (see Chapter 2). Large molecules of polluting substances are now thought merely to cross the placenta more slowly than molecules that are small. Added to this are the constant risks that are taken by prolonged use of chemicals, such as food additives, without adequate knowledge of the effects they will have. The ongoing use of diethylstilbesterol in meat animals is but one example of this kind of error. Another example is the mercury pollution of water and fish that resulted in the poisoning of numerous Japanese; women who ate the poisoned fish gave birth to blind and paralyzed children.[9] Laboratory evidence suggests that a major air pollutant, sulfur dioxide, may cause genetic damage.[10]

Since standard test systems for many chemical pollutants are extremely insensitive, it would seem reasonable to take as few chances as

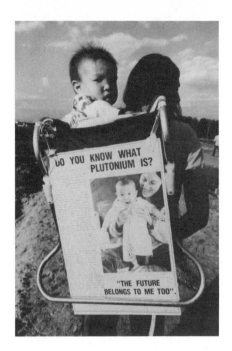

possible. Strict regulations should be imposed on chemicals that may possibly affect human beings in an adverse way. And those regulations should be in effect not after, but before human harm occurs.

Noise

It is known that undue noise can have a negative effect on animal reproduction.[11] The effect it has on the unborn or newborn human is still being researched. One hospital study found that "under the plastic hood of the incubators the noise spectrum fell well above the recommended acceptance level and, due to the prolonged exposure time, very close to the danger area."[12]

Japanese scientists have made an interesting observation. Studying 307 babies, they noticed that the way a baby reacted to aircraft noise depended on the length of the mother's stay in noisy Itami City,

which is near the Osaka International Airport. When a woman spent the second half of her pregnancy or the period directly after the birth of the child in Itami, the child was much more likely to be disturbed by the aircraft noise. Why? The child could hear the noise. When the women moved to Itami before conception, so that the babies spent their entire fetal life near the airport, 58 percent of the babies slept soundly during airplane noise, and only 6 percent awoke and cried. Apparently most of the babies could not hear the noise. A possible explanation, therefore, for the babies who are apparently less disturbed by airplane noise is that they are born partially deaf and that the damage to their delicate developing hearing structure occurred in the early months of pregnancy.

Endocrine Gland Influences

Insulin, a product of specific cells within the pancreas, helps regulate carbohydrate metabolism. Without enough insulin, one form of diabetes develops (see pages 476–479). Diabetic mothers have malformed children ten times more frequently than the average.

The Rh Factor

In 1968, in this country, 941 babies reportedly died of **Rh hemolytic disease**, a condition resulting from too much destruction of red blood cells. Since that time that number has greatly decreased. Before examining the reasons, let's consider the disease itself. The condition is also known as *erythroblastosis fetalis* (Greek *erythros*, "red," +

blastos, "germ," + *osis*, "increase"). The increase in red "germ" cells refers to the numerous immature primitive red blood cells seen in the circulation of the affected child. Their development in the fetus accounts for the term *fetalis*. Why do they occur? To make up for the excess number of red cells that are destroyed. Why are the normal red blood cells destroyed? In this the Rh factor is involved. What is Rh?

Rh is a chemical substance. Its exact structure is unknown. It sits on the surface of the red blood cells of 85 percent of all people. They are then *Rh positive*. The 15 percent who do not carry it are *Rh negative*. Why is it called Rh? The *Rh*esus monkey also has the factor. Has Rh a known purpose? No. It just causes trouble. How?

In one of eight marriages, the woman is Rh negative and the man is Rh positive. If the child is Rh negative, like the mother, there is no problem. But the child may inherit the Rh-positive factor from the father. The Rh-negative mother thus carries an Rh-positive child. Erythroblastosis fetalis occurs when the Rh-positive blood of the child enters the mother's blood. The baby's Rh-positive factor is foreign to the mother. It is an *antigen*, an antibody generator. To neutralize her baby's Rh-positive antigens, the mother produces antibodies in her blood. When these antibodies enter the child, they destroy red blood cells.

There are two ways in which the child's antibody-stimulating Rh-positive factor reaches the mother's circulation. One way is through the placenta during pregnancy. Normally, only small amounts of baby antigen reach the mother in this fashion. During the time that she is carrying her first child, these minimal amounts are usually not enough to cause the mother to manufacture antibodies. The second way that the child's Rh antigen enters the mother occurs during delivery. Indeed, most of the child's Rh-positive blood reaches the mother during delivery, since, at that time, the afterbirth loosens and bleeds. Therefore, it is after delivery that she manufactures most of her antibodies. Once she has manufactured such antibodies, she will be restimulated, in future pregnancies involving an Rh-positive fetus, to produce antibodies with only the small amount of antigen that enters through the placenta. That is why erythroblastosis fetalis usually affects the child of a later pregnancy more severely than an earlier one; a third child, for example, will be more adversely affected than a second; a fourth child, more than a third; and so on.

To repeat, then, in most cases the mother usually does not produce enough antibodies to harm the child during a first pregnancy. During the actual delivery of her first child, however, she receives enough Rh-positive blood to manufacture a high level of antibodies. These antibodies remain in the mother's blood. With the second child, harm is likely. As with the first child, the second may inherit the father's Rh-positive blood factor. The mother's antibodies, formed in response to the Rh-positive antigen of the first baby, now pass through the placenta of the second baby. The antibodies destroy the unborn second child's red blood cells. To recoup, the child hastily makes new cells. These are the primitive red blood cells of erythroblastosis fetalis. But, as immature cells, they do not make up for the destroyed mature red blood cells. Anemia results. Products from the child's red cell destruction seep into the skin. Jaundice occurs.

The 941 U.S. babies who reportedly died of Rh hemolytic disease in 1968 resulted in a death rate (deaths per 100,000 live births) of 2.72. By the end of 1976 these had decreased to 233 deaths, and a death rate of 0.74. And there is continued hope for even greater improvement.[13]

Three new procedures are responsible for the declining death rate associated with Rh hemolytic disease: (1) Complete replacement by transfusion of the baby's blood; (2) transfusion of the baby with Rh-negative blood while still in the uterus; and (3) the *preventive* injection of Rh immunoglobulin containing antibodies against Rh-positive blood to Rh-negative women following *abortion*, *amniocentesis* (defined later in this chapter), and the delivery of an Rh positive infant.

The Mother's Age

As a rule, young mothers (under thirty) provide a relatively safer intrauterine environment for their children than do older mothers. Perhaps older women do not produce adequate endocrine secretions to guarantee proper development of ova. With increase in the mother's age, for example, the frequency of Down's syndrome as well as some other rare abnormalities increases.

It should not be concluded, however, that the younger mother needs less medical attention than the older mother. Indeed, as has been already stated, more younger mothers are known to have children with Down's syndrome than was formerly thought. Genetic counseling must change to account for this fact. Child marriage and pregnancies in the country are but a small percentage of the total, but they are by no means rare. The young teenage mother presents special problems (see page 408).

Drugs

In 1961 and 1962, thousands of children whose mothers had taken a German-made tranquilizer containing the drug thalidomide early in pregnancy were born severely malformed. This calamity will long be a mournful reminder of the danger of using inadequately tested drugs. The complexity of testing drugs can be illustrated by the fact that humans are sixty times more sensitive to thalidomide than mice, one hundred times more sensitive to it than rats, two hundred times more than dogs, and seven hundred times more than hamsters. Thus, enormous doses, given to several species, might not indicate the danger to the human embryo and fetus.[14] When one considers the real scientific problems that exist in establishing toxicity in controlled laboratory-produced substances, the extreme foolhardiness of the abuse of illicit, unmeasured, untested, and grossly impure street drugs becomes even more apparent.

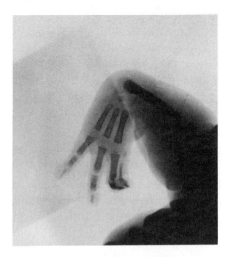

X-ray photograph showing the deformed arm of a one-year-old child whose mother had taken the drug thalidomide during early pregnancy.

Whether drugs will affect the unborn child depends on the stage of the child's development. During the first four weeks, the embryo cells undergo extremely rapid multiplication. Any drug that can attack rapidly multiplying cells may cause changes that are significant enough to cause loss of the embryo. If this

occurs between menstrual periods, the woman does not even know of her pregnancy. Drug action at a more advanced stage (the fifth to the eighth week) can cause abnormal tissue and organ differentiation. There are critical periods in the development of the human embryo during which various structures are being differentiated and thus during which some drugs may have the most profoundly deleterious effects. Some of these are the nervous system, days fifteen to twenty-five; eyes, days twenty-four to forty; heart, days twenty to forty; legs, days twenty-four to thirty-six.[15] By the eighth week of pregnancy, differentiation of these body parts is basically complete. After that, the hazard to the fetus diminishes greatly. It should, however, be understood that some drugs not responsible for immediately apparent effects may nevertheless retard growth and development. Some of the possible effects of specific drugs on the unborn child were discussed in Chapter 7.

Birth Defects

More babies die of defective development before they are born than after. Such defective embryos account for most of the million miscarriages in this country every year. Most occur early in pregnancy—the period of greatest vulnerability of the developing child. Some miscarriages occur so early that the woman may never have known she was pregnant. Others occur after a few months. Many of these deaths are nature's way of getting rid of an abnormally developing fetus so that a new and better one can be started. Of every sixteen babies born alive in

this country, one is found to be defective within the first year. (Some birth defects, such as gout and diabetes, may not be apparent for years.) This amounts to about a quarter of a million babies a year. Eighteen thousand of these die in the first year of life.

Of course, as the birthrate increases, so do the number of babies born with birth defects. Moreover, modern surgery, newer drugs, and more research combine to keep many defective children alive to adolescence and maturity. Though this kind of effort will always be a

basic purpose of medicine, such survival nevertheless means problems for individuals and society. (Table 14–1 lists and provides information on the more common birth defects.)

How to Avoid Some Birth Defects

1. A physician should be seen as soon as pregnancy is suspected because the fetus is most vulnerable during early pregnancy (the first twenty weeks), and delay in-

creases the chances of premature birth and, therefore, a defective child.

2. No medication, not even vitamins, should be taken unless prescribed by the family doctor. Drugs may pass through the placenta and the child may be injured. Alcohol should be avoided. Even moderate drinking of alcohol may damage the unborn child.

3. Except in emergencies, abdominal X-rays early in pregnancy should be avoided. Any physician about to X-ray a female patient, therefore, will want to know if she is pregnant.

4. Cigarette smoking should be discontinued. The possible ill effects of cigarette smoking on an unborn child were discussed on page 224.

5. If possible, elective surgery should be delayed until after pregnancy. Abrupt changes to high altitudes should be avoided. In both instances, even temporary oxygen depletion might injure the embryo. In commercial airliners this is not ordinarily a problem.

6. An adequate diet must be followed.

7. Relatives should never marry. Even rare hereditary disorders occur much more commonly among the children of such unions.

8. Under some circumstances, the advice of a genetic counselor is indicated. The family physician will know if such help is necessary.

9. The mental retardation of the child with untreated **phenylketonuria** (**PKU**)[16] (see Table 14–1) is always tragically obvious. However, one aspect of the condition has frequently been overlooked. Successful treatment of PKU during infancy and childhood has enabled many women to have normal children. However, treatment is not often maintained into adolescence. Untreated maternal PKU may result in a damaged fetus; indeed, the fetus can be adversely affected even in a woman of normal intelligence with unsuspected PKU. Dietetic treatment of a woman known to have PKU should be started before the onset of pregnancy. To discover unknown cases, sisters of all phenylketonuric patients should be examined, regardless of their intelligence. Also, when a woman has had one or more retarded children without obvious cause, PKU must be considered. Some physicians recommend screening for PKU of all women before pregnancy occurs.[17]

TABLE 14–1 The More Common Birth Defects				
TYPE OF DEFECT	APPROXIMATE FREQUENCY	DESCRIPTION	CAUSES AND TREATMENT
Birthmarks	Very common.	The disfiguring ones are red or wine-colored patches of small dilated blood vessels.	Cause unknown. Treatments include plastic surgery, skin grafts, or tattooing of normal skin colors over the purple area.
Cleft lip (harelip)	About 1 in 1,000 babies born in the U.S. has a cleft lip; two-thirds of these also have a cleft palate. Frequency seems lower in blacks than in whites.	If embryonic swellings that will become the upper lip do not fuse at the right time, the gap remains and the baby will have a cleft lip.	Sometimes related to genetic defects. Influence of intrauterine environment and of some drugs given during pregnancy is being studied. Harelip can be repaired in the first few weeks after birth, and cleft palate before age fourteen months in most cases.
Cleft palate	About 1 in every 2,500 babies has a cleft palate without cleft lip. The two conditions are not genetically related.	A cleft palate is a hole in the roof of the mouth.	

TABLE 14-1 (*continued*)

TYPE OF DEFECT	APPROXIMATE FREQUENCY	DESCRIPTION	CAUSES AND TREATMENT
Clubfoot	1 in 300.	The foot turns inward (usually) or outward and is fixed in a tip-toe position.	Possibly due to position of child in uterus or to maldevelopment of the limb bud. Treatments include shoe splints, braces, corrective shoes, plaster casts, or surgery. Tends to recur, so treatment must begin early and is often prolonged.
Congenital heart disease	1 in 125.	Some are so slight as to cause little strain on the heart; others are fatal. In some abnormalities, the baby appears blue.	German measles during pregnancy is one cause. Many heart conditions can now be repaired by surgery, saving lives and preventing invalidism.
Congenital urinary tract defects	1 in 250.	May involve kidneys, ureters, bladder, and genitalia. Organs may be absent, fused, or obstructed.	Causes include certain hormones given during pregnancy. Some hereditary tendency. Most conditions are correctable by surgery.
Diabetes	The prevalence of diabetes increases with advancing age, varying from about 1 case per 625 persons under age 25 to 1 in 15 persons age 65 to 75.	A metabolic disorder. The body cannot handle sugar normally, and high glucose levels in the blood and urine result. This familial condition is related without any question to abnormal utilization of insulin. Long-standing diabetics may develop complications involving blood vessels, kidneys, heart, eyes, and peripheral nerves. Obesity predisposes individuals to the disease.	Marked hereditary tendency. Persons with family history of diabetes should seek periodic check-up. Doctors can recognize symptoms, make positive diagnosis, and prescribe specific treatment. Special diets, oral medication, and injections of insulin are measures that will usually keep condition under control and permit normal activity. Good prenatal care is especially important for known or suspected diabetics.
Erythroblastosis fetalis (Rh hemolytic disease)	Prior to use of Rh immune globulin, hemolytic disease of the fetus and newborn occurred in 1 in every 150 to 200 pregnancies. About 15 percent of whites and 5 percent of blacks in the United States are Rh negative.	Without treatment or early prevention baby is often yellow soon after birth. Anemia is a common symptom. Mental retardation may be severe. Erythroblastosis is a common cause of stillbirth.	Baby inherits Rh-positive gene from his father, and the mother is Rh negative. Red blood cells of fetus reach mother's blood, causing her blood to form antibodies that pass back through the placenta to the baby and destroy his red cells in varying degrees. First pregnancy is usually uneventful. Rh immune globulin prevents sensitization of mother, if given soon after birth of each baby. Intrauterine or exchange transfusion, replacing baby's blood with compatible blood right after birth, prevents severe damage to babies of sensitized mothers.

TABLE 14–1 *(continued)*

TYPE OF DEFECT	APPROXIMATE FREQUENCY	DESCRIPTION	CAUSES AND TREATMENT
Extra fingers and toes (polydactyly)	Extra digits are twice as frequent as fused digits. Incidence is 1 in 100 among blacks; 1 in 600 among whites.	Extra fingers or toes.	Cause unknown; frequently hereditary. Cure is amputation of the extra digits. This can often be done at birth or at about age three.
Fused fingers and toes (syndactyly)	Fused digits do not have such racial variation.	Too few digits.	Surgery can improve the function and appearance of the hand or foot.
Fibrocystic disease (cystic fibrosis)	About 1 in 1,000 births. Rare among blacks; infrequent in Orientals.	A sickly, malnourished child with persistent intestinal difficulties and chronic respiratory problems. Death usually due to pneumonia or other lung complications.	Hereditary. New tests detect carriers. Mucus blocks the exit of digestive juices from the pancreas into the intestinal tract. Excess mucus is also secreted by lungs. Treatments have extended life.
Galactosemia	Somewhat more rare than PKU (see below).	Causes eye cataracts and severe damage to liver and brain, resulting in mental retardation.	Hereditary. Caused by absence of an enzyme required to convert galactose to glucose. Experiments show that early recognition and dietary treatment can arrest the disease. Diagnosis can be made at birth.
Hydrocephaly (water on the brain)	1 in 500.	Enlargement of the head due to excessive fluid within the brain. Fluid's pressure often causes compression of the brain with resulting mental retardation.	Cause unknown. May result from prenatal infection or abnormality in development. Treatment is an operation to lead fluid from brain into bloodstream or some other body cavity. Frequently fatal if not treated.
Missing limbs	Very rare.	One to four limbs missing or seriously deformed.	Cause unknown. A large international outbreak was due to thalidomide used by pregnant mothers. Great strides have been made in prosthetic (artificial) devices.
Down's syndrome (Mongolism)	1 in 600. Women twenty-five years old have about 1 chance in 2,000 of producing a Mongoloid child. Women of forty-five have about 1 chance in 50.	Short stature, slightly slanted eyes, and varying degrees of mental retardation.	All patients have an extra chromosome or its equivalent. Causes can be hereditary or environmental. No known cure, but IQ can be improved by special training.
Open spine (spina bifida)	Approximately 1 in every 500 births. More common among whites than blacks. About half of the patients are also victims of hydrocephaly (see above).	Failure of the spine to close permits the protrusion of spinal cord or nerves; often leads to total dysfunction of legs, bladder, and rectum. Often the child has other serious defects.	Cause unknown. Sometimes surgery in the early months of life can correct or arrest the condition, preventing other complications. Several new surgical techniques are being used on the bladder, rectum, and spinal cord.

TABLE 14-1 *(continued)*

TYPE OF DEFECT	APPROXIMATE FREQUENCY	DESCRIPTION	CAUSES AND TREATMENT
Phenyl-ketonuria (PKU)	Approximately 1 in 20,000 whites. Extremely rare in blacks.	Child appears normal at birth, but the mind stops developing during the first year. Retardation is severe. One-third never learn to walk; two-thirds never learn to talk. Pigment of skin and hair is decreased.	Hereditary metabolic defect. The liver enzyme that changes the protein phenylalanine to tyrosine is inactive or absent; phenylalanine accumulates. PKU can be detected within the first few days of life. Treatment is special low-phenylalanine diet for the infant, which can prevent further retardation. Early treatment important. Some experiments show that after a few years PKU children can be fed normal diets.
Sickle-cell anemia	One in 10 American blacks has trait; 1 in 400 has anemia. Low among whites.	Red blood cells of people with this disease periodically become crescent- or sickle-shaped, clump together, and prevent transport of needed oxygen to body organs, causing painful sickle-cell "crises."	Hereditary. When both parents have the trait, each child has 1 chance in 4 of inheriting sickle-cell anemia. Careful management can help prevent crises; research to develop medications is promising.

SOURCE: Adapted from a booklet published by the National Foundation—March of Dimes, White Plains, New York.

Genetic Counseling

Second cousins want to marry. They share three diabetic parents. What are the genetic dangers? A couple has a second child who has Down's syndrome. Can they hope for a normal child? A young man's sister has been incapacitated for ten years with severe muscular dystrophy. The young man is engaged to be married and is deeply troubled about the chances of his future children having the disease. An adoption agency has a potential home for a pretty child, the product of an incestuous union. What are the risks to the adopting parents? Parents are worried about their baby. Something is wrong, and the family doctor has suggested they seek genetic counseling.

These are some of the intensely human problems brought to genetic counselors. They can help as no one else can. They discuss risks with those who inquire. In the event a diagnosis of a possible genetic illness is required, more detailed work is necessary. Genetic counselors can best be located through local medical societies, hospitals, and medical schools of universities.

At this point, it would be well to differentiate between two frequently confused terms. The word *congenital* does not have the same meaning as *genetic*. **Congenital** means only "present at birth." It does not signify the cause of a condition. Some congenital conditions are not genetic, and many genetic conditions are not congenital. Huntington's chorea is an illness marked by irregular movements, speech disturbances, and mental deterioration. Although a genetic disease, it is not manifested until adulthood. However, maternal infection with German measles virus in the first trimester of pregnancy may result in the infection of the unborn child. The child may then manifest the congenital rubella syndrome.

The mere fact that an illness occurs in more than one member of a

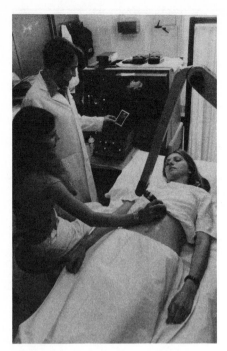

FIGURE 14-12
Ultrasound is a valuable technique for detecting abnormalities in any body part—whether bone or tissue. Here it is being used to check the development of a fetus.

family is not necessarily an indication that it is hereditary. Family members often share similar environments and habits; more likely, a combination of environment and genetic predisposition is responsible. During a person's first visit to a geneticist (who is usually, but not necessarily, a physician), a complete family history is taken. In order to obtain a complete family history, more than one family member may have to be interviewed. The geneticist must obtain information about both the paternal and maternal grandparents, parents, siblings, uncles, aunts, and first cousins. Miscarriages, stillbirths, and infant deaths are carefully noted. The inquiry may, but usually does not, extend beyond the first cousins.

From the family history, the geneticist constructs a *pedigree chart*. Blood samples and cell studies provide body material for study. These are taken from the patient, both parents, and other relatives likely to be carrying an abnormality.

Diagnosis of the Unborn

In competent hands, **amniocentesis** is a safe procedure in which a needle is inserted through the walls of both the abdomen and the pregnant uterus in order to withdraw for examination the amniotic fluid in which the fetus floats. When indicated, amniocentesis should be done between the fourteenth and sixteenth week of pregnancy. Before amniocentesis, ultrasound studies should be done.[18] Ultrasound studies are carried out by machines that pass soundlike waves (sounds that cannot be heard by the human ear) through the body until they hit an organ or a child within the body. These waves are then reflected back

as echoes and are recorded on a picture called an *echogram* (see Figure 14-12).

Amniocentesis is useful in assessing the maturity as well as the condition of the fetus; it can be of aid in genetic counseling; it is often of assistance in foretelling problems with the Rh factor; and it may be valuable in determining some fetal malformations. As pregnancy advances, the amniotic fluid becomes a rich source of information about the unborn child. Enzymes, amino acids, and a variety of other normal and abnormal products may be added to the fluid as a result of the child's excretion of urine. Among the sources of cells in the amniotic fluid may be the amnion itself, the fetal skin, urine, windpipe, bronchi, and the lining of the gastrointestinal system. The living cells from the fluid multiply in cell culture. Examination of connective tissue cells from cultured cells of the amniotic fluid can reveal the existence of chromosomal abnormalities. Cells may also be studied for enzyme activity or for the presence (or absence) of various substances.

Thus, the amniotic fluid is useful for diagnosing and possibly preventing a variety of conditions. For example, in a test that requires only an hour of laboratory work, the amniotic fluid, drawn after the thirty-fourth week of pregnancy, can be tested for the maturity of the lungs of the fetus. In this way the physician can determine the likelihood of a serious condition called the *respiratory syndrome of the newborn*. After the twentieth week of pregnancy, the cells of amniotic fluid may be tested for Rh blood disease. The cells of the amniotic fluid inform the geneticists of the genetic sex of the fetus, while both the fluid and the cells within it are useful in determining the age of the unborn

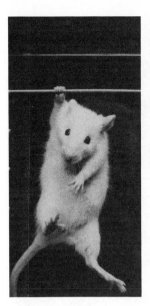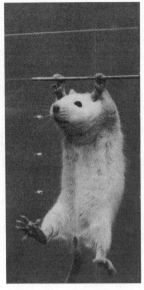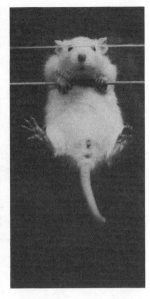

This laboratory rat is participating in a study at Batelle Pacific Northwest Laboratories in Richland, Washington. It is being tested to see whether exposure to ultrasound in the womb affects physical development after birth.

child. In addition, amniocentesis is valuable in the diagnosis of a growing number of genetic disorders. At least two to three weeks are required to grow enough cells and to complete the karyotype, or to demonstrate an enzymatic defect. In some cases, an even longer time is required, and the waiting period is a trying time for the anxious parents-to-be.

Amniocentesis for the determination of genetic sex is never done merely to satisfy parental curiosity about whether their child will be a boy or a girl. It may be done so that a woman who is a carrier of an X-linked disorder can elect to permit abortion of a male fetus. (An X-linked disorder is one in which the female X chromosome carries the harmful gene, which affects only male children. Such a woman will transmit the X-linked disorder to only one-half of her sons.) Unfortunately, the more common X-linked disorders, such as hemophilia, still cannot be diagnosed before birth.

The same is true of genetic disorders that result in abnormal body metabolism. Cystic fibrosis, for ex-

ample, the greatest genetic killer of white children, cannot yet be diagnosed before birth. However, research may soon remedy this situation. There is now some evidence that a deficiency of a particular component of a certain enzyme may be responsible for cystic fibrosis.[19]

Sickle-cell anemia remains among the metabolic genetic disorders that cannot be diagnosed directly by amniocentesis. One way to discover whether the disease is present is to obtain fetal blood, but the risk to the life of the unborn child is between 5 and 10 percent. Now a safer way has been developed. First cells are obtained by amniocentesis. Then chromosomes are analyzed to see where particular genes are placed on the chromosomes. This type of analysis is called **gene mapping**. The techniques of gene mapping first require the discovery of certain chemical *restriction enzymes*. These chemical enzymes cut up DNA at definite sites on a gene. A restriction enzyme cuts a gene involved with sickle-cell anemia into two different lengths. The shorter fragments are present in people without sickle-cell anemia. Both

long and short fragments are present in people with only the sickle-cell trait. Only the longer fragments are present in people with sickle-cell anemia. Such discoveries promise to make the diagnosis of genetic diseases before birth much less hazardous.[20]

An important metabolic genetic disorder that *can* be diagnosed by amniocentesis is **Tay-Sachs disease**. This tragic condition, characterized by blindness and severe mental retardation and certain death during early childhood, can be diagnosed as early as the sixteenth week by the detection of the absence of an enzyme. Tay-Sachs disease is most commonly found among this country's Ashkenazie Jews—that is, those Jews who originally settled in northern and central Europe (as distinguished from the Sephardic Jews, who settled in Spain and Portugal). Preliminary results of a recent survey suggest that one of twenty-five U.S. Jews may be a carrier of Tay-Sachs disease.[21] People who are not Jews also may carry the disease, although less frequently. Carriers may be found by a simple blood test.

The most common chromosomal

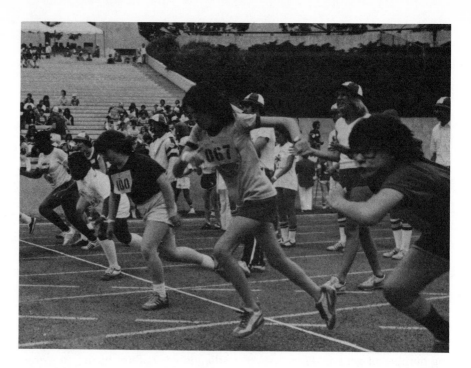

The Special Olympics is for mentally retarded people. The challenge of competitive sports affords them a unique opportunity to gain belief in themselves.

aberration that can be detected by amniocentesis is that causing Down's syndrome. The frequency of this disorder increases with the mother's age: between ages thirty-five and thirty-nine, the risk is about one in three hundred; between forty and forty-four, it is one in one hundred; at age forty-five or older, it is one in forty. Although only 13 percent of all pregnancies occur in women over thirty-five years old, more than one-half of all children with Down's syndrome are born to women in this age group. It should be remembered, however, that the father may also be responsible for Down's syndrome.

Clearly there is work to be done. And only from this work can there be hope to conquer hereditary disorders. Not so long ago it was written that "The most incomprehensible thing about the world is that it is incomprehensible."[22] But much longer ago it was written in the Bible, "For nothing is secret that shall not be made manifest."

Summary

Genetics should be studied for several reasons. (1) There is some concern that scientists will "tamper with heredity." By altering human chromosomes, humanity can be changed. (2) We have already made steps toward synthesizing life by use of recombinant DNA techniques. It is feared that this knowledge will be used unwisely. (3) Atomic radiation can have harmful effects on genes. (4) Birth defects are an important cause of human illness.

An understanding of genetics begins with the cell. The two major parts of the cell are the *nucleus*, an organelle, and the surrounding *cytoplasm*.

A *plasma membrane* envelops the cytoplasm. Within the nucleus are the *chromosomes*, and within these are the *genes*—the units of heredity. Infoldings of the plasma membrane form a cell transport network called the *endoplasmic reticulum*. Clustered along the endoplasmic reticulum are the *ribosomes*, the sites of protein synthesis. In the cytoplasm are organelles known as *mitochondria*, which convert the chemical energy of nutrients into *adenosine triphosphate* (ATP). Other organelles, *lysosomes*, digest complex nutrients, bacteria, and worn-out cellular materials.

There are two basic kinds of cells in the human body: *germ cells* or gametes (ova and spermatozoa), which reproduce the species, and *somatic cells*, or all other cells of the body. Primordial sex cells and the somatic cells have forty-six chromosomes, or twenty-three pairs. If a *zygote* is to have forty-six chromosomes, then the ovum and sperm that fuse to form it can have only twenty-three each. Twenty-two of these are nonsex chromosomes, the autosomes. The remaining one is either an *X* or a *Y sex chromosome*. The ovum can only carry an X sex chromosome, while the sperm may have either an X or a Y. If a sperm having an X chromosome fertilizes the ovum, the result is a female (XX). If the sperm has a Y chromosome, a male (XY) results.

The germ cells attain their twenty-three single chromosomes through the process of *meiosis*. The zygote and all subsequent somatic cells, which will all normally have forty-six chromosomes, increase by a division process known as *mitosis*.

The original single cell of the zygote differentiates into trillions of widely varying cells under the direction of the material of the genes, *deoxyribonucleic acid (DNA)*, within which is stored the genetic information. From the nucleus, the DNA acts as a blueprint for *ribonucleic acid (RNA)*. As the RNA forms, it leaves the nucleus in segments, which join together as a ribosome on the endoplasmic reticulum in the cytoplasm. In a similar way, a template, or mirror copy, of part of the DNA—*messenger RNA*—and a smaller type of RNA—*transfer RNA*—are formed. Now the cell can manufacture protein. Each type of transfer RNA picks up from the cytoplasm its particular amino acid—the chemicals from which proteins are made. These transfer RNAs bring their amino acids to the ribosome-messenger RNA association. Meanwhile, the ribosome is moving along the messenger RNA, which is in the form of a string of chemicals. These chemicals are arranged in sequences of three, or *codons*, which specify a particular amino acid. As the ribosome "reads" each codon on the messenger RNA, it picks up the correct amino acid from a transfer RNA. Each new amino acid is attached to the previous one, until the new protein is complete. The nuclear DNA, through these proteins, directs the make-up and function of all the cells of the body.

Genetic disorders may occur either because of an error in the physical or chemical structure of a chromosome—a *mutation*—or because of an error in the amount of chromosomal material in the cell. Mutations may come about because of a change in the cellular environment (as happens with German measles virus) or for no apparent reason (a spontaneous mutation). Chromosome breaks may result in translocation, in which part of a chromosome becomes attached to another, or deletion, in which the piece becomes lost. Errors in the amount of chromosomal material generally take the form of an incorrect number of chromosomes. This can happen during either meiosis or mitosis. Meiotic nondisjunction, in which a pair of chromosomes fails to separate, results in a gamete with either one chromosome too few or one too many. The zygote formed by the union of this gamete with a normal gamete will have either a condition called monosomy (forty-five chromosomes) or trisomy (forty-seven chromosomes). Trisomy of the twenty-first autosome results in *Down's syndrome*, characterized by physical and mental retardation. If nondisjunction occurs in an early mitotic division of the zygote, mosaicism results, in which some body cells have forty-seven chromosomes, some have forty-five, and, perhaps, some are normal.

It is theorized that because maleness is determined by only one Y chromosome, while femaleness is governed by two X chromosomes, the male is more susceptible to disease.

Certain illnesses have been found to occur more frequently in some races than in others. While environment has a role in this, certain illnesses are known to be genetically determined. Sickle cell disease, which affects the shape of the hemoglobin molecule, largely affects the Negro population.

The cellular environment of the developing embryo can be disturbed by many factors. Some of these are improper nutrition, infection (for instance, by German measles or syphilis), radiation, chemical pollution, noise, endocrine gland disorders, the Rh factor, the mother's age, and drugs (such as thalidomide). These and other factors can cause a variety of birth defects. Controlling harmful environmental factors can help prevent both congenital ("present at birth") and genetic defects. In addition, relatives should not marry, and, if genetic disease is suspected in one's family, a genetic counselor should be consulted. Through the process of *amniocentesis*, a variety of conditions and abnormalities (including Down's syndrome, sickle-cell disease, and *Tay-Sachs disease*) can be diagnosed in the unborn infant. If a disease or abnormality is present, or if the fetus is a male and the mother is a carrier of an X-linked disorder, abortion is then an alternative the parents may wish to choose.

References

1. Quoted in Paul Ramsey, "Shall We 'Reproduce'?" *Journal of the American Medical Association*, Vol. 220 (June 12, 1972), p. 1483.
2. "Gene Transplant in Mammalian Cells," *Science News*, Vol. 118 (October 28, 1978), p. 292.
3. Barbara J. Culliton, "Cell Membranes: A New Look at How They Work," *Science*, Vol. 175 (March 24, 1972), p. 1350.
4. John Lear, "Spinning the Thread of Life," *Saturday Review* (April 5, 1969), pp. 63–64.
5. Marshall W. Nirenberg, "The Genetic Code, II," *Scientific American*, Vol. 208 (March 1963), p. 82.
6. Theodosius Grigorievich Dobzhansky, *Heredity and the Nature of Man* (New York, 1964), pp. 49–50.
7. Ibid., pp. 50–51.

8. Lewis Holmes, "How Fathers Can Cause the Down Syndrome," *Human Nature*, Vol. 1 (October 1978), pp. 70–72.

9. Neville Grant, "Mercury in Man," *Environment*, Vol. 13 (May 1971), p. 3. An excellent account of a recent and tragic outbreak of mercury poisoning in this country is given in Paul E. Pierce et al., "Alkyl Mercury Poisoning in Humans," *Journal of the American Medical Association*, Vol. 220 (June 12, 1972), pp. 1439–1441.

10. "Facts on Pollution's Genetic Hazards," *Medical World News*, Vol. 13 (September 29, 1972), p. 10.

11. Krishna B. Singh, "Effect of Noise on the Female Reproductive System," *Journal of Obstetrics and Gynecology*, Vol. 112 (April 1, 1972), pp. 981–991.

12. Frank L. Seleney and Michael Streczyn, "Noise Characteristics in the Baby Compartment of Incubators," *American Journal of Diseases of Children*, Vol. 117 (April 1969), p. 450.

13. Center for Disease Control, "Rh Hemolytic Disease, United States, 1968–1977," *Morbidity and Mortality Weekly Report*, Vol. 27 (December 8, 1973), p. 2.

14. Paul Sampson, "A Warning About Introducing New Teratogens," *Journal of the American Medical Association*, Vol. 221 (August 21, 1972), p. 853.

15. Bernard L. Mirkin, "Effects of Drugs on the Fetus and Neonate," *Postgraduate Medicine*, Vol. 47 (January 1970), pp. 91–95.

16. An excellent review of PKU is given by David Yi-Yung Hsia, "A Critical Evaluation of PKU Screening," *Hospital Practice*, Vol. 6 (April 1971), pp. 101–112.

17. "Maternal Phenylketonuria," *British Medical Journal*, Vol. 4 (October 24, 1970), p. 192.

18. Andrew Milunsky, "Prenatal Diagnosis of Genetic Disorders," *The New England Journal of Medicine*, Vol. 295 (August 12, 1976), p. 377.

19. Gail McBride, "Prenatal Diagnosis: Problems and Outlook," *Journal of the American Medical Association*, Vol. 222 (October 9, 1972), p. 134.

20. Jean L. Marx, "Restriction Enzymes: Prenatal Diagnosis of Genetic Disease," *Science*, Vol. 202 (December 8, 1978), pp. 1068–1069.

21. "Estimates of Tay-Sachs Gene Carriers May Be Low," *Journal of the American Medical Association*, Vol. 220 (May 15, 1972), p. 915.

22. Jack Folsom & Friends, *The Endless Mirror* (New York, 1974), p. 130.

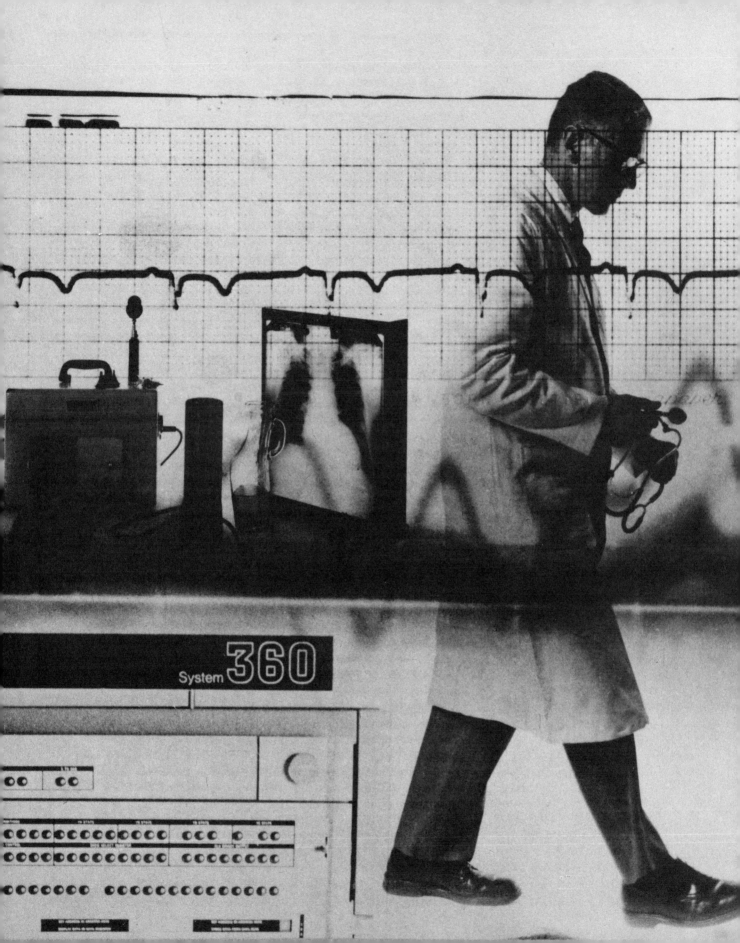

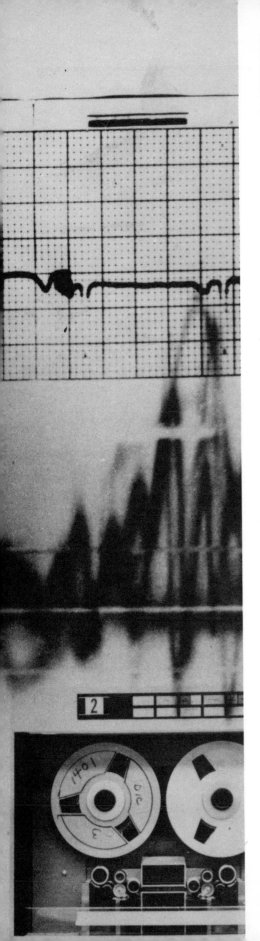

15

The U.S. Health Care Industry

The Past As Prologue

The U.S. Health Care Industry: Increasing Cost and Structure
Why Have Health Care Costs Risen?

Programs That Organize to Provide Health Services
Hospitals: A Vast U.S. Investment
Nursing Homes
Physicians
Free Clinics: Ambulatory Care for the Alienated
Dentists

Programs That Finance Health Services: Profit and Nonprofit
The Private Health Insurance Industry
Public Health Insurance
Compulsory National Health Insurance

Programs That Both Organize and Finance Health Services
Comprehensive Prepaid Group Practice Plans
Neighborhood Health Centers
Health Maintenance Organizations

Advancing One's Thoughts on Some Health Problems
The Rising Costs of Medical Care
The Unavailability of Medical Care
The Quality of Health Care
On Being Penny-Wise and Pound-Foolish

Fakers and Phonies
Early Medicine Shows
Early Showmen of Nutrition
Kidney Quacks
Why Are Quacks So Successful?
How to Identify Quacks

Summary

The Past As Prologue

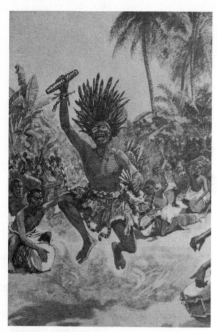

Advantaged by the tribespeople's lack of medical knowledge and by their absolute faith in him, the witch doctor exerts a powerful influence over his "patients." (Recall from the discussion on page 156 just how powerful his influence can be.)

"The first cry of pain in the primitive jungle was the first call for a physician."[1] Whether that first call was ever answered will never be known, but we do know that tribal witch doctors have been practicing medicine—however primitively—for a long time. Sometimes the fee for their services was a weapon or some poultry; it has even been known to be a daughter.[2] Primitive people also had some form of health insurance. A witch doctor would often receive gifts in advance, not only from those who thought they might need his services but also from those who feared his art.[3] No doubt there were times when the primitive physician would rather have done without payment, for if he failed to cure his patient, there was always the possibility he would be put to death.[4] Such rough treatment of physicians, however, was not limited to primitives. Four thousand years ago, the Babylonians paid ten shekels of silver for a major operation on a freeman and two shekels for the same operation on a slave. If the freeman died, the surgeon's hands were cut off; if the slave died, the surgeon merely had to replace him.[5] During the medieval era, even the teaching of medicine was sometimes risky. A candidate for examinations in medicine at the University of Paris had to swear he would not avenge himself on his teachers if he failed.[6]

Some citizens of ancient times enjoyed government health insurance. The Greek historian Diodorus wrote in the first century before Christ that, in Egypt, "all [the sick] are taken care of without giving pay privately. For the physicians receive support from the community."[7] During the Middle Ages, groups of workers who had banded together in guilds (or "unions") would help one another in case of sickness. Thus, the guild of Birmingham, for example, provided a rent-free home to "the common midewyffe" in return for obstetrical care.[8]

Early European hospitals were most often built by the wealthy, not as places to go to get well, but as refuges to protect themselves from the sick. On the other hand, during the seventeenth century, in the French hospital Hôtel-Dieu, three or four sick persons occupied each bed while as many lay on the floor beside it. Every six hours, those on the floor exchanged places with those in the bed.[9] In a single bed, one person might be ill, another dying, a third already dead. "By 1787 the practice was to put two or three at the head of a bed, while between their faces were two or three pairs of reciprocal feet."[10] The English were more considerate; at the Manchester Infirmary, in 1771, strict regulations required that "every new admission had clean sheets, to be changed every three weeks."[11]

In this country, medical care did not get off to a particularly good start. True, the Massachusetts Bay Colony hired a tax-paid physician to care for the poor who became sick, and almost a century later Benjamin Franklin helped establish the first general hospital, but the people seemed to prefer quacks and cultists. The general suspicion of physicians was demonstrated by the "Doctors' Riot" that occurred in New York between April 13 and 15, 1788, after a human arm or leg tumbled out of a hospital window onto some people in the street.

"The cry of barbarity . . . was soon spread," and the Doctors' Riot ensued. "An innocent Person got beat & abused, for being *only dressed in black*." As a result of the riot four people died.

In the early years of the Republic, U.S. physicians were trained in Europe. Soon, however, medical schools began to open in this country, providing training both for physicians and medical teachers. But even by as late as 1860, Oliver Wendell Holmes, one of the great physicians of the nineteenth century, in an address before the Massachusetts Medical Society, tartly observed that, with a few exceptions, "if the whole *materia medica*, as now used, could be sunk to the bottom of the sea, it would be all the better for mankind—and all the worse for the fishes." Such forthright self-criticism set the stage for what followed. U.S. health workers began a long journey of spending and achievement that was to make the health care industry of this nation among the most respected in the world. Yet despite its achieve-

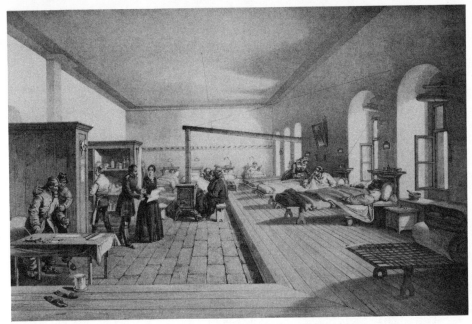

A hospital for soldiers wounded in the Crimean War (1854–1886). It is clean, well-ventilated, light, and spacious — largely as a result of the efforts of Florence Nightingale to improve hospital conditions. Nightingale's life was a testament to the importance of the relationship between ecology and health.

ments, its benefits have not been made equally available to all citizens. That fact remains a basic problem of today's health care industry in the United States, and it is the subject of this chapter.

The U.S. Health Care Industry: Increasing Cost and Structure

The moral test of government is how it treats those who are in the dawn of life, the children; those who are in the twilight of life, the aged; and those who are in the shadows of life, the sick, the needy and the handicapped."[12]
HUBERT H. HUMPHREY, JR. (1911–1978)

The health care industry is this nation's third largest business. Between 1960 and 1977, the amount spent for health services rose from $26.4 billion to $165 billion. The es-

timated amount for 1980 is $230 billion.[13] Figure 15–1 shows how this money is spent. An increasing proportion of this amount is being spent by the federal government (see Figure 15–2). In addition, the cost of an average hospital stay increased from $311 per patient in

FIGURE 15–1
How the United States spends its money on health. (Based on an estimated fiscal 1978 health spending of $182 billion.)

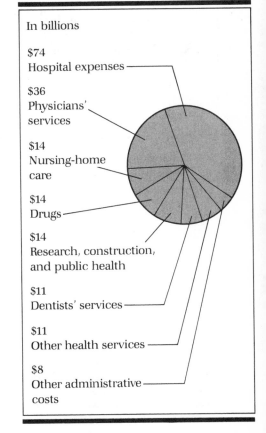

In billions

$74
Hospital expenses

$36
Physicians' services

$14
Nursing-home care

$14
Drugs

$14
Research, construction, and public health

$11
Dentists' services

$11
Other health services

$8
Other administrative costs

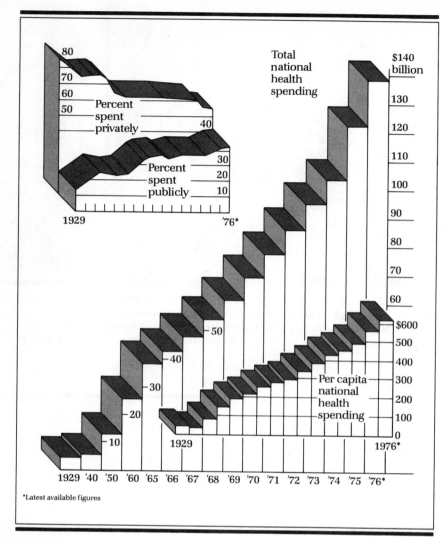

FIGURE 15-2
How much does health cost?

*Latest available figures

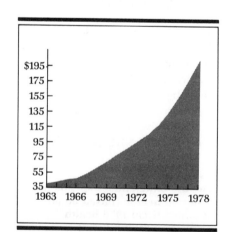

FIGURE 15-3
The cost of one day in the hospital. In 1978, the average patient paid $203 a day, more than half of which covered staff salaries. Not included are fees for outside physicians.

1965 to $1,017 in 1975 and is still rising (see Figure 15-3). As is to be expected, the cost per person (per capita) is also steadily increasing.

The gross national product (GNP) of a nation is the total market value of the nation's goods and services. In recent years the health care system of this country has accounted for an increasingly larger portion of the GNP. In 1960, the United States spent less than 6 percent of the GNP on health care; in 1978 it was nearly 9 percent and going up. In 1978 more than 12 percent of every federal dollar went to the health industry. In sum, from 1960 to 1978, yearly U.S. health expenditures increased almost 700 percent.

Why Have Health Care Costs Risen?

There is no shortage of opinion from which to supply answers to this question. There are blizzards of articles and frequent debates on the subject. Of course, general inflation is one of the causes, but it cannot be the only one because for about fifteen years the total dollar amount of U.S. health bills has risen about twice as fast as other prices. True, most health care is better than ever, and the older population—who most need health care—is increasing yearly. (Both these factors may be considered as part of the price of success.) But it cannot be denied that another reason for the dramatic increase in costs has to do with the very small minority of physicians, hospitals, and nursing homes that are reaping huge and unjustified profits.

To make matters more expensive, by 1978, doctors' incomes were rising faster than the cost of living, and the number of doctors per population had increased considerably since 1970. This increase, however, has not resulted in lower fees. Some reasons for this are that doctors powerfully influence the demand for their services. One can give up some needs of life, but one can hardly forgo a needed operation that is recommended by a family doctor and consultants. However, it should be understood that the physician is also caught in the inflationary trap. The costs of office space and equipment have risen enormously, and malpractice insurance premiums are often exhorbitant.

To these reasons for the increasing cost of health care must be added the fact that present-day life styles have contributed significantly to an increased need for medical attention.

One study in California showed the significance of just seven habits: eating moderately, eating regularly, eating breakfast, no cigarette smoking, at least some exercise, moderate or no use of alcohol, and seven to eight hours of sleep. Men at age 45 who followed only three or fewer of these habits had a further longevity of 22 years; four to five of the habits, 28 years; and six to seven habits, 33 years. There is a difference of 11 years in longevity, for men beginning at 45 years of age."[14]

Furthermore, the high medical costs associated with automobile accidents and cigarette smoking point to the importance of discovering *why* people drive carelessly or smoke cigarettes. *Prevention* of avoidable medical care is essential to lowering health care costs. Still there remains a sizable gap between medical knowledge of preventive medicine and people's willingness

to implement that knowledge. For instance, despite widely publicized reports on the hazards of cigarette smoke to smokers and nonsmokers alike, a law that would separate smokers from nonsmokers in public places was badly beaten at the polls in at least one state. The campaign cost to cigarette manufacturers to defeat the proposed law was only $5 million, a fraction of what they spend yearly on cigarette advertising.

If people can so easily be dissuaded from voting in a law to protect their own health, it is clear that public health programs must often fight an uphill battle to gain community support and acceptance. Moreover, there has been the accusation that the high cost of medical care is increased by unnecessary surgical and medical procedures. In short, *cost* and *need* are not always synonymous. In some instances this is no doubt true, though to what extent is difficult to say. One thing is certain, however. The cost of operating highly expensive new medical machinery is high—but so is the need for the machinery and the costly personnel to operate it and to interpret its results.

The Program Area Committee on Medical Care Administration of the American Public Health Association has classified medical care programs in the United States into three general types.[15] These are

1. programs that organize to provide health services,
2. programs that finance health services, and
3. programs that both organize and finance health services.

The basic structure of much of the remainder of this chapter is built around these program categories.

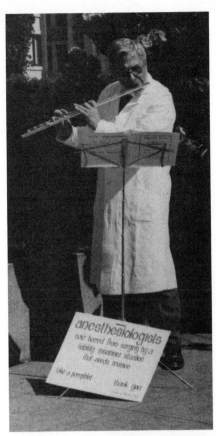

No physician can practice medicine without some risk. Premiums for insurance against lawsuits have risen tremendously. Here, a trained specialist calls attention to the problem in his own special way.

Programs That Organize to Provide Health Services

Hospitals: A Vast U. S. Investment

Material resources (hospitals, nursing homes, equipment) and health personnel (such as physicians, nurses, and technicians) are organized in such a way as to provide services directly to those who need them. These services are provided on an outpatient (ambulatory) or inpatient basis, or some may be provided in the home or elsewhere.

In 1979 hospitals in the United States numbered almost eight thousand, contained some two million beds, and were worth billions of dollars. The scope of their activity was similarly huge: About 2.5 million hospital employees were involved in handling more than 33 million admissions as well as millions of outpatient visits.

Hospitals are either *public* or *private*. Somewhat more than a third of all hospitals are publicly owned; of these, federal hospitals receive most of their funds from government agencies. To a lesser extent, this is true of state and local government hospitals. On the other hand, private hospitals generally receive their funds from patients, third parties (insurance carriers), and government programs such as Medicare and Medicaid (see pages 458–459). By far the greatest majority (almost 90 percent) of the private hospitals in the United States are operated on a nonprofit basis. Thus, their profits are reinvested in improvement of services and facilities. The remaining private hospitals are run for profit. On the average, profit-making hospitals net more money per patient-day than do nonprofit hospitals. Profit-making hospitals are smaller institutions and seem to be the focus of much of the concern about the quality of hospital care.

THE HILL–BURTON ACT

Since 1946, the federal government has assisted local areas in the building of hospitals. This cost-sharing program was made possible by passage of the Hill-Burton Hospital Survey and Construction Act. The original purpose of this act was to improve the distribution of hospitals, with particular emphasis on needy rural areas. However, rural populations have diminished in the past quarter-century, and it may well be that the more than $6 billion spent in providing 300,000 hospital beds has resulted in too many rural hospitals. Because old urban hospitals were not much helped by the original act, it was later amended to provide the states with federal money for the improvement of urban hospitals.

It has been claimed that hospitals play an important part in the high cost of health care. They are, it is pointed out, not influenced by the laws of supply and demand. The decision for hospitalization and treatment in the hospital is mostly made by the supplier—the physician. It is the doctor who usually decides if hospitalization is needed and what hospital will be used, what tests and treatments are performed, and how long the hospital stay will be. It is emphasized by some that many hospitals generally have more beds than they actually need. Empty rooms cost money. There is thus little or no incentive in many hospitals to economize or to reduce the patients' costs.[16]

ACCREDITATION OF HOSPITALS

Accreditation is the mechanism by which the U.S. medical community seeks to establish high standards of hospital care. Hospitals are accredited by a Joint Commission on Accreditation of Hospitals sponsored by the American Medical Association, the American Hospital Association, the American College of Surgeons, and the American College of Physicians. The commission judges a hospital on the basis of its physical plant, governing body, administration, staff, and the extent and types of service it offers. Accreditation is sought by most hospitals; today, about two-thirds of U.S. hospitals, containing well over three-fourths of the nation's hospital beds, are accredited. Accreditation is one means by which prospective patients can choose a reliable hospital.

Nursing Homes

Nursing homes are institutions that provide health services for people, particularly the elderly, who must be inpatients but who do not need hospital care. Nursing homes developed as a result of the 1935 Social

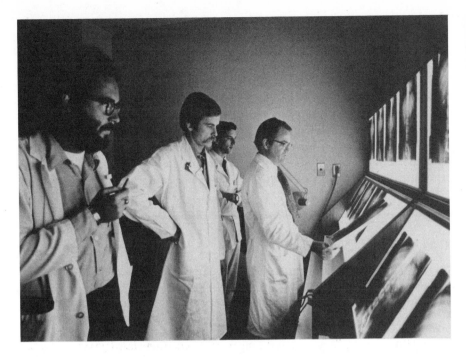

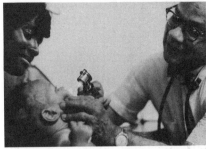

Family doctors (like the one shown above) have a broad, general knowledge of medicine. They assume continuing responsibility for the health care of all family members, regardless of age. Specialists (such as the ones at left) are, as the name implies, experts in a particular field of medicine. They are consulted by family doctors when the need arises and provide medical help or conduct research in their area of specialization.

Security Act. Understandably, the framers of the act did not wish to perpetuate the grim public poorhouses of the time. Consequently, public institutions were originally excluded from the act, and privately owned nursing homes became immensely profitable. Today there are more than thirteen thousand nursing homes in the United States.

The average age of the people who live in this nation's nursing homes is eighty. Often the medical and nursing care they receive is minimal. They spend their wintry years surviving feebly in drab and cheerless surroundings. However, recently passed Medicare legislation (page 458), by stipulating that funds be withheld unless certain standards are met, has had a beneficial effect on the quality of care available in nursing homes. Medicare has also stimulated the formation of the Joint Committee on Accreditation of Nursing Homes, which is designed to improve their quality.

Physicians

Physicians and hospitals are at the core of programs that organize health services. Most physicians are in solo or in group practice; they maintain offices and make financial arrangements with patients on a private basis.

Doctors of medicine (M.D.) are graduates of accredited medical schools (see below). They cannot legally practice in a state until they have passed the state board examination and been issued a license by the state. (You will find definitions of other practitioners, such as chiropracters, in the Glossary of this book under the heading "specialties.")

GENERALISTS AND SPECIALISTS

Engaging in general medical practice as family physicians, *generalists* care for all family members, of all ages and for all conditions that do not require specialists. They rec-

ommend a specialist when needed. Fortunately, a great deal of postgraduate training is available to family physicians. In this technological age of rapid advancements in knowledge, the modern physician without such training does not remain modern for long.

In this country, medical schools must meet the requirements of the Committee on Medical Education, which represents both the American Medical Association and the Association of American Medical Colleges. It was not always so. Even by the turn of this century, most medical instruction was still wretched. Medical diploma mills were common,[17] a situation that became generally known as a result of the Flexner Report of 1910.[18] The advice that Abraham Flexner set forth in his report revolutionized medical teaching for the better in this country. One of his recommendations, however, also significantly changed the direction of medical care. Flexner recommended that medical school courses be divided into major specialty areas and that intensive education be given in each area. This concept was adopted, and new knowledge that developed in each medical area was eagerly applied to the appropriate specialty.

Inevitably, this system of medical education, based on technological advance, began to produce an increasing number of *specialists*. This development served a purpose: As medical practice became more complex the physician could hardly continue to practice only out of a little black bag. After the Second World War, the emphasis on specialization was accelerated. Through the National Institutes of Health, the federal government poured millions of dollars into an attack on health problems that required the services of specialists. In 1931, four out of five physicians in this nation were general practitioners. Today, only about one out of five is a generalist.

Unfortunately, although specialists are certainly important for adequate health care, such intensive specialization is not basically what the people of this nation need. The overwhelming majority need, not

A *M*A*S*H* Note for Docs

*The man who may be everybody's favorite doctor never dissected a frog in med school, never made rounds as an intern, never even earned an M.D. degree. No matter. When Actor Alan Alda, 43, known to millions of televiewers as Army Captain Hawkeye Pierce of the Korean War-era 4077th Mobile Army Surgical Hospital (M*A*S*H), spoke at the Columbia University College of Physicians and Surgeons commencement last week, he was absolutely right in telling the class, "In some ways you and I are alike. We both study the human being. We both try to reduce suffering. We've both dedicated ourselves to years of hard work. And we both charge a lot." Alda, named an honorary member of P and S's 210th graduating class, also offered some heartfelt advice to the new doctors as they prepared to pick their way through "the minefield of existence." Excerpts:*

Be skilled, be learned, be aware of the dignity of your calling. But please don't ever lose sight of your own simple humanity.

Unfortunately, that may not be so easy. You're entering a special place in our society. People will be awed by your expertise. You'll be placed in a position of privilege. You'll live well, people will defer to you, call you by your title, and it may be hard to remember that the word doctor is not actually your first name.

I ask of you, possess your skills, but don't be possessed by them. You are entering a very select group. You have a monopoly on medical care. Please be careful not to abuse this power that you have over the rest of us.

Put people first. And I include in that not just people, but that which exists *between* people.

Let me challenge you. With all your study, you can read my X-rays like a telegram. But can you read my involuntary muscles? Can you see the fear and uncertainty in my face? Will you tell me when you don't know what to do? Can you face your own fear, your own uncertainty? When in doubt, can you call in help?

Will you be the kind of doctor who cares more about the case than the person? ("Nurse, call the gastric ulcer and have him come in at three.") You'll know you're in trouble if you find yourself wishing they would mail in their liver in a plain brown envelope.

Where does money come on your list? Will it be the sole standard against which you reckon your success? Where will your family come on your list? How many days and nights, weeks and months, will you separate yourself from them, buried in your work, before you realize that you've removed yourself from an important part of your life? And if you're a male doctor, how will you relate to women? Women as patients, as nurses, as fellow doctors—and later as students?

Thank you for taking on the enormous responsibility that you have—and for having the strength to have made it to this day. I don't know how you've managed to learn it all. But there is one more thing you can learn about the body that only a non-doctor would tell you— and I hope you'll always remember this: the head bone is connected to the heart bone. Don't let them come apart.

SOURCE: *TIME* (May 28, 1979), p. 68. Reprinted by permission from TIME, The Weekly Newsmagazine; Copyright Time Inc. 1979.

more specialists, but more primary physicians through whom they can gain entrance into a medical care system. Given the opportunity, people will go to a generalist much more often than to a specialist. Undoubtedly, generalists will continue to be major providers of health care in the future—as they were in the past.

On the other hand, specialists are extremely important to high-grade medical care. Even in ancient times, physicians specialized. In the fifth century B.C., the Greek historian Herodotus, called the Father of History, wrote that the Egyptians had "a treater of the teeth, and a guardian of the colon." In this country, modern specialty training is a far cry from what it was in the 1890s, before the Flexner Report. Writing about some of the abdominal and pelvic surgeons of that time, the *Journal of the American Medical Association* editorialized that they were "as restless and ambitious a throng as ever fought for fame on the battlefield."[19] Today, U.S. specialty training ranks with the world's best.

To become a specialist, the physician must undertake three to five years of extra resident training in a hospital that is approved for that purpose. Upon completion of the rigorous residency, the physician may be certified as a specialist by passing a written and oral examination that takes several days. The burden of proof of special competence is upon the applicant. The American Examining Board for each specialty must be approved by the Council on Medical Education of the Department of Medical Education of the American Medical Association and the Advisory Board for Medical Specialists. If a high-school student of eighteen decides to become a certified medical specialist,

he or she may not accomplish this mission until past the age of thirty. Specialty training is not for those who have great difficulty in deferring gratification.

Physicians may engage in *medical* or *surgical* specialties or in others that are allied to either or both. Moreover, various subspecialties have been created. For example, treatment of allergies has become a subspecialty of internal medicine. (Listings of medical specialties and subspecialties appear in the Glossary.)

ON CHOOSING A PHYSICIAN

Although most local medical societies and hospitals have an emergency call system that can provide a physician in case of a crisis, a family physician should be selected before sickness strikes. True, a "crisis physician" may be life saving, but he or she cannot serve the patient best. For maximum-quality care, a thorough past knowledge of the patient is required.

To find a suitable physician one may begin by telephoning the local Medical Society, which will provide names of several physicians whose offices are in the neighborhood. If there is no Medical Society in the community, inquiries may be made of close friends or a local hospital.

The physician may be checked in the *American Medical Directory* found in most public libraries and hospitals. This volume provides basic information on all licensed physicians, such as where they received their training, date of licensure, type of practice, office location, teaching positions held, and hospital and scientific associations.

During the first visit to a new physician, fees and home calls should be frankly discussed. The

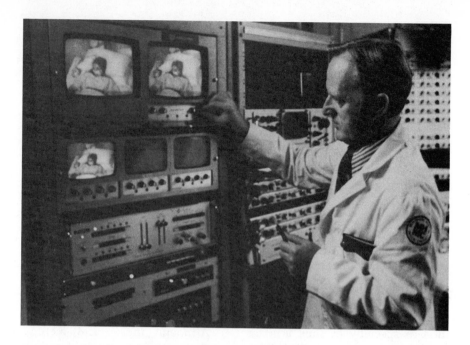

Physicians' assistants provide many valuable services. Here, a trained technician keeps a watchful, and knowledgeable, eye on the equipment monitoring a surgery patient.

physician will give information on basic fees, the cost of special services, methods of payment, acceptable medical protective insurance programs, usual consultation fees by other physicians of his or her acquaintance, as well as some idea of hospital fees.

Many physicians will not make house calls. They feel that a patient who is too ill to come to the office is best treated in a hospital, where more adequate equipment is available. Typically, the physician will meet the patient at the hospital, or if for some reason he or she cannot be there, a competent physician will be on duty there to take over.

If after several visits the patient is not satisfied with his or her doctor, this should be frankly discussed. Most physicians will recommend one or more other physicians that may be more suitable.

HELP FOR THE HARRIED PHYSICIAN

One way in which some physicians have been trying to ensure ef-

ficient and effective patient care is by using a *physician's assistant*. Though the idea of having lay assistants perform some of a physician's functions is an old one, dating back to the seventh century B.C. in Greece, the recent upsurge of interest was sparked in 1965 by Dr. Eugene A. Stead, Jr., former chairman of medicine at Duke University Medical Center. Tapped for the program were newly discharged Army and Navy corpsmen who already had two years of training in patient care. Their function was not to diagnose or determine treatment but to serve the physicians in a variety of other ways, such as taking medical histories, giving injections, taking X-rays, doing preliminary physical examinations, repairing sensitive electronic equipment, and suturing minor wounds.

The idea took hold. In 1968, the World Health Organization issued its Technical Report No. 385 on the training of medical assistants and similar personnel. It became a model for many later programs.[20] In 1969, the University of Washing-

ton initiated the Medex Project, in which practicing physicians taught medical corpsmen. Here, three months of university training were followed by nine to twelve months of training under the future employer. Despite problems and opposition, which often greet new programs, the physician's assistant movement is mushrooming. So far, those most pleased with the physician's assistants are the physicians and the patients they serve: recommendations that bear witness to the program's effectiveness.

GROUP PRACTICE

Group practice has been defined as "any group of three or more physicians (full-time or part-time) formally organized to provide medical services, with income distributed according to some prearranged plan.[21] Most group practitioners are specialists in the various fields of medicine; occasionally one or more family physicians may be included in a group.

The history of group medical

practice in the United States is not without significance. In 1932, the Committee on the Costs of Medical Care published its disturbing findings about the unavailability of medical care to vast segments of the population. Among the recommendations made by the majority of the committee was that medical personnel be organized into units. Each unit would include physicians, dentists, nurses, and other technical personnel, and each would preferably be directly associated with a fully equipped hospital.[22] In an editorial, the official journal of the American Medical Association referred to those who had made the recommendation as "medical Soviets."[23] A week later another editorial read: "There is the question of Americanism versus Sovietism for the American people."[24] Today, group practice is commonplace enough to make such editorial opinion seem quaint.

Nevertheless, group practice has not thus far proved to be without drawbacks:

> The results of group practice for the patient have not been as impressive as the advantages enjoyed by the group; frequently the patients do not receive the benefits of reduced medical costs. Many groups have been drawn together by their professional, economic, and intellectual interests rather than by a desire to meet the diversified needs of the clientele.[25]

Free Clinics: Ambulatory Care for the Alienated

Free clinics have been opened in some major cities throughout the nation; a few serve people in rural areas. They occupy abandoned homes, storefronts—any place where the rent is cheap and the location convenient. Most of the costs of a free clinic are borne by private donations, and most of the help is voluntary. Perhaps the first of these was San Francisco's Haight-Ashbury Free Medical Clinic. In 1967, that city's "hippie invasion" created an emergency medical care crisis of huge dimensions. Within three months, more than twenty thousand young people sought help from the clinic. "Sickness and drugs were two things they all had in common."[26] Three years later most of the "flower children" were gone. A majority of them presumably had returned home and gone back to school; some left for other parts of town; others went wandering and hallucinating along the Pacific Coast. A few were in communes. Today, although "the Haight" is an upper-middle-class neighborhood, the free clinic is still there, and it is still a busy place.

Dentists

The academic requirements for the degrees of *doctor of dental surgery* (D.D.S.) and *doctor of dental medicine* (D.D.M.) are essentially the same. Dental training is not limited to study of the teeth. Since dental health is part of body health, the introductory years of dental school are today quite similar to those of medical school. Most dental schools in the United States are attached to a major university and must be approved by the Council on Dental Education of the American Dental Association. Upon completion of dental school, the graduate must pass a state board examination before he or she can practice. (Listings of dental specialties appear in the Glossary.)

COMPREHENSIVE DENTAL HEALTH CARE

Almost a decade ago a five-committee Task Force of the American Dental Association stated:

> The average child is a dental cripple by the time he graduates from high school. . . . The time has come for the nation to apply the dental knowledge and technology at hand through an organized national dental health program. . . . The most efficient and economic approach to improving the status of the nation's dental health is to prevent and control dental disease beginning with children.[27]

The task force made numerous recommendations, most of which have yet to be implemented. Two of the most important were

1. *comprehensive dental care for children*, beginning with pre-school-age children and progressively expanding the program by age groups until all children through the age of seventeen are included.
2. *the provision of emergency dental services to all persons*. Although many practicing dentists give freely of their time to university teaching clinics, their services do not meet the recommendations. Recommendations are not programs.

Programs That Finance Health Services: Profit and Nonprofit

People cannot predict when they will be ill; consequently, they cannot know in advance when they will need money for medical care, or now much they will need. Health insurance programs are based on the concept that the amount of money that a large group of people will need to pay for health services can be predicted reasonably accurately. Therefore, money is collected from the individuals of the group. These pooled funds are then used to pay part or all of the costs of the unpredictable individual illnesses of the group. Thus, in effect, the individuals of the group budget for sickness in advance, and they share the risk. Such financing is done through the private health insurance industry or through the federal government, as with Medicare.

The Private Health Insurance Industry

The private health insurance industry is made up of three broad categories: (1) Blue Cross and Blue Shield, (2) independent insurance plans, and (3) commercial insurance companies.

BLUE CROSS AND BLUE SHIELD

Blue Cross plans provide health insurance for over seventy-one million people in all the states. Insurance plans that wish to use the Blue Cross symbol must meet the approval of the American Hospital Association's Blue Cross Commission. One requirement that a plan must meet in order to be approved by the Commission is a nonprofit method of operation—that is, profits must go into improving the plan. Blue Cross plans pay a large proportion of hospital, surgical, laboratory, and other medical costs.

Blue Shield plans in the fifty states insure over sixty-three million people. Like Blue Cross plans, they are nonprofit and provide free choice of physicians. Blue Shield plans must be approved by local medical societies. Like Blue Cross plans, Blue Shield plans operate outside the regular insurance laws in most states, and the benefits and provisions of both plans vary among the states. Both Blue Cross and Blue Shield plans are sold to individuals as well as to groups, and both have been attacked. Why? They have lost their independence, being now controlled not by the receivers of health care but by the providers. The receivers, willing or not, must often pay—through higher premiums—for increasing costs. Some of these costs may well be excessive. This hardly reduces health care waste and inflationary costs.[28]

INDEPENDENT AND COMMERCIAL INSURANCE PLANS

About eight million people are enrolled in the five hundred *independent insurance* plans in the nation. Some are joint ventures between employees in unions and management. Others provide benefits through comprehensive prepaid group practice plans (see pages 460 and 461). Also among these are nonprofit service corporations, which permit a free choice of dentists and also provide service benefits.

In the United States, about a thousand profit-making *commercial insurance* companies write group and individual health insurance policies covering about 122 million persons for hospital care. Some of these companies offer "package insurance." Added to hospital coverage are life and disability insurance as well as other benefits. Another innovation made by these companies is *major medical insurance.* Major medical policies are not designed to pay for sickness costs that can be handled by ordinary insurance. Instead they cover the costs of illnesses that run into thousands of dollars. The section below suggests how a major medical insurance claim may be computed.

COMPUTING MAJOR MEDICAL INSURANCE BENEFITS[29] Major medical policies have maximum benefits that range from $2000 to ten or even twenty times that figure. Usually they contain both a *deductible* and a *coinsurance* clause. As with most automobile insurance, the insured pays the deductible amount before the company pays anything. The cost of the premium affects the size of the deductible; a higher deductible means a lower premium. A coinsurance clause provides that a stated percentage of the cost must be borne by the insured *after* the deductible amount has been subtracted.

For example, a person has two types of sickness insurance policies: One pays total basic hospital and surgical benefits up to $1200; the second is a major medical policy paying a maximum benefit of $10,000, with a deductible clause of $500 and a coinsurance clause of 20

percent. The person is diagnosed as having an operable brain tumor. Costly surgery and months of aftercare bring the total expenses to $9700. The insured's calculated benefits would be as follows:

Total cost of the illness	$9700
Total benefit paid by basic plan	−1200
Balance covered by major medical	8500
Minus the deductible amount	− 500
Balance subject to coinsurance (20 percent)	8000
Minus coinsurance	−1600
Amount paid by major medical	$6400

So:

The basic insurance paid	$1200
The major medical insurance paid	6400
The patient paid ($9700 − $7600)	$2100

Of course, these figures are theoretical and would be higher or lower depending on the premiums paid and the hospital and physician fees. Unfortunately, patients are often trapped between an inflation that has increased all three and an income that has not kept up with inflation.

DISABILITY INSURANCE

In circumstances such as those of the imaginary patient above, disability (loss-of-income) insurance would be most helpful. During such a long illness, months without employment means that money is being spent but none is being earned. The patient may have accumulated sick leave with pay, but that source of income is limited. Family security is thus threatened.

With the exception of death benefits, no insurance has a longer history than that covering loss of income. As early as the fourteenth century, the Gild* of the Smiths of Chesterfield in England provided that "If any brother is sick, and needs help, he shall have a half penny daily from the common fund of the gild until he has got well."[30]

The cost of disability insurance premiums varies greatly. Of course, group policies are far less expensive than an individual policy. The amount paid in case of need and the length of time that payments are made will depend on the cost of the premiums to the insured.

ON KNOWING WHAT ONE IS BUYING

Whether an individual buys medical expense insurance or disability insurance, it is his or her responsibility to know what is in the policy and to review it annually. If "fine print" in the policy is not understood, clarification in writing should be received from the company. Policies should be compared with others. Some basic questions should be answered. What risks are covered? Which are specifically excluded? Some policies cost very little, which may well be because they offer so little; they exclude all but the most unusual risks. Referring to this type of policy, a comedian once joked: "I have health insurance. If a giraffe bites me on the shoulder, I get $18, provided I am pregnant at the time."[31] The risks that should be covered are those that are most likely to happen and to cost the most.

Among other questions to ask about insurance coverage are these: Is the policy cancelable by the com-

*The modern spelling is "guild."

pany during the life of the contract? If so, when? At what age of the insured may the policy be canceled? Do the premium costs increase as the insured gets older? By how much? In the event the insured becomes ill and collects benefits, do payments continue during the time of disability? Is there a waiting period before benefits are paid? If so, how long is it? If the insured becomes ill and collects benefits, and in the same year (or any other time) falls ill again with the same or another illness, will the company continue to pay benefits? If so, for how long? If the insured is hurt and then dies, how much time must elapse before the company pays a death benefit? Does the policy cover complete or partial disability or both, and, in any case, for how long? Exactly what does the policy pay for, and how does it compare with policies that cost slightly less or more? Are all the costly benefits in the policy really needed now? Might they be needed later? Are there less expensive policies with a more practical list of benefits? Can the policy be changed to meet the changing needs of the insured?

SHORTCOMINGS OF PRIVATE INSURANCE PLANS

This nation's private health insurance industry does not meet the needs of great numbers of people. True, about 80 percent of the U.S. population is covered by some form of health insurance. However, in many cases the amount and type of coverage are inadequate. For example, although the vast majority of the people have at least some hospital-associated coverage, nonhospital-associated coverage (such as nursing-home care) is held by a much smaller percentage.

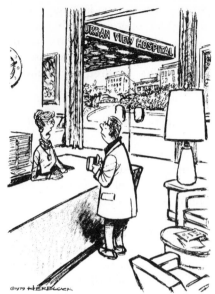

"IF YOU HAVE TO ASK, YOU CAN'T AFFORD IT"

In addition, for many people private health insurance is too expensive. The lower a person's income, the less likely he or she is to be insured. Yet it is the poor who are most likely to be sick. Children of the poor are particularly disadvantaged.

Public Health Insurance

MEDICARE AND MEDICAID

Our political institutions do not match the scales of economic and social reality. The national state has become too small for the big problems of life and too big for the small problems.[32]

In 1965, Congress amended the Social Security Act to include Title 18 (Medicare), which provided a program of health insurance for persons sixty-five years of age or older. Title 18 established two programs:

1. *Compulsory hospital insurance* financed by Social Security taxes paid by workers and their employers. The hospital insurance program helps to pay the costs of hospital care, extended-care facilities (such as nursing homes), and outpatient diagnostic services.
2. *Voluntary medical insurance* financed by the voluntarily paid premiums of the insured and matching funds from the government's general revenues. The medical insurance program helps to pay for doctor bills and certain other services not covered by the hospital insurance.

Congress also amended the Social Security Act to include Title 19 (Medicaid). This provides for federal grants to the states for the following purposes:

1. Operating a medical assistance program for those persons who are already receiving public assistance from the federal government: Included in this group are the aged, blind, disabled, and families with dependent children.
2. Helping those who have enough money to live on, but not enough to pay for medical expenses.
3. Providing assistance for all children under the age of twenty-one whose parents are unable to pay their medical bills.

Today, both Medicare and Medicaid are in financial trouble. Certainly part of the problem lies in the general inflation of the economy. And although employee contributions have increased greatly, the increase has not been met with a comparable increase in service or with an adequate regulation of costs. Worse, unless radical changes are made, the cost will continue to increase because the system often rewards waste and discourages thrift. Despite constant government efforts at control and limitation of payment, many health economists feel that there remains much "bill padding" in the form of unnecessary tests and other procedures.

PROFESSIONAL STANDARDS REVIEW ORGANIZATIONS: PEER EVALUATION

In 1972 a significant amendment to the Social Security Act mandated review by physicians of the quality of other physicians' services and the reasonableness of fees charged for institutional Medicaid and Medicare services. Effective in 1975, this legislation has prompted much discussion among physicians. Some evaluation of the quality of a physician's services had long been a part of the medical scene. Physicians whose quality of service was deemed low or whose fees were outrageous were "talked to" privately by a committee of their peers. Punitive action was a possibility; it could, for example, take the form of loss of hospital privileges—a disaster for any modern medical practitioner. Most physicians in organized medicine seemed prepared to accept peer review of their professional care; it was peer review of their fees that brought about powerful opposition.

The leaders of the American Medical Association realized the difficulties in repealing the law, however. So they suggested a long-range goal of public education that would better acquaint people with the dangers of government intervention in health care. The leaders of the American Medical Association have long opposed the encroachment of government into what they consider to be a private relationship between physician and patient. It was hoped by some that people would be sent to Congress who would support their opposition to the law. Meanwhile, "while the law remains on the books, professional leadership would have to be exerted to assure that its deleterious effects be kept at a minimum."[33] Nevertheless, the U.S. Department of Health, Education, and Welfare has established hundreds of Professional Standards Review Organization (PSRO) areas throughout the nation. Some PSROs have taken on an increased responsibility for the surveillance of the quality of medical and hospital care. This includes such specifics as length of stay in the hospital and whether hospitalization was necessary in the first place.

Compulsory National Health Insurance

Some form of compulsory national health insurance for the people of the United States seems inevitable. Many factors are causing an increasingly educated population to demand that serious consideration be given to compulsory national health insurance. Among these are the popularity (despite its problems) of Medicare, the spiraling costs of health care, the unequal distribution of health care personnel and facilities, the inaccessibility and unavailability of health care for millions of the most needy citizens, the wasteful emphasis on diagnosis and treatment rather than on the more sensible and economical prevention of sickness, the lack of continuity of health care for the individual, the disproportionately high rates of sickness and death among the poor, and the high national rates of sickness and death in this country as compared with other industrialized countries.

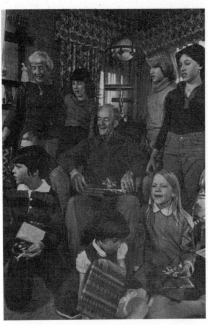

The late Senator Hubert H. Humphrey, shown here with his family, was one of the nation's most outspoken proponents of national health-care legislation.

POSSIBLE CRITERIA
FOR A NEW VENTURE

Planners generate projections,
Doctor-critics make
*   corrections.*
Outcome? Programs, targets,
*   ranges —*
But patients don't see any
*   changes.* [34]

Despite such cynicisms various plans for compulsory national health insurance are receiving constant and serious consideration. The United States is the only modern industrialized country in the world without such a program. From the conservative American Medical Association to the somewhat more liberal labor unions, various groups have put forth a profusion of avidly discussed plans. Many are at odds with the plans that have been put forth by every president since Franklin Roosevelt. The very number of proposed plans has led to confusion. It is well, therefore, to consider this basic question: What criteria may be used in evaluating national health insurance proposals? The criteria may change with the times. However, they represent general concepts that will need to be considered by Congress before it passes further national health insurance legislation.

Robert Eilers[35] has suggested the following criteria for evaluating a national health insurance proposal:

1. The program must guarantee that adequate health coverage will be within financial reach of everyone.

2. Arrangements for the delivery of health services should be understandable and acceptable to the consumer.

3. The program should provide for the most comprehensive health care with the most efficient use of resources.

4. Whether by taxation or coinsurance payments, most of the consumers covered by national health insurance should help pay for it. This cannot include those below the poverty level, who must, nevertheless, be covered.

5. The program should include and impose standards for the quality of care. These should be reviewed periodically. Consumers as well as professional people should be involved in establishing and maintaining high standards of health care.

Programs That Both Organize and Finance Health Services

Comprehensive Prepaid Group Practice Plans

People who enroll in a comprehensive prepaid group practice plan purchase the assurance that they will receive complete medical care, including hospitalization, when it is needed. Comprehensive medical care is assured by the payment of a fixed annual amount. If the cost of the actual care provided is greater than anticipated, the physicians in the group absorb the excess. If the cost is less, the physicians share a bonus. In any event, the plan must operate on a fixed budget.

Thus, two factors are at work: *the incentive to economize, and the responsibility for providing complete care to the clientele* of the plan. For this reason, expensive specialists are consulted only when necessary; *primary physicians* (these include the general practitioners, internists, and pediatricians) furnish the basic medical services. Hospital care is provided only when absolutely necessary, thus eliminating a major source of needless expense.

For members of the Kaiser Foundation Medical Care Program in California, Hawaii, and the Portland-Vancouver area, the cost of comprehensive care is between 20 and 30 percent less than the private physicians' fee-for-service system.[36] The Health Insurance Plan of New York is another example of a comprehensive prepaid group practice plan, as are the Ross-Loos Medical Group in Los Angeles, the Community Health Organization of Detroit, the Group Health Association in Washington, D.C., and the Group Health Cooperative of Puget Sound. All have provided good medical care with as little economic waste as possible.

Neighborhood Health Centers

The purpose of a neighborhood health center is to bring comprehensive health services to people in low-income urban areas. The person does not need to go from one place to another to receive care for more than one organ or ailment. Diagnosis and treatment of disease are but part of comprehensive health care; also included is an active program for the prevention of illness.

Neighborhood health centers are federally supported; dozens of such centers are in operation throughout the country. Representatives of the community have an important voice in the planning, development, and management of neighborhood health centers. Some people claim that the poor are not knowledgeable enough to contribute to so sophisticated a project. They forget two things: first, that many of this nation's greatest hospital and beneficial health societies were founded by poor immigrants, and, second, that without the active participation of community representatives, the people of the community do not think of the health center as their own. Instead, they resent it as just another project, planned by outsiders who have no real feeling for their needs.

Health Maintenance Organizations

Established by law in 1973, a health maintenance organization (HMO) is one that delivers comprehensive health care to a voluntarily enrolled population at a prenegotiated *annual rate*. The HMO concept developed from the proven success of prepaid group practice plans, such as the Kaiser Foundation program and the Group Health Cooperative of Puget Sound (noted earlier). Such organizations meet the definition of an HMO most completely. However, other kinds of groups also may form HMOs. These include either providers of health services, such as physicians, hospitals, and medical societies, or consumers of health services, such as labor unions or business firms.

Any HMO must meet the four basic requirements that are inherent in the definition: that is, it must be (1) a system of health care (including personnel and facilities) organized to serve all the health needs of (2) a defined population that chooses to enroll, and for which the HMO assumes responsibility twenty-four hours a day, seven days a week, in return for (3) payment for total services that is made on a previously established, prepaid, per-person or per-family basis and that is handled by (4) an adequate managing organization dedicated to the best medical service without waste.

Because the annually prepaid amount is fixed, the HMO is economically motivated to maintain the subscriber's health, to expedite his or her recovery when sick, and to perform these services with maximum efficiency. Added costs of inefficient service are not borne by the subscriber. Since HMOs compete with one another for subscribers, consumers are in a good bargaining position to receive the most for their money. However, this being the case, might not HMOs tend to cut costs by decreasing services and serving only low-risk populations? To avoid that possibility, the federal government's plans for HMOs include a system of controls. If, for example, an HMO contracts with the federal government under Medicare, the HMO management must provide mechanisms for government monitoring. Federal financial help, in the form of loans, grants, and contracts, is now expanding existing HMOs and establishing new ones. In 1978, there were 178 HMOs operating in the United States and more were being planned.

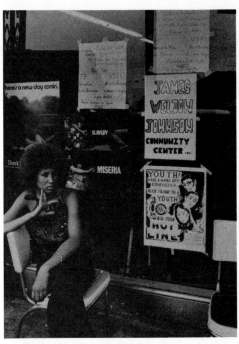

A neighborhood health center.

Advancing One's Thoughts on Some Health Problems

The Rising Costs of Medical Care

That health care costs are continuously rising has already been shown, and some of the reasons for this have been discussed. As has been pointed out, one reason for the enormously increased cost is medical progress. Technological advances have made possible an expensive array of new diagnostic and treatment facilities that were unheard of a generation ago. Yet this knowledge must be tempered by the fact that only too often these facilities are not economically used. Also causing spiraling costs of medical care is an increasingly urbanized and educated populace demanding better preventive, curative, and rehabilitative care. Ironically, people often ignore a preventive life style, yet they consider health a right rather than a privilege.

In addition, a changed population is now being attacked by illnesses that were not so common a generation ago. Recall from earlier discussions that the increased control of many communicable diseases has afforded people a longer life span. Thus more survive to develop chronic and more costly ailments. Since the turn of the century, the proportion of the elderly to the rest of the population has more than quadrupled. And for an aged person the average hospital stay costs more than eleven times that for a youth and more than twice that for a middle-aged patient. Doctor bills for the elderly are three times those for the young and twice those for the

middle-aged. Moreover, people over sixty-five are twice as likely to suffer chronic disease as are those under sixty-five; they are admitted to hospitals more often and stay longer.

On the one hand, hospitals are faced with increased demands for more expensive and prolonged care; on the other hand, they are forced to meet inflated payroll and other expenses. The results: Hospital bills have skyrocketed, and so have health insurance premiums. Unfortunately, increased costs have not been translated into an increased availability of medical care.

The Unavailability of Health Care

The present organization and method of distributing health care in the United States is, like any business, based on competition. Physicians in private practice compete with one another for the consumer who can afford to pay. The physician relishes independence and economic competition. The same is true of the private hospital, which, as an independent institution, is responsible only to a board of trustees. Both private physicians and private hospitals go where the money is and, aside from much charity work, serve those with money (see Figure 15–4 illustrating physician distribution). Those without money must seek care in public hospitals.

Are public hospitals as desirable as private hospitals? The medical care they offer may be as good; nevertheless, those who have enough money do not ordinarily go

to them. It has been said that the sick son of one of the most persistent U.S. Senate champions of public health care was seen by twelve specialists in a private hospital. It would be cruel to criticize the Senator for buying the best health care for his son. It is no less cruel, the Senator would be first to agree, to deprive the needy of superlative health care because they cannot afford it.

The availability of health care is further diminished because hospital beds are not distributed according to population needs. North Dakota has 6.3 hospital beds per one thousand residents—more hospital beds per person than any other state; yet that is an average of less than 0.8 hospital beds per one

FIGURE 15–4
Where the doctors are.

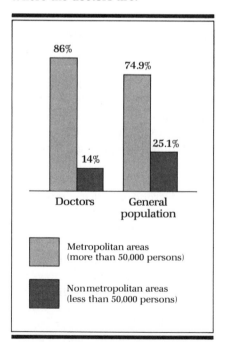

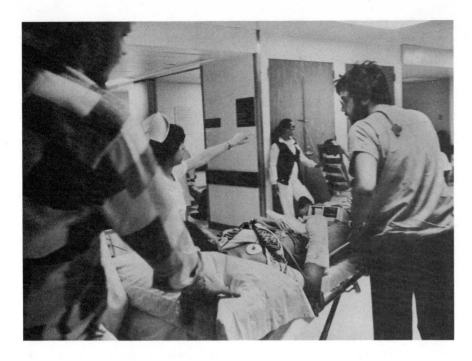

The emergency room has become the busiest section of most hospitals, often because patients have learned that they can get quick, competent care there—even when they do not consider themselves to be an emergency case.

thousand square miles. The discouraging inconvenience to the sick is obvious. Massachusetts has twice as many hospital beds per one thousand square miles.

Physicians are also unevenly distributed. In Mississippi, there are only sixty-nine physicians for every 100,000 people; in New York, the ratio is two hundred physicians for every 100,000 people. Half a million people in the United States live in counties without a single practicing physician. For example, in Missouri, 96,300 people in fifteen counties have no physician.[37] It is becoming increasingly difficult to entice physicians, nurses, and other medical personnel to rural parts of the country. How serious is this situation? The rates of infant and postnatal mortality are higher in rural than in urban areas, armed-forces volunteers from rural areas are rejected on health grounds more often than their urban counterparts, and a considerable number of the adults on farms suffer from such chronic ailments as hypertension, arthritis, and heart disease, all of which limit their ability to work.

The Quality of Health Care

The overspecialization, high cost, and maldistribution of health care cannot help but affect its quality. Comprehensive care and continuity of service are increasingly difficult to obtain. Patient service is fragmented. It has been wryly remarked that many an ambulatory patient avoids entering the front door of a hospital for fear of getting lost in a maze of specialists' offices. It is only in the emergency room that patients can be sure of obtaining medical care at all times. Visits to emergency rooms in the United States have increased enormously. However, only a small proportion of these could be classified as true emergencies. Nevertheless, emergency-room visits continue to increase.

Hospital emergency rooms are mostly equipped to handle only ur-

gent problems. They may provide provisional diagnoses leading to admission to the hospital for firm diagnoses and treatment. But for most patients hurried treatment in a crowded emergency room is a poor substitute for a thorough, time-consuming approach to each patient as a whole person with interrelated problems. Preventive medicine and follow-up care are not generally practiced in emergency rooms. Thus, emergency-room care for the ambulatory patient is seldom more than medical piecework. Continuity of care, so desirable for both physician and patient, is rarely achieved.

In recent years, however, effort has been successfully exerted to overcome many of these shortcomings. In an increasing number of hospitals the emergency "room" has been replaced by an emergency "department." Emergency medicine is rapidly gaining the status of a specialty. Indeed, even emergency psychiatry is being successfully practiced.

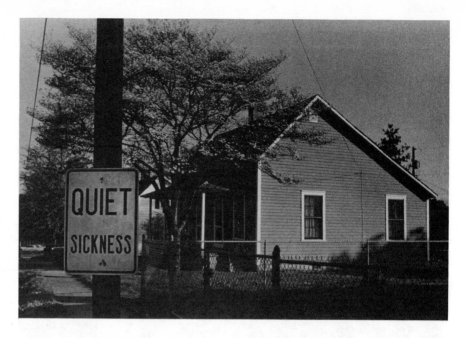

This sign poignantly calls attention to the sick men and women of a town—sick, in this case, with brown-lung disease because of their occupation as mill workers in cotton-bale-opening rooms. As with other medical problems, occupational illness may someday be prevented as a result of research.

On Being Penny-Wise and Pound-Foolish

Some years ago a physician addressed the regular meeting of the city council of a large Midwestern city. A deliberate man, he developed his theme carefully: to cure a child cost more than to prevent the disease. The physician's audience, largely composed of business people, regarded him with curious interest. Unaccustomed to this approach, some listeners were not sure they liked it. They were more comfortable with sentiment. Someone had brought a crippled child of seven to the previous meeting. The child's eyes were enormous and reproachful. A lot of money had been raised that afternoon for a crippled children's clinic.

Now the physician told them that contributions were needed to support a psychiatrist for the crippled children's clinic. Treatment was needed for the mental limp. A child, benefited by such treatment, would be less likely to inhabit costly psychiatric wards, would be less

prone to populate prisons, would more likely work and pay taxes someday. Such a child would cost now but repay later. Health was an investment. Contributions to it, deductible from personal income tax this year, would lower taxes in the future. They did not need to be told of their obligations to children, the physician told them. But had they realized that health was good business? It was a bargain.

His theme was not new, he admitted. At the turn of the century, summer was the season of death in the New York tenements. Thousands of babies died of summer diarrhea. Physicians, hurrying to beat the undertaker to the tenement baby, had a slogan: "It costs $25 to save a baby, but $75 to bury it."

"Let us take another example you all know about," the physician continued. "Recently, we vaccinated 100,000 children against measles. At $1.50 per vaccination, the cost was $150,000. This means, however, that 100,000 children won't get the disease. But without the vaccine, just about all the children would have

contracted measles. One measles case out of 1,000 develops encephalitis. This is a brain inflammation. Had we not vaccinated the 100,000 children, we would have had 100 cases of measles encephalitis. Of these, 25 children would have died and 40 would have been permanently retarded physically and mentally, or both. We won't talk now about the 25 children who would have been lost. But to care for one retarded child during his or her lifetime costs $250,000. It is simple arithmetic. Forty children times $250,000 equals $10,000,000. Subtract the $150,000 cost of the vaccination program from the $10,000,000. The net profit: $9,850,000."

The speaker sat down. There was a pause and then a murmur of approval. The chairman asked for comments. One after another the audience members rose to support the speaker. Saving a child appealed to their emotions; saving a dollar, to their business sense. It was a good way to be good.

The physician's talk had convinced the business people of the community that preventive health measures were indeed good business. By unanimous vote, adequate funds for the psychiatrist were made available.

In such instances, the facts are clear, the arithmetic obvious. Preventive action will save money and lives. But sometimes money is spent to support scientific research that does not seem to be beneficial. Consider this example. At an eastern university a bespectacled professor spent long hours in his laboratory studying microbes in soil. He was obeying the ancient exhortation of Job: "Speak to the earth, and it shall teach thee." It was enough work for his lifetime. "A handful of soil contains as many microorganisms as there are human beings in the world."[38] The scientist's budget was small; he was more interested in microbes than money—and particularly in a certain microbe called *Streptomyces griseus*. He discovered that this microbe produced an antibiotic substance, *streptomycin*, which is effective against the bacillus that causes tuberculosis. For the scientist, words uttered by an ancient scholar long ago had come true: "The Lord created medicines out of the earth and he that is wise shall not abhor them."[39]

Soon streptomycin was being widely used. Other effective anti-tuberculosis drugs were soon discovered. In the United States, many tuberculosis sanitariums closed. Thousands of tuberculosis patients went home and were treated on an ambulatory basis. In about twenty-five years, savings in hospitalization costs have amounted to more than $4 billion.

Basic research is good economics. It may begin with curiosity about a fruit fly or a forgotten microbe in a heap of soil. But it often ends with the prevention of human suffering and death, and the saving of vast amounts of money.

Fakers and Phonies

Before you take his drop or pill
Take leave of friends and make
your will.[40]

So wrote one critic of a famous eighteenth-century English quack named Joshua Ward. The cruelty of quackery still persists. Cruel, because it cheats and impoverishes the sick and, worst of all, often delays treatment until the possibility of cure is lost.

Early Medicine Shows

Show business and fake medicine share hardy ancestors. The medieval mountebank (quack) would mount a bench and, by act and costume, strive to gain the attention of the market crowd. The medicine show drew a gullible audience, which then bought phony remedies. Quackery* rolled on in tandem with

*"Quacksalver" is an old word for a medical phony; the word "quack" is an abbreviation of the term and dates from 1638.

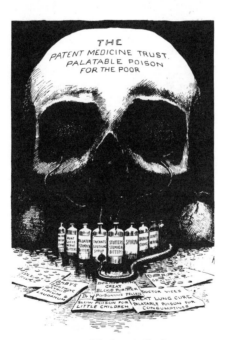

Impact was added to a furious magazine crusade against patent medicines by cartoons like this one, drawn by E. W. Kemble for *Collier's*. The dim lettering on the casks in the eye sockets reads "Laudanum" and "Cheap Poisonous Alcohol." A second skull lurks within.

performance, and in the eighteenth century, London actor-author David Garrick immortalized the playwright-quack John Hill this way: "For physic and farces, his equal there scarce is/His farce is his physic, his physic a farce is."[41]

In the New World, early California quacks also playacted. During the Gold Rush days, "they bought diplomas from physicians' widows, thereafter assuming the name of the deceased as a professional alias . . ." and published advertisements advising that their services were "*not for the pregnant woman.*"[42] It was a good, if not too subtle, way of getting abortion business.

Such widely disparate Americans as "The Hoosier Poet," James Whitcomb Riley, and William Avery Rockefeller, the father of financier John D. Rockefeller, spent years as traveling medicine men. Billed as the "Hoosier Wizard," Riley did everything from playing the violin and drums to giving poetic readings.[43]

An engaging entrepreneur, Rockefeller often feigned being deaf and dumb. He attracted crowds by using his talents as a marksman.[44]

Early Showmen of Nutrition

P.T. Barnum said, "There's a sucker born every minute." He was not short of followers. Many showmen have parlayed the digestive system into successful financial enterprises. Among these were Bernarr Macfadden and Gaylord Hauser. Both Eleanor Roosevelt and George Bernard Shaw contributed to Macfadden publications. Shaw, a vegetarian, perhaps was at home with the Macfadden diets of carrot strips and nuts and fruits. Macfadden had, incidentally, borrowed his philosophy of chewing from another food faddist, Horace Fletcher. Thirty-two teeth inhabit the human mouth. It followed that food had to be chewed no fewer than thirty-two times. So Fletcher rhymed: "Nature will castigate/Those who don't masticate."[45]

The Duchess of Windsor wrote the introduction to the French edition of a Gaylord Hauser book.[46] What prompted her? Certainly not poverty. Was it the lure of show business? Did she not, after all, merely join such other luminaries of the day as Greta Garbo and Paulette Goddard? They, too, were Hauser fans. How were they to know the use of blackstrap molasses was nutritional nonsense? And that the M.D. on Hauser's stationery was a mistake?

Hauser took a degree in naturopathy early in his career; a typographic error that transformed "N.D." into "M.D." on his stationery led to understandable difficulties with the American Medical Association; in recent years he has been careful to dis-

claim medical status and to state that his "wonder foods" are to be regarded only as diet supplements.[47]

Long before Hauser, during the nineteenth century, a stream of medicines had flooded the market, concocted to "open men's purses by opening their bowels."[48] Arnold Ehret, the "professor," claimed that "every disease is constipation." He urged a rigorous regimen of fruits and nuts, fasting, and air bathing. This regimen, he claimed, offered the added dividends of relief from sterility, impotence, masturbation, and prostitution. Women followers were even offered immaculate conception. As Barnum would have predicted, there were plenty of takers.

It was the sheer absorptive qualities of the gut that alcohol peddlers found so useful—that, and human taste. At her death in 1883, Lydia Pinkham was a respected member of the Woman's Christian Temperance Union. Little, if anything, was said of the 18 percent alcohol content of her "vegetable compound." (Most present-day table wines are 12 percent alcohol.) Was it not, after all, "added solely as a solvent and preservative"? The recommended dosage was, nevertheless, more than generous. A full, even overflowing, tablespoon, four times daily, was not too much for "a falling of the womb." For Lydia's devoted customers, prohibition was no hardship. The Pinkham people were part of a pattern. For seventy years, Kansas voted for prohibition, meanwhile merrily tippling such spirited drink as Wild Cherry Tonic and Dr. Worme's Gesundheit Bitters.[49] Another cure-all, called Hostetter's Bitters, originally contained 39 percent alcohol. It was often dispensed in saloons by the shot.[50]

There were quacks who were

mechanically inclined, and they did not limit their machines to the gut. Perhaps inspired by the Industrial Revolution, many got off to an early start in this country. By the end of the eighteenth century, the Chief Justice of the Supreme Court, numerous legislators, and even George Washington had been hoodwinked. From a Colonial medical humbug, Elisha Perkins, they all bought a pair of brass and iron rods that was supposed to cure all ills. Such wholehearted governmental support helped Perkins become rich.[51] He was but one of the first of a long line. Some years ago, for example, Dinsha P. Ghadiali, the man with "fifteen college degrees," invented the Spectro-Chrome. It was a metal box housing a one-thousand-watt bulb. In front of the bulb, he could slide panes of colored glass. For each disease, he had a different colored glass. Ruth Drowns fixed herself the Drowns Radio Vision Instrument. A drop of blood (any drop would do) was all she needed for a diagnosis. The patient could be miles away. The tragedy of all such fraud remains with the sick. By phony tests and treatment, individuals with early treatable disease, such as operable cancer, may be delayed from seeking competent help until their condition has progressed to incurable.

Kidney Quacks

The kidney rivals the intestine for the number of quacks who have exploited it. If not an actual kidney quack, Ann Moore, the "Fasting Woman of Tutburg," certainly gave the phonies of her time something to think about. She solemnly swore, in 1809, to have neither eaten nor drunk a thing for five years. Many a credulous Englishman believed her. A doubting Dr. Alexander Hender-

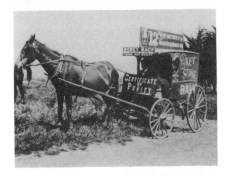

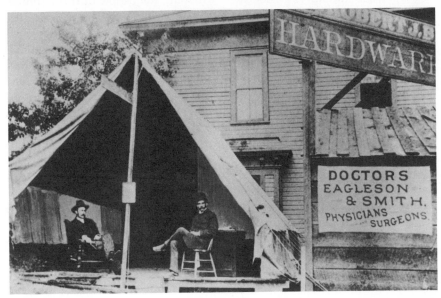

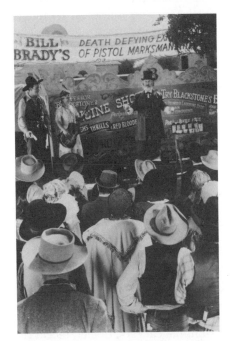

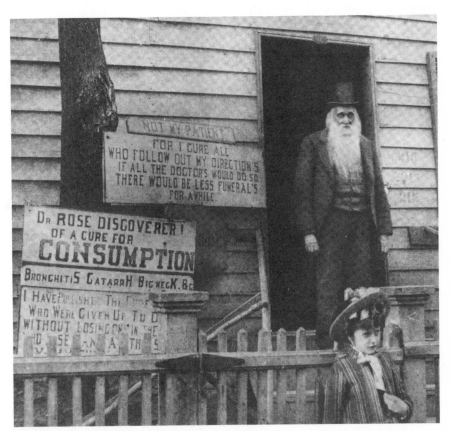

PHOTO ESSAY
The U.S. health care industry has a long and often colorful history.

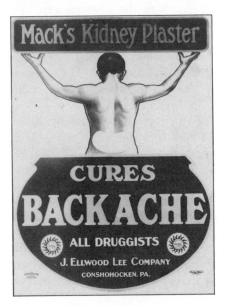

son revealed the fraud when he noted her sweating skin. Nor did he help Ann Moore's claim when "chance contact of his foot with an earthenware vessel hidden under the bed left him in no doubt that her kidneys were functioning very much as other people's."[52]

Quacks used to diagnose illness not by examining the patient, but merely by inspecting the urine. "What says the doctor to my water?" asks Sir John Falstaff in Shakespeare's *The Second Part of King Henry the Fourth*. His page answers: "He said, sir, the water itself was a good healthy water, but for the party that owned it, he might have more diseases than he knew for."

Modern quacks have been no less imaginative than their predecessors. Unproved cancer cures are among the most profitable. The kidneys, too, are moneymakers for the phonies. But the kidneys are a grim choice for quackery. Chronic kidney disease affects the entire body. Heart disease and hypertension often accompany the kidney's inefficiencies.

Why Are Quacks So Successful?

Many ailments go away without treatment; many require treatment; others resist all valid modern treatment. Quackery takes advantage of all three circumstances, and the imagination of those who practice it has kept pace with the increasing complexity of health sciences. Modern quacks, like their predecessors, are still selling smoke, but modern science is so greatly advertised that one would think today's quacks would have a harder time. More rigid government action has helped protect the public to a degree, but health quackery is now a many-faced fraud, an illegitimate giant robbing the people of this nation of billions of dollars every year. The medicine shows of yesterday have been replaced by modern methods of advertising.

There are only two general ways of defeating the quack. One is the *law*; the other, *education*. Both must work together and as persistently as the persistent quack. The Public Health Service, the U.S. Postal Service, and the Food and Drug Administration are just three major federal government agencies legally able to fight quackery. On the state and local levels other agencies also join in the fight against quackery. Voluntary (or nongovernmental) organizations, such as the American Medical and Dental Associations, the American Public Health Association, and the American Cancer Society, are but a few national organizations with local chapters that can promote education against health cheaters.

But the job of these agencies is not an easy one. There are quacks who feed off the profits of sure cures for such chronic diseases as cancer, arthritis, and emotional problems. One can understand the plight of the patient. A cancer victim, for example, honestly told that modern medicine has little to offer for a cure, will desperately seek and listen to anyone who holds out hope. Perhaps the most disgraceful modern example of this is a substance derived from apricot pits called Laetrile. By 1978 Laetrile had been legalized in fourteen states. Oklahoma's U.S. District Court judge has played doctor, supporting the rights of individual patients to receive Laetrile. The National Health Federation (nobody can object to the name) and the Committee for Freedom of Choice in Cancer Therapy, Inc., are powerful pro-Laetrile citizens' lobbies. The federal National Cancer Institute has been forced, not by scientists but by politicians, into an expensive study of Laetrile.

Yet Laetrile (also known as amygdalin), advertised as an "anticancer vitamin," is neither a vitamin nor an anticancer drug. The largest series of animal tests on Laetrile has been carried out by scientists at one of the nation's major private research centers—the Sloan Kettering Institute. The mouse breast-cancer tests in particular were the most thorough and conclusive ever conducted. The conclusion: Laetrile has no effect on cancer.

Some people argue that Laetrile should be legalized so that it might be given to terminally ill patients, since there is no harm in deceiving people whose lives are ending. But this would mean government deception by implying that the drug has some value as a cancer cure. That very implication would lure others who might be saved by medical treatment to certain death.

Here are some of the presently known facts about Laetrile:

1. Unlike all other cancer drugs, it has never been proved effective on animal cancers. In fact, recent research at the Northeastern University Medical School strongly suggests that Laetrile is poisonous and can lead to enlargement of the cancer and even to death—apparently from cyanide poisoning.[53]

2. People promoting Laetrile claim that the substance is available in twenty-three other countries. Yet the incidence of cancers and death rates from them in those countries are not better, and they are often worse, than those in the United States.

3. Mexico is a mecca for U.S. citizens seeking Laetrile for their cancers, despite the fact that in

1976, the Mexican government canceled its approval of the substance because no hopeful results were obtained from their research.

4. People who are pro-Laetrile spread the lie that the United States is keeping the substance off the market because of economic greed. However, the Soviet Union, with neither private enterprise nor profit motive, and with a splendid cancer research work program, declared Laetrile useless. Moreover, to suggest that over a quarter of a million physicians are conspiring together to keep the drug off the market is simply absurd.

5. Supporters of Laetrile insist that cancer is caused by modern food-processing methods. It is, they claim, a deficiency disease caused by the absence of a vitamin. Yet Laetrile is not a vitamin, and cancer was prevalent long before food-processing was part of the U.S. way of life.

6. Studies of the leaders of the Laetrile movements reveal that many have questionable histories. Some have posed as physicians and other professional people. Others have made fortunes out of Laetrile—some as high as $150,000 to $200,000 monthly.

7. Drug manufacturers must meet strict federal standards that demonstrate effectiveness before they may sell their medicines. Laetrilists seek to make their "product" an exception.

8. The "freedom of choice" argument of Laetrile supporters is simple nonsense. People can freely choose their doctors. A cancer patient has freedom of choice in deciding whether or not to take the over three dozen anticancer drugs approved by the federal Food and Drug Adminis-

tration. Does not the freedom of choice argument of the Laetrile supporters really mean a license to steal?

9. Perhaps the saddest aspect of many Laetrile supporters is their association with bigoted groups, such as the White People's Party, who claim the opposition to Laetrile stems from a "Rockefeller-Jewish clique." Such rubbish deserves little answer. The Rockefeller Foundation has done too much for world health to deserve such insult. So have scientists of all faiths—including those who are Jewish.

Diet quackery is also a major industry in this country. Perhaps the most lucrative diets are those designed to reduce weight. However, there is no better example of modern quack diets than the Zen macrobiotic diet that flourished about a decade ago.

Fortunately, for most people food fads are of brief duration. Unfortunately, their consequences often persist. Scurvy, rickets, anemia, low protein and calcium blood levels, emaciation from sheer starvation, and loss of kidney function have been among the costs of this diet. Macrobiotic diets even killed some people. They were supposed to create a spiritual awakening, but apparently excluded from such an awakening were the small children of macrobiotic dieters. An inadequate diet during early childhood diminished the number and size of cells. Added to the danger of childhood rickets and scurvy was the serious risk of mental retardation. But the possible cruelties of macrobiotic dieting did not end there. Consider this statement by the originator: "No illness is more simple to cure than cancer (this also applies to mental disease and

heart trouble) through a return to the most natural eating and drinking: Diet No. 7."[53] A similar recommendation is given for appendicitis. Following such advice could delay proper diagnosis and treatment. It could cost the life of a macrobiotic dieter. The diet has been rejected by Zen Buddhists. It deserves rejection by everybody and is, thankfully, no longer popular.

But quackery continues. There are still phony devices, such as respirators, vaporizers, and vibrators, that have made false claims and have been put off the market. The arthritis quacks have a vast population to cheat. An estimated fifty million people in this country suffer from the various forms of the condition. It is the greatest crippler of this nation's people. It is one of the most common and oldest recorded ailments in human history. Vibrators may harm the person with arthritis; they are excellent for massage (when needed) and are often helpful in relieving muscular aches and pains and stiffness. But they do not cure arthritis. Aspirin is a valuable drug in the treatment of the condition. But it is the "aspirin plus" compounds that are more heavily advertised and that cost U.S. consumers about a quarter of a billion dollars yearly. Nor is aspirin quite so harmless as is generally thought. A few aspirin will cause about a teaspoon of harmless bleeding of the stomach. But it should be used with caution for children and by people with possible stomach ulcers and allergic conditions.

Aspirin must join many other over-the-counter drugs that need greater controls. Along with aspirin and vibrators, more control is needed for full-scale treatment resorts that promise to cure arthritis with mineral springs, radiation, special diets, and machines. These do not cure arthritis, but they do make a lot of money.

And the list could go on. The number of quacks and their devices is as great as human suffering.

How to Identify Quacks

Quacks can often be spotted by the number of characteristics they have in common. Several of the more obvious things to look for are listed below.

1. They always have something to sell.

2. They offer quick cures on a money-back basis.

3. They proclaim themselves experts with vastly important "professional" associations.

4. Testimonials and phony case histories, rather than responsible studies published in reputable journals, are their stock in trade.

5. Scientific data are distorted rather than reported.

6. They often condemn one's present way of eating.

7. They claim that such institutions as the American Medical Association and the Food and Drug Administration are "corrupted"

by "big business" and conspire to persecute them to hide the "truths" that they alone possess.

How may quacks be defeated? By dispelling the fear on which they breed. And this can best be accomplished through enlightenment and understanding. In an entirely different context, a great physicist once quoted still another scientist in a manner appropriate to the present subject. "Marie Sklodowska-Curie said: 'Nothing in life is to be feared —it is only to be understood! Now is the time to understand more—so that we may fear less.'"[54]

Summary

The health care industry is the third largest business in the United States, and the amount spent for health services keeps increasing. General inflation accounts in part for rising health costs. However, unjustifiable increases in some physicians' fees and in hospital and nursing home costs, and unnecessary tests and surgery, are also responsible. In addition, the general public contributes to the problem through life styles that cause them to need more medical care. Finally, newer and better types of medical equipment are expensive and further add to the cost of health services.

Medical care programs in the United States have been classified into three general categories. First are programs that organize to provide health services. Hospitals and nursing homes offer medical equipment and health personnel, with services given on an inpatient or outpatient basis. Free clinics also provide health services in some places. Hospitals may be either public, receiving most of their funds from the government, or private, receiving their funds from patients, insurance carriers, and such government programs as Medicare and Medicaid. The Hill-Burton Hospital Survey and Construction Act emphasized the building of rural hospitals; it is today sensibly amended to provide federal money for improving urban hospitals. Prospective patients should make sure the hospitals they choose are accredited by the Joint Commission on Accreditation of Hospitals. Nursing homes, which developed as a result of the 1935 Social Security Act, are generally privately owned and immensely profitable. Recent Medicare legislation has been aimed at improving their quality.

Physicians may practice alone or in groups. Each doctor of medicine, or M.D., must graduate from an accredited medical school, pass a state board examination, and receive a license from the state in which he or she will practice. Physicians may be either generalists, treating all family members for all conditions, or specialists, providing special competency in specific areas of health. A person should select a family physician before sickness strikes. Recently, training of physicians' assistants has begun to provide help for doctors by freeing them from various routine duties.

Dentists may be either doctors of dental surgery (D.D.S.) or doctors of dental medicine (D.D.M.). Although dentists treat mainly the teeth, the dental school training they receive covers general body health, which is inseparable from dental health. Dentists must pass a state board examination after graduating from dental school. Comprehensive dental care for all people, beginning in childhood, is a goal toward which some concerned dentists are working.

The second type of medical care programs are those that finance health services. Health insurance programs use funds collected from groups of people to pay for the illnesses of individuals within the groups. There are three types of private health insurance. Blue Cross provides coverage for hospital care, physicians' services, laboratory tests, and drugs; Blue Shield covers physicians' fees and, in some states, hospital costs. Health insurance may also be provided by *independent insurance* plans, such as those set up by unions and management. Finally, there are the *commercial insurance* plans, which often provide—besides basic health insurance—life and disability insurance and major medical coverage, which helps pay for extraordinary medical costs. Before choosing any type of insurance, individuals should carefully investigate which type will best serve their needs.

Congress has taken action to provide health insurance for those who cannot afford private coverage. Recently, there has been much talk of compulsory national health insurance. Until that becomes a reality, though, coverage will continue to be available to certain groups of people through Medicare and Medicaid, which were provided for by amendment to the Social Security Act. Medicare covers persons sixty-five years of age and older; Medicaid covers those already receiving public assistance and those who simply cannot afford to pay medical bills. Both programs are in financial trouble, and "bill padding" by unscrupulous physicians adds to the difficulty. Professional Standards Review Organizations (PSROs) may help somewhat through their surveillance of the quality of medical and hospital care.

Finally, the third type of medical care programs are those that both organize and finance health services. Included under this category are comprehensive prepaid group practice plans, the health maintenance organizations (HMOs) that developed out of them, and neighborhood health centers.

Several health care problems deserve particular attention. The rising costs of medical care have already been discussed. Another problem, the unavailability of health care, is manifested by the serious lack of hospital beds and physicians in some areas of the country. And many people simply cannot afford the health services that are available. Finally, the quality of health care is often poor, in part due to lack of comprehensive and continuous care.

Fakers and phonies abound in the health field. Showmen hawking ineffective remedies, nutritional faddists, and kidney quacks are all part of the history of phony medicine. The danger here is not only to one's pocketbook. If proper medical treatment is put off in favor of quack remedies, a treatable condition may become incurable. This possibility is at the center of the controversy over Laetrile. This drug is claimed to cure cancer, but no research has ever been able to prove that it can. Food fads present another danger—that previously healthy people will become ill from nutritional deficiency. This danger was very evident in the host of ills that persisted in people, especially children, who adhered to the Zen macrobiotic diet popular a decade ago. Only law and education can defeat those who make their living from such quackery.

References

1. Victor Robinson, *The Story of Medicine* (New York, 1931), p. 1.
2. Jonathan Wright, "Medical Fees Among Primitive Man," *New York Medical Journal* (December 16, 1916), p. 4.
3. Ibid., p. 6.
4. Jonathan Wright, "The Responsibilities and the Dangers of Medical Practice Among Primitive Men," *New York Medical Journal* (February 24, 1917), p. 4.
5. Sir Weldon Dalrymple-Champneys, "An Examination of the Place of the Doctor in the State from Ancient Times to the Present Day," *Royal Society of Medicine Proceedings*, Vol. 37 (January 1944), pp. 89–100.
6. David Reisman, *The Story of Medicine in the Middle Ages* (New York, 1935), p. 155.
7. Ibid., pp. 12–13, citing Diodorus Siculus, *History*, Vol. 1, tr. by C.H. Oldfather et al. (London, 1935), p. 82.
8. J. Toulmin Smith, *English Guilds* (London, 1870), p. 249.
9. E. B. Hoag, "Diseases as Regarded by the Ancients," *Los Angeles Medical Journal* (May 1904), p. 5.
10. Lawrence Wright, *Warm and Snug* (London, 1962), pp. 292–293.
11. Ibid., p. 293.
12. "The Happy Warrior," *Newsweek*, Vol. 91 (January 23, 1978), p. 23.
13. Robert Claiborne, "Why We Can't Afford National Health Insurance," *Saturday Review*, Vol. 5 (May 13, 1978), p. 12.
14. Lester Breslow, *LACMA Physician, Bulletin of the Los Angeles County Medical Association*, Vol. 108 (September 21, 1978), p. 29.
15. Beverlee A. Myers, *A Guide to Medical Care Administration*, Vol. 1: *Concepts and Principles*, prepared for the Program Area Committee on Medical Care Administration, American Public Health Association, (revised, 1969), pp. 42 and 43.
16. Robert Claiborne, "The Great Health Care Rip-Off," *Saturday Review*, Vol. 7 (January 7, 1978), pp. 10–16, 50.
17. Rosemary Stevens, *American Medicine and the Public Interest* (New Haven, Conn., 1971), p. 67, citing Carnegie Foundation for the Advancement of Teaching, *Medical Education in the United States and Canada*, Bulletin No. 4 (New York, 1910).
18. Ibid., citing *Medical Education in the United States and Canada*.
19. Ibid., p. 50, citing *Journal of the American Medical Association*, Vol. 17 (1891), p. 947.
20. Edwin F. Rosinski, "'Doctor's Assistant' Has Grown to Be a World-Wide Skill with Various Degrees of Responsibilities," *California's Health*, Vol. 30 (October 1972), pp. 15–16, citing *World Health* (June 1972).
21. Myers, *A Guide to Medical Care Administration*, Vol. 1, p. 42.

22. *Medical Care for the American People: The Final Report of the Committee on the Costs of Medical Care* (Chicago, 1932).
23. *Journal of the American Medical Association*, Vol. 99 (December 3, 1932), p. 1950.
24. "The Report of the Committee on the Costs of Medical Care," an editorial in the *Journal of the American Medical Association*, Vol. 99 (December 10, 1932), p. 2035.
25. Committee for Economic Development, *Building a National Health-Care System* (New York, 1973), p. 49.
26. David E. Smith, John Luce, and Ernest A. Dernburg, "The Health of Haight-Ashbury," *Transaction*, Vol. 7 (April 1970), p. 43.
27. "Task Force/Priorities," *Journal of the American Dental Association*, Vol. 83 (September 1971), p. 577.
28. Claiborne, "The Great Health Care Rip-Off."
29. The discussion in this section is based on Fred T. Wilhelms, Raymond P. Heimerl, and Herbert M. Jelley, *Consumer Economics*, 3rd ed. (New York, 1966), pp. 278–279.
30. Smith, *English Guilds*, p. 169.
31. Stevens, *American Medicine and the Public Interest*, p. 427, citing Richard Carter, *The Doctor Business* (New York, 1958), p. 96, quoting Phil Leeds.
32. Daniel Bell, quoted in John Herbers, "Deep Government Disunity Alarms Many U.S. Leaders," *The New York Times* (November 12, 1978), p. 1.
33. "The AMA Charts Its Course for PSRO," *American Medical News*, Vol. 16 (December 10, 1973), p. 4.
34. Michael M. Stewart, *Hospital Tribune*, Vol. 7 (January 1, 1973), p. 22.
35. Robert D. Eilers, "National Health Insurance: What Kind and How Much?" *New England Journal of Medicine*, Vol. 284 (April 22, 1971), pp. 881–886, and Vol. 284 (April 29, 1971), pp. 945–954.
36. Donald L. Madison, "The Structure of American Health Care Services," *Public Administration Review*, Vol. 31 (September–October 1971), p. 522, and footnote 25, p. 527.
37. Staff of the Committee on Ways and Means, *Basic Facts on the Health Industry* (1971), pp. 76–78.
38. Kenneth V. Thimann, *The Life of Bacteria* (New York, 1963), p. 3.
39. From the Book of Ben Sirach in the *Apocrypha*.
40. Quoted in the *American Journal of Public Health*, Vol. 60 (November 1970), p. 2196, from *History of Medicine* (London, 1970).
41. Quoted in C.J.S. Thompson, *The Quacks of Old London* (New York, 1928), p. 325.
42. George W. Groh, *Gold Fever* (New York, 1966), p. 285.
43. James Harvey Young, *The Toadstool Millionaires* (Princeton, N.J., 1961), p. 194.
44. Allan Nevins, *John D. Rockefeller*, Vol. 1 (New York, 1940), Chapters 2 and 3.
45. Ronald M. Deutsch, *The Nuts Among the Berries* (New York, 1961), p. 91.
46. Ibid., p. 163.
47. *M.D., Medical Newsmagazine*, Vol. 3 (May 1959), p. 160.
48. James Harvey Young, *The Medical Messiahs* (Princeton, N.J., 1967), p. 21.
49. Gerald Carson, *One for a Man, Two for a Horse* (Garden City, N.Y., 1961), p. 44.
50. Hostetter V. Sommers, cited in Young, *The Toadstool Millionaires*, p. 130.
51. Morris Fishbein, *Fads and Quackery in Healing* (New York, 1932), p. 12.
52. Alexander Henderson, *An Examination of the Imposture of Ann Moore*, quoted in J.C. Drummond and Anne Wilbraham, *The Englishman's Food* (London, 1939), pp. 343–344.
53. "Laetrile 'poisoning,' " *Science News*, Vol. 116 (July 21, 1979), p. 39.
54. Quoted in Council on Foods and Nutrition of the American Medical Association, "Zen Macrobiotic Diets," *Journal of the American Medical Association*, Vol. 218 (October 18, 1971), p. 397.
55. Glenn T. Seaborg, "Need We Fear Our Nuclear Future?" *Bulletin of the Atomic Scientists*, Vol. 24 (January 1968), p. 42.

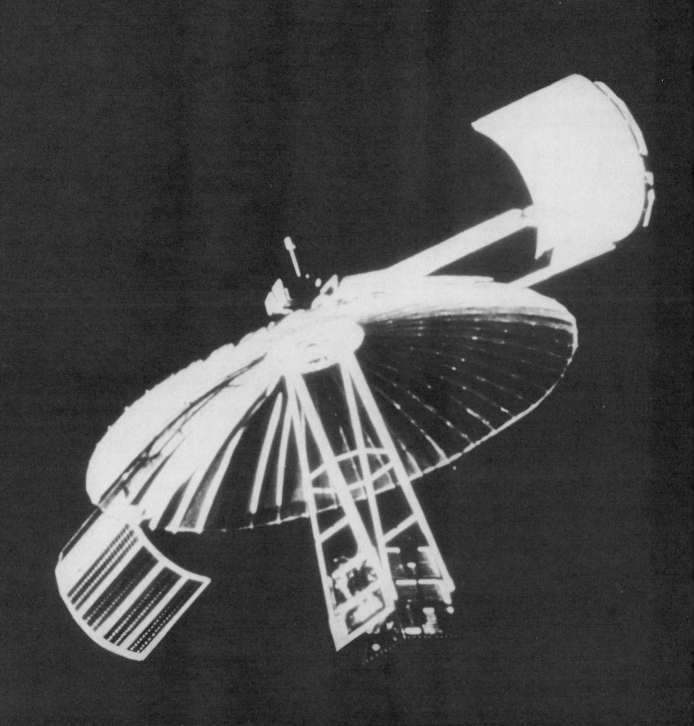

Epilogue

For nothing is secret that shall not be made manifest.

LUKE 8:17

In recent years miraculous achievements have taken place in the field of human health. Accidentally severed limbs and parts of limbs have been successfully replanted. Blocked arteries have been replaced with grafts that take over the function of channeling blood to critical body parts. Kidneys, hearts, and other organs have been transplanted with various degrees of success, and the techniques are improving.[1] In one extraordinary case, with the aid of diplomacy and computers, a rarely compatible kidney of a fourteen-year-old girl who died in a hospital in Norfolk, Virginia, was implanted fifty hours later into a thirty-six-year-old man in Moscow in the Soviet Union.[2] Nor was this the first of such exchanges between the two countries.

On other fronts, computer-controlled stimulation of electrodes placed against the brain's visual cortex has enabled totally blind people to see patterns of light. Artificial hearing devices are becoming ever more sophisticated. Ultrasonics (a technique discussed in Chapter 14) can, for example, tell the physician if a patient is carrying a grossly abnormal fetus. The ultrasound travels through the water in the amniotic sac in the uterus to bounce off the contents within it (the fetus and placenta). These "echoes" are recorded as echograms. CAT scanners (refer to page 481) provide cross-sectional pictures of various body parts, which allow physicians to make diagnoses that were once possible only during surgery. Computers aid physicians in deciding the best methods of treatment, and satellites may someday provide instant health information to people everywhere. Active DNA and RNA have both been synthesized from ordinary laboratory chemicals. Bacteria can be induced to manufacture such chemicals as insulin, somatostatin, and growth hormone by a process that results in the genes for these abilities being inserted into a unique part of the bacterial DNA. Electrical currents, delivered through electrodes implanted in certain areas of the brain, can relieve intolerable pain for some terminally ill cancer patients. Technological aids, such as fetal monitoring devices and computers, are being enlisted to save the lives of thousands of babies who might otherwise have died from such problems as the Sudden Infant Death Syndrome or Rh hemolytic disease.

Test-tube fertilization of human ova by human sperm has been accomplished, and, not surprisingly, a "test-tube conceived" baby is now a delightful member of a happy family. Also, it is possible to transplant a nucleus containing the chromosomes of a skin cell of one frog into the denucleated ovum of another frog. The ovum, containing a full set of chromosomes, is "tricked" into fertilization and divides, and a frog develops without the aid of sperm.

The photograph (opposite) is of an Applications Technology Satellite (ATS-6), which enables health workers in remote regions of the globe to communicate with physicians and hospitals in more centrally located areas.

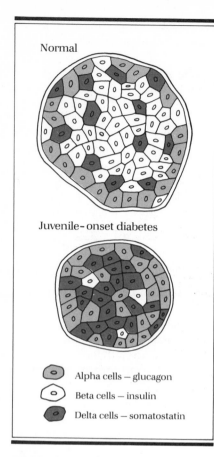

FIGURE E-1
Normally, the major cells of the islets of Langerhans are the insulin-producing beta cells. In Type I, or juvenile-onset, diabetes, the beta cells are almost entirely destroyed. In Type II (maturity-onset) diabetes, there is no massive destruction of beta cells. The islets shown here are about 280 times life size.

In less than fifty years, the same scientific trickery is predicted for humans.

Yet with all these remarkable discoveries, health problems continue to beset vast numbers of people. Tuberculosis, leprosy, malnutrition, diarrheal diseases, malaria, and cholera are among the plagues that still torment people. One complex dysfunction of part of the endocrine system, diabetes mellitus, affords us a good model for tracing medical progress—past, present, and future—toward the conquering of serious human health problems.

Diabetes Mellitus: Riddle of the Past, Challenge of the Present, Hope in the Future

The effects of diabetes mellitus,* a chronic condition, have been recorded for almost forty centuries. Ancient physicians knew that there was more than one type of the condition, the urine tasted sweet, patients suffered thirst, and there was excessive urination. But not until 1869 did Paul Langerhans, a German medical student, discover the *islets of Langerhans*, special islands of cells scattered throughout the pancreas. By the turn of the century it was known that clusters of cells, called *beta cells*, were grouped in the islets of Langerhans (see Figure E-1). Normally, the beta cells produce *insulin*, a chemical hormone that is released directly into the blood, which lowers glucose (blood sugar) by helping most of the body's cells take up this sugar. Other types of cells in the islets of Langerhans also help maintain the delicate balance of sugar in the body. *Alpha* cells produce a chemical hormone called *glucagon*. When the glucose level falls, glucagon is secreted directly into the blood to raise the level up to normal. *Delta* cells produce the hormone *somatostatin*, which inhibits the release of both insulin and glucagon according to the body's needs.

As will be seen, when the destruction of beta cells results in an insufficient amount of insulin, or when there is an insensitivity of body cells to insulin, too much sugar accumulates in the blood, and the result is the condition called *diabetes mellitus*.

In 1921, Canadian surgeon Frederick G. Banting and his medical-student assistant Charles H. Best discovered that purified natural insulin could be injected to treat some cases of diabetes mellitus.[3] Yet Banting, newly knighted and the recipient of a Nobel prize, understood that there was still more to be known. Impatient with formal-dress events held in his honor, he

Diabetes mellitus must not be confused with *diabetes insipidus*, a disease of the pituitary gland in which large amounts of almost colorless, tasteless urine are passed.

grumbled, "No one has ever had an idea in a dress suit."

Diabetic children who received insulin in the 1920s were kept alive for many years. But by the 1940s and 1950s it was clear that the problem of diabetes mellitus was far from solved. Research continued, and in the 1960s it was proved that only about 20 percent of diabetics are almost totally insulin deficient and that the onset of these cases occurs suddenly and mostly (but not always) among juveniles. This condition is called *Type I*, or *juvenile-onset, diabetes mellitus*.

What about the remaining 80 percent of the cases, which are called *Type II*, or *maturity-onset, diabetes mellitus*? It was found that most (but not all) Type II diabetics are adults and overweight. Their beta cells produce some, but usually not enough, insulin and, often, produce it too slowly. Moreover, people with Type II diabetes have a problem not characteristic of Type I diabetes. Elegant techniques revealed that for people with Type II diabetes, specific receptor molecules on their cell membranes do not recognize enough of the insulin that is being produced by the beta cells. Recognition of insulin is necessary before the cells can go through the beginning chemical processes that enable them to take up the sugar glucose from the blood. Thus, in Type II diabetes, cells may starve in the midst of plenty, and the resulting high blood-sugar level is believed to cause some of the complications that shorten the lives of those who suffer from this disorder.[4]

It is these complications, which are described in the following section, that explain why even treated diabetes mellitus of both types is a major killer of people in the United States today. Generally, Type I diabetes is more severe than Type II because its victims have had the disorder longer.

Complications of Diabetes Mellitus

Insulin for injection is today prepared from the pancreatic tissue of pigs and cattle. Since the advent of prepared insulin, people with Type I diabetes mellitus now commonly live to adulthood. Nevertheless, they are more prone to develop a serious condition called *ketosis* than are Type II diabetics. What happens is that with the absence of cellular glucose—a primary energy source —the body begins to rely on muscle and fat tissue for its energy. Fat is then used in excess by the liver, resulting in the production of an excessive amount of substances called ketone bodies, which accumulate in the blood. Should the concentration of these ketone bodies rise to a high enough level, the blood becomes acidic. Moreover, the already existing problem of a loss of too much water from the body adds to the patient's distress. The person can sink into a diabetic coma and die unless insulin is promptly injected. This process of excessive production of ketone bodies is called *ketosis.*

Other complications that frequently occur with both types of diabetes mellitus are believed to be most commonly the result of an excess of sugar in the blood. These complications are of three types:[5]

1. *Degeneration of large blood vessels*, as seen with atherosclerosis (see pages 97–99), which leads to strokes, heart attacks, disease of the arteries near the body surface, and gangrene. (Should the latter occur, amputation of the gangrenous body part is often necessary.)

2. *Degeneration of the small blood vessels* which leads to kidney failure, disease of the retina resulting in blindness (diabetes mellitus is today the most common cause of blindness in the United States), and blood circulatory problems.

3. *Degeneration of the nervous system*, which leads to loss of sexual potency; loss of sensation in and ability to move the limbs, hands, and feet; and a wide variety of other problems including indigestion, nausea, diarrhea, inability to control urination or bowel movements, and rapid heartbeat.

Efforts to Control Destructive Diabetes Mellitus

Control of diabetes mellitus depends on the maintenance of a *constant* level of glucose in the blood. Why constant? A fundamental problem for diabetics being treated with insulin is that the blood glucose level varies too greatly during a single day. In nondiabetics, the normal manufacture of insulin maintains the body's blood glucose level within narrow limits (see Figure E–2). The wide variations in the glucose level of diabetic patients is believed to contribute to the onset of complications of the condition.[6]

There is a commonly used test for diabetes mellitus and several new ones. One new test is able to measure the proportion of sugar that attaches to the hemoglobin within the red blood cells; another measures the ability of the receptor molecules of red blood cells to take up insulin.[7]

But despite these sophisticated new techniques, the central problem remains the inability to main-

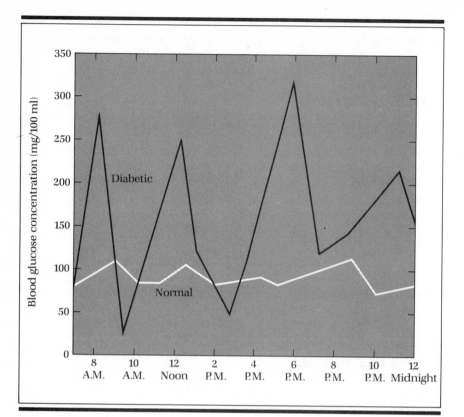

FIGURE E-2
Even with insulin therapy, diet, and exercise, the diabetic's blood glucose exhibits wide variations from the normal range. In healthy people, insulin and glucagon maintain the stability of blood glucose shown here, despite variations in food intake and exercise. The wide swings in a diabetic's glucose level are thought to contribute to the development of the complications of the condition.

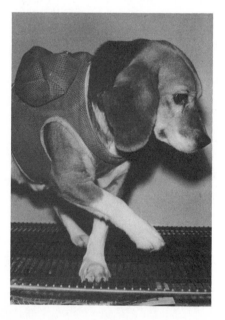

FIGURE E-3
This dog is wearing an artificial pancreas in a backpack. The apparatus consists of an insulin pump and a microcomputer which is programmed to control the injection of adequate amounts of insulin. At present, investigators are substituting these computer-controlled devices for others that supply insulin in response to an implanted glucose sensor.

tain blood sugar within a normal range. Thus complications associated with prolonged diabetes mellitus still occur.

However, two experimental approaches toward solving the problem have been made. One method is to find a way to transplant normal human pancreatic tissue into the body of a person with diabetes. By 1980 the problem of short-term rejection of such tissue by the immune system had not been solved. Current research with nonhumans is directed toward attempts to alter islet tissue before transplantation in ways that frustrate the immune response. This may be the beginning of a breakthrough in the rejection problem of islet tissue of the pancreas.[8] In addition, particular efforts are being directed at transplanting beta cells.

The second experimental approach employs complex mechanical devices that control the concentration of glucose in the blood while regularly delivering a measured amount of insulin into the blood.[9] Figure E-3 shows a dog wearing an artificial pancreas in a backpack. The device consists of an insulin pump and a microcomputer that is programmed to control the injected supply of insulin. The goal of research with this device is to have it supply insulin in response to an implanted sensor that monitors the body's glucose levels.

In another area of research, there is promising work directed at obtaining limitless amounts of insulin using recombinant DNA technology. Reasons for the need are twofold: some people with diabetes mellitus are allergic to pig and cattle insulin (the chief sources), and there is the threat of a shortage of these traditional sources. Also, it is now possible to isolate the genes that are responsible for the production of human insulin. When these genes are inserted into a *plasmid* (a small circular DNA molecule) of a bacterium, the bacteria with changed plasmids will go on to produce human insulin. So far the yield is low and the long-term effect is unknown. However, enthusiasm for the process is justified, and pharmaceutical companies are vying for patents to produce this scientific wizardry.[10]

Health: New Frontiers

The Computer in Health Work

The microcomputer on the dog in Figure E–3 is indeed tiny. New technologies, particularly miniaturization, have combined with mass production to produce computers that twenty years ago occupied a large room but that today are no larger than a file cabinet and cost less than $10,000.

In Seattle, for example, the Harborville Medical Center has a computer that automatically and precisely adjusts the amount of life-giving fluid administered to a burn patient. Blood pressure, urine output, and other important body functions are also computer monitored and modified so that the patient receives the exact amount of fluid needed. Computers can also provide local and nationwide health data and teach health personnel in the process. More than ten years ago two physicians began to gather detailed long-term data on rheumatism to learn how this group of diseases progressed during the life spans of patients. Several years later the American Rheumatism Association widened these efforts. In 1974, the U.S. National Arthritis Act was passed. One result was a pilot national data system operating from the Stanford University Medical Center, which receives information from half a dozen medical centers. By the end of 1978 some 6,000 pa-

tients, seen more than 30,000 times, provided material for many articles on this major crippling condition.[11] The ability to gather and quickly disseminate so much information is a giant step forward in efforts to conquer disease.

Health via Satellite

In a remote Alaskan village some years ago, eleven-year-old Sally Sam lay critically ill. Contact by satellite was made with a physician in Seattle. The diagnosis was acute appendicitis. Within fifteen minutes the girl was picked up by an aircraft and taken to a hospital. At Seattle's University of Washington is a satellite communication and television broadcasting headquarters. The university houses the only medical school in the combined states of

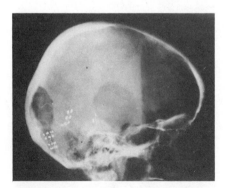

FIGURE E–4
X-ray showing electrodes implanted on the surface of the cerebellum of the brain. Electrical stimulation of the area controls epilepsy.

Washington, Montana, Idaho, and Alaska, and it also serves as a source of consultation and education for health workers in other states.[12]

Replacing, Replanting, Repairing

Although it requires great skill and patience, the replacement of a severed hand, foot, or arm is no longer an unusual feat for a team of skilled surgeons. Replacement of toes and fingers is almost commonplace. The success of such replacements and of kidney transplants, and the limited success of heart transplants, have encouraged surgeons to extend their efforts in biomedical engineering.

Heart-lung machines, pacemakers, and artificial heart valves, arteries, and joints are but some of the successes that biomedical scientists have successfully engineered. It is now possible to change personalities and control epilepsy by the implantation in the brain of electrodes that can be stimulated by the patient by pressing a controlling button (see Figure E–4).

At the University of Utah an imaginative group of researchers from many fields are working together on a variety of projects that promises much for humanity.[13] They have already developed a wearable artificial kidney that offers added years of comfort to those who must routinely cleanse their blood of poisons because their own kidneys have failed. Artificial limbs are also within the interests of this active group. As early as 1961 Russian scientists had perfected a technique whereby people with severed hands were able to will electrical signals from the brain via nerves leading to muscle stumps to open and close an artificial hand. At the University of Utah an artificial arm has been refined and a hand engineered so that a forefinger and thumb can grasp objects that require delicate handling. The arm can lift four pounds and withstand static loads of fifty pounds. And the user merely needs to will the movement of the extremity. Information is sent from the cerebrum to the enervated stump of the arm. Although weakened, the muscle stump still contains useful nerve endings. A microcomputer in the artificial arm gets and processes electrical signals to deliver the right message to the proper parts of the arm. Still being perfected in the laboratory, the "Utah arm" will soon be a boon to many amputees.

Both at Columbia University and at the University of Utah, a variety of specialists are occupied with research into artificial hearing and seeing mechanisms. Artificial hearing programs involve implanting electrodes in the cochlea of the inner ear. These electrodes enable sound sensations, called "audenes," to be heard by the patient. In one case, a woman who had been deaf for many years was able to recognize melodies of her childhood. Although still in its infancy, a beginning has been made. Somewhat more advanced is the artificial seeing program.

The brain's cerebrum is a mass of white matter covered by a layer of gray matter. In the back (or posterior) portion of the cerebrum is a section that is responsible for sight. This section of the brain is called the *visual cortex.* The techniques involved in artificial sight completely bypass the entire eye and its optic nerve. Ordinarily, the impulses of what is seen are relayed by the optic nerve to the brain for interpretation. In artificial sight programs, electrodes are directly implanted into the visual cortex of a blind volunteer. It was found that when these implanted electrodes are stimulated

Artificial devices that bioengineers are developing offer head-to-toe replacements for an array of malfunctioning body parts. Many are in an early stage and are being tested on laboratory animals.

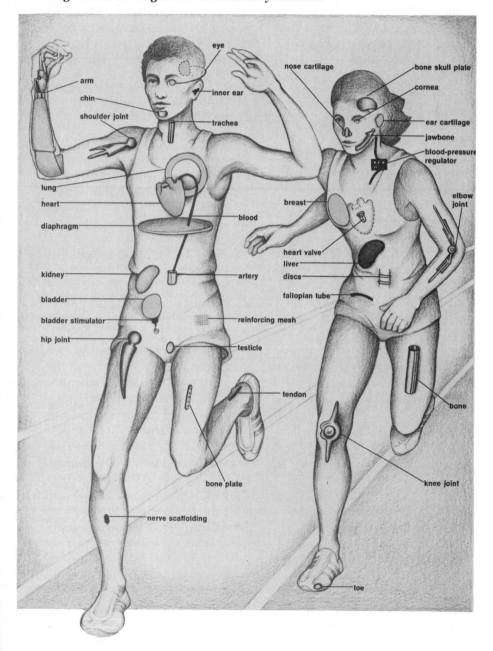

by a mild electric current, points of light are seen. These are called "phosphenes."

The next step was to arrange the phosphenes into meaningful shapes. In 1974, scientists at the universities of Utah and Western Ontario stimulated the visual cortex of blind volunteers with electrical currents which were passed through electrodes. (Refer back to Figure E–4 to see what brain-implanted electrodes look like through an X-ray.) The volunteers saw letters of the alphabet. Next, against the visual cortex of the brain of a totally blind Vietnam veteran, the researchers placed an array of electrodes that were coupled to a television camera. Computer-controlled stimulation of the electrodes produced patterns of light (the phosphenes) that the veteran recognized and was able repeatedly to reproduce.[14] The electrodes were then stimulated to form the image of letters of the Braille alphabet. In December 1978, two new volunteers who had received implants were able to read the Braille images much faster than they could with their fingers.[15]

Now plans are underway for a miniature television camera to be implanted into a glass eye. Powered by a battery, this television camera would be connected to hundreds of tiny electrodes in the brain. An image of a blind volunteer's visual cortex would be obtained by a Computerized Axial Tomography (CAT) scanner. (Like ultrasound, CAT scanners are among the major diagnostic inventions of this age. CAT scanners can provide a great number of special X-rays, called *tomograms*, that show cross-sectional images of any body part, as shown in Figure E–5. The information gleaned from such images could previously be obtained only through exploratory surgery.) With the cross-sectional X-rays of the volunteer's visual cortex for reference, physicians would then implant about five hundred individually designed electrodes into the designated area. The miniature camera in the glass eye or the eyeglasses could then send information about light patterns (or phosphenes) to the brain, which, it is hoped, would translate the patterns into familiar images. Early work in this field is quite encouraging.

The Bible is full of accounts of miraculous reimplantations of severed body parts by various saints.[16] Today, *microsurgery* is a modern miracle requiring a microscope capable of magnifying nerves and blood vessels as much as forty times their original size. The surgical thread is so thin that it generally is not visible to the naked eye. Microsurgery has opened whole new vistas in surgical endeavors that vary from the removal of tiny pituitary tumors to the repair of nerves to restore muscle action. Incredibly delicate eye surgery has also been made possible by microsurgery. But one of the most fruitful achievements of microsurgery promises to be in the area of *stroke prevention.* On pages 109–110, mention was made of "little" strokes that are often warnings of a more massive stroke. If a CAT scan reveals an operable condition, and the obstruction is in an artery in the brain, microsurgery may be life-saving. A hole about the size of a silver dollar is drilled in the skull. Under the high magnification of the microscope, the surgeon is able to gently grasp a healthy artery with a tiny forceps, bypass the occluded one, and sew the clear artery to a healthy artery nearby. Patients who have had the advantage of such microsurgery are less inclined to have deadly strokes than people who have not had it.[17]

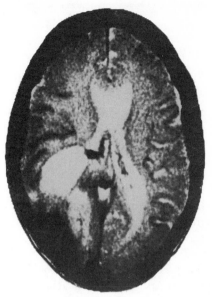

FIGURE E–5
A CAT scanner works on the principle of computerized axial tomography. The patient remains immobile while the device rotates around the area to be X-rayed. An X-ray beam source on one side works in conjunction with a crystal X-ray detector directly opposite to automatically create a cross-sectional image of body parts, as shown above. These images then appear on a television screen for viewing. The CAT scanner has been hailed by doctors as the greatest revolution in diagnostic medicine since the discovery of X-rays.

In Conclusion

There is no doubt that the scientific achievements of recent years have made possible standards of health care beyond the most optimistic expectations of those who worked toward similar goals only ten years ago. Yet despite remarkable progress, the task that faces future health-care workers is at least as monumental as that which has been accomplished to date. Health care and food supplies are poorly and unequally distributed throughout the world. The World Health Organization is laboring to meet general and specific shortages with inadequate funds and personnel. Particular efforts are being made to stop the increase of barren desert lands in the world. In this country, there are agencies that fight disease constantly. On a federal level, the Public Health Service joins with state and local health departments in the continuing struggle to provide better health care. Voluntary agencies, such as the American Cancer Society and the Planned Parenthood Foundation, to name just two, play vital roles in promoting health.

But people must care as individuals, as active participants in the venture that affects us all. Without enough individual participation, the best health organization is enfee-

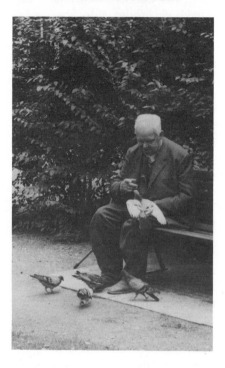

bled. In the individual lies the basic responsibility for health. That is what this book has been about. A parable from the Talmud, very old yet completely modern, sums it up.

There was once a rabbi who had the reputation for knowing what was in a man's mind by reading his thoughts. A wicked boy came to see him and said: "Rabbi, I have in my hand a small bird. Is it alive, or is it dead?"

And the boy thought to himself: If he says it is dead, I will open my hand and let it fly away; if he says it is alive, I will quickly squeeze it and show him it is dead. And the boy repeated the question: "Rabbi, I have in my hand a small bird. Is it alive, or is it dead?" And the rabbi gazed steadily at him, and said, quietly: "Whatever you will; whatever you will."[18]

Unlike the little bird, people are neither victims nor innocent bystanders. We are more than a casual collection of chromosomes. The French philosopher Jean-Paul Sartre has written that people are "condemned to be free."[19] Sartre continued:

Everything takes place as if I were compelled to be responsible . . . engaged in a world for which I bear the whole responsibility without being able, whatever I do, to tear myself away from this responsibility for an instant. For I am responsible for my very desire of fleeing responsibilities."[20]

So freedom means responsibility. It is a responsibility that must be learned. This is the paradox of the freeperson. It is an inescapable reality. It is the road to health.

References

1. Paul S. Russell and Benedict Cosimi, "Transplantation," *The New England Journal of Medicine*, Vol. 301 (August 30, 1979), pp. 470–479.
2. Joseph H. Fried, "Efforts of Kidney Transplanters Transcend International Borders," *The New York Times*, Vol. 128 (July 1, 1979), pp. 1 and 18.
3. F.G. Banting et al., "Pancreatic Extracts in the Treatment of Diabetes Mellitus," *Canadian Medical Association Journal*, Vol. 22 (March 1922), pp. 141–146.

4. "Diabetes Therapy to Match the Cause," *Science News*, Vol. 115 (March 24, 1979), p. 182.

5. Julie Wei, "The 'Disease' Diabetes: The Basic Facts," Part II, *Research News*, University of Michigan, Vol. 30, p. 13.

6. Gina Bari Kolata, "Blood Sugar and the Complications of Diabetes," *Science*, Vol. 203 (March 16, 1979), pp. 1098–1099.

7. T. J. Robinson et al., "Erythrocytes: A New Cell Type for the Evaluation of Insulin Receptor Defect in Diabetic Humans," *Science*, Vol. 205 (July 13, 1979), pp. 200–202.

8. Alice Chenault Maurer, "The Therapy of Diabetes," *American Scientist*, Vol. 67 (July–August 1979), p. 430, citing P.E. Lacy et al., "Prolongation of islet allograft survival following in vitro (24 C) and a single injection of ALS," *Science*, Vol. 204 (1979), p. 312.

9. Julio V. Santiago et al., "Closed-loop and Open-loop Devices for Blood Glucose Control in Normal and Diabetic Subjects," *Diabetes*, Vol. 28 (January 1979), pp. 71–81.

10. "Human Insulin: Seizing the Golden Plasmid," *Science News*, Vol. 114 (September 16, 1978), p. 195.

11. Beverly J. Montgomery, "Computers in Medicine," *Journal of the American Medical Association*, Vol. 240 (December 8, 1978), pp. 2613 and 2617.

12. Beverly J. Montgomery, "Medical Communication Via Satellite," *Journal of the American Medical Association*," Vol. 240 (November 17, 1978), pp. 2239–2240.

13. Maya Pines, "Modern Bioengineers Reinvent Human Anatomy with Spare Parts," *Smithsonian*, Vol. 9 (November 1978), pp. 50–56.

14. W.H. Dobelle, M.G. Mladejovsky, and J.P. Girvin, "Artificial Vision for the Blind: Electrical Stimulation of Visual Cortex Offers Hope for a Functional Prosthesis," *Science*, Vol. 183 (February 1, 1974), pp. 440–443.

15. Laurence Cherry, "Medical Technology: The New Revolution," *The New York Times Magazine* (August 5, 1979), Section 6, p. 16.

16. "Replants Have Saintly Origin and Tradition," *Journal of the American Medical Association*, Vol. 237 (April 4, 1977), p. 1417.

17. Laurence Cherry, "Medical Technology: The New Revolution," *Journal of the American Medical Association*, Vol. 237 (April 4, 1977), p. 16.

18. Quoted in Daniel Bell, "The Year 2000—The Trajectory of an Idea," *Daedalus*, Vol. 96 (Summer 1967), p. 697.

19. Jean-Paul Sartre, *Of Human Freedom* (New York, 1966), p. 94.

20. Ibid., p. 97.

Further Readings

Chapter 1

Gaisford, John. *Atlas of Man*. New York: St. Martin's Press, 1978.

A superb book describing the different people inhabiting the world today. Beautifully illustrated.

Anderson, Carl L. *Community Health*. St. Louis, Mo.: C.V. Mosby, 1978.

Orman, A.R., C.C. Standley, and J.E. Azar, eds. *Family Formation Patterns of Health*. Geneva: World Health Organization, 1976.

An international study done in five countries.

Smith, Anthony. *The Seasons*. New York: Harcourt Brace Jovanovich, 1970.

Chapter 2

Bernarde, Melvin A. *Our Precarious Habitat*. New York: W.W. Norton, 1973.

Fritsch, Albert J. *The Household Pollutants Guide*. New York: Anchor Books, 1978.

Discusses harmful substances found in the home, which to avoid, some precautions to take when using them, and safe substitutes.

Fuller, John G. *The Poison That Fell from the Sky*. New York: Random House, 1977.

Griesel, Irma, and Peter Jensch. *Investigating Our Ecosystem*. Boston: Houghton Mifflin, 1976.

An easy-to-read balanced view of the human and social aspects of the ecosystem, with an interesting approach to environmental problems.

Harrington, Michael. *The Vast Majority*. New York: Simon & Schuster, 1978.

A book about the poor.

Lawrence, Kenneth. *Noise Control in the Workplace*. Germantown, Md.: Aspen Systems Corp., 1978.

McPhee, John. *The Curve of Finding Energy*. New York: Farrar, Straus, and Giroux, 1978.

The author discusses the fairly simple technique, available in declassified government documents, of how one person working alone can build an atomic bomb at home.

Merrill, Richard, and Thomas Gage, eds. *Energy Primer: Solar, Water, Wind, and Biofuels*. New York: Dell Publishing, 1978.

A guide for those interested in small-scale renewable energy sources. Contains articles, source listings, and hundreds of illustrations.

Milne, Lorus J. and Margery. *Ecology Out of Joint*. New York: Charles Scribner's Sons, 1977.

Hundreds of cases of human recklessness with nature are described and discussed. Highly recommended.

Young, Louise B. *Earth's Aura*. New York: Alfred A. Knopf, 1978.

The author's purpose is to tell the reader about the atmosphere—for example, about ozone as both hero and villain in battles over air pollution.

Chapter 3

Benenson, Abram S. *Control of Communicable Diseases in Man*. An official Report of the American Public Health Association. New York: American Public Health Association, 1970.

Dixon, Bernard. *Invisible Allies: Microbes and Man's Future*. London: Temple Smith, 1976.

Dowling, Harry F. *Fighting Infection*. Cambridge, Mass.: Harvard University Press, 1978.

A review of almost two centuries of treatment of infectious disease.

Fisher, Richard B. *Joseph Lister*. New York: Stein and Day, 1978.

A full biography of the surgeon who introduced antiseptic techniques to medicine.

Glasser, Ronald J. *The Body Is the Hero*. New York: Random House, 1976.

Skinner, F.A., P.D. Walker, and H. Smith. *Gonorrhea Epidemiology and Pathogenesis*. New York: Academic Press, 1978.

This volume covers, among other topics of current research, the method of attachment of gonococci to mucous surfaces, phagocytosis, and immunology.

Zuckerman, Avivah. *Dynamic Aspecs of Host-Parasite Relationships*. New York: Halsted Press, 1978.

Chapter 4

Brophy, Jane E., and Arthur I. Holleb. *You Can Fight Cancer and Win*. New York: Quadrangle, 1977.

A practical guide to handling common problems faced by the cancer patient. It discusses potential solutions not only to medical, but also to financial, employment, and social problems faced by the person living with cancer.

Cantor, Robert Chernin. *And a Time to Live: Toward Emotional Well-Being During the Crisis of Cancer*. New York: Harper & Row, 1978.

The author discusses vital emotional issues: faith in the physician; fear of abandonment; process of restitution; failure of treatment; handling depression; and much more.

Eisenberg, M. Michael. *Ulcers*. New York: Random House, 1977.

A lay guide to a disease afflicting over ten million people a year. The author discusses myths, false assumptions, and conflicting medical opinion. Contains an "ulcer susceptibility test."

Evans, Peter. *Mastering Your Migraine*. New York: E.P. Dutton, 1979.

Israel, Lucien. *Conquering Cancer.* Trans. by Joan Pinkham. New York: Random House, 1978.

Based on hard facts and authoritative opinion, the author's outlook is optimistic. The book takes a stand against the despair that the diagnosis of cancer evokes.

Levitt, Paul M., and others. *The Cancer Reference Book.* New York: Paddington Press, 1979.

Sands, Harry, and Frances C. Minter. *The Epilepsy Fact Book.* Philadelphia: F.A. Davis, 1977.

This book is written for people with epilepsy, their families, friends, and employers. It presents detailed, empathic answers to questions about seizures.

Star, Cima. *Understanding Headaches.* New York: Monarch Press, 1977.

Investigations of the causes of headaches and how to treat them effectively.

Whelan, Elizabeth. *Preventing Cancer.* New York: W.W. Norton, 1978.

The book presents the latest findings that link cancer to such factors as diet, smoking, drinking habits, and exposure to chemicals and radiation. Included are recommendations that can reduce your chances of developing cancer.

Chapter 5

Biegel, Leonard. *The Best Years Catalogue.* New York: G.P. Putnam's Sons, 1978.

This source book offers information about the problems, pleasures, and potentials of growing older.

Caine, Lynn. *Lifelines.* New York: Doubleday, 1978.

A book to help women cope with the loss of a husband, loneliness, and moments of new crisis.

Feibleman, James K. *Understanding Human Nature.* New York: Horizon Press, 1978.

The book traces human nature from its known origins through the evolution in ideas about its present character.

Glickman, Beatrice M., and Nesha B. Springer. *Who Cares for the Baby?* New York: Schocken Books, 1978.

A book for young parents needing guidance in seeking the best kind of other-than-mother care in this society.

Howard, Jane. *Families.* New York: Simon & Schuster, 1978.

Covers the customs, likes, dislikes, jokes, and traditions of American families. The author finds that families are not dying out but "in flamboyant and dumbfounding ways are changing their size and their shape and their purpose."

Keniston, Kenneth, and the Carnegie Council on Children. *All Our Children: The American Family Under Pressure.* New York: Harcourt Brace Jovanovich, 1978.

A report of the Carnegie Council's study of the way children grow up in the United States, including questions they explore and conclusions they reach.

Mee, Charles L., Jr. *Seizure.* New York: M. Evans, 1978.

The book takes the reader into the strange and complex human brain. It is also the account of a patient's struggle against a brain tumor and of the dedicated neurosurgeon into whose hands her life was placed.

Rosenberg, Samuel. *Why Freud Fainted.* New York: Bobbs-Merrill, 1978.

A provocative explanation of Freud's colorful behavior.

Simon, Bennett. *Mind and Madness in Ancient Greece: The Classical Roots of Modern Psychiatry.* Ithaca, N.Y.: Cornell University Press, 1978.

The author shows how diverse views of mind and madness of modern psychiatry were foreshadowed in works of ancient Greeks.

Veatch, Robert M. *Death, Dying and the Biological Revolution: Our Last Quest for Responsibility.* New Haven, Conn.: Yale University Press, 1976.

The author addresses the variety of new judgments about death and dying that have been necessitated by modern biomedical and technical advances.

Wax, Judith. *Starting in the Middle.* New York: Holt, Rinehart and Winston, 1979.

Includes reports about marital crisis, economic stress, career options, new sexual attitudes of women, and anecdotes about the joys and sorrows of middle age.

Chapter 6

The Boston Women's Health Book Collective. *Ourselves and Our Children.* New York: Random House, 1978.

The book explores each stage of parenthood and urges parents to be aware of their own concerns. Focuses on needs of *parents*.

Brown, Barbara. *Stress and the Art of Biofeedback.* New York: Bantam Books, 1977.

Biofeedback as a technique to reduce stress and treat stress-related illness is explored. The exciting possibilities of biofeedback in controlling disorders such as high blood pressure, migraines, and ulcers are discussed.

Caplan, Frank. *Parents' Yellow Pages.* New York: Doubleday, 1978.

The book lists museums for children, approved day-care centers, mail-order houses for wooden toys, and other subjects for the concerned parent.

Comfort, Alex. *A Good Life.* New York: Simon & Schuster, 1976.

Alex Comfort approaches the aging process with an attitude of vigor, honesty, and depth of perception. Topics covered are retirement, exercise, sexuality, leisure, and death. This book is not only for those who are now old, but for people of all ages.

Halpern, Howard M. *Cutting Loose.* New York: Simon & Schuster, 1979.

This is a practical and readable book that gives helpful advice for "coming to terms with your parents."

Hamilton, Marshall L. *Fathers' Influence on Children.* Chicago: Nelson-Hall, 1978.

Pelletier, Kenneth R. *Mind as Healer, Mind as Slayer.* New York: Dell Publishing, 1977.

Three major sections in this book deal with sources of stress, guidelines for the evaluation of one's own stress levels, and profiles of various disease-prone personalities. A practical section also deals with the prevention of stress-related diseases through techniques such as biofeedback and meditation.

Selye, Hans. *The Stress of Life*. New York: McGraw-Hill, 1978.

The author describes how endocrine glands and the nervous system help the body adjust to changes.

Smith, Manuel J. *Kicking the Fear Habit*. New York: Dell Publishing, 1977.

The author discusses the use of the natural Orienting Reflex (OR) as the fundamental instinct that automatically sorts out what we see, hear, and feel according to priorities. The book includes workbooks of OR instructions for conquering specific fears.

Chapter 7

Estes, Nada J., and M. Edith Heinemann, eds. *Alcoholism: Development, Consequences, and Interventions*. St. Louis, Mo.: C.V. Mosby, 1977.

The book explains care, treatment, and diagnosis of alcoholism from both psychological and physiological perspectives.

Evans, Wayne O., and Jonathan O. Cole. *Your Medicine Chest*. Boston: Little, Brown, 1978.

This is an accurate and comprehensive review of information about drugs, how commonly used medicines work in your body, and the effects and side effects of various drugs.

Graedon, Joe. *The People's Pharmacy*. New York: Avon Books, 1979.

A complete almanac of over-the-counter and prescription drugs, dangerous drug interactions, and brand-name medications.

Grinspoon, Lester. *Marijuana Reconsidered*. Cambridge, Mass.: Harvard University Press, 1977.

This is about some of the medical, psychological, social, personal, and legal significances of marijuana use in the United States today.

Haberman, Paul W., and Michael M. Baden. *Alcohol, Other Drugs and Violent Death*. New York: Oxford University Press, 1978.

Hafen, Brent Q. *Alcohol: The Crutch That Cripples*. St. Paul, Minn.: West Publishing, 1977.

Paupst, James. *The Sleep Book*. New York: Collier Books, 1975.

This book explores the effects of alcohol and drugs on sleep, dream research, and insomnia and other sleep disorders.

Stafford, Peter. *Psychedelics Encyclopedia*. Berkeley, Calif.: And/Or Press, 1977.

A chronicle of the history, botany, pharmacology, and effects of hallucinogens.

Walker, Sydney, III. *Help for the Hyperactive Child*. Boston: Houghton Mifflin, 1977.

The author discusses the so-called "miracle" cures for hyperactivity, who becomes hyperactive and why, where to get help, and what to do to prevent hyperactivity.

Chapter 8

Cooper, Kenneth H. *The Aerobics Way*. New York: M. Evans, 1977.

With the author's aerobic point system, the reader can determine how much exercise is needed to provide the vigor and zest desired. Included is the method for measuring progress toward a pre-set goal.

Daniels, Jack, Robert Fitts, and George Sheehan. *Conditioning for Distance Running*. New York: John Wiley & Sons, 1978.

This is not a "how-to condition" book but one that explains the physiological and biochemical considerations in strenuous conditioning. For the more technically oriented person.

Eden, John. *The Eye Book*. New York: Penguin Books, 1978.

Explains in clear language how eyes work, how to maintain their health, what can go wrong with them, and how to deal with ocular difficulties and disease. Also included is information on the newest innovations in first-aid techniques, surgical procedures, and contact lenses.

Elrick, Harold, and others. *Living Longer and Better: Guides to Optimal Health*. Mountain View, Calif.: World Publications, 1979.

A book about living habits that can give substantial protection against the major killers—heart attacks, strokes, and other degenerative diseases. The idea of preventing disease is stressed.

Fahey, Thomas D. *The Good Times Fitness Book*. New York: Butterick Publishing, 1979.

This is a book that shows how to get the most out of running, swimming, biking, tennis, golf, and other activities.

Fixx, James. *The Complete Book of Running*. New York: Random House, 1978.

The book contains illustrations with 125 line drawings.

Goldstein, Norman. *The Skin You Live In*. New York: Hart Publishing, 1978.

How to recognize and prevent skin problems and how to care for your skin are discussed. New techniques for prevention of problems and new treatments are explained.

Kiell, Paul J., and Joseph S. Frelinghuysen. *Keep Your Heart Running*. New York: Winchester Press, 1978.

A health/physical fitness manual. Vigorous physical activity is stated as the cornerstone of improving the length and quality of life. Physical activity programs are described, and information on nutrition is presented.

Kuntzleman, Charles T., and the Editors of Consumer Guide. *Rating the Exercises*. New York: William Morrow, 1978.

An evaluation of exercise programs.

Rosenthal, Richard. *The Hearing Loss Handbook*. New York: Schocken Books, 1978.

This is a handbook for those with inherited, congenital, or acquired hearing-loss problems. It explains hearing functions, aids that are used and their suitability to various hearing problems, guarantees to check on, and proper ways to obtain the best services.

Wilmore, Jack H. *Athletic Training and Physical Fitness: Physiological Principles and Practices of the Conditioning Process*. Boston: Allyn and Bacon, 1979.

The book explores the myths and realities of muscle-building aids. Includes measurement and assessment techniques.

Chapter 9

Beller, Anne Scott. *Fat and Thin: A Natural History of Obesity.* New York: Farrar, Straus, and Giroux, 1977.

For thousands of years an ample figure was attractive and desirable. The author discusses the guilt and anxiety that society has imposed on fat people. The book includes information on body size, diet, evolution, and personality traits of the obese, normal, and lanky.

Department of Agriculture. *Family Fare: A Guide to Good Nutrition.* Washington, D.C.: U.S. Government Printing Office, 1978.

Eisenberg, M. Michael. *Ulcers.* New York: Random House, 1978.

Evans, Michele. *Fearless Cooking For Men.* New York: Van Nostrand Reinhold, 1977.

The book covers many recipes from famous men. An easy-to-use cookbook.

Rhein, Reginald W., Jr., and Larry Marion. *The Saccharin Controversy.* New York: Monarch Press, 1977.

An introduction to the arguments for and against the use of saccharin, and the people and politics involved in that controversy.

Shannon, Ira L. *Sugar: Brand Home Guide.* Chicago: Nelson-Hall, 1977.

The book gives the sucrose content of over one thousand foods and beverages, including baby food, gum, cereals, bread, and many others.

Smith, Lendon. *Feed Your Kids Right.* New York: McGraw-Hill, 1979.

This book draws on the latest scientific findings and the author's wide experience to explore the relationship between what children eat and how they feel and behave. Provides a planned and tested nutritional program aimed at preventing illnesses and behavior problems from birth through adolescence.

Winick, Myron. *Malnutrition and Brain Development.* New York: Oxford University Press, 1976.

The effects of prenatal and postnatal malnutrition on brain structure and function.

Chapter 10

Adams, Jane. *Sex and the Single Parent.* New York: Coward, McCann and Geoghegan, 1978.

An exploration of the questions that arise based on the author's own candidly described experiences and those of friends whom she interviewed.

Allred, G. Hugh. *How To Strengthen Your Marriage and Family.* Provo, Utah: Brigham Young University Press, 1976.

This is a commonsense approach to developing better human relationships between husband and wife, parents and children.

Daley, Eliot A. *Father Feelings.* New York: William Morrow, 1978.

The author suggests that fathers should set guidelines, not spoil children at holiday time, spend time separately with each child, consult children about vacation plans, and display warmth and understanding.

Eisler, Diane. *Dissolution.* New York: McGraw-Hill, 1977.

A well-documented book on no-fault divorce, child custody, and alternatives for women.

Gittelson, Natalie. *Dominus.* New York: Farrar, Straus, and Giroux, 1978.

The book translates with clarity and compassion the effects of women's emerging consciousness on the male ego.

Kelley, Robert K. *Courtship, Marriage, and the Family*, 2nd ed. New York: Harcourt Brace Jovanovich, 1974.

Lynch, James J. *The Broken Heart.* New York: Basic Books, 1977.

Noble, June and William. *How to Live with Other People's Children.* New York: Hawthorne Books, 1978.

The focus of the book is on step-relationships and adjustments.

Seligson, Marcia. *Options.* New York: Random House, 1978.

The author writes of her personal expedition across the country to look at open marriages, group marriages, and other experimental living arrangements.

Wassmer, Arthur C. *Making Contact.* Pinebrook, N.J.: The Dial Press, 1978.

The author introduces step-by-step learning techniques for every kind of shyness: behavior changing skills; the "script" to make you at ease on the phone; the use of body language; and many other ways to overcome shyness.

Chapter 11

Bell, Alan P., and Martin S. Weinberg. *Homosexualities: A Study of Diversity Among Men and Women.* New York: Simon & Schuster, 1978.

This official publication of Kinsey's Institute for Sex Research is a comprehensive study of homosexuality in which the range of lifestyles in the homosexual population is examined.

Brownmiller, Susan. *Against Our Will.* New York: Bantam Books, 1975.

This book deals with the psychology of rape, victims of rape, rape and the law, and how women can protect themselves against this violent crime.

Fuchs, Estelle. *The Second Season.* New York: Anchor Press, 1978.

Discusses the sexual life of women in the middle years.

Katchadorian, Herant A., and Donald T. Lunde. *Fundamentals of Human Sexuality*, 2nd ed. New York: Holt, Rinehart and Winston, 1977.

Keane, Philip S. *Sexual Morality: A Catholic Perspective.* Ramsey, N.J.: Paulist Press, 1978.

An examination of sexual morality and problem areas that create anguish and uncertainty—for example, homosexuality, varieties of heterosexual expression, contraception, sex education, celibacy, and others.

Levinson, Daniel J., and others. *The Seasons of a Man's Life*. New York: Alfred A. Knopf, 1978.

The book reveals a great hidden pattern that underlies and shapes every man's life.

Magee, Bryan. *The Gays Among Us*. New York: Stein and Day, 1978.

Explores the lifestyles of female and male homosexuals, the causes of homosexuality, and the law in relation to homosexuality.

Pietropinto, Anthony, and Jacqueline Simenauer. *Beyond the Male Myth*. New York: Times Books, 1978.

The result of a nationwide survey, the book takes an extensive look at sexual attitudes and practices of American men. Documents men's feelings about sex, women, marriage, and love.

Sarnoff, Suzanne and Irving. *Sexual Excitement and Sexual Peace*. New York: M. Evans, 1978.

The book discusses masturbation, a last sexual taboo, as the most hidden and suppressed form of sexual expression. The authors franky discuss the significance of feelings of guilt, and the ways in which parents can deal with their children.

Silverstein, Charles. *A Family Matter*. New York: McGraw-Hill, 1977.

A parents' guide to homosexuality.

Yates, Alayne. *Sex Without Shame*. New York: William Morrow, 1977.

The author shows parents how to preserve a child's healthy erotic response, and offers concrete ways to encourage, enrich, and expand the child's sexuality from birth through puberty to marriage.

Chapter 12

Francke, Linda Bird. *The Ambivalence of Abortion*. New York: Random House, 1978.

The book contains personal stories of abortions of hundreds of men and women of all ages from all sections of the country.

Keniston, Kenneth, and the Carnegie Council on Children. *All Our Children*. New York: Harcourt Brace Jovanovich, 1978.

Llewellyn-Jones, Derek. *Everywoman: A Gynaecological Guide for Life*. Salem, N.H.: Faber & Faber, 1978.

The author answers questions and clarifies the "business of being a woman" from menstruation to menopause.

Our Bodies, Ourselves. New York: Simon & Schuster, 1976.

This book, written by and for women, seeks to promote growth and change in women and men. It was written in response to an imperative need for women to learn about their bodies in order to have control over them and their lives. A few of the topics discussed are the anatomy and physiology of sexuality, reproduction, rape, birth control, abortion, and parenthood.

Rose, Louisa, ed. *The Menopause Book*. New York: Hawthorne Books, 1977.

The book explains what happens to most women during menopause and also prepares women to cope with their own menopausal pattern. The eight doctor-authors are specialists in gynecology, psychiatry, and internal medicine.

Tunnadine, David, and Roger H. Green. *Unwanted Pregnancy—Accident or Illness?* New York: Oxford University Press, 1978.

An in-depth look at psychological factors of unwanted pregnancies. Discusses characteristics common to many women requesting abortion.

Chapter 13

Annis, Linda Farrill. *The Child Before Birth*. Ithaca, N.Y.: Cornell University Press, 1978.

A concise account of the nine months from conception to birth and factors influencing development and learning.

Dick-Read, Grantly. *Childbirth Without Fear*. New York: Harper & Row, 1978.

The essence of this book is natural childbirth, the psychological problems connected with childbearing, and a step-by-step guide for expectant parents, their teachers, and attendants.

Hausknecht, Richard, and Joan Rattner Heilman. *Having a Caesarean Baby*. New York: E.P. Dutton, 1978.

This volume details the entire Caesarean birth experience from pregnancy until the mother and baby are safely home. It deals with reasons for Caesarean birth, pros and cons of anesthesias, psychological and physical impacts on the mother and baby, and recovery.

Leboyer, Frederick. *Birth Without Violence*. New York: Alfred A. Knopf, 1976.

The revolutionary and simple techniques for easing an infant's birth trauma are presented.

Macdonald, Charlotte. "The Stunted World of Teen Parents." *Human Behavior*, Vol. 8 (January 1979), pp. 53–55.

Zelnik, Melvin, and John F. Kanter. "Contraceptive Patterns and Premarital Pregnancy Among Women Aged 15–19 in 1976." *Family Planning Perspectives*, Vol. 10 (May–June 1978), pp. 135–142.

Nilsson, Lennart. *A Child Is Born*. New York: Delacorte Press, 1978.

A revised edition with 125 color photographs and written text for prospective parents.

Chapter 14

Goodfield, June. *Playing God: Genetic Engineering and the Manipulation of Life*. New York: Random House, 1977.

The author discusses the creation of new species, based on the need to preserve genetic stocks of plants and animals and to produce disease-resistant varieties.

Hendin, David, and Joan Markes. *The Genetic Connection: How to Protect Your Family Against Hereditary Diseases*. New York: William Morrow, 1977.

A guide to how knowledge of genetic diseases can be applied. Lists genetic counseling and treatment centers in each state.

Judson, Horace Freeland. *The Eighth Day of Creation*. New York: Simon & Schuster, 1979.

The author traces the history of the discovery of DNA through his interviews with biologists, physicists, and other scientists; the manufacture of proteins through the information in the DNA molecule; and the discovery of messenger RNA.

Lear, John. *Recombinant DNA: The Untold Story.* New York: Crown Publishers, 1978.

A report of a twenty-month study of the recombinant DNA controversy. The public issue concerns whether scientists are to continue manipulating the discovery or whether the people are to say how funds will be spent.

Portugal, Franklin H., and Jack S. Cohen. *A Century of DNA.* Cambridge, Mass.: MIT Press, 1978.

A history of the structure and function of the genetic substance. The authors discuss the false starts and wrong turns that have been made and the obstacles to progress.

Wade, Nicholas. *The Ultimate Experiment: Man-Made Evolution.* New York: Walker and Company, 1977.

Describes how recombinant technology was developed and is used. Discusses the concerns expressed by scientists and the public.

Chapter 15

Carroll, Charles R., and Warren E. Schaller. *Health, Quackery, and the Consumer.* Philadelphia: W.B. Saunders, 1976.

Cornacchia, Harold J. *Consumer Health.* St. Louis, Mo.: C.V. Mosby, 1976.

Health insurance, health care economics, consumer protection, and psychological factors in consumerism are among the areas covered in this book.

Dicker, Ralph Leslie, and Victor Royce Syracuse. *Consultation with a Plastic Surgeon.* New York: Warner Books, 1977.

A simple, straightforward question-and-answer exchange covering face lifts, nose surgery, dermal abrasion, sex changes, and many other medical procedures.

Ginzberg, Eli. *The Limits of Health Reform: The Search for Realism.* New York: Basic Books, 1977.

Reforms in the last thirty years have resulted in no significant improvements in quality, equity, or availability of this nation's health care system. The author takes the stand that reforms should be aimed at containing costs and providing care to those who most need it.

Gots, Ronald, and Arthur Kaufman. *The People's Hospital Book.* New York: Crown Publishers, 1978.

Contains information on obtaining maximum comfort, safety, and care before, during, and after a hospital stay.

Kovner, Anthony R., and Samuel P. Martin, eds. *Community Medicine and Health Care Delivery.* New York: Grune and Stratton, 1978.

A basic textbook for health professions by which medical and nursing students and practitioners view their work in a wider span of organization, finance, and government regulation.

Law, Sylvia, and Steven Polan. *Pain and Profit: The Politics of Malpractice.* New York: Harper & Row, 1978.

This is a careful, thoughtful review of the malpractice situation. It includes reports on the legal system, insurance system, and medical system in the United States.

Lipp, Martin R. *The Patient Is Human.* New York: Harper & Row, 1977.

The book covers the common psychiatric problems encountered in practice, particularly in a hospital setting but also in an ambulatory setting.

Newman, Ian M. *Consumer Behavior in the Health Marketplace.* Lincoln, Neb.: Health Education Department, School of Health, Physical Education and Recreation, 1978.

This is a record of proceedings from a symposium on consumerism that examines the forces that affect consumer behavior in the purchase of health-related products and services. Ten scholars in the health field address consumer behavior from a variety of perspectives.

Quinlan, Joseph and Julia. *Karen Ann.* New York: Doubleday, 1977.

A record of a tragedy that became a medical dilemma and a legal landmark.

Epilogue

Galton, Lawrence, *Medical Advances.* New York: Crown Publishers, 1977.

The book covers a broad range of problems that affect the entire family, and it includes information on the latest discoveries in the field of medicine.

Learning To Live With Diabetes. Austin, Tex.: Texas Department of Health Resources, 1978.

A seventy-page book to help patients manage and understand this life-long disease. A practical guide with humorous illustrations.

Packard, Vance. *The People Shapers.* New York: Little, Brown, 1978.

The author offers the idea that human engineers are at work increasing the capacity of a small number of people to control and manipulate the lives of a large number of people. Techniques used include programming behavior, manipulating genes, altering the beginning and ending of life, controlling and surveillance, and others.

Swazey, Judith P., and Karen Reeds. *Today's Medicine, Tomorrow's Science.* Essays on Paths of Discovery in the Biomedical Sciences. Washington, D.C.: U.S. Department of Health, Education, and Welfare, 1978.

This publication is an examination of the ways in which categorical or disease-oriented research has contributed to the fundamental biological phenomena and processes.

Wechsler, Henry, Joel Givun, and George F. Cahill, Jr., eds. *The Horizons of Health.* Cambridge, Mass.: Harvard University Press, 1977.

How to Understand Your Doctor

Medical terms seem complicated, but if they are broken up into their Greek and Latin parts they become comparatively simple. The following list includes the elements of almost all the terms that will be mentioned by your doctor, or that will be met with in your reading. All of these terms, whether complete words or combining forms, are either directly or eventually from the Greek, with the single exception of *denti-*, which is of Latin origin.

–ALGIA means "pain." It occurs in neur*algia*, the technical term for "pain" along the course of a nerve. (*neuron*, "nerve")

ARTHRO– means a "joint."
*Arthr*itis is an inflammation of the "joints." (*-itis*, "inflammation")

CARDIO– means "heart."
*Cardi*ac refers to the state of the "heart."
A *cardio*graph is a device that makes a graph of the heartbeat on paper. (*grapho*, "write")
The man who is expert in the diagnosis and treatment of disorders of the "heart" is a *cardio*logist. (*-logy*, "science of")

CYSTO– means a "sac" or "bladder."
*Cyst*itis is inflammation of the "bladder."
A *cysto*scope is an instrument that enables the doctor to examine the interior of the "bladder." (*skopeo*, "look")
*Cysto*tomy refers to cutting into the "bladder." (*-tomia*, "cutting")
A *cyst* is a "sac" containing morbid matter within the body.

DENTI– means "tooth."
*Dent*ure is a word that describes false "teeth."
A *denti*frice is the powder or paste with which we clean our "teeth." (*frico*, "rub")
*Dent*ine is the ivory-like material of which "teeth" are made.

–DERM, DERMAT– means "skin."
Epi*derm*is is the name for the outermost layer of "skin," so called because it is on top. (*epi-*, "on")
A *dermat*ologist is a "skin" specialist. (*-logy*, "science of")

DYS– means "disordered," "difficult," "faulty."
*Dys*pepsia is "faulty" digestion. (*peptos*, "cook")
*Dys*entery is a "disorder" of the intestines. (*enteron*, "intestine")

"How to Understand Your Doctor" (pp. 400–404) in WORD ORIGINS AND THEIR ROMANTIC STORIES by Wilfred Funk (Funk & Wagnalls). Copyright 1950 by Wilfred Funk Inc. Reprinted by permission of Harper & Row, Publishers, Inc.

–ECTOMY means a "cutting out" and comes from the Greek *ek*, "out," and *-tomia*, "cutting."
Append*ectomy* is the "cutting out" of the appendix.
Tonsill*ectomy* is the "cutting out" of the tonsils.
Gast*rectomy* is the "cutting out" of the stomach. (*gastros*, "stomach")

ENTERO– means "intestine."
*Entero*stomy is the surgical term for making an opening in the small "intestine." (*stoma*, "mouth")
*Enter*itis is the inflammation of the "intestine." (*-itis*, "inflammation")

GASTRO– means "stomach."
*Gastr*ic juices operate upon the contents of the "stomach."
*Gastr*itis is inflammation of the "stomach."

HEMO– means "blood."
*Hemo*globins are the coloring matter in the red "blood." (*globus*, "globe")
*Hemo*philia is a hereditary condition characterized by a tendency to excessive "bleeding" from the slightest wound. (*philia*, "fondness")

HEPATO– means "liver."
*Hepat*itis is inflammation of the "liver." (*-itis*, "inflammation")
A *hepat*ic is a medicine one takes for the "liver."

HYPER– means "excessive."
*Hyper*acidity is a condition of "excessive" acidity.
*Hyper*tension is a state of overtension.
A *hyper*thyroid condition is caused by overactivity of the thyroid gland.

HYPO– means "under" or "insufficient."
*Hypo*acidity is a "lack" of acid in some part of the body.

HYSTERO– means the "uterus."
*Hyster*ectomy: an operation performed on women for the removal of the "uterus." (*-ectomy*, "a cutting out")

–ITIS means "inflammation."
Appendic*itis* is an "inflammation" of the appendix.

NEPHRO– means the "kidney."
*Nephr*itis is the medical name for Bright's disease, which, of course, is an inflammation of the "kidneys." (*-itis*, "inflammation")

OPHTHALMO– means "eye."

An *ophthalmo*logist is a doctor who treats the "eyes" and their diseases. (*-logy*, "science of")

–OSIS means a "diseased" or "abnormal" condition.

Neur*osis* is a "disorder" of the nervous system. (*neuron*, "nerve")

Psych*osis* is a "disease" of the mind. (*psyche*, "mind")

Thromb*osis* is the formation of a clot in the circulatory system. (*thrombos*, "clot")

Hali*tosis* refers to unpleasant breath. (*halitos*, "breath")

OSTEO– means "bone."

*Oste*itis is inflammation of the "bones." (*-itis*, "inflammation")

*Osteo*pathy is based on the theory that disease is caused by some maladjustment of the "bone" structure and can be cured by manipulation. (*patheia*, "suffering")

OTO– means "ear."

*Oto*logy is the medical name given to the study and treatment of the "ear."

An *oto*scope is the instrument the doctor uses when he looks into the "ear." (*skopeo*, "look")

PHARYNGO– means "throat."

*Pharyng*itis is an inflammation of the "throat." (*-itis*, "inflammation")

*Pharyng*ology is that branch of medical science that treats the "throat" and its diseases.

PHLEB– means "vein."

*Phleb*itis is the inflammation of a "vein" that in women is sometimes called "milk leg." (*-itis*, "inflammation")

PNEUM– means "lung."

*Pneum*onia is primarily an inflammation of the "lungs."

PSYCHO– means "mind."

*Psych*iatry is a specialized branch of medical science that treats "mental" disturbances and diseases. (*iatreia*, "healing")

*Psycho*analysis is a method developed by Sigmund Freud for analyzing the "mental" life of a person in preparation for treating "mental" ills.

*Psycho*logy is the study of the "mind." (*-logy*, "study of")

RHEA means a "flowing" or a "discharge."

Diar*rhea* is literally a "flowing" through. (*dia-*, "through")

Gonor*rhea* has as one symptom a "discharge" from the reproductive organs. (*gonos*, "generation")

Pyor*rhea* is a purulent inflammation of the sockets of the teeth characterized by a "discharge" of pus. (*pyon*, "pus")

RHINO– means "nose."

*Rhin*al infection is "nasal" infection.

*Rhin*itis is inflammation of the mucous membranes of the "nose." (*-itis*, "inflammation")

Glossary

A

acoustic nerve The nerve leading from the inner ear to the brain.

active immunity Long-lasting resistance to infection acquired either through the production of antibodies by the body after invasion by disease-causing organisms or through injection of a vaccine composed of organisms that have been weakened or killed. Compare *passive immunity*.

adenoids An increased amount of tissue containing white blood cells, often situated (particularly in children) at the back of the nose and above the throat.

adenosine triphosphate (ATP) A chemical compound that contains high-energy chemicals that when broken down yield the energy necessary for muscular contractions, production of proteins, maintenance of body heat, and other energy-requiring reactions.

aerobic exercises Exercises that require muscular contractions so that there is an increased use of oxygen.

afferent arteriole A very small artery that leads to an organ.

afterbirth The placenta and membranes expelled from the uterus following childbirth.

agitation The state of being perturbed or disturbed.

Al-Anon An organization for spouses of alcoholics to help them cope with the problems that accompany alcoholism.

Alateen An organization for children of alcoholics to help them cope with the special problems they face.

Alcoholics Anonymous An organization composed of alcoholics who, through group support, attempt to help themselves and other alcoholics overcome their dependence.

allergen A substance capable of inducing a specific and acquired overreaction of the immune response.

allergic rhinitis Inflammation of the nasal mucous membranes caused by any effective allergen.

allergy Abnormal body reactions resulting from undue sensitivity to a wide variety of substances, including various foods, dusts, and pollens.

amino acid One of a group of nitrogenous organic compounds that serve as the basic units of proteins.

amnesia Loss of memory.

amniocentesis A procedure to obtain a sample of amniotic fluid by puncturing the intrauterine amniotic sac through the abdominal wall. Used to diagnose certain genetic disorders.

amnion The membranes forming the fluid-filled sac that protects the embryo.

amniotic fluid The fluid within the amniotic sac surrounding the fetus.

anemia A condition characterized by less than a normal amount of red blood cells and hemoglobin.

anesthesia Loss of sensation induced by anesthetic agents.

Antabuse A chemical used in the treatment of alcoholism.

antibody A protein substance produced by plasma cells in response to a specific antigen; it combines with and, in effect, neutralizes the antigen.

antigen A substance, usually protein, that when foreign to the body stimulates the formation of a specific antibody.

anvil The middle bone in the middle ear.

anxiety An emotional state characterized by apprehension and tension.

anxiety state A feeling of apprehension or tension that is not restricted to particular events or persons.

aorta The artery that transports oxygenated blood from the left ventricle of the heart to the rest of the body.

aqueous humor The fluid filling the space between the cornea and lens of the eye. It is thought to be secreted by the ciliary body.

arteriole A very small artery.

artery A tubular vessel through which the blood passes away from the heart to other parts of the body.

arthritis Inflammation of a joint.

asthma Respiratory symptoms that result from particle irritation, infection, or an allergic reaction. These symptoms include recurrent attacks of labored breathing, wheezing, coughing, and a sense of constriction in the chest.

astigmatism A visual defect that results when two adjacent portions of the cornea of the eye have different curvatures and thus prevent the image from being clearly focused on the retina.

atherosclerosis A circulatory disease process of large- and medium-sized arteries, marked by deposits of yellow plaques containing cholesterol and other fatty substances.

atrium (pl. **atria**) One of the pair of smaller chambers of the heart; it receives blood from the veins and passes it to the ventricles.

attenuated A weakened or reduced virulence of a virus of pathogenic organism.

auditory canal The passage beginning with the acoustic meatus (opening) that leads to the eardrum. It is about $1^{1}/_{4}$ inches long in the adult. The glands of the canal produce earwax.

auditory tube The mucous-membrane-lined canal that connects the pharynx with the middle ear.

auricle The ear flap, or external ear.

autosome A chromosone that is not a sex chromosome. In humans there are forty-four autosomes (twenty-two pairs).

aversion experience A form of treatment for alcohol or drug dependence that connects an unpleasant experience with use of the drug.

axon The extension of a nerve cell that transmits impulses from the central nervous system to the other nerve cells, muscles, glands, or blood vessels.

B

B lymphocyte A type of white blood cell; it plays the major role in the antibody immune response. See *lymphocyte*; *T lymphocyte*.

bacillus A rod-shaped bacterium.

bacteria (sing. **bacterium**) One-celled microorganisms, some of which cause disease; the main groups are bacilli, cocci, and spiral-shaped.

barbiturate A depressant drug used as a hypnotic (causing sleep) or a sedative (producing a quieting effect on the central nervous system).

Bartholin's gland One of the two small bodies embedded in the labia minora on either side of the opening of the vagina; it produces a lubricating material during prolonged sexual stimulation.

benign Not malignant; not recurrent.

birth control Intentional limitation of the number of children by preventing conception through such means as contraceptives, the rhythm method, tubal ligation, and vasectomy.

bouton A small knob located at the end of each axon; it almost touches the neuron to which an impulse is being sent.

bursa A small sac lined with synovial membrane (within a joint) and filled with synovial fluid; it is found between parts that move upon each other, such as the bursa above the bone in front of the kneebone (patella).

C

Caesarean section A surgical operation for the delivery of a fetus performed when birth by natural means is dangerous or impossible. It is accomplished by means of an incision through the walls of the abdomen and uterus.

calculus A solid mass that is found in ducts, cysts, and on the surface of teeth. It is composed mainly of salts and minerals.

calorie The amount of heat necessary to raise the temperature of one gram of water one degree Centigrade. More commonly used is the *kilocalorie*, which is one thousand times greater than the calorie.

cancer A malignant cellular tumor.

capillary A minute blood vessel connecting an arteriole and a venule.

capillary bed The capillaries of a given area or organ.

carbohydrates Any of certain organic compounds, including starches, sugars, and cellulose, that are made up of carbon, hydrogen, and oxygen.

carcinogenic A cancer-producing substance.

carcinoma A cancer of epithelial cells such as those in glands, skin, and the lining membranes of organs. It tends to infiltrate surrounding tissues and to spread to other parts of the body.

cardiovascular system The part of the body's circulatory system composed of the heart and blood vessels.

caries Decay of bone or teeth.

cell body A living cell minus the processes of that cell.

central nervous system The brain and spinal cord.

cerebrovascular accident (CVA) Neurological deficits, seizures, or alterations in consciousness caused by cerebral hemorrhage or embolism of the cerebral vessels.

cerebrovascular disease A disease related to the blood supply of the cerebrum.

cerebrum The main portion of the brain, located in the upper cranium and forming the largest part of the human central nervous system. It is believed to control conscious and voluntary processes.

cervix The constricted portion of the uterus; it is the neck of the uterus and its lower portion.

chancre The primary sore or ulcer that is the first sign of syphilis.

character disorder Socially unacceptable patterns of behavior that are not combined with the anxiety often seen in other neuroses.

chemotherapy The use of chemical agents to prevent or treat disease.

chlamydia A group of microorganisms that can cause parrot fever, trachoma, and two kinds of sexually transmitted diseases.

cholesterol A chemical substance found in the fatty parts of animal tissue. It may be involved in atherosclerosis.

choroid The vascular structure of the eye.

chomosome One of the several more or less rod-shaped bodies that appear in the nucleus of a cell. They are constant in number for each species and contain the genes, or hereditary factors. The normal number in humans is forty-six: twenty-two pairs of autosomes, and two sex chromosomes.

chronic bronchitis A persistent inflammation of the mucous membrane of the bronchi.

chronic degenerative diseases Lasting diseases that cause tissues to become increasingly less functional.

circadian rhythm The cyclic repetition of certain phenomena in living organisms at about the same time every twenty-four hours.

climacteric The bodily, glandular, and sometimes emotional changes that occur at the end of the reproductive period in the woman and that usually result in some diminution of sexual activity in the man. In the woman, menstruation ceases; in both sexes, there is a reduction in the production of sex hormones.

cocaine A stimulant drug derived from coca leaves; it causes excitability and loss of fatigue and hunger.

coccus A sphere-shaped bacterial cell.

cochlea The spirally wound portion of the bone containing the inner ear.

codeine An analgesic and a respiratory sedative.

codon An informational unit of chemicals making up genetic material.

colon The part of the large intestine that begins at the cecum and ends at the end of the sigmoid flexure.

communicable Any infection that can be transferred from one individual to another.

community A group of individuals who share the same environment, interests, and privileges.

complement A substance in the normal blood serum that combines with antigen-antibody complexes to destroy the antigen.

conception The fertilization of an ovum by a spermatozoon.

conducting system A network of specialized cells in the heart responsible for keeping the heart beating rhythmically.

conductive deafness Partial or total deafness due to interference with transmission of sound through the outer or middle ear.

congenital Existing at birth.

congenital defect A defect existing at birth, regardless of its cause; resulting from or developing in the prenatal environment.

congestion Excessive or abnormal accumulation of blood in a body part.

conjunctiva The mucous membrane covering the front portion of the eyeball.

conscience Morality, or the sense of right and wrong.

contagious See *communicable*.

contraceptive A device designed to prevent conception.

conversion reaction The form of neurosis in which the anxiety-causing impulse is converted into a physical symptom.

cornea The transparent portion of the eyeball.

coronary artery One of the arteries that supply the heart muscle with blood.

corpus luteum A yellow body on the ovary formed by an ovarian follicle that has matured and released its ovum; it secretes the hormone progesterone.

cross-tolerance The effect of tolerance to one drug producing a tolerance to another, similar drug, as heroin to morphine. Compare *tolerance*.

culture The sum of what people have learned and transmitted from generation to generation.

cyanosis A bluish discoloration of the skin due to reduced hemoglobin in the capillaries.

cyotoplasm All the protoplasm (the essential substance of the cell) contained within a cell except the nucleus.

D

decibel (dB) A unit of sound measurement, or of loudness.

deciduous teeth The twenty primary (or "baby") teeth that are later replaced with permanent teeth.

delusion A belief held in spite of incontrovertible evidence to the contrary. A characteristic of certain psychotic disorders.

dendrite The portion of the neuron that carries nerve impulses to the cell body.

dental cavity A localized, progressive disintegration of a tooth.

dental plaque Transparent films on the surface of the teeth secreted by the salivary glands; bacteria multiply in the plaque to promote cavity formations.

dentin The tissue that forms the major part of the tooth. It is covered by enamel over the crown of the tooth.

deoxyribonucleic acid (DNA) A chemical substance found in the nucleus of cells; it is the material of the gene and, thus, of heredity; along with proteins, it makes up the chromosomes. DNA is also found in mitochondria and in cytoplasm.

depressant Any of a group of drugs that depresses the central nervous system.

depressive reaction A psychoneurotic disorder in which depression is used to partially relieve anxiety.

depressive state An emotional disorder characterized by extreme depression.

detoxification The process of changing a chemical or compound within the body to one that is more easily excreted or that is less poisonous.

dialysis machine A mechanical device that purifies uremic blood by filtration.

diastole The rhythmic period of relaxation and dilation of a heart chamber as it fills with blood. Compare *systole*.

diastolic pressure The lowest blood pressure during relaxation of the ventricles.

dissociative reaction A psychoneurotic disorder in which the person's conflicting attitudes, emotions, or personality parts are disconnected from one another, such as in multiple personality or amnesia.

Down's syndrome A congenital condition associated with a chromosomal abnormality; it is characterized by a somewhat flattened skull and nose, eyes that appear slanted, and other physical abnormalities; there is usually moderate to severe mental retardation. Also called *Mongolism* or *Trisomy 21*.

drug abuse According to the World Health Organization, "persistent or sporadic excessive drug use inconsistent with or unrelated to acceptable medical practice."

drug dependence A state of reliance —physical, psychological, or both— on a drug, arising from ingestion of that drug on a continuous or periodic basis.

duct A tube, especially one for conveying glandular secretions.

duodenal ulcer A peptic ulcer in the duodenum, or the first part of the small intestine.

E

eardrum The tympanic menbrane.

ecology The shared interaction between living things and their environment.

ecosystem The systematic, orderly combination or arrangement of living organisms reacting with one another in a shared environment.

ectoparasite A parasite that lives on its host's exterior.

eczema An acute or chronic disease of the skin; it is itchy, inflammatory, and noncommunicable.

edema The swelling of tissues caused by an abnormal accumulation of excess fluids.

ego-identity A term used by Erikson and other psychologists to describe the sense of self that emerges as part of the development process.

ejaculation The expulsion of semen that usually occurs at the climax of sexual stimulation; it is accomplished by peristaltic contractions of parts of the male genital system.

embolus A clot or other obstruction that travels through the bloodstream until it lodges in a blood vessel and plugs it.

embryo The early stage of development of an organism in the uterus. In the human, the term describes the period of development from one week after fertilization to the end of the second month of pregnancy.

emphysema A lung condition marked by abnormal increase in the size of the air spaces in the lungs. It causes destruction of the walls of the alveoli (air sacs) of the lungs.

enamel The calcified covering over the crown of a tooth.

endocrine gland A gland that secretes its hormone directly into the bloodstream rather than into a duct. Compare *exocrine gland*.

endometrium The inner lining of the uterus.

endoplasmic reticulum A membranous transportation system of canals within the cytoplasm of cells; it is formed by inward folds of the plasma cell membrane that surrounds the cell. Materials needed by the cell move through these canals. The endoplasmic reticulum also connects with the nuclear membrane. On part of the endoplasmic reticulum are the ribosomes.

endorphins A group of chemical compounds produced by the brain and pituitary gland that have the pain-killing effects of morphinelike drugs.

environment The sum total of all the factors that make up one's surroundings.

enzyme An organic compound, usually a protein, that acts as a catalyst, starting or speeding up specific chemical reactions of other compounds without itself taking part in those reactions.

erogenous zone An area of the body that is especially sensitive to sexual stimulation. Some of these are the mouth, lips, tongue, breasts and nipples, buttocks, and genitals.

erythrocyte See *red blood cell*.

essential hypertension Hypertension that is unrelated to any other disease and for which the cause is unknown.

estrogen The female sex hormone. Also, a general term for compounds produced by ovarian hormonal activity resulting in secondary sex characteristics and cyclic genital changes.

Eustachian tube See *auditory tube*.

exocrine gland A gland that secretes its products into a duct rather than directly into the bloodstream. Compare *endocrine gland*.

F

Fallopian tube The tube that extends from the ovary to the uterus and through which the ovum (egg) travels. Also called *oviduct*.

farsightedness A visual disorder marked by the ability to see far objects more clearly than near ones. It is caused by a loss of elasticity in the lens that causes images to fall in back of the retina. Also called *hyperopia*.

fats Substances high in caloric value and found in some form in most foods.

fetus In humans, the developing child in the uterus from the beginning of the third month of pregnancy until birth.

flexor muscle A muscle that flexes a limb or a body part.

fluoride A salt used in the control of dental caries.

follicle-stimulating hormone (FSH) One of the gonadotropic (gonad-stimulating) hormones produced by the anterior lobe of the pituitary gland under the direction of the hypothalamus. FSH promotes the maturation of the Graafian follicle in the female and maturation of spermatozoa in the testes of the male.

foreskin See *prepuce*.

fraternal twins Twins resulting from the simultaneous fertilization of two ova. Compare *identical twins*.

frequency In sound, the number of periodic vibrations or waves that occur during a given period of time, usually seconds.

fungus A parasitic, low form of plant life.

G

gallbladder A hollow organ situated underneath the liver for the storage of bile and secretion of mucus.

gamete A secondary sex cell. In humans, either a male spermatozoon or a female ovum.

gastric ulcer An ulcer of the mucous lining of the stomach.

gene The basic unit of hereditary and genetic information. Each gene is self-producing and is located at a specific place on a chromosome.

gene mapping Sorting and categorizing chromosomes to obtain knowledge of the order of genes and their relative distance. Important for understanding hereditary diseases.

General Adaptation Syndrome (G.A.S.) A term, postulated by Hans Selye, denoting three stages of reaction to stress: (1) alarm, (2) resistance, and (3) exhaustion.

genital herpes A sexually transmitted disease caused by genital herpesvirus 2.

genotype The particular assortment or combination of genes of an individual. Compare *phenotype*.

germ cell A spermatozoon or an ovum.

gingivitis Inflammation of the mucous membrane and soft tissue surrounding a tooth.

gland A group of cells that separates elements from the blood and produces from them a specific substance for the body to use.

glans The sexually sensitive body at the end of the clitoris or penis. It is the head of either organ.

glomerulus (pl. **glomeruli**) One of the numerous tiny capillary coils or tufts in the kidney, each projecting into the expanded end, or capsule, of a uriniferous tubule, and from which blood wastes are filtered into the tubule.

gonad A gland that produces gametes; the ovary or testis.

gonadotropic hormone Any hormone that influences a gonad.

gonorrhea A sexually transmitted disease caused by gonococci bacteria.

Graafian follicle A tiny sac or pouch in the ovary that contains the maturing ovum, releasing it at ovulation.

granulocyte A type of white blood cell that patrols the circulating blood and sticks to the walls of veins.

H

hallucination The perception of sights or sounds that are not actually present.

hallucinogen An agent or drug that produces hallucinations.

hammer The first bone of the middle ear. Also called the *malleus*.

hashish A drug derived from the plant *Cannabis sativa*. It is the concentrated resin of the leaves of the female plant and is five to ten times stronger than marijuana.

hay fever A condition of watering eyes, itching nose, and sneezing; it is caused by pollen antigens in the air.

health foods A vague term commonly used to refer to natural or organic foods.

helminth A worm or wormlike parasite.

hemoglobin The pigment that is the primary constituent of red blood cells and that carries oxygen and carbon dioxide.

hemophilia A hereditary disease in which the blood cannot clot.

hemorrhage The loss of large quantities of blood.

hepatitis A Infectious hepatitis, a viral disease.

hepatitis B Serum hepatitis, a viral disease.

hermaphrodite An organism in which both male and female sex organs exist. In the human, it is characterized by the presence of both ovarian and testicular tissue and reproductive organs that are not typical of one gender.

histamine A chemical released by body tissues in allergic reactions; it causes capillaries to dilate.

hives A skin rash characterized by itching welts with raised centers.

Hodgkin's disease A progressive, formerly fatal enlargement of the spleen, lymph nodes, and general lymphoid tissue.

hormone A chemical substance that is secreted by an endocrine (ductless) gland into the circulatory system and that has a specific effect on a certain target organ.

host An animal or plant that harbors or nourishes another organism (a *parasite*).

hymen The membrane that partly or entirely covers the external opening of the vagina in some virginal females. It is usually broken by sexual intercourse, but its absence may be due to many other reasons.

hyperkinetic Pertaining to abnormally increased mobility or activity.

hypertension Persistent, abnormally high blood pressure.

hypertensive heart disease Enlargement of the heart caused by the heart beating against increased blood pressure (hypertension).

hysteria A neurotic response to an anxiety-provoking situation, characterized by conversion or dissociative reactions.

I

identical twins Twins developed from a single ovum. Compare *fraternal twins*.

immunity See *active immunity* and *passive immunity*.

immunoglobulin An animal protein that helps create an immune reaction as an antibody for a specific antigen.

impact statement A description of the potential effects on the environment of a proposed major action or project.

infertility The inability to conceive.

intensity In sound, the amount of force per volume, measured in decibels.

interferon A protein formed by animal cells during their interaction with viruses. It has the ability to confer on fresh animal cells of the same animal species resistance to infection by other viruses.

ionizing radiation Energy released from unstable atomic nuclei in the form of waves or tiny bits of matter.

iris The colored disk suspended in the aqueous humor of the eye. It separates the front and rear eye chambers and is perforated by an adjustable pupil.

ischemia Lack of sufficient blood to a body part, due to obstruction of a blood vessel.

ischemic heart disease A condition caused by a less than adequate supply of nourishing blood to the heart.

isometrics Contractions in which muscles cannot shorten. Tension develops but it is dissipated as heat. Neither movement nor work is performed.

isotonics Contractions in which a muscle shortens against a load, leading to work and movement.

K

karyotype A chart showing the typical characteristics (such as number, size, and form) and systematic arrangement of the chromosomes of a cell of an individual or species.

kilocalorie See *calorie*.

L

large intestine The portion of the intestine that extends from the ileum to the anus and consists of the cecum, colon, and rectum.

lens The crystalline, transparent, solid body of the eye. It is suspended behind the iris between the front chamber and the vitreous body (the transparent substance that fills the eyeball between the retina and lens).

leukemia A cancer of the blood-forming organs that may be either chronic or acute and that is marked by a great increase in the number of white blood cells and by enlargement of the lymphatic tissue and bone marrow.

leukocyte See *white blood cell*.

leukocytosis An increase in leukocytes, which occurs with most bacterial infections.

ligament A fibrous connective tissue that holds bone joints together or supports organs.

lipid Fat.

lipoprotein A group of chemicals in the blood that are composed of a protein combined with a fat.

liver A glandular organ located on the upper right side of the abdominal cavity. It is the body's largest gland.

London-type smog Caused by the burning of fossil fuels, such as coal. Sulfur dioxide, a product of incomplete combustion of the fuel, is oxidized in the air to form sulfur trioxide, which is very irritating to the breathing apparatus. When combined with fog, an irritating acid is formed.

longitudinal arch The lengthwise arch of the foot.

Los Angeles-type smog Also called "oxidizing" or "photochemical" smog, it is rarely associated with fog. It is the product of automobile emissions, which, when mixed with sunlight, cause a variety of irritating, even poisonous, substances, such as oxides of nitrogen and ozone.

loudness A characteristic of sound. See *intensity*.

luteinizing hormone (LH) The hormone manufactured and released by the anterior (front) lobe of the pituitary gland. It plays an important role in the release of the ovum from the ovary (ovulation). The LH, like FSH, is under the control of a releasing hormone from the hypothalamus.

lymph A clear yellowish liquid collected from the tissue spaces. Once it has entered the lymph vessels, it transports molecules back to the blood protein from where they seep into the extracellular spaces. It also contains white blood cells loaded with wastes that are filtered out by the lymph nodes.

lymph node One of a number of masses of lymphoid tissue situated along the course of lymphatic vessels. They filter cellular debris and other wastes from lymph. In them, lymphocytes are situated and plasma cells make antibodies, which aid in immunity.

lymphocyte A type of white blood cell on which the body's immune response depends. Manufactured largely in the bone marrow, lymphocytes enter the bloodstream to be differentiated into *B lymphocytes* and *T lymphocytes*.

lymphoma A new growth, usually cancerous, of lymphatic tissues.

lysosome Tiny organelles found inside a cell that contain digestive enzymes capable of breaking down complex nutrients into simpler substances that the cell can use.

M

macrophage A type of cell that assists T lymphocytes in the cell-mediated immune response; it functions as a phagocyte, engulfing and ingesting foreign particles or cells (such as bacteria) that harm the body.

malignant Cancerous; dangerous to health or life.

malocclusion Improper alignment of the upper and lower rows of teeth.

manic-depressive psychosis A psychotic disorder marked by extreme mood swings from elation to depression.

manic reaction A psychological disorder marked by extreme excitement.

marijuana A drug derived from the plant *Cannabis sativa*.

meiosis A type of cell division that occurs only in the maturation process of sex cells; each daughter nucleus receives one-half the number of chromosomes normally found in a somatic (body) cell. See also *mitosis*.

menarche The onset of menstruation.

menopause The cessation of menstruation in the female, usually occurring between the ages of forty-five and fifty.

menstruation A periodic discharge of blood and fluids from the uterus during the childbearing years.

messenger RNA A type of ribonucleic acid that transfers information from a portion of the nuclear DNA to a ribosome of a cell, where proteins are formed.

metabolism All the chemical and physical processes by which living substances are produced and maintained; the process by which energy is made available to the cell.

metastasize To transfer a disease (usually cancer) from one organ to another.

methylmercury An organic chemical that can be harmful because it remains in the body for long enough periods of time to attack the brain and spinal cord.

microorganism A microscopic organism, especially a bacterium or a one-celled protozoan.

Minamata disease Organic methylmercury poisoning causing signs and symptoms of nervous system damage, including blindness, deafness, inability to speak, paralysis, and mental retardation.

mitochondria Any of the organelles in the cytoplasm of a cell that convert the chemical energy of cellular nutrients into a high-energy compound called adenosine triphosphate (ATP). They also contain their own DNA.

mitosis A type of cell division in which each daughter nucleus receives the exact number and complement of chromosomes that the parent somatic (body) cell has. See also *meiosis*.

mold Any of a group of very small fungi that live on living, decaying, or dead matter.

morphine The principal alkaloid of opium; it is used as an analgesic (painkiller).

morphinelike drug Any opium-derived drug that has the effect of morphine.

multiple personality Extremely rare form of dissociation in which two or more distinct personalities exist within the same individual.

multiple sclerosis A chronic degenerative disease of the central nervous system.

mutation A change in form or other characteristic; often refers to a spontaneous change in the genetic makeup of an organism.

mycoplasma Minute microorganisms, lacking rigid cell walls, that will grow to small colonies on an enriched medium such as serum. Among the illnesses they cause is a form of inflammation of the lungs and their linings.

myelin The white, fatty covering of some nerves.

myocardium The heart muscle.

N

narcolepsy A rare disorder marked by an uncontrollable desire for sleep or by sudden attacks of sleep.

narcotic Any of the opium-derived drugs. Used medically to relieve pain and produce sleep.

natural foods Products that contain no artificial additives or preservatives.

nearsightedness A visual disorder marked by the ability to see near objects more clearly than far ones. It is caused by a lengthening of the diameter of the eye from front to back, which causes images to fall in front of the retina. Also called *myopia*.

nephritis Kidney inflammation.

nephron One of the very small filtering units of the kidney that produce urine. It is composed of a glomerulus (a capillary tuft) and a kidney tubule.

nerve impulse A change in the membrane of a nerve fiber, which triggers excitation in other nerves, muscles, or gland cells.

neuron A complete nerve cell, including all its projections and terminations; regarded as the basic structural unit of the nervous system.

neurosis (pl. **neuroses**) An emotional disorder that variously interferes with an individual's ability to deal effectively with reality. It is marked by anxiety and impairment of functioning in some areas of life. Compare *psychosis*.

neurotic disorder See *neurosis*.

neurotransmitters Chemical substances that are responsible for the transmission of nerve impulses between synapses.

non-A, non-B hepatitis A recently identified viral inflammation of the liver; it seems to constitute most of the after-transfusion hepatitis common in the United States today.

nongonococcal urethritis A sexually transmitted disease whose cause is unknown.

nonspecific general resistance The body's defense mechanisms that are not directed against any particular invader. Compare *specific resistance*.

nucleus A spherical body found within a cell and consisting of several characteristic organelles, such as a nuclear membrane, nucleoli, granules of chromatin, and diffuse protoplasm. Also within the nucleus are the chromosomes.

O

obsessive-compulsive reaction A psychoneurotic disorder characterized by persistent, irrational thoughts (obsessions) and by the repeated performance of ritualistic behaviors (compulsions).

oogonium The primordial, or original, cell from which an ovum derives; its divisions produce oocytes.

opium A drug derived from the opium poppy.

optic nerve The main nerve that connects the retina of the eye with the brain.

organ of Corti A spiral-shaped organ located within the cochlea of the inner ear; it contains the ciliated cells and the nerves that carry sound vibrations to the auditory nerve and thus to the brain.

organic foods Foods grown without pesticides and that contain no artificial substances.

osteoarthritis A chronic joint disease marked by the deterioration of cartilage and bone.

oval window An opening in the wall between the middle ear and the bony cochlea into which the stirrup fits.

ovary The female gonad; the reproductive gland of the female in which the ova (eggs) develop.

ovulation The discharge of a mature ovum from the Graafian follicle of the ovary.

ovum (pl. **ova**) The mature female reproductive cell, or egg, which, after fertilization by a spermatozoon, develops into a new individual of the same species.

P

pacemaker An area of the heart tissue specialized to trigger rhythmic contractions of the heart muscle. Also, a mechanical device that does the same thing.

pancreas A gland whose secretions digest proteins, fats, and carbohydrates. It also contains the islets of Langerhans, the cells of which control sugar metabolism in the body.

Papincolaou (Pap) test A painless diagnostic test for cancer of the uterine cervix. The test can also be applied to other easily accessible areas to detect cancer cells.

paralysis Loss or impairment of movement or feeling due to a lesion of the muscular or nerve mechanism.

paranoia A psychotic disturbance marked by the gradual development of suspicions or systematized delusions of persecution or grandeur that affect only a part of the personality.

parasite An animal or plant that lives within or upon another living organism (the host), at whose expense the parasite may obtain some advantage.

passive immunity Immunity that is acquired by the administration of preformed antibody; it is borrowed immunity and does not last long. Compare *active immunity*.

penis The external male organ of sexual intercourse and the organ of urination.

peptic ulcer An ulcer chiefly in areas of the digestive tract that are exposed to the acidic gastric juice. These areas include the esophagus, stomach, and first portion of the duodenum.

peptide A combination of two or more amino acids having one or more peptide groups present.

pericardial sac A sac enveloping the heart containing lubricating fluid.

periodontal disease Disease of the tissues surrounding the teeth.

periodontitis Inflammation of the supporting tissue surrounding a tooth.

peripheral nervous system The portion of the nervous system not included in the brain and spinal cord. It consists, in part, of the twelve pairs of cranial nerves and the autonomic (involuntary) nervous system.

permanent teeth The adult teeth that replace the deciduous teeth.

peyote An intoxicant derived from a variety of the Mexican cactus plant.

phagocytosis The ingestion of foreign particles by certain white blood cells.

phenotype The physical appearance of the individual that results from the interaction of the genotype and the environment. Compare *genotype*.

phenylketonuria (PKU) A genetic disorder of the metabolism of phenylalanine, an amino acid essential for growth in infants, caused by the absence of the enzyme necessary to metabolize this amino acid. The disorder may be associated with mental retardation.

phobia An irrational fear.

pitch The quality of sound measured by its frequency of vibration.

placenta The organ in the uterus through which the fetus is nourished and wastes are removed. It connects the fetus to the mother by means of the umbilical cord.

plaque A fatty deposit on the lining of the arteries, characteristic of atherosclerosis. Also, a deposit of hardened debris on the surface of a tooth, which may serve as a medium for the growth of bacteria and thus play a role in tooth decay.

plasma The fluid portion of the blood.

plasma membrane The porous organelle that surrounds a cell and allows only certain kinds and amounts of materials to enter and leave it.

platelet A colorless disk present in blood and involved in the coagulation of blood and the formation of blood clots.

plumbism Lead poisoning.

prepuce In the uncircumcised male, the fold of skin that covers the head of the penis (glans); in the female, the fold formed by the labia minora that covers the glans of the clitoris. Also called *foreskin*.

progesterone The hormone secreted by the corpus luteum; its basic function is to ready the uterus for the reception and development of a fertilized ovum.

properdin A protein in the blood that combines with invading bacterial cells to activate the complement; it is necessary to the action of the immune system.

protein One of a group of compounds made up mostly of amino acids that are the main component of protoplasm.

protoplasm A semiliquid, translucent material that is the essential matter of all plant and animal cells.

protozoan Any of a group of one-celled animals, such as an amoeba.

psychoneurosis See *neurosis*.

psychopathic personality A character disorder marked by chronic antisocial behavior.

psychosis (pl. **psychoses**) A severe emotional disorder characterized by a general inability to distinguish between objective reality and subjective hallucinations, delusions, and distortions. Compare *neurosis*.

pulp The soft part of the interior of an organ.

pupil The perforation in the iris of the eye through which light passes.

pyorrhea A discharge of pus; it is a sign of advanced dental disease.

Q

quality A characteristic of sound. See *timbre*.

R

receptor A molecule or a combination of molecules on the surface of cells.

recycling Disposing of solid wastes through reuse.

red blood cell A very small, nonnucleated disk that contains hemoglobin and carries oxygen to and carbon dioxide away from the tissues. Also called *erythrocyte*.

renal artery Artery leading to the kidney.

resistance The ability of an organism to ward off harmful effects of toxic agents, such as poisons and, especially, disease-causing microorganisms.

respiratory system All the structures and passages, including the lungs, diaphragm, and muscles, that are concerned with breathing.

retina The back part of the eyeball; it receives images, formed by the lens, that are then carried to the brain via the optic nerve.

Rh hemolytic disease An anemia of the newborn infant or fetus, caused by transfer through the placenta of maternal antibodies that are usually formed because of an incompatability between the blood group of the mother and the child.

rheumatoid arthritis A chronic disorder that usually affects the joints and connective tissue of the body.

rheumatoid factor A group of antibodies in the blood of people who have rheumatoid arthritis; they combine with other antibodies to form antigen-antibody combinations.

ribonucleic acid (RNA) A substance that is a template of portions of the DNA and that functions in the cytoplasm of a cell. There are three types of RNA: messenger RNA (mRNA), ribosomal RNA (rRNA), and transfer RNA (tRNA).

ribosome A cellular organelle at which the proteins are constructed or synthesized. It is not believed to be stationary and is thought to actively participate in protein formation. It is formed as ribosomal RNA under the direction of DNA.

rickettsia A type of microorganism that causes such diseases as typhus and Rocky Mountain spotted fever.

root The part of an organ that is embedded in tissue.

round window The opening into the bony cochlea below the oval window. It is covered by a membrane.

rubella (German measles) A highly contagious viral infection common among young people. It is usually mild in nature. Signs and symptoms include rash, fever, and swollen nodes in the back of the neck. It lasts about three days. When a pregnant woman is exposed in the first trimester, the danger is to the unborn child.

rubeola (regular measles) A potentially dangerous viral infection that, despite an effective vaccine, is still common in children. It is marked by a sore throat, nasal discharge, and rash.

S

sarcoma A cancer arising in connective tissue such as bone, cartilage, or muscle.

scabies A contagious skin disease caused by a mite; the most prominent symptom is itching. Also called "the itch."

schizophrenia Any of a group of psychotic disorders characterized generally by disturbed thinking patterns.

sclera The fibrous outer layer of the eyeball.

scrotum The external pouch or sac that contains the male testes and related organs.

seminal vesicle The paired pouches attached to the urinary bladder that join the vas deferens to form the ejaculatory duct.

seminiferous tubule The passage in the testis in which sperm develop and through which they leave the testis.

senile dementia A chronic organic brain syndrome associated with the elderly. The person may behave childishly and have difficulty handling new information.

septum A wall that divides two spaces. In the nose, it is the partition separating the two nostrils.

sexually transmitted diseases A group of diseases most commonly transmitted through sexual contact.

sickle-cell anemia A chronic genetic disorder occurring mostly in blacks and in some whites. It is marked by acute attacks of abdominal pain, severe anemia, and ulcerations of the lower extremities. It is caused by a defective chemical arrangement of the hemoglobin in the red blood cells. Insufficient oxygen causes the red blood cells to be sickle-shaped.

sickle cell disease See *sickle-cell anemia*.

sinoatrial (SA) node Located within the wall of the right atrium, the SA node is responsible for the rhythmic beating of the heart. Also called the *pacemaker*.

skeletal muscle A voluntary muscle; one attached to a bone and concerned with body movements.

small intestine The part of the digestive tube extending from the pylorus to the junction with the large intestine at the cecum.

smooth muscle An involuntary muscle consisting of nonstriated spindle-shaped muscle fibers. It appears in such structures as the intestines and the blood vessels. Compare *striated muscle*.

somatic cells The cells of the body except the germ cells.

specialties
  Medical:
  allergy The treatment of abnormal body reactions resulting from undue sensitivity to a wide variety of substances, including various foods,

dusts, and pollens. A recently defined area of study is *pharmacogenetics*—the study of inherited sensitivities to drugs.

anesthesiology The administration of general and local anesthetics before and/or during an operation or medical procedure.

cardiovascular disease The study, diagnosis, and treatment of illnesses of the heart and blood vessels.

dermatology The science of the skin and its diseases.

endocrinology The study of the endocrine glands and their secretions.

gastroenterology The study of diseases of the stomach and intestines.

hematology The treatment of blood diseases.

internal medicine The diagnosis and nonsurgical treatment of diseases of the internal organs; it encompasses many of the subspecialties defined here.

neurological surgery A surgical specialty that concentrates on operations on the brain and nervous system.

neurology The treatment of disorders of the nervous system.

obstetrics and gynecology *Obstetrics* is the care of women during pregnancy, labor, and immediately after childbirth; *gynecology* is concerned with disorders of the female reproductive system and sexual organs.

ophthalmology The study of the eye; ophthalmologists diagnose and treat eye disorders and prescribe eyeglasses or contact lenses.

orthopedic surgery The treatment of disorders of the bones, muscles, and joints.

otology, laryngology, and rhinology The treatment of diseases of the ear, nose, and throat.

pathology The study of the causes, nature. and effects of disease. The pathologist does not see patients but works in a laboratory.

pediatrics The care and treatment of children from infancy to middle teens.

physical medicine The physical reconditioning and rehabilitation of diseased and disabled persons, including the use of physical and occupational therapy, massage, exercise, heat, and other methods for restoring physical condition.

plastic surgery The restoration or reconstruction of a body structure damaged by disease or injury or for cosmetic reasons.

proctology The science of the structure, function, and diseases of the anus and rectum.

psychiatry The study and treatment of mental and emotional disorders.

public health The field of community or population health.

pulmonary disease The diagnosis and treatment of diseases of the lungs.

radiology and roentgenology The diagnosis and treatment of diseases by means of X-rays, radium, and other radioactive substances.

surgery (general) The performance of operations on any part of the body; it encompasses many of the subspecialties defined here.

thoracic surgery Operations performed on the chest.

urology The study and treatment of diseases and abnormalities of the urinary trace of both males and females and of the male genital organs.

Dental:

endodontics The prevention, diagnosis, and treatment of diseases that affect the tooth pulp and the tissues surrounding the tooth root.

oral pathology The diagnosis and treatment of tumors and other lesions of the mouth.

oral surgery Operative procedures on the teeth, mouth, and adjacent structures.

orthodontics Correction of poorly positioned teeth so that they make proper contact during chewing.

periodontics Treatment of diseases of the tissues that surround and support the teeth.

prosthodontics The art and science of making dental appliances and substitutes, such as artificial dentures, bridges, and crowns.

specific resistance A part of the body's defense mechanism that is directed against a definite, particular invader. Compare *nonspecific general resistance*.

sperm, spermatozoon (pl. **spermatozoa**) A mature male germ or sex cell that is capable of fertilizing an ovum.

spleen An organ situated in the upper abdomen immediately below the diaphragm on the left side. It destroys old red blood cells, thus setting hemoglobin free; it also produces lymphoid cells.

spore A highly resistant organism developed by some bacilli in response to unfavorable living conditions. It can remain dormant until it comes in contact with a more favorable ecosystem, at which time it produces bacteria that multiply and release poisons, thus causing disease.

sterility See *infertility*.

stimulant A drug or agent that temporarily increases the activity of some organ or vital process.

stirrup The third bone of the middle ear. Also called the *stapes*.

striated muscle A voluntary skeletal muscle consisting of muscle fibers that appear striped under a microscope. When it contracts, it produces movement of bones. Compare *smooth muscle*.

subfertility The state of being relatively sterile or less than normally fertile.

synapse The region of contact between projections of two adjacent neurons; it forms the area where a nervous impulse is transmitted from one neuron to another.

syndrome A group of signs or symptoms that occur together.

syphilis A sexually transmitted disease caused by spirochete bacteria.

systole The period of contraction of the heart. Compare *diastole*.

systolic pressure The highest blood pressure during contraction of the ventricles.

T

T lymphocyte A type of white blood cell (called "killer cell") that is active in the cell-mediated immune response, directly attacking and destroying many organisms that invade the body. In this activity, they are joined by another type of white blood cell, the *macrophage*. See *lymphocyte, B lymphocyte*.

tartar A hard salt and mineral deposit found on teeth.

Tay-Sachs disease A hereditary childhood disease characterized by blindness and mental retardation. It is most commonly found among Ashkenazie Jews—Jews who originally settled in central Europe rather than in Spain and Portugal. The condition is always fatal.

temperament An individual's emotional disposition.

temperature inversion A layer of warm air trapping a layer of cold air beneath it. The result is a lack of vertical air motion, which is important for cleansing ground-level air.

tendon A strong, fibrous cord at the end of a muscle that attaches the muscle to a bone.

testis (pl. **testes**) The male gonad, which produces spermatozoa; it is an egg-shaped gland contained in the scrotum. Together the testis and epididymis make up the testicle.

testosterone The hormone produced by the testes that induces and maintains the male secondary sex characteristics.

thrombus A plug or clot in the blood vessel or in the heart.

timbre The peculiar characteristic of sound that, along with pitch and intensity, makes a tone distinctive.

tolerance The adaptation of the body to a specific drug so that increased doses of the drug are necessary to produce the original effect.

tonsils Two spongy lymph tissues situated in the back of the mouth on either side of the throat and believed to supply the mouth and pharynx with bacteria-destroying phagocytes.

toxoid A toxin antigen that, with its poisonous properties inactivated, can stimulate the production of antibody-antitoxin when injected into the body.

trace element A substance that, though found in extremely small amounts in the body, is necessary to life.

tranquilizer A drug or agent used as a depressant in controlling and relieving various emotional disturbances.

transfer RNA A type of ribonucleic acid that, instructed by DNA, combines with a specific amino acid and transfers it to a ribosome in the process of protein synthesis.

transverse arch The arch that crosses the width of the foot. It is composed of ligaments, muscles, and tendons.

traumatic neurosis Transient personality changes that occur during periods of acute stress.

Trisomy 21 See *Down's syndrome*.

triglyceride A fatty substance in the blood that is necessary for life. An excess of triglycerides will promote atherosclerosis.

tumor A swelling or abnormal mass resulting from excessive cell growth.

U

umbilical cord The long cord containing the arteries and vein that connects the fetus with the placenta.

uremia A biochemical abnormality that occurs during kidney failure.

uterus The womb, which receives and holds the fertilized ovum during fetal development and becomes the principal agent in expelling the fetus at birth.

V

vaccine A preparation given in order to cause immunity in a person or an animal.

vagina The canal-like organ in the female that extends from the neck (lowest part) of the uterus to the vulva (external genital region) and that receives the penis in sexual intercourse.

vein A vessel through which blood passes from an organ or body part back to the heart.

venereal diseases See *sexually transmitted diseases*.

ventricle One of the lower pair of heart chambers, with thick, muscular walls, that compose the bulk of the heart.

venule A small vein.

Vincent's angina An infection involving the pharynx and tonsils that is caused by a specific microorganism.

virulence The degree to which a microorganism is able to produce disease.

virus A very small (usually ultramicroscopic) infective agent that is characterized by a lack of its own metabolism; it can multiply only within living cells.

vulva The female external genital organs.

W

white blood cell A small, colorless cell found in the blood, lymph, and tissues. It is responsible for the destruction of disease-causing organisms. Also called *leukocyte*.

withdrawal symptoms A collection of acute physical and psychological illnesses that occur when there is an absence of a specific drug in the body of a person who is dependent on that drug.

X

X sex chromosome The sex chromosome carried by one-half of the male gametes and all of the female gametes. The male carries one X chromosome; the female, two.

Y

Y sex chromosome The sex chromosome carried by one-half of the male gametes and none of the female gametes. The male carries one Y chromosome; the female, none.

yeast A type of fungus that germinates and multiplies in the presence of sugar or starch.

yolk sac A sac that becomes quite large in the early stages of cell division but that withers within a few months after providing cells that are destined to become lymphocytes. It may be thought of as a temporary accessory organ of the embryo.

Z

zygote The single-celled fertilized ovum that results from the union of the male and female gametes.

Illustration Credits

Chapter 1: p. 2, Gerry Cranham, Rapho/Photo Researchers, Inc.; 5, Chermayeff and Geismar; 9*tl*, Yoram Lehmann/©Peter Arnold, Inc.; 9*tr*, Roger-Viollet; 9*cl*, ©Jim Kalett/Photo Researchers, Inc.; 9*bl*, ©Jim Kalett/Photo Researchers, Inc.; 9*br*, Marcia Weinstein; 10, M.W.F. Tweedie from National Audubon Society, Photo Researchers, Inc.; 11, WHO; 12, *New York Daily News*; 13, Michael Putnam/©Peter Arnold, Inc.; 14, Billy E. Barnes; 16, Taurus Photos; 17, Gemeentemuseum's Gravenhage; 18*t*, W. Luthy/De Wys, Inc.; 18*b*, American Museum of Natural History; 19, Radio Times Hulton Picture Library; 20, USDA.

Chapter 2: p. 22, Bill Robinson; 25*t*, ©Sylvia Johnson/Woodfin Camp and Asso.; 25*b*, John Running/Stock, Boston; 27, Charles Gatewood; 29, Charles Gatewood; 30*t*, Art Reference Bureau; 30*b*, Art Reference Bureau; 31, Figure 2–1, From INTRODUCTION TO GEOGRAPHY, Fifth Edition, by Henry M. Kendall et al., copyright ©1976 by Harcourt Brace Jovanovich, Inc. Reproduced by permission of the publisher; 33, Jim Coit; 34, UN; 35*t*, Wide World Photos; 35*b*, Corning Glass Works; 37, Fred Forbes/Humbird Hopkins, Inc.; 38, Harmer Rooke; 39, UPI; 40, Wide World Photos; 41, WHO; 42, UPI; 45, Dan Miller; 47, Michael Hayman/Corn's Photo Service; 49, Charles Gatewood.

Chapter 3: p. 52, Institute for Cancer Research, Philadelphia, Pa.; 54, N.Y. Academy of Medicine; 55*l*, E.R. Squibb & Sons; 55*c*, Upjohn Company; 55*r*, Courtesy of Drs. G.B. Chapman, L.M. Drusin, and W.J. Wicbe, Department of Biology, Georgetown University; 56*l*, HEW; 56*r*, U.S. Public Health Service; 57,

R.M. Albrecht; 60, Aaron Polliack, M.D.; 61, King Features Syndicate; 62, Smithsonian Institute; 67, Christopher Stewart; 68, The Jacob A. Riis Museum of the City of New York; 71*t*, Institute for Cancer Research, Philadelphia, Pa.; 71*l*, Dr. R.W. Horne; 71*r*, Dr. R.W. Horne; 73, Copyright 1980 by Sidney Harris; 75*tl*, Dr. R.W. Horne; 75*tr*, Department of Pathology, University of Bristol; 75*bl*, Dr. Albert J. Dalton/National Cancer Institute; 75*br*, Dr. R.W. Horne/Dr. Jack Nagington; 76*t*, NIH; 76*c*, Dr. June Almeida, The Wellcome Research Laboratories; 76*b*, Dr. Daniel W. Bradley, Hepatitis Laboratories Division, Center for Disease Control; 79*l*, E.R. Squibb & Sons; 79*r*, Society of American Bacteriologists.

"Disease and Destiny": p. 1, Woodcut by Michael Wohlgemuth, 1493; 3, WHO; 5, British Museum; 6, Mansell Collection; 9, Mansell Collection; 10, Bodleian Library; 11, Mansell Collection; 13*t*, N.Y. Academy of Medicine; 13*b*, County of Los Angeles Health Department; 18, Mansell Collection; 19, Mansell Collection.

Chapter 4: p. 86, Wide World Photos; 90, Courtesy Eugene L. Gottfried, M.D.; 91, Courtesy Dr. Keith R. Porter, The Rockefeller Institute for Medical Research; 95, Carl A. Smith, M.D.; 97, Figure 4–9, From the National Heart, Lung, and Blood Institute's FY1976 Fact Book; 99, American Heart Assn.; 101, Ron Sherman, *Medical World News*; 104, New York University Medical Center; 109, EKM-Nepenthe; 110, Tiburon, From THERE IS A RAINBOW BEHIND EVERY DARK CLOUD, Copyright 1978 Center for Attitudinal Healing, reprinted by permission of Celestial Arts, Millbrae, CA 94030; 112*tr*, R.D. Ullmann/Taurus Photos; 112*bl*, Areo Service; 112*br*, ©George Gardener, 1979; 112*tl*, Marc and Evelyne Bernheim/Woodfin Camp & Asso.; 112*bc*, American Cancer Society; 113, Ewing Galloway; 116, Figure 4–13, Courtesy of the American Cancer Society, Inc.; 118, Figure 4–14, from End Results Group, National Cancer Institute, HEW.

Chapter 5: p. 122, Charles Gatewood; 126, Ted Polumbaum; 127, Erika Stone; 128, Bruno Bettelheim; 129, Michael Weisbrot; 130, Lennart Nilsson; 131, Billy E. Barnes; 132, Charles Gatewood; 133, Shirley Zieberg; 134*tl*, Erika Stone; 134*tr*, Wide World Photos; 134*bl*, Shirley Zieberg; 134*br*, Mark Haven; 135*tl*, Marcia Wienstein; 135*tr*, Erika Stone/©Peter Arnold,

Inc.; 135*bl*, Francia Russell, Associate Artistic Director, Pacific Northwest Ballet, Seattle, Wash.; 135*br*, Shirley Zieberg; 136, Gloria Karlson; 141, Globe Photos; 142*l*, The Columbus, Ohio, *Dispatch*; 142*r*, The Columbus, Ohio, *Citizen Journal*; 143, U.S. Army photo; 145*l*, Clay-Adams, Inc.; 145*r*, UPI; 147, Brown Brothers.

Chapter 6: p. 154, Harvey Stein; 156, Courtesy Hans Selye, International Institute of Stress; 157, *Minneapolis Tribune*; 158, Harvey Stein; 161, ©Wendy Watriss/Frederick Baldwin 1979/Woodfin Camp & Asso.; 163, Jim Coit; 165, Shirley Zeiberg; 166, Robert Eckert/EKM-Nepenthe; 167, David Covey; 169, Robert Eckert/EKM-Nepenthe; 170, George W. Gardener; 172, John R. Maher/EKM-Nepenthe; 173, Culver Pictures; 174, Marion Bernstein; 177*l*, University of Wisconsin, Regional Primate Research Center; 177*r*, WHO; 178, Wide World Photos.

Chapter 7: p. 186, David Scharf/©Peter Arnold, Inc.; 189, Figure 7–1, ©1978 by The New York Times Company. Reprinted by permission; 191, Foldes/Monkmeyer Press Photo Service; 193, ©Robert Goldstein 1977; 195, Archie Lieberman/Black Star; 196, Eric Kroll/Taurus Photos; 200, Culver Pictures Inc.; 201, Charles Gatewood; 203*tl*, Charles Gatewood; 203*tr*, ©Peeter Vilms/Jeroboam, Inc.; 203*cl*, Charles Gatewood; 203*cr*, ©Jeffrey Blankfort/Jeroboam, Inc.; 203*bl*, Jim Coit; 203*br*, Jim Coit; 204, Michael Denny; 205, Kenneth L. Jones; 207, ©George W. Gardener; 208, North Carolina Department of Mental Health; 211, Smithsonian Institute; 215, Charles Marden Fitch/Taurus Photos; 223, American Cancer Society.

Chapter 8: p. 230, Roger Malloch/©1969 Magnum Photos, Inc.; 232*l*, Jim Coit; 232*r*, Wide World Photos; 233, Manfred Kage/©Peter Arnold, Inc.; 236, Melanie Kaestner; 237, Erika Stone; 238, Bruce Curtis/©Peter Arnold, Inc.; 243, Bob Sanchez; 244, ©Karen R. Preuss/Jeroboam, Inc.; 247, Peter Müller/©Peter Arnold, Inc.; 249, National Society to Prevent Blindness Service, Inc., Chicago; 251*t*, Historical Pictures Service, Inc., Chicago; 251*b*, St. Louis Art Museum.

Chapter 9: p. 260, WHO; 262, Charles Marden Fitch/Taurus Photos; 263*t*, Erika Stone; 263*b*, Mark N. Boulton/Photo Researchers, Inc.; 266, Erika Stone; 267, Karen Gottstein; 269*tl*, Marilyn Silverstein/©Peter Arnold, Inc.;

269*tr*, Ben Ross; 269*cr*, Eugene Gordon/Taurus Photos; 269*br*, Michael Putnam/©Peter Arnold, Inc.; 269*bl*, Hazel Hankin; 270, Jim Coit; 275, Photo Almasy; 276, ©1979 Peter Menzel; 277, WHO; 279, Marion Bernstein; 280, Courtesy Dr. Neal E. Miller; 282, Erika Stone; 284, Ben Ross; 287*t*, photo by Anthony M. Kuzma from *Medical Tribune*; 287*bl*, *br*, Johnson L. Thistle, M.D., from the *New England Journal of Medicine*.

Chapter 10: p. 292, John R. Maher/EKM-Nepenthe; 294, Jean Prevost; 295, Photo Researchers, Inc.; 296, ©James Motlow/Jeroboam, Inc.; 298*tl*, UPI; 298*tr*, John R. Maher/EKM-Nepenthe; 298*c*, Peter Simon/Stock, Boston; 298*bl*, Robert Eckert/EKM-Nepenthe; 298*br*, Charles Gatewood; 300, Robert Eckert/EKM-Nepenthe; 302, ©Thomas Hopker 1978/Woodfin Camp & Asso.; 304, Charles Gatewood; 305, Erika Stone; 307, ©Karen R. Preuss/Jeroboam, Inc.; 309, J. Kohl & *Saturday Review*; 310, Kenneth Siegel; 312, Jeff Jacobson/Magnum Photos, Inc.

Chapter 11: p. 316, ©David Sandoz, 1979/Humbird Hopkins, Inc.; 319, Photo Researchers, Inc.; 320, ©Sepp Seitz/Woodfin Camp & Asso.; 321*l*, ©David Hume Kennerly, 1979/Contact Press Images; 321*r*, Giraudon, Paris, and ©S.P.A.D.E.M., Paris/V.A.G.A., New York; 323, ©Karen R. Preuss/Jeroboam, Inc.; 324, ©Joanne Leonard 1979/Woodfin Camp & Asso.; 325, Karen Halvorsen Gilborn; 327, Charles Gatewood; 331, ©Susan Ylvisaker/Jeroboam, Inc.; 333, Charles Gatewood; 335, Charles Gatewood; 338, Photographs by David Finn, from *Embrace of Life, The Sculpture of Gustav Vigeland*, published by Harry N. Abrams, Inc., 1968.

Chapter 12: p. 346, Landrum B. Shettles, M.D.; 353, L.J.D. Zaneveld, K.G. Gould, W.J. Humphreys, and W.L. Williams, *Reproductive Medicine*, 6:13, 1971; 363, ©Paolo Koch, Rapho/Photo Researchers, Inc.; 364, Ben Ross; 365, from INTERCOM, the monthly newsmagazine of the Population Reference Bureau, Inc., Washington, D.C.; 368*tl*, Paress/Magnum Photos, Inc.; 368*tr*, WHO Photo by P. Almasy; 368*c*, ©Marcia Weinstein; 368*bl*, Billy E. Barnes; 368*br*, UPI; 369, Jean-Claude Lejeune/Stock, Boston; 375, ©Roland et Sabrina Michaud, Rapho/Photo Researchers; 377, ©Optic Nerve/Jeroboam, Inc.

Chapter 13: p. 386, Elliott Erwitt/Magnum Photos, Inc.; 389, ©Harvey Stein, 1979; 391, Martin M. Rotker/Taurus Photos; 392*tl*, Martin M. Rotker/Taurus Photos; 392*tr*, Martin M. Rotker/Taurus Photos; 392*lb*, Carnegie Institute of Washington, 392*lt*, Carnegie Institute of Washington; 392*lc*, Carnegie Institute of Washington; 392*br*, Donald Yeager/Camera MD Studios; 394, Paul Y. Keating; 395, Erika Stone; 397, Erika Stone; 398, Photos courtesy Museum of Science and Industry, Chicago; 399, Paul Dix/reflejo; 400, Allen Green/Visual Departures; 401, Jim Coit; 402, ©Kay Lawson/Jeroboam, Inc.; 403, Lewis P. Lipsitt; 404, Wide World Photos; 405, Erika Stone; 406, Steve Hansen/Stock, Boston; 408, Wide World Photos.

Chapter 14: p. 412, Courtesy Dr. Carl B. Mankinen; 415, Courtesy Albert E. Vatter, M.D.; 416*tl*, Dr. Dorothy Warburton, Columbia University, N.Y.: 416*tr*, The Upjohn Company; 416*b*, courtesy Jon Beckwith, M.D., and Lorne MacHattie, M.D.; 420*l*, Courtesy O.L. Miller, Jr., and Barbara R. Beatty, Biology Division, Oakridge National Laboratory; 420*r*, O.L. Miller, Jr., and Aimee H. Bahken, Biology Division, Oakridge National Laboratory; 422, Courtesy Albert E. Vatter, M.D.; 423, from Masayasu Nomura, "Ribosomes," copyright 1969 by Scientific American, Inc., all rights reserved; 425, Courtesy Eva McGilvray, M.D.; 426, UPI; 427, Bruce Roberts/Photo Researchers, Inc.; 429*t*, R.F. Baker, Department of Microbiology, Univ. of Southern Calif., School of Medicine; 429*b*, Sam Falk/Monkmeyer; 431, Ira Wyman/Sygma; 433, Courtesy David H. Baker, M.D.; 438, Ben Ross; 439, Photos by Linda Linfesty, Battelle-Pacific Northwest Laboratories, Richland, Washington; 440, California Special Olympics.

Chapter 15: p. 444, ©1975 David Attie; 446, Historical Pictures Service, Inc., Chicago; 447, Library of Congress; 448, Figure 15–2, ©1976 by The New York Times Company. Reprinted by permission; 449, Robert Eckert/©EKM-Nepenthe; 451*l*, ©William Rosenthal/Jeroboam, Inc.; 451*r*, Billy E. Barnes; 454, Ben Ross; 458, Copyright 1979 by Herblock in *The Washington Post*; 459, AP; 461, Marion Bernstein; 462, Figure 15–4, ©1975 by The New York Times Company. Reprinted by permission; 463, Ben Ross; 464, Earl Dotter; 467*tr*, Seattle Historical Society; 467*bl*, Culver Pictures, Inc.; 467*tl*, Denver Public Library, Western History Department; 467*cl*, Brown Brothers; 467*br*, Brown Brothers.

Epilogue: p. 474, NIH; 478, A.M. Albisser, Hospital for Sick Children, Toronto, Canada; 479, Courtesy *Medical Tribune*; 480, Patricia Wynne; 481, David Norman, M.D., University of California, San Francisco, School of Medicine, Department of Radiology; 482, E. Mandelmann/WHO.

Index

Page numbers preceded by "SI" refer to the "Disease and Destiny" special insert.
Page number in *italics* refer to illustrations.

Somatic cell, 417, 419, 421
Somatostatin, 475, 476
Sound, 253
Sperm, *see* Spermatozoa
Spermatozoa, 44, 45, 318, 324, 329, 350, 352, *353*, 356, 357, 374, 388, 405, 417, *418*, 419
Sphincter, *see* Muscles
Spleen, 96, *281*
Spores, 55
Stapes, *see* Stirrup
Stimulants, 190 (table), 206–212
  amphetamine type of, 206–208, 209
  cocaine, 211–212
  hallucinogens, 209–211
Stirrup, of ear, 251, *252*
Stress, 159 (table), 169–170, 245, 277
  aging and, *156*
  change and, 158–160
  dealing with, 160–162
  divorce and, 159 (table), 310
  emotional, 125, 140, 143, 144, 156
  overcrowding and, 363, 364
  signs of, 156–157
Striated muscles, *233*, 233–234, 236
Subfertility, 404, 405
  causes of, 404, 405
Sudden Infant Death Syndrome (SIDS), 402, 402*n*, 403
Suicide, 178–180
Swine flu, 67
Synapse, *145*, 146
Syndrome, 156, 426*n*
Synesthesia, 209
Syphilis, 54, 55, 56, *79*, 428
  causes of, 78
  complications from, 81
  history and, 83
  symptoms of, 79, 81
Systole, 93
Systolic pressure, 108

T

Tartar, 257, 258
Tay-Sachs disease, 439
Teeth, 254–258, 283
  care of, 256–257
  problems with, 256–258
  structure of, *255*
Temperament, 174
Temperature inversion, 30, *31*
Tendons, *242*
Testes, 318, 323, 324, 349 (table), 350, *351*, 352, 417
Testicle, 352
Testosterone, 320*n*, 350
Tetanus, 55, 77–78
Thalidomide, 433
Thrombus, 99, 101, 109, 372

Thymus gland, 348
Thyroid gland, 348, 349 (table)
Tobacco, 217–225
  diseases and, 218, 219, 220, 222–224
  pregnancy and, 224
  respiratory system and, 217, *218*
Tolerance:
  to alcohol, 199
  to drugs, 190 (table), 191, 193, 194, 213
Tomogram, 481
Tonsils, 96
Toxemia of pregnancy, 394
Toxin, 58, 69, 77–78
Toxoid, 69
Trace elements, 268
Trachea, *218*
Tranquilizers, 198, 199
Transcendence, 209
Transfer RNA, 422, *423*
Transverse arch, *242*, 243
Traumatic neuroses, 143
Triglycerides, 97, 372
Trisomy, 426
Trisomy 21, *see* Down's syndrome
Tubal ligation, 376
Tuberculosis, 20, 68
Tumescence:
  in female, 322, 341
  in male, 323
Tympanic membrane, *see* Eardrum
Typhus, 19, 20, 40, 56

U

Ultrasonics, *438*, 475
Ultrasound, *see* Ultrasonics
Umbilical cord, 389, *390*, 393, 399
Uremia, 108
Urethra, 350, *351*, 352, *355*, 361
Urinary bladder, *351*, 352
Urogenital system, 56
U.S. Atomic Energy Commission (Energy Research and Development Administration), 46
U.S. Food and Drug Administration, 40, 43, 270, 273 (table)
U.S. health care industry, 447–465
  increasing costs of, *447*, *448*, 449, 462
  medical care programs in, 449–461
  quality of health care and, 463
  unavailability of health care and, 462, 463
Uterus, 318, 322, *353*, 354, *355*, 356, 357, *358*, 359, 388, 389, *390*, 397, 419
Uvula, 283

V

Vaccine, 58, 64, 65 (table), 66, 67
  for influenza, 66, 67, 68

for rabies, 14
for rubella, 66
for rubeola, 13, 66, 69
Vagina, 318, 322, 328, 336, 341, 353, 354, *355*, 356, 357, 361
Vaginismus, 336
Valium, 198, 199
Van Leeuwenhoek, Anton, 54
Vas deferens, 323, 350, *351*, 352, 376
Vasectomy, 376
Vegetarianism, 279–280
Veins, 91, *93*
Ventricle, 92, *93*
Venules, 91, *92*
Villi, 287, *288*
Virulence, 54
Viruses, 5, 6, 55, 71, 72, 73, 74, 75, 76
  affecting fetus, 73
  drugs and, 72
  structure of, *70*, *71*
Visual cortex, 480, 481
Vital amines, *see* Vitamins
Vitamins, 263, 264 (table), 265–267, 268, 273 (table), 279, 280
  niacin, 266, 267
  vitamin B, 266
  vitamin C, 265, 266
  vitamin D, 267
  vitamin E, 267
  vitamin K, 267
Vulva, 354

W

Water, 263, 268
  functions of, in body, 268
Weight, 270, 273, 274 (table)
  dieting and, 275–276
  obesity, 273, 274–276
  problems of, 275
  underweight, 277
Withdrawal symptoms, 190 (table), 191, 194, 195, 197, 199
World Health Organization, 482

X

X-chromosome, 417, *418*, 428
XYY-chromosome, 425

Y

Y-chromosome, 417, *418*, *419*, 428
Yeasts, 55
Yellow fever, 24, 40
Yolk sac, 59

Z

Zygote, 358, 388, 389, 417, 419, 426